Case Studies of Postoperative Complications after Digestive Surgery

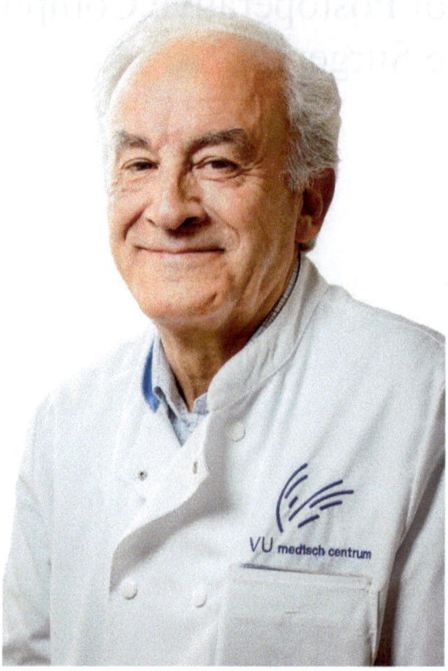

Miguel A. Cuesta

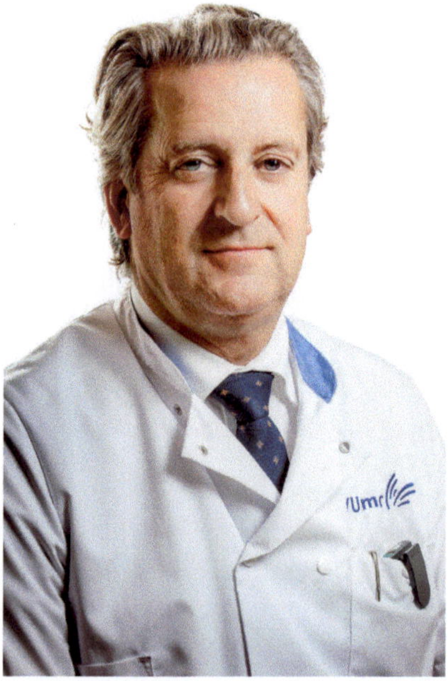

H. Jaap Bonjer

Miguel A. Cuesta • H. Jaap Bonjer
Editors

Case Studies of Postoperative Complications after Digestive Surgery

Springer

Editors
Miguel A. Cuesta
Department of Surgery
VU University Medical Center
Amsterdam
The Netherlands

H. Jaap Bonjer
Department of Surgery
VU University Medical Center
Amsterdam
The Netherlands

ISBN 978-3-319-01612-2 ISBN 978-3-319-01613-9 (eBook)
DOI 10.1007/978-3-319-01613-9
Springer Heidelberg New York Dordrecht London

Printed on acid-free paper

Springer is part of Springer Science+Business Media (www.springer.com)

Preface

Surgeons continually strive to provide the best care possible to their patients. Employing smaller incisions to reduce postoperative pain and lower the risk of wound infection and incisional hernia, improving technology of surgical instruments to facilitate safer dissection of tissues, and utilizing imaging techniques during surgery to perform more precise resections are some examples of the focus on enhancing quality of surgery. Major progress has been realized during the past decades; diagnostic invasive surgical procedures have been replaced by a variety of imaging techniques which provide high resolution three-dimensional insight in the anatomical aspects of the disease allowing surgical teams to refine their surgical approach; large abdominal incisions have been replaced by stab incisions allowing patients to ambulate very early after surgery and resume their activities within days instead of long postoperative stays in the hospital; and endoluminal and image-guided percutaneous placement of stents or drains to relieve obstructions or fluid collections which impede recovery of the patient.

Quality of surgery has increased greatly but many surgical interventions are still hampered by imperfect outcomes coined "complications," a term the definition of which is subject to debate. Francis D. Moore described in his book "A miracle and a privilege" the introduction by Ernest Amory Codman of a system for classifying imperfect outcomes, as being due to errors in diagnosis, technique, or judgment. Moreover, these were sharply differentiated from a group identified as patient's disease. This classification provides an excellent platform for further improvement. Intricate knowledge of the disease the patient presents with is of paramount importance.

The natural course of the disease, the impact of the disease on other organ systems, and the expected changes after surgical intervention are front and center during assessment of the patient and determination of a plan on how to best manage the patient. This complex process requires collective intelligence of all those healthcare professionals who have profound knowledge of various aspects of the disease and participate in the care of the patient. These multidisciplinary meetings are the gold standard of surgical practice of the twenty-first century.

Preparation and anticipation are key to successful surgery. In depth understanding of the anatomy, carefully determining the positioning of the patient, surgical approach, exposure and dissection, transection and ligation techniques, and, of great importance, discussing these with all members of the surgical and anesthesiological team are some of the elements that will determine the course of the surgery and the recovery after surgery.

Structured checklists have been implemented progressively to standardize and document the complex preoperative, intra-operative, and postoperative processes.

Management of the patient after surgery requires a team of healthcare professionals that assesses the patient frequently and provides the knowledge and skills required to accelerate recovery on one hand and detect factors interfering with recovery on the other hand.

The objective of this second book, Cases Studies of Postoperative Complications after Digestive Surgery, is to describe and discuss case by case, major complications after Digestive Surgery, diagnosed and treated in our practice. This book is closely related to the other volume, titled Treatment of Postoperative Complications after Digestive Surgery. These two volumes share the expertise of more than 50 highly dedicated and experience surgeons and surgical residents to allow the reader to learn the lessons learnt by their teachers and colleagues. The first volume, the main textbook, comprises 25 chapters with the focus on prevention and treatment of major complications by carefully proceeding through assessment, planning, and preparation, performing surgery, and managing the patient after surgery.

In this second part, a more practical and descriptive volume comprises more than 100 case studies bringing daily surgical practice to the reader and provide a wealth of learning opportunities. Extensive imaging documentation of the different cases is provided along with drawing pictures of the pathology with great attention to anatomical detail. In this digital age, there appears to be some hesitation to choose pencil over mouse. However, translating images and anatomical experience into drawings is invaluable in preparing the surgeon's mind and that of the other members of the surgical team. Wendy Vetter, Dana Hamers, and Miguel Cuesta have illustrated selected cases which provide great insight and hopefully inspire the reader to pick up colored pencils.

We hope that this book will enrich the knowledge and understanding of surgeons and surgical residents around the world and will inspire them to contribute to improving surgery continually.

Amsterdam, The Netherlands

Miguel A. Cuesta
H. Jaap Bonjer

Contents

List of Contributors

Isaias Alarcón Department of Surgery, Virgen del Rocio Hospital, Sevilla, Spain

Antonio Barranco Department of Surgery, Virgen del Rocio Hospital, Sevilla, Spain

Willem A. Bemelman, M.D., Ph.D. Department of Surgery, Academic Medical Center, Amsterdam, The Netherlands

Frits J. Berends, M.D. Department of Surgery, Rijnstate, Arnhem, The Netherlands

Mark I. van Berge Henegouwen Department of Surgery, Academic Medical Center, Amsterdam, The Netherlands

Carlos Bernardos Department of Surgery, Virgen del Rocio Hospital, Sevilla, Spain

Marc Besselink, M.D., Ph.D. Department of Surgery, Academic Medical Center, Amsterdam, The Netherlands

Surya S.A.Y. Biere, M.D. Department of Surgery, VU University Medical Center, Amsterdam, The Netherlands

Adriaan A. van Bodegraven Department of Gastroenterology, VU University Medical Center, Amsterdam, The Netherlands

H. Jaap Bonjer, M.D., Ph.D., F.R.C.S.C. Department of Surgery, VU University Medical Center, Amsterdam, The Netherlands

Klaske A.C. Booij Department of Surgery, Academic Medical Center, Amsterdam, The Netherlands

Jorg de Bruin, M.D. Department of Surgery, VU University Medical Center, Amsterdam, The Netherlands

Oliver R.C. Busch, M.D., Ph.D. Department of Surgery, Academic Medical Center, Amsterdam, The Netherlands

Rebecca P.M. Brosens Department of Surgery, VU University Medical Center, Amsterdam, The Netherlands

Maria Dolores Casado, M.D. Department of Surgery, Virgen del Rocio Hospital, Sevilla, Spain

Miguel A. Cuesta, M.D. Department of Surgery, VU University Medical Center, Amsterdam, The Netherlands

Gwen M.P. Diepenhorst, M.D. Department of Surgery, VU University Medical Center, Amsterdam, The Netherlands

Juan de Dios Franco Department of Surgery, Hospital de Jerez, Cadiz, Spain

Michael F. Gerhards, M.D. Department of Surgery, OLVG Hospital, Amsterdam, The Netherlands

Suzanne S. Gisbertz, M.D. Department of Surgery, Academic Medical Center, Amsterdam, The Netherlands

Ramon Gorter, M.D. Pediatric Surgery, VU University Medical Center, Amsterdam, The Netherlands

Dirk J. Gouma Department of Surgery, Academic Medical Center, Amsterdam, The Netherlands

Thomas M. van Gulik Department of Surgery, Academic Medical Center, Amsterdam, The Netherlands

Nike M. Hanneman, M.D. Department of Surgery, Medisch Centrum, Alkmaar, The Netherlands

Birgitta M.E. Hansson, M.D. Department of Surgery, Canisius Hospital, Nijmegen, The Netherlands

Koen Hartemink, M.D. Intensive Care, Department of Surgery, VU University Medical Center, Amsterdam, The Netherlands

Anthony J. Healey, M.D. Department of Surgery, St Mark's Hospital, London, UK

Maarten A.J.M. Jacobs Department of Gastroenterology, VU University Medical Center, Amsterdam, The Netherlands

Ignace M.C. Janssen, M.D. Department of Surgery, Rijnstate, Arnhem, The Netherlands

Wenceslao Vasquez Jimenez, M.D., Ph.D. Department of Surgery, Gregorio Marañon Hospital, Madrid, Spain

Geert Kazemier, M.D. Department of Surgery, VU University Medical Center, Amsterdam, The Netherlands

Bastiaan R. Klarenbeek Department of Surgery, MC Leeuwarden, Leeuwarden, The Netherlands

Niels de Korte, M.D. Department of Surgery, Spaarne Hospital, Hoofddorp, The Netherlands

Rutger J. Lely, M.D. Department of Radiology, VU University Medical Center, Amsterdam, The Netherlands

Kirsten Maas, M.D. Department of Surgery, VU University Medical Center, Amsterdam, The Netherlands

Jack L. Martin Department of Surgery, St Mark's Hospital, London, UK

Sonsoles Martinez Lopez, M.D. Department of Surgery, Gregorio Marañon Hospital, Madrid, Spain

Cristina Mendez, M.D. Department of Surgery, Virgen del Rocio, Sevilla, Spain

Akash M. Metha, M.D. Department of Surgery, VU University Medical Center, Amsterdam, The Netherlands

Herold J. Metselaar Department of Gastroenterology, Erasmus Medical Center, Rotterdam, The Netherlands

Salvador Morales-Conde, M.D. Department of Surgery, Virgen del Rocio Hospital, Sevilla, Spain

R. Jeroen van Moorselaar Department of Urology, VU University Medical Center, Amsterdam, The Netherlands

Marta Gutierrez Moreno, M.D. Department of Surgery, Virgen del Rocio, Sevilla, Spain

Chris J.J. Mulder Department of Gastroenterology, VU University Medical Center, Amsterdam, The Netherlands

Francisco Nevárez Noboa, M.D. Department of Surgery, Hospital del Sureste, Madrid, Spain

Hugo W. Nijhof, M.D. Department of Surgery, Kennemer Gasthuis, Haarlem, The Netherlands

J. Wolter Oosterhuis Department of Surgery, VU University Medical Center, Amsterdam, The Netherlands

Donald L. van der Peet Department of Surgery, VU University Medical Center, Amsterdam, The Netherlands

Jan Peringa, M.D. Radiology, OLVG Hospital, Amsterdam, The Netherlands

Marijn Poelman, M.D. Department of Surgery, VU University Medical Center, Amsterdam, The Netherlands

Alfredo Alonso Poza, M.D., Ph.D. Department of Surgery, Hospital del Sureste, Madrid, Spain

Jelle P. Ruurda Department of Surgery, University MC, Utrecht, The Netherlands

Jose L. Garcia Sabrido, M.D. Department of Surgery, Gregorio Marañon Hospital, Madrid, Spain

Laura Gonzalez Sanchez, M.D. Department of Surgery, Hospital J. Negrin, Tenerife, Spain

María Sánchez Ramírez Department of Surgery, Virgen del Rocio, Sevilla, Spain

Teresa Sanchez Rodriguez, M.D. Department of Surgery, Virgen del Rocio, Sevilla, Spain

Maria Conde Rodriguez Department of Surgery, Hospital Clinico, Universidad de Madrid, Spain

Joris J.G. Scheepers, M.D. Department of Surgery, Ranier de Graaf Hospital, Delft, The Netherlands

Gianluca Sciannamea, M.D. Department of Surgery, Virgen del Rocio Hospital, Sevilla, Spain

María Socas, M.D. Department of Surgery, Virgen del Rocio Hospital, Sevilla, Spain

Manon C.W. Spaander Department of Gastroenterology, Erasmus MC, Rotterdam, The Netherlands

Jurriaan B. Tuynman Department of Surgery, VU University Medical Center, Amsterdam, The Netherlands

Alexander A.F.A. Veenhof, M.D. Department of Surgery, VU University Medical Center, Amsterdam, The Netherlands

Mariëlle L.A.W. Vehmeijer-Heeman, M.D. Department of Surgery, VU University Medical Center, Amsterdam, The Netherlands

Elisabeth A. te Velde Department of Surgery, VU University Medical Center, Amsterdam, The Netherlands

Victor J. Verwaal Department of Surgery, Antoni v Leeuwenhoek Hospital, Amsterdam, The Netherlands

Cornelius G. Niels Vos, M.D. Department of Surgery, VU University Medical Center, Amsterdam, The Netherlands

Bas P.L. Wijnhoven, M.D. Department of Surgery, Erasmus MC, Rotterdam, The Netherlands

Henri A.H. Winters Department Plastic Surgery, VU University Medical Center, Amsterdam, The Netherlands

Chan Yuan, M.D. Department of Surgery, VU University Medical Center, Amsterdam, The Netherlands

Chapter 1
Case on Suspicion of an Anastomotic Problem After Esophageal Resection for Cancer

Surya S.A.Y. Biere

Keywords Postoperative • Complications • Anastomotic leakage • Esophageal resection

Diagnosis and Indication for Surgery

A 60-year-old male was evaluated for dysphagia of 3 months duration and was consequently diagnosed for having an adenocarcinoma of the distal oesophagus.

Endosonography, CT scan of thorax and abdomen, and PET-CT staged this carcinoma as cT3N1M0. The patient had initially been treated by neoadjuvant chemoradiotherapy. Six weeks later he underwent an Ivor Lewis two-field lymphadenectomy esophageal resection.

Postoperative Course: Identification and Treatment of the Complication

On the 6th postoperative day, he developed fever and dyspnoea and became respiratorily insufficient requiring intubation and mechanical ventilation. A CT scan of the thorax and abdomen revealed an anastomotic leakage with a thoracic empyema (Fig. 1.1). A re-thoracotomy was performed, showing a mediastinitis, and an empyema as a consequence of a leakage of one-third of the circumference of the

S.S.A.Y. Biere, M.D.
Department of Surgery, VU University Medical Center, Amsterdam, The Netherlands
e-mail: s.biere@vumc.nl

M.A. Cuesta, H.J. Bonjer (eds.), *Case Studies of Postoperative Complications after Digestive Surgery*, DOI 10.1007/978-3-319-01613-9_1,

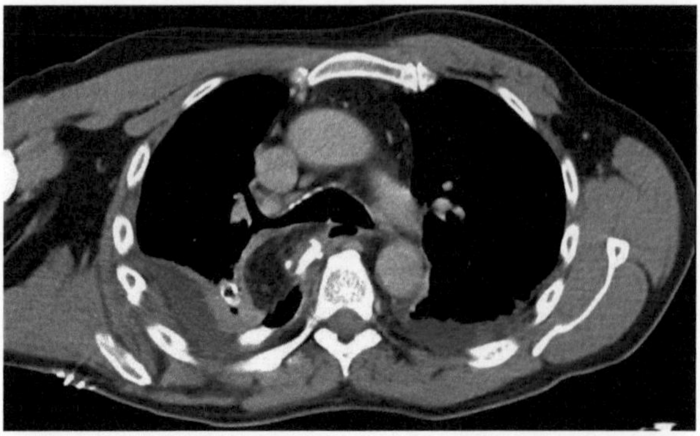

Fig. 1.1 CT scan: leakage of anastomosis and empyema

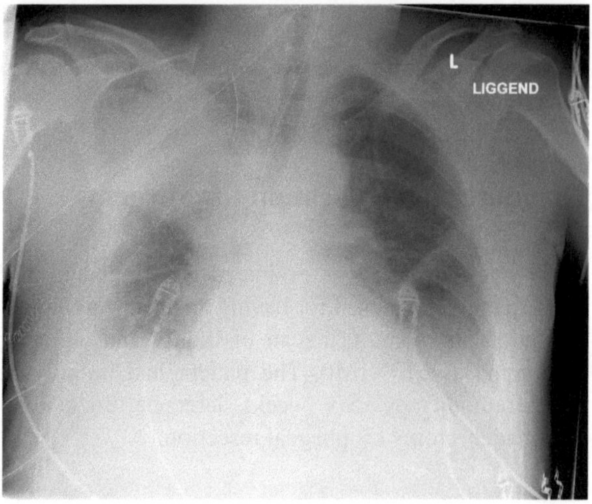

Fig. 1.2 Postoperative Thorax X-ray, with contour of the serratus plasty on the *right* hemithorax

anastomosis. After drainage and decortication of the right lung, the ischemic part of the anastomosis was resected, and the anastomosis reconstructed in end-to-end fashion, protected by a serratus anterior muscle plasty that was introduced through the third intercostal space after rib resection. The patient was admitted postoperatively to the ICU with sepsis, athelectasia of lower lobes on both sides, and patchy images of both lungs, this being considered as the respiratory distress syndrome (Fig. 1.2). After stabilization with a positive end-expiratory pressure (PEEP) of 10 cm H_2O and a fraction of inspired oxygen (FiO_2) of 60 %, he could be detubated after 2 days. Nevertheless, re-intubation was necessary on the following day due to the recurrence of fever and respiratory insufficiency. After a slow process of recovery for 19 days, being treated with mechanical ventilation, antibiotics, and enteral feeding through the jejunostomy, the patient could again be detubated, and subsequently being discharged to the medium care unit. In the meantime he developed jaundice (due to medication and sepsis), hypernatremia, and delirium. On the 26th postoperative day, the patient could be discharged to the ward. A slow process of recovery followed without complications, and he could finally be discharged to a revalidation center on the 44th postoperative day.

Discussion

This case of intrathoracic anastomotic leakage following an Ivor Lewis procedure was suspected clinically because of a worsening of the clinical situation with sepsis and respiratory insufficiency. Leakage of the anastomosis with empyema and mediastinitis was further confirmed by means of a CT scan. After assessment of the situation when the patient clinically deteriorated, adequate action was immediately taken resulting in a re-thoracotomy with drainage of mediastinitis, empyema, and reconstruction of the anastomosis. Decortication is necessary to treat the empyema and to obtain an adequate expansion of the lung. Reconstruction of an anastomosis after leakage remains a controversial issue. Some oesophageal surgeons will make a plea for disconnection of the anastomosis, cervical esophagostomy, and gastrostomy, especially if a long segment of ischemic gastric conduit is present. Afterwards, a long period of time for recovery is needed, before engaging in reconstruction by means of colon interposition. But if a short segment of ischemia is involved, others will prefer preservation of the anastomosis, by stenting the leakage and draining the empyema or reconstructing the anastomosis after necrotectomy of the ischemic part and protection of the new anastomosis by a vital muscle plasty (Illustration 1.1). A muscular plasty increases the likelihood of optimal results, avoiding the risks of disconnection and reoperations. Nevertheless, if the situation of the patient in this case had worsened after his reoperation and after confirmation of leakage of the anastomosis or necrosis of the muscle plasty, then a disconnection procedure would have been indicated. Concerning the type of plasty to perform in the case of anastomotic leakage, there are different possibilities such as a pleura plasty, a pericardial patch plasty, an intercostal muscle, and pectoral or serratus muscle plasty. The choice here for serratus anterior plasty can be deemed logical because the intercostal muscle at the level of the thoracotomy was not available.

In the case that patient has been approached by thoracoscopy, surgeon has to decide to approach the patient by re-thoracoscopy or open. Thoracoscopic approach of the empyema leaving enough drains and the possibility of closure of the leakage is a good option [1].

Other possibilities such as the less invasive three-tube insertion approach needs more study [2].

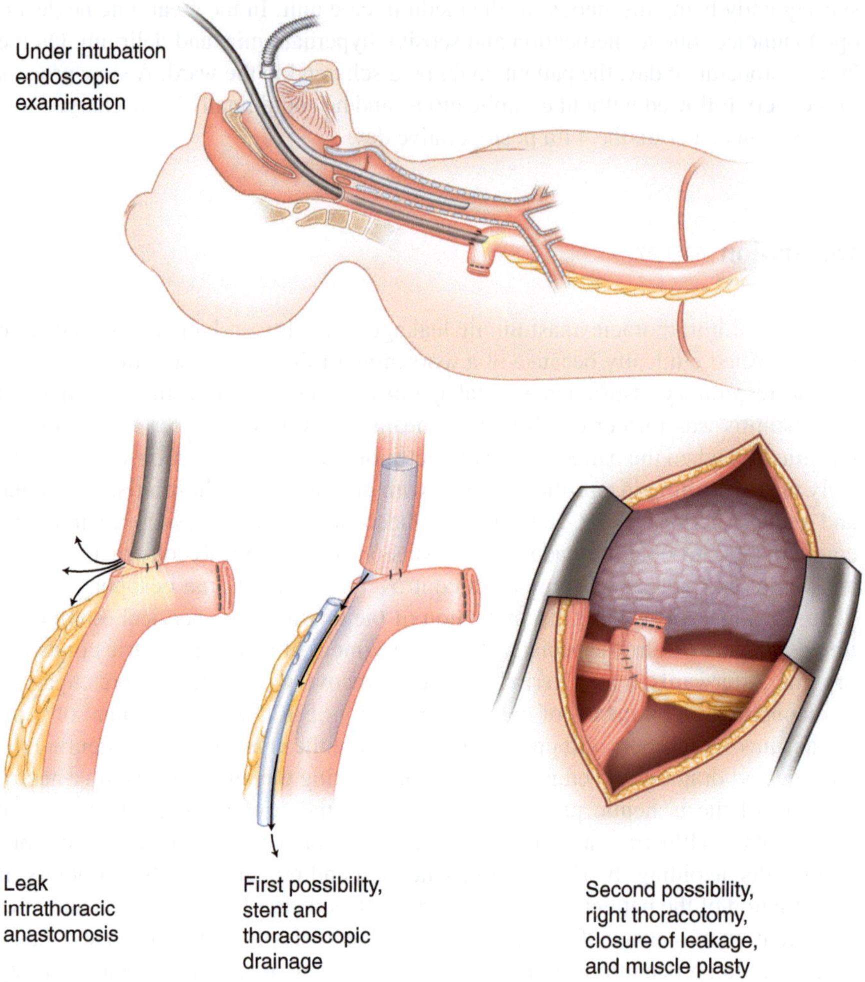

Illustration 1.1 If anastomosis leakage after oesophageal resection for cancer is diagnosed with mediastinitis or empyema, there are two treatment possibilities. During endoscopy, stent with covering of the leakage and local adequate drainage or right thoracotomy, anastomosis revision, and muscular plasty

References

1. Li XH, Hu Y, Rong TH, et al. Medical thoracoscopy and gastroscopy for the treatment of intrathoracic anastomotic leakage following esophagectomy. Oncol Lett. 2012;5:198–200.
2. Yin G, Xu Q, Chen S, et al. Fluoroscopically guided three-tube insertion for the treatment of postoperative gastroesophageal anastomotic leakage. Korean J Radiol. 2012;13:182–8.

Chapter 2
Case on Cervical Leakage of an Esophago-gastric Conduit Anastomosis

Surya S.A.Y. Biere

Keywords Cervical leakage • Anastomosis • Dysphagia • Transthoracic esophagectomy • Cervical stent

Diagnosis and Indication for Surgery

A 64-year-old female was evaluated for dysphagia, revealing a squamous cell carcinoma of the mid-esophagus. Endosonography, CT scan of thorax and abdomen, and PET-CT staged this carcinoma as cT3-4N2M0. The patient was treated by neoadjuvant chemoradiotherapy. This resulted, clinically and on the PET CT scan, in a significant reduction in tumor size and regional lymph nodes.

After a period of 6 weeks, she underwent a three-stage two-field lymphadenectomy thoraco-laparoscopic esophageal resection in prone position with a cervical anastomosis.

Postoperative Course: Identification and Treatment of the Complication

The patient started oral feeding the 5th day after the operation; on the 8th day she developed an infection of the cervical wound. Because of the aspect of the drained saliva and leak of air, a cervical anastomosis leakage was obvious. The patient was initially treated by care of the wound and jejunostomy feeding, but

S.S.A.Y. Biere, M.D.
Department of Surgery, VU University Medical Center, Amsterdam, The Netherlands
e-mail: s.biere@vumc.nl

M.A. Cuesta, H.J. Bonjer (eds.), *Case Studies of Postoperative Complications after Digestive Surgery*, DOI 10.1007/978-3-319-01613-9_2,

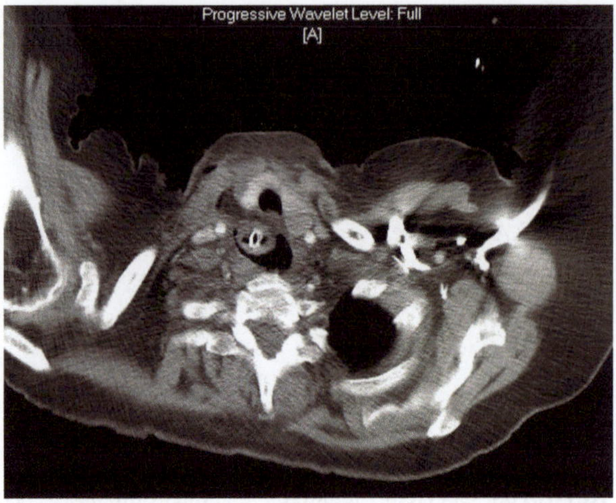

Fig. 2.1 CT scan with persistent cervical-proximal mediastinum leakage

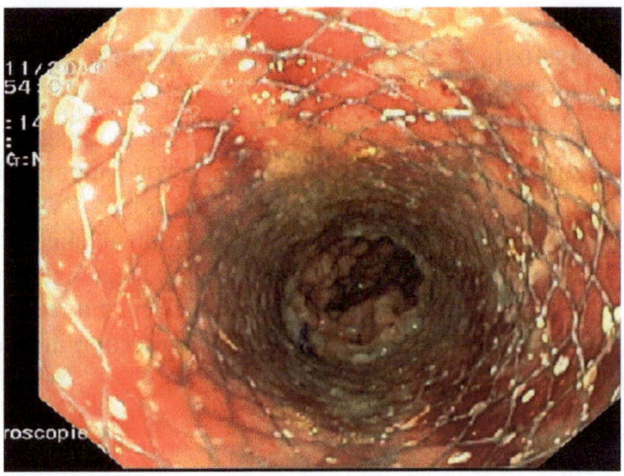

Fig. 2.2 Stent to cover the leakage

persistence of leakage for more than 10 days was reason to perform a CT scan that showed an adequately drained leakage from the proximal mediastinum (Fig. 2.1). Because of continuous leakage a stent was inserted at the level of the anastomosis. After placing the first stent, the wound continued to leak and a swallow X-ray showed dislocation of the stent and the presence of leak. A new endoscopy was performed, the old stent removed, and a new stent placed (Fig. 2.2). The leakage disappeared immediately and the patient could start step-by-step oral feeding. On the 31st postoperative day, she was discharged on condition of oral feeding and 1 L feeding through the jejunostomy. The stent was removed at the outpatient clinic 2 weeks after a confirmation by endoscopy that the anastomotic defect was closed.

Pathological outcome showed no vital rest of a tumor in the specimen, and all 15 lymph nodes scored negative for cancer.

Discussion

Treatment of a cervical leakage of an esophago-gastric conduit anastomosis is mostly conservative and consists of drainage of the wound, followed by care of the wound, and jejunostomy feeding. By doing so, a controlled fistula is created and leakage will stop in several days. There are two exceptions to this treatment (Illustration 2.2).

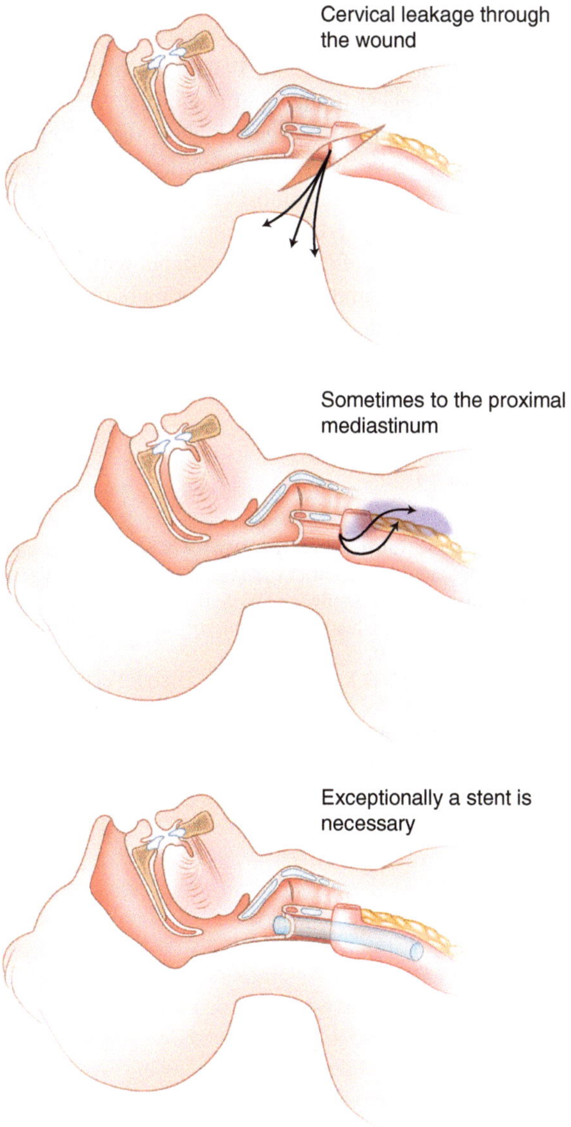

Illustration 2.2 Cervical anastomotic leakage after esophageal resection. Sometimes, it leaks to proximal mediastinum. Exceptionally, a stent is considered necessary

First, if the leakage descends into the mediastinum with mediastinitis and second, if the cervical fistula lasts for a long period of time, perhaps longer than 10 days with persistence of a high production.

Indication for the use of a cervical stent was in the present case the persistence of the leakage and the imaging on the CT scan of the presence of a leak, adequately drained in the high mediastinum. There was a relative indication for placing a stent; probably the continuation of the conservative treatment had lead to closure of the fistula. One of the possible advantages of the stent over conservative treatment is the possibility of avoiding late stenosis. Dislocation of the stent is a well-known complication, especially because the space to place the stent distal of the crycopharingeus muscle is very small. Placement of the stent will permit patient from the beginning to ingest liquids and bland diet. The question arises how long the stent will be kept in place in order to close the leakage and avoid stenosis—probably between 4 and 6 weeks [1]. The incidence of anastomotic leakage after esophagectomy with cervical anastomosis is reported to be around 14 % [2]. A recent meta-analysis of randomized trials comparing cervical with thoracic anastomosis showed a higher incidence of leakage in patients with cervical anastomosis [3]. A report of 242 patients who underwent transthoracic esophagectomy with a cervical anastomosis, demonstrated an incidence of leakage in 11.1 % of the patients and only 50 % of the patients with leakage developed mediastinitis [4].

References

1. Scheepers JJ, van der Peet DL, Veenhof AA, et al. Systematic approach of postoperative gastric conduit complications after esophageal resection. Dis Esophagus. 2010;23:117–21.
2. Hulscher JBF, van Sandwick JW, de Boer AG, et al. Extended transthoracic resection compared with limited transhiatal resection for adenocarcinoma of the esophagus. N Engl J Med. 2002;347:1662–9.
3. Biere SSAY, Maas KW, Cuesta MA, van der Peet DL. Cervical or thoracic anastomosis after esophagectomy for cancer: a systematic review and meta-analysis. Dig Surg. 2011;28:29–35.
4. Korst RJ, Port JL, Lee PC, Altorki NK. Intrathoracic manifestations of cervical anastomotic leaks after transthoracic esophagectomy for carcinoma. Ann Thorac Surg. 2005;80:1185–90.

Chapter 3
Case on Postoperative Chyle Leakage

Alberto Martinez Isla, Jack L. Martin, and Anthony J. Healey

Keywords Chyle leakage • Cervical anastomosis • Thoracic duct • Chylothorax

Diagnosis and Indication for Surgery

A 63-year-old female was diagnosed with a squamous cell carcinoma of the mid esophagus, staged as T3N1M0. She was treated by chemoradiotherapy and supported by enteral feeding through a duodenal feeding tube. After complaints decreased, the patient could reinitiate oral feeding prior to intervention.

Operation

A three-stage two-field lymphadenectomy esophageal resection was performed with a cervical anastomosis. Intervention was difficult because of fibrosis around the tumor and it was not clear that the thoracic duct was resected at the place of the tumour. Moreover, at the level of the hiatus there were several small branches of the thoracic duct, which were ligated.

Pathology

Radically resected T3N1 squamous cell carcinoma.

A.M. Isla, M.B.B.S., M.Sc., F.R.C.S. (✉) • J.L. Martin • A.J. Healey, M.D.
Department of Surgery, St Mark's Hospital, London, UK
e-mail: a.isla@imperial.ac.uk

M.A. Cuesta, H.J. Bonjer (eds.), *Case Studies of Postoperative Complications after Digestive Surgery*, DOI 10.1007/978-3-319-01613-9_3,

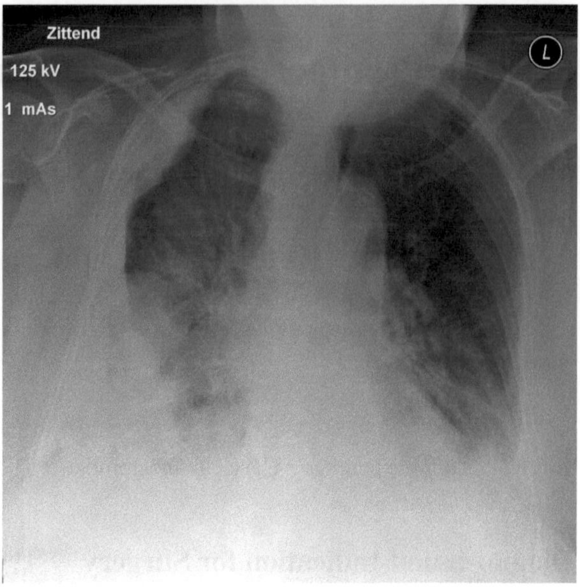

Fig. 3.1 Thorax X-ray with chylothorax

Postoperative Course: Identification and Treatment of the Complication

Postoperatively, the patient developed a chylothorax, at first with a daily production of 0.5 L, but in the next days the production increased above 1 L (Figs. 3.1 and 3.2). The diagnosis of chyle was confirmed by the milky aspect and by high levels of triglycerides in the fluid. A mid chain T (MCT) diet was administered and even though the color became less white, the production was still higher than 1 L (Fig. 3.3). The patient was doing well and after deliberation, it was proposed to do a thoracoscopy in order to identify the leakage and to ligate the thoracic duct, if necessary by thoracotomy. Before the operation, cream was orally given to the patient. At thoracoscopy the leak could be identified—not at a distal level, but at the mid area of the mediastinum. The thoracic duct was clipped at this level and the thorax again was drained. Postoperatively, drain fluids were sanguinolent and no more chylous of aspect. At the third postoperative day, the drain was removed.

Discussion

The thoracic duct is the principal collecting channel of the lymphatic system. It carries intestinal chyle and lymph from the whole body, except from the right side of the head and neck, right upper limb, right lung, right side of the heart, and the

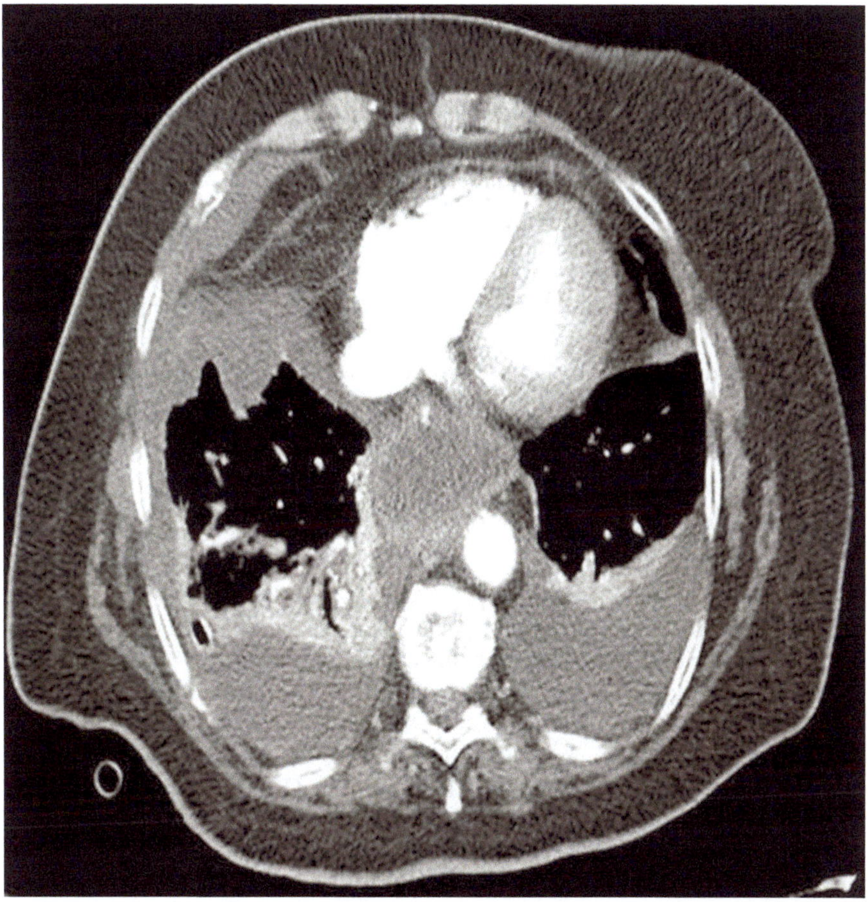

Fig. 3.2 CT scan with image of chylothorax

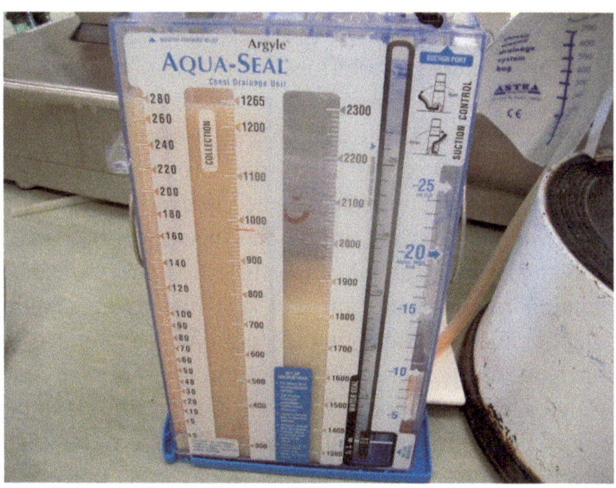

Fig. 3.3 Aspect of chyle in the thorax drain system

convex surface of the liver [1, 2]. The thoracic duct originates at the cisterna chyli that lies at the body of the second lumbar vertebrae. Varying in length from 37 to 45 cm, the thoracic duct ascends into the thorax through the diaphragmatic hiatus, posterior to the median arcuate ligament, between the azygos vein and the aorta. It crosses to the left side of the thorax at a variable level between the sixth and fourth thoracic vertebrae to continue its ascent to the left of the esophagus. It passes posterior to the aortic arch and then anterior to the subclavian artery to enter the neck via the superior thoracic aperture to join the left subclavian vein at its junction with the internal jugular vein [2]. While this is the classical course, considerable variation may be found, which are reported to occur in approximately half of the population [3]. There are numerous valves throughout the length of the duct and at the lymphatico-venous junction with the left subclavian vein.

Complications of Chyle Loss

Local pressure effects of a chylothorax can produce cardiorespiratory compromise. Following appropriate drainage, prolonged leakage can result in wide ranging metabolic, nutritional, and immunological complications [1–3]. Maintaining adequate intravascular volume and accurate fluid replacement is difficult in patients with chyle leaks. The most frequently observed electrolyte abnormalities are acidosis, hyponatraemia, and hypocalcaemia [1, 2]. Patients rapidly become nutritionally deplete and require nutritional support. Cell-mediated immunity and humoral responses are both impaired by ongoing chyle loss due to the loss of lymphocytes and immunoglobulins [1, 2].

Mechanism of Thoracic Duct Injury

The thoracic duct is notoriously difficult to visualize at both open and thoracoscopic surgery. Blunt dissection associated with a traditional open transhiatal oesophagectomy, for example, can produce shearing forces that injure the fragile thoracic duct. It is now a well-recognized complication of thoracic and esophageal surgery with a reported incidence in esophagectomy of approximately 2–4 % [1]. However, inadvertent injury has been reported in cardiothoracic surgery, neck surgery, trauma, central venous insertion, and radical nephrectomy [1]. Preoperative administration of an oral diet rich in fat (e.g., double cream) can enable easier identification of the thoracic duct and may reduce the chance of injury through inadvertent transection or laceration [4]. Thoracic duct injury may present with a right or left chylothorax. The side may be a guide to the location of the injury, as an injury below T5-T6 usually presents with a right-sided chylothorax and that above this level presents with a left-sided chylothorax [3, 5].

Prevention of Thoracic Duct Injury

Various preventative strategies have been employed to avoid chyle leaks. The only randomized trial of preventive techniques involved the application of fibrin glue to the mediastinal dissection. Interestingly, this actually demonstrated a significant increase in the lymph leakage. Others have attempted routine ligation of the thoracic duct. Systematic ligation of mass ligation proved safe and effective. It minimized the risk of postoperative chylothorax in patients who underwent transthoracic esophagectomy for cancer [6].

Diagnosis

In the majority of postoperative patients, a chyle leak presents as excessive drainage (more than 500 mL) of straw or cream-colored fluid from the chest drain (or abdominal drain in patients who have undergone transhiatal oesophagectomy). In patients without a postoperative chest drain in situ, signs and symptoms of a pleural effusion with progressive cardiorespiratory deterioration are the most common presentation [1]. There is frequently a refractory period of 2–10 days before the presence of chyle in the drains. The diagnosis may be further delayed as straw-colored chest drain fluid is a normal occurrence, and the classical milky chyle may not be apparent in a fasting patient. The diagnosis therefore requires a high index of suspicion. It is the authors' experience that if there is persistent and excessive drainage from the thorax, enteral administration of double cream may turn the drain output milky, thereby confirming the diagnosis [4]. High concentration of lymphocytes and triglycerides is highly suggestive of a chyle leak, and diagnosis can be confirmed by the finding of chylomicrons on electrophoresis of the drain fluid [1].

Treatment Options

Conservative Treatment

Traditional conservative management of chylothorax involved drainage of the pleural cavity, measures to reduce chyle flow, adjunctive treatments such as somatostatin analogues, nutritional support, and prompt management of septic complications. Chyle flow can be substantially reduced by withholding dietary fat intake, with the exception of medium chain triglycerides (absorbed directly into the circulation, bypassing the lacteal system). Total parental nutrition is an alternative method of nutritional support, favored in patients with on-going high chyle losses or foregut reconstructive surgery [1]. Nevertheless, there is a high mortality associated with conservative management with patients frequently succumbing to overwhelming

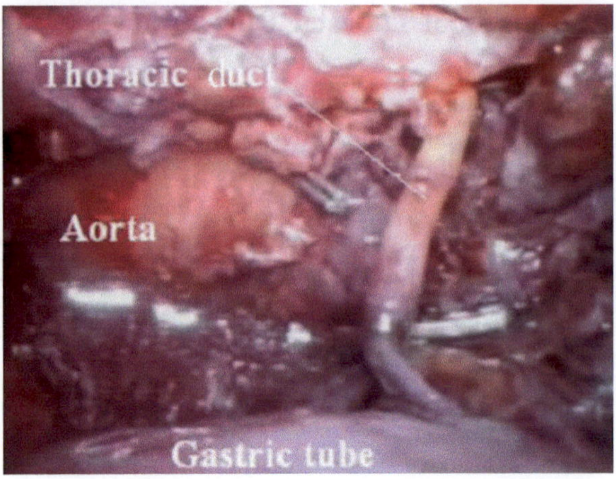

Fig. 3.4 Thoracic duct crossing the aorta showing place injury and clipped proximally

infection. The thoracic duct has numerous lymphatico-venous anastomoses with the azygos, intercostal, and lumbar veins. This allows for surgical intervention with ligation above and below a thoracic duct injury at any point in the neck or chest without concern. While a brief period of conservative management may be appropriate for relatively low output chyle leaks, drain outputs >10 mL/kg/day are unlikely to resolve and therefore surgical intervention should be undertaken.

Surgical Treatment

Preoperative imaging may be of value in the assessment of the thoracic duct injury and various methods are advocated, including computed tomography, magnetic resonance imaging, lymphoscintigraphy, and lymphangiography [1, 4]. The traditional surgical approach was via a thoracotomy. The mainstay of surgical treatment is now with a minimally invasive thoracoscopic approach. Preoperative double cream administration aids identification of the thoracic duct. Following identification of the leak, control is achieved by application of a laparoscopic clip to the thoracic duct (Fig. 3.4, Illustration 3.1). In patients in whom the leak cannot be isolated, it has been recommended that the duct be identified and ligated more proximally, at the level of the diaphragm, while some authors advocate pleurodesis, pleurectomy, or pleura-peritoneal shunting [7].

Complications of Chyle Leaks

Conservative approaches to the management of chyle leaks had a mortality of approximately 50 %. Surgical ligation of the duct dramatically reduced this mortality, and minimally invasive, thoracoscopic approaches have further reduced

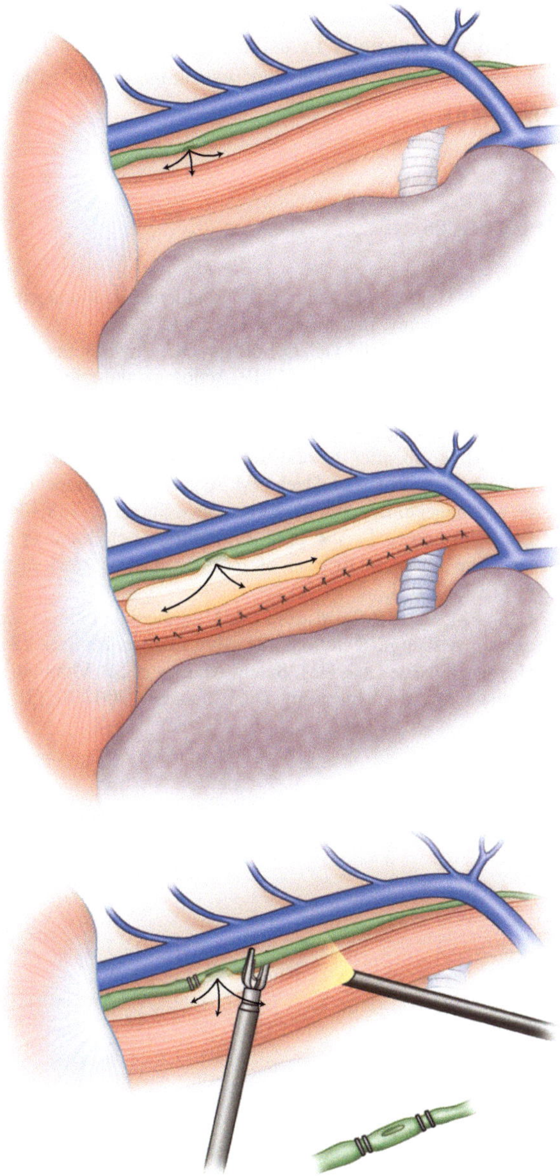

Illustration 3.1 There are different mechanisms for lesion of the thoracic duct. Once indication for surgery is made, thoracoscopic identification of the leakage and clipping of the duct is the treatment of choice

the associated mortality. A review of the reported cases in the literature from 2007 demonstrated an overall mortality of 18 %, 23 % for conservative management (range 0–57 %), and 15 % for surgical intervention (by thoracotomy) [4]. A case series of thoracoscopic intervention reported no mortality and minimal morbidity with this approach [2]. Percutaneous catheterization and embolization of the thoracic duct is a modern interventional approach, and though still in its infancy, good results have been reported [8]. However, the failure rate of this technique is approximately 30 %, and the procedure can delay definitive surgical management [8]. Hence, minimally invasive surgical ligation for thoracic duct remains a vital tool in the armory for the esophageal and thoracic surgeon in managing chylothorax.

References

1. Wemyss-Holden SA, Launois B, Maddern GJ. Management of thoracic duct injuries after oesophagectomy. Br J Surg. 2001;88:1442–8.
2. Merrigan BA, Winter DC, O'Sullivan GC. Chylothorax. Br J Surg. 1997;84:15–20.
3. Nair SK, Petko M, Hayward MP. Aetiology and management of chylothorax in adults. Eur J Cardiothorac Surg. 2007;32:362–9.
4. Valenti V, Martinez-Cecilia D, Gil A, Martinez-Isla A. Thoracoscopic treatment of post surgical chylothorax after the oral administration of a fat-rich diet. Cir Esp. 2008;84:51–2.
5. Orringer MB, Bluett M, Deeb GM. Aggressive treatment of chylothorax complicating transhiatal esophagectomy without thoracotomy. Surgery. 1988;104:720–6.
6. Lai FC, Chen L, Tu YR, et al. Prevention of chylothorax complicating extensive esophageal resection by mass ligation of thoracic duct: a random control study. Ann Thorac Surg. 2011;91:1770–4.
7. Denk PM, Gatta P, Swanstrom LL. Multimedia article. Prone thoracoscopic thoracic duct ligation for postsurgical chylothorax. Surg Endosc. 2008;22:2742.
8. Hayden JD, Sue-Ling HM, Sarela AI, Dexter SP. Minimally invasive management of chylous fistula after oesophagectomy. Dis Esophagus. 2007;20:251–5.

Chapter 4
Case on Postoperative Hiatal Herniation After Esophageal Resection

Surya S.A.Y. Biere

Keywords Postoperative hiatal herniation • Esophageal resection • Esophageal cancer • Cervical anastomosis • Esophagectomy

Diagnosis and Indication for Surgery

A 56-year-old female was evaluated for dysphagia, revealing an adenocarcinoma of the distal esophagus. The tumor could not be assessed with endosonography because of luminal stenosis. A CT scan and PET-CT scan stage the tumor as cTxN1M0. The patient received neoadjuvant chemoradiotherapy.

Operation

Subsequently, a three stage open transthoracic esophagectomy with a cervical anastomosis was performed.

Pathology

Radically resected T3N1 adenocarcinoma. Two out of 17 lymph nodes showed metastasis. The circumferential resection margin was 3 mm.

S.S.A.Y. Biere, M.D.
Department of Surgery, VU University Medical Center, Amsterdam, The Netherlands
e-mail: s.biere@vumc.nl

M.A. Cuesta, H.J. Bonjer (eds.), *Case Studies of Postoperative Complications after Digestive Surgery*, DOI 10.1007/978-3-319-01613-9_4,

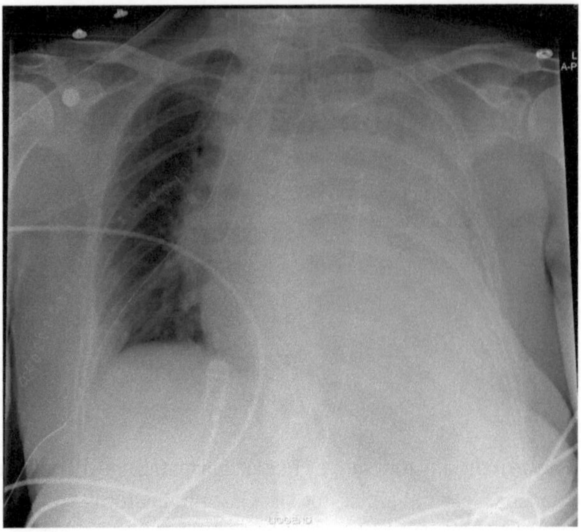

Fig. 4.1 Aspect of the bowel herniation on the Thorax X-ray

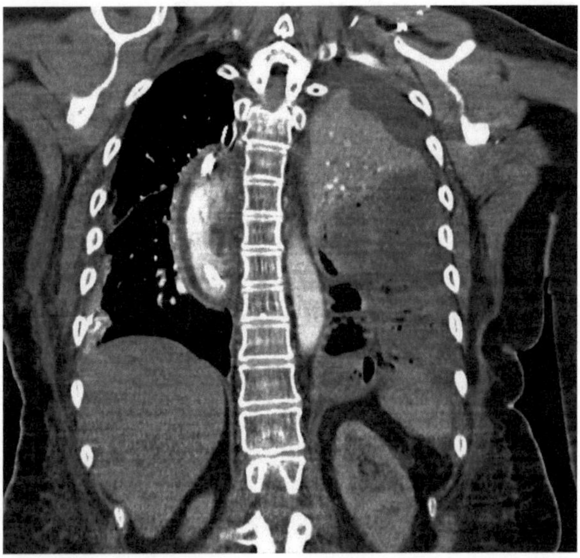

Fig. 4.2 CT scan thorax and herniation

Postoperative Course: Identification and Treatment of the Complication

Progressively, during the first two postoperative days, the patient developed an increasing pleural effusion of the left hemithorax on the chest radiograph (Fig. 4.1). A CT scan on the 3rd day revealed a hiatal herniation of the small bowel, renouncing the image on the chest radiograph (Fig. 4.2). A relaparotomy was performed.

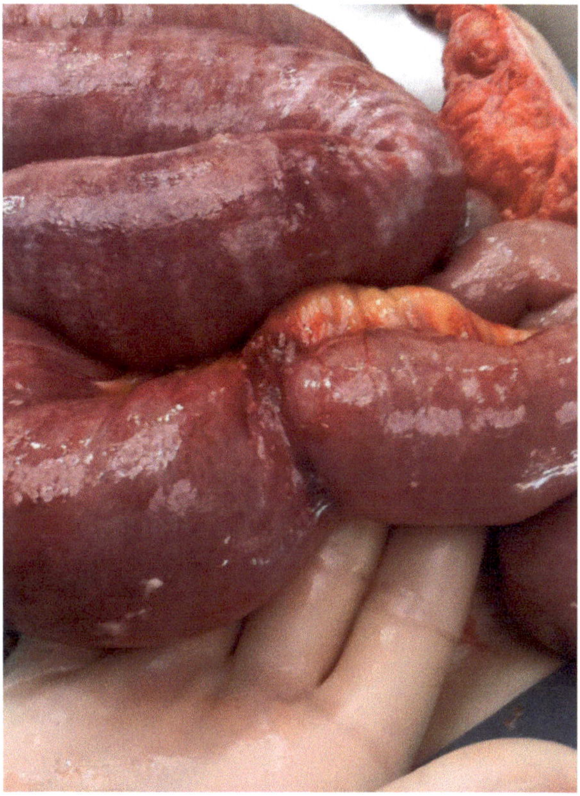

Fig. 4.3 Aspect of the herniated bowel during laparotomy after reposition

The bowel was reduced, being vital and a hiatal plasty was performed (Fig. 4.3). The patient could be discharged on the 30th postoperative day.

Discussion

Hiatal herniation is a rare complication after transthoracic esophageal resection for cancer. A report of 355 patients demonstrated an incidence of hiatal herniation of 3.5 % [1]. The median time to diagnosis was 8 months. Another series of 218 patients showed an incidence of hiatal herniation of 4 % of which only 2 % occurred during the first week after surgery [2]. In the case presented above, the hiatal herniation occurred at the third day postoperatively and was associated with intestinal obstruction and strangulation. Radiological assessment such as a chest radiograph and a CT scan are essential in the diagnosis of hiatal herniation, although in this case the chest radiograph was misleading. Management should include reduction of the hernia by laparotomy and approximation of the hiatal defect with—if necessary—a mesh, which is rarely necessary (Illustration 4.1a, b) [2]. An important factor is the enlargement of the hiatus performed during the operation, although this is not a standard procedure in transthoracic esophagectomy compared to transhiatal esophagectomy [3]. Prevention of this complication by narrowing of the diaphragmatic opening and some form of fixation of the gastric conduit to the hiatus may be indicated to avoid this complication. Awareness of its possible occurrence may help prevent the development of intestinal obstruction and strangulation.

a

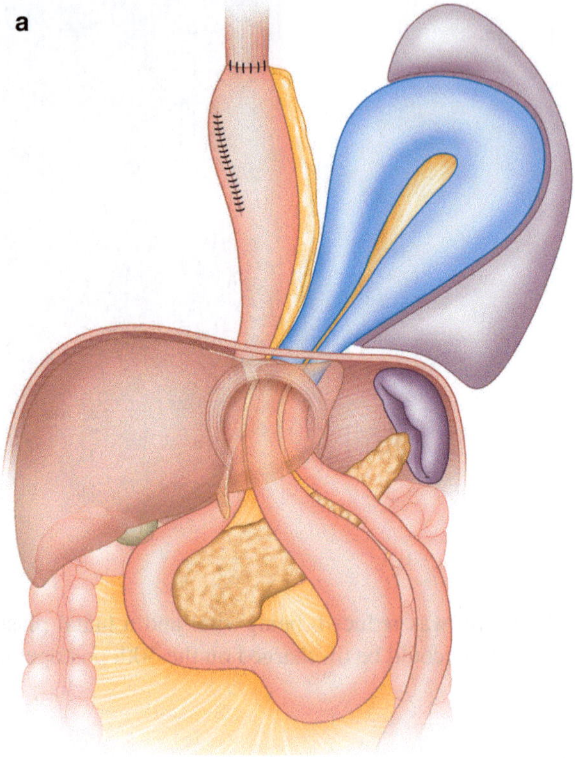

Illustration 4.1
(**a**, **b**) Hiatal herniation with incarceration of small bowel in the *left* hemithorax. Reduction by laparotomy with approximation of the hiatus

Illustration 4.1 (continued)

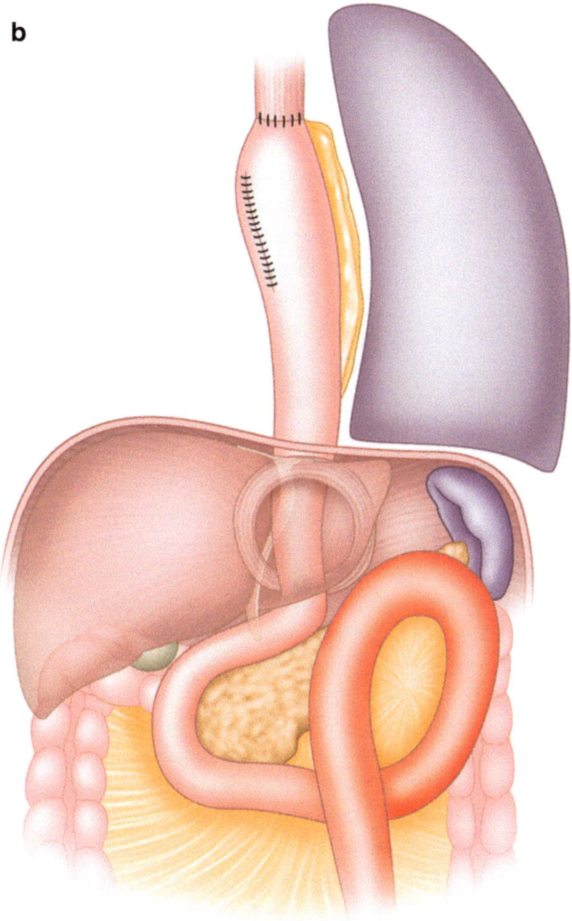

References

1. Vallböhmer D, Hölscher AH, Herbold T, et al. Diaphragmatic hernia after conventional or laparoscopic-assisted transthoracic esophagectomy. Ann Thorac Surg. 2007;84:1847–52.
2. Schieman C, Grondin SC. Paraesophageal hernia: clinical presentation, evaluation, and management controversies. Thorac Surg Clin. 2009;19:473–84.
3. van Sandick JW, Knegjens JL, van Lanschot JJ, Obertop H. Diaphragmatic herniation following oesophagectomy. Br J Surg. 1999;86:109–12.

Chapter 5
Case on Benign Stenosis of the Intrathoracic and Cervical Esophagogastric Anastomosis After Esophagectomy

Kirsten Maas, Bas P.L. Wijnhoven, and Manon C.W. Spaander

Keywords Esophageal cancer • Esophagectomy-Stenosis anastomosis • Endoscopic dilatation

First Patient (Intrathoracic Anastomosis)

Diagnosis and Indication for Surgery

A 60-year-old female was seen in the outpatient clinic because of dysphagia and 10 kg weight loss. Endoscopic and pathologic evaluation revealed squamous cell carcinoma of the distal esophagus. Further investigation by CT scan, endoscopic ultrasound together with PET-CT revealed a T2N0M0 squamous cell carcinoma of the esophagus. She was treated with neoadjuvant chemotherapy. No concurrent radiotherapy was given because of previous radiation for treating breast cancer. Chemotherapy was followed by curative esophagectomy.

K. Maas, M.D. (✉)
Department of Surgery, VU University Medical Center, Amsterdam, The Netherlands
e-mail: k.maas@vumc.nl

B.P.L. Wijnhoven, M.D.
Department of Surgery, Erasmus MC, Rotterdam, The Netherlands
e-mail: b.wijnhoven@erasmusmc.nl

M.C.W. Spaander
Department of Gastroenterology, Erasmus MC, Rotterdam, The Netherlands

M.A. Cuesta, H.J. Bonjer (eds.), *Case Studies of Postoperative Complications after Digestive Surgery*, DOI 10.1007/978-3-319-01613-9_5,

Operation

An Ivor Lewis procedure included laparoscopy and thoracoscopy to create the gastric conduit, a dissection of the intrathoracic esophagus, engagement of a two-field lymphadenectomy, and intrathoracic anastomosis. Conversion to thoracotomy was needed because of adhesions in the right thorax probably due to pneumonia a few weeks before surgery. The intrathoracic anastomosis was performed end-to-side by means of a 25 mm circular stapler.

Pathology

Radically resected T2N0 adenocarcinoma of the esophagus.

Postoperative Course: Identification and Treatment of the Complication

During the postoperative course, the patient suffered from dysphagia because of pyloric spasm, which was treated with a 20 mm balloon dilatation. After this dilatation, she could increase her oral intake and was subsequently discharged with combined feeding (oral and by jejunostomy). The jejenunostomy could be retired 4 weeks later because of optimal oral intake. Yet, 6 months later, she was suffering from progressive dysphagia and lost 3 kg of her weight. Swallow X-ray showed a relative stenosis at the site of anastomosis of the esophagus, treated by endoscopic dilatation (Fig. 5.1). Five dilatations with Savary dilatators up to 20 mm were needed to successfully treat the stenosis. After the last dilatation, the patient could swallow normally and regained weight. No more dilatations were needed.

Discussion

The major reason for midterm morbidity after esophagectomy with esophagogastric anastomosis is the development of benign anastomotic strictures [1]. An incidence of 48 % for hand sewn anastomoses and 35 % for semi-mechanical anastomoses in the neck is described [2]. It is important to distinguish two types of anastomotic strictures: the early strictures responding to few dilatations without restenosis and the so-called refractory stenosis, where over ten dilatations are needed on a frequent basis to treat and to avoid restenosis. Risk factors for refractory stenosis are anastomotic leakage, neoadjuvant chemoradiotherapy, and diagnosis of the stricture within

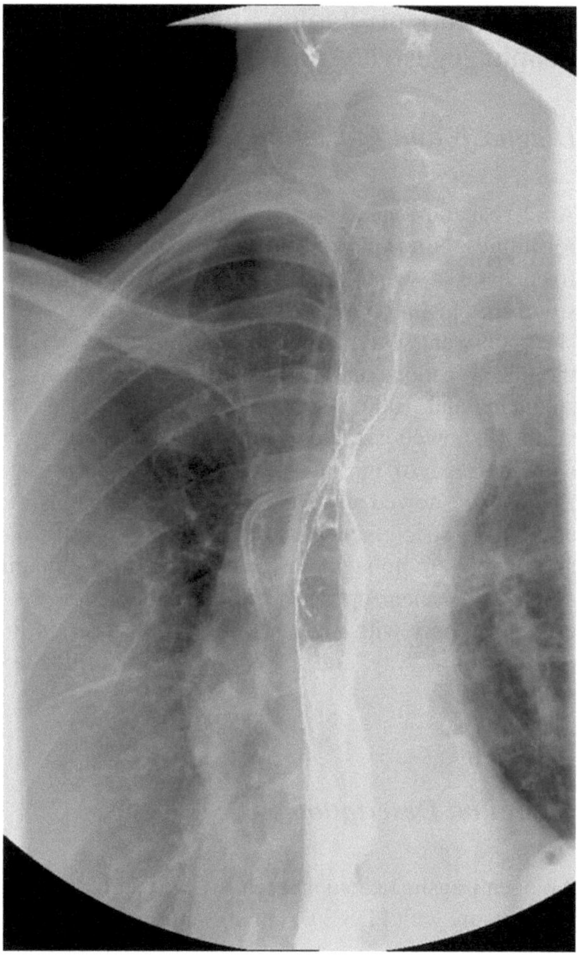

Fig. 5.1 Swallow X-ray showing stenosis of the anastomosis at intrathoracic level

90 days after surgery [1]. In the above-mentioned case there was no leakage of the anastomosis in the postoperative period. The patient had received neoadjuvant chemotherapy only because of previous radiotherapy for breast cancer. Chemotherapy alone has not been mentioned as a risk factor for stenosis. Strictures developed over 1 year postoperatively are usually malignant strictures [3].

Cervical anastomoses are described to be risk factors for benign strictures [3]. However, a recent review showed no differences in anastomotic strictures between cervical and intrathoracic anastomosis [4].

We conclude that despite the improvement of survival after esophagectomy over the last years, the long-term complications still importantly influence the quality of life of these patients. More focus is needed on the improvement of the esophagogastric anastomosis techniques in order to decrease postoperative anastomotic complications.

Second Patient: Benign Stenosis of the Cervical Esophagogastric Anastomosis After Esophagectomy

Diagnosis and Indication for Surgery

A 62-year-old female presented to the gastroenterologist with severe dysphagia for liquids. Nine years before she had undergone a laparoscopic cardiomyotomy for achalasia, which was converted to a laparotomy due to perforation of the stomach. No fundoplication was added to the procedure. The years following, she underwent several dilatations for recurrent dysphagia and peptic stenosis of the distal esophagus. Manometry showed a hypotensive lower esophageal sphincter and 100 % simultaneous contractions of the esophagus. A barium swallow showed a dilated esophagus (but no mega- or sigmoid esophagus) and slow passage of contrast across the esophagogastric junction after 10 min. Endoscopy showed no peristalsis of the esophagus, stasis of gastric juice, and the esophagogastric junction could be easily passed. No Z-line could be determined, and there were no signs of hiatal hernia or esophagitis. After discussing all the surgical treatment options with the patient, she was determined to undergo an esophagectomy with a gastric tube reconstruction in order to relieve dysphagia in a definitive way, and the endosopic surveillance of the esophagus could be abandoned.

Operation Description

An open transhiatal esophagectomy was performed with an end-to-end esophagogastrostomy with PDS 3/0 running suture.

Postoperative Course: Identification and Treatment of the Complication

The postoperative course was uncomplicated and the patient was discharged on day 7.

Seven weeks after discharge, the patient reported dysphagia for solids and liquids; subsequently, an endoscopy showed at 20 cm from the incisors a stenosis of the anastomosis with edema and inflammation. At week 10, she underwent a dilatation over a guidewire with Savary dilators up to 9 mm (Fig. 5.2). The weeks following, she underwent one to two weekly dilatations up to 16 mm, but the stenosis recurred and dysphagia persisted. At week 17, three longitudinal short incisions (precut) at the site of the persistent stenosis were made, followed 1 week

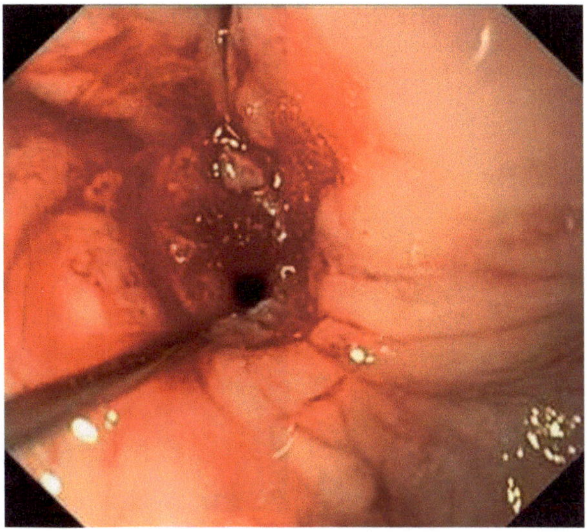

Fig. 5.2 Stenosis of anastomosis with guide wire in place. Precut was done and the stenosis was dilated till 17 mm with Savary dilators. At the end of the procedure Kenacort 1 cc was injected at the stenosis

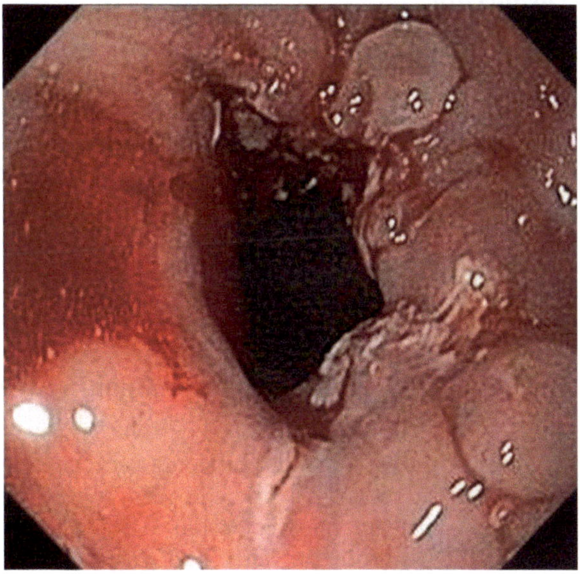

Fig. 5.3 Refractory stenosis of the esophagogastrostomy 17 weeks after the operation after multiple dilatations. Precut of benign stenosis

later by a dilatation up to 16 mm (Fig. 5.3). This was again followed by four more endoscopic sessions in which precut and dilatation ware performed. Despite these interventions, symptomatic stenosis recurred within a few days following treatment. At week 30, another precut was done at three sites of the stenosis followed by dilatation up to 17 mm and injection of 1 cc steroids in the submucosa (Kenacort® 10 mg/mL) One more dilatation was performed 4 weeks later and since then the anastomosis remained wide open and easy to be passed with an endoscope (Fig. 5.4).

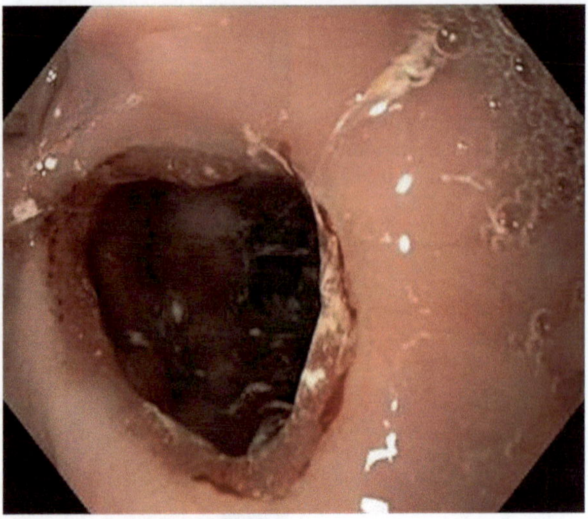

Fig. 5.4 Optimal result after 39 weeks with multiple dilatations

Discussion

This case shows that benign stenosis of the esophagogastrostomy can be refractory to repeated dilatation and incisional therapy. During the treatment the patient was intermittently unable to swallow solid foods and had remained on a liquid diet. Weight loss and decreased quality of life were reported by the patient and generate important issues to address. By adding a corticosteroid injection to the precut and dilatation session, we observed that the restenosis was resolved and the patient is well 2 years after surgery.

Incidence and Risk Factors for Benign Stenosis

Benign strictures of a cervical anastomosis occur frequently and incidence rates of 26–42 % are reported [1]. Strictures seem to be more common and more severe after gastric pull up when compared to colon interposition. Most strictures are becoming symptomatic and referred for treatment around 2–3 months after the surgery. Factors involved in the development of benign strictures are diverse: postoperative anastomotic leakage, neoadjuvant therapy, and a history of cardiac disease are reported to increase the risk. The location of the anastomosis (neck versus chest) does not seem to play a major role. But since anastomoses in the neck tend to leak more often this might induce anastomotic stricture with time. There are also some reports that relate stricture formation with the use of stapler devices and in particular with the size of the staple device employed [5]. A meta-analysis comparing hand-sewn and stapled anastomosis for the development of strictures however found no difference between the two techniques [6]. When performing a hand-sewn anastomosis, the end-to-side anastomosis is associated with a lower anastomotic stricture rate, compared to the end-to-end anastomosis. However, prevention of stricture formation was at high costs with increased anastomotic leakage and longer in-hospital stay [7].

Treatment

The preferred treatment of benign strictures is endoscopic mechanical dilatation, which is an established and safe treatment option (Illustration 5.1a,b). Most strictures respond well to dilatation and need three to eight dilatations for successful treatment. A proportion of patients with benign cervical strictures, however, suffer from a refractory stricture requiring more than ten and sometimes up to 30 dilatations. Possibly, patients at increased risk (neoadjuvant treatment, leakage, early stricturing [<90 days]) for refractory strictures might benefit from routine

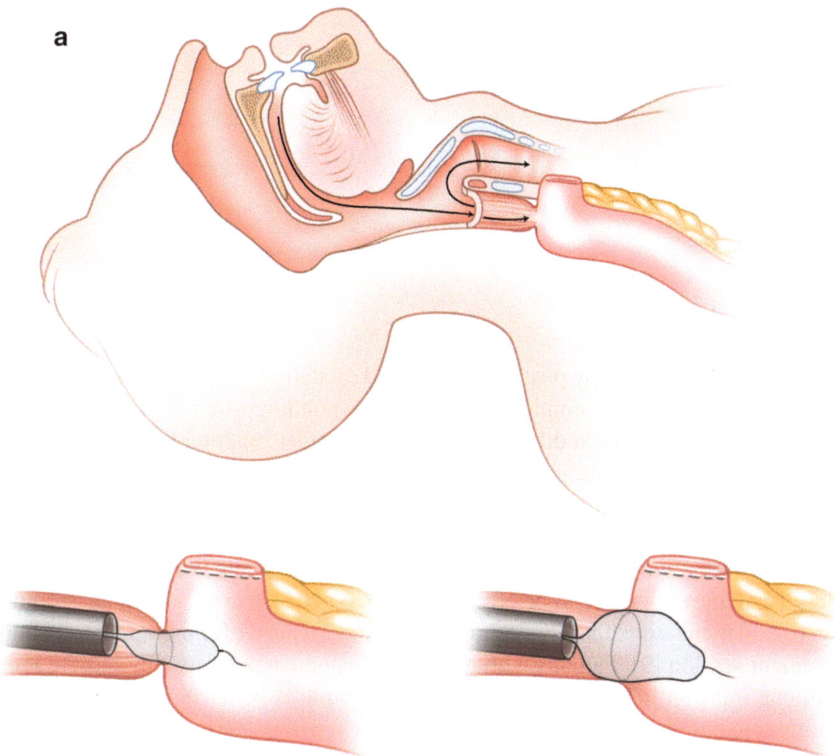

Illustration 5.1 (**a, b**) Cervical and intrathoracic anastomosis stenosis after esophageal resection. Dysphagia and risk for bronchoaspiration. Dilatation by means of Savary dilators or pneumodilatation

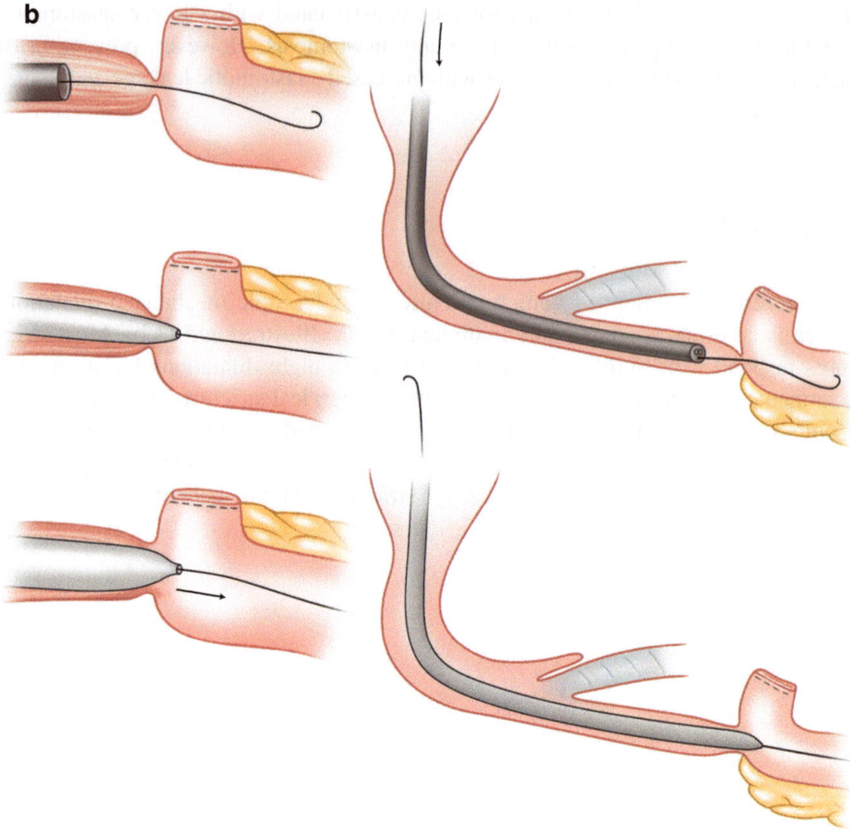

Illustration 5.1 (continued)

performance of endoscopy postoperatively and dilatation in an earlier stage. In case of complex strictures or simple strictures not responding to wire-guided bougie or through-the-scope balloon dilatation, one can consider other endoscopic treatment techniques such as intralesion steroid injection, incision therapy, argon plasma, or placement of a temporary self-expandable stent. Steroid injection in the stenosis combined with dilatation may be effective for refractory strictures with longer dilatation-free time intervals and decreased overall number of dilatations [8]. Incision therapy appeared to be effective—especially in short-segment anastomotic stenosis. Patients remained symptom-free during 1-year of follow-up after a single treatment session [9]. Patients with a longer-segment stenosis usually require more than one incision treatment. Whether this technique is better in combination with steroid injection in the stenosis or alone has not yet been clarified. The third option is placement of a temporary self-expandable stent, where the stent remains in place for 6–8 weeks. Long-term resolution of refractory stenosis up to 80 % has been described [10]. By placement of a plastic or fully covered metal stent, the stent can easily and non-traumatically be removed. However, stent migration remains a concern and is seen in up to 20 % of the patients.

Prevention

The use of a semi-mechanical side-to-side cervical anastomosis has been suggested for significantly reducing the development of strictures, possibly due to the larger cross-sectional surface area of the anastomosis [2, 11]. However, the drawback of this technique is that by using a linear stapler a longer esophageal remnant is needed in order to perform the side-to-side anastomosis. Therefore, patients with tumors located at the higher upper third of the esophagus might not be appropriate for this technique. Second, when the esophageal lumen is already obviously dilated at operation, it is not necessary to apply this technique for enlarging the anastomotic orifice further. Besides less stenosis, applying a semi-mechanical technique with use of the linear stapler also seems to decrease the leakage rates. Orringer has reported a decrease of clinical significant leaks from 10 to 15 % (manually sewn anastomosis) to 2.7 % after introduction of the linear stapling technique in over 100 patients [2].

A recent randomized study in 291 patients comparing the wrapping of the omental pedicle flap around the esophagogastric anastomosis with a stapled technique, reported only a decreased incidence of anastomotic leakage and strictures in the omental wrapping group [12]. The theory behind this phenomenon is that adhesions form between the omentum and the gastric tube, thereby helping to seal microscopic leaks and aid in tissue remodeling. The pool of histiocytes, monocytes, and granulocytes in the omentum may also contain the local infective process, thereby protecting the anastomosis. Gastric ischemic conditioning prior to esophagogastrostomy might improve gastric perfusion and hence decrease the rate of leakage and strictures [13]. But this has still to be proven in randomized controlled trials. There are more techniques and modifications of existing techniques described, such as the mucosal tube technique and supercharge technique. However, there is a paucity of trials that compare one with the other technique. The best surgical technique and location of the anastomosis (neck versus chest) therefore remains to be determined. Recently, it was hypothesized that benign anastomotic stricture formation is related to reflux of erosive gastric contents from the gastric tube. In the 40 patients randomized to receiving proton pump inhibitors (PPIs) after a circular stapled anastomosis in the chest, benign anastomotic strictures developed in 13 % as compared to 45 % of patients not on PPIs [14].

References

1. van Heijl M, Gooszen JA, Fockens P, et al. Risk factors for development of benign cervical strictures after esophagectomy. Ann Surg. 2010;251:1064–9.
2. Orringer MB, Marshall B, Iannettoni MD. Eliminating the cervical esophagogastric anastomotic leak with a side-to-side stapled anastomosis. J Thorac Cardiovasc Surg. 2000;119:277–88.
3. Sutcliffe RP, Forshaw MJ, Tandon R, et al. Anastomotic strictures and delayed gastric emptying after esophagectomy: incidence, risk factors and management. Dis Esophagus. 2008;21: 712–7.

4. Biere SSAY, Maas KW, Cuesta MA, van der Peet DL. Cervical or intrathoracic anastomosis after esophagectomy for cancer: a systematic review. Dig Surg. 2011;28:29–35.
5. Dresner SM, Lamb PJ, Wayman J, et al. Benign anastomotic stricture following transthoracic subtotal oesophagectomy and stapled oesophago-gastrostomy: risk factors and management. Br J Surg. 2000;87:362–73.
6. Urschel JD, Blewett CJ, Bennett WF, et al. Handsewn or stapled esophagogastric anastomoses after esophagectomy for cancer: meta-analysis of randomized controlled trials. Dis Esophagus. 2001;14:212–7.
7. Nederhof N, Tilanus HW, Tran TC, et al. End-to-end versus end-to-side esophagogastrostomy after esophageal cancer resection: a prospective randomized study. Ann Surg. 2011;254: 226–33.
8. Kochhar R, Makharia GK. Usefulness of intralesional triamcinolone in treatment of benign esophageal strictures. Gastrointest Endosc. 2002;56:829–34.
9. Hordijk ML, Siersema PD, Tilanus HW, Kuipers EJ. Electrocautery therapy for refractory anastomotic strictures of the esophagus. Gastrointest Endosc. 2006;63:157–63.
10. Repici A, Conio M, De Angelis C, et al. Temporary placement of an expandable polyester silicone-covered stent for treatment of refractory benign esophageal strictures. Gastrointest Endosc. 2004;60:513–9.
11. Xu QR, Wang KN, Wang WP, et al. Linear stapled esophagogastrostomy is more effective than hand-sewn or circular stapler in prevention of anastomotic stricture: a comparative clinical study. J Gastrointest Surg. 2011;15:915–21.
12. Dai JG, Zhang ZY, Min JX, Huang XB, Wang JS. Wrapping of the omental pedicle flap around esophagogastric anastomosis after esophagectomy for esophageal cancer. Surgery. 2011;149: 404–10.
13. Varela E, Reavis KM, Hinojosa MW, Nguyen N. Laparoscopic gastric ischemic conditioning prior to esophagogastrectomy: technique and review. Surg Innov. 2008;15:132–5.
14. Johansson J, Oberg S, Wenner J, et al. Impact of proton pump inhibitors on benign anastomotic stricture formations after esophagectomy and gastric tube reconstruction: results from a randomized clinical trial. Ann Surg. 2009;250:667–73.

Chapter 6
Case on Recurrent Nerve Lesion (Double) as a Consequence of Esophageal Resection for Cancer

Ramon Gorter

Keywords Esophageal resection • RLN • Laryngoscopy • Cordotomy • Arytenoidectomy

Diagnosis and Indication for Surgery

A 79-year-old male with complaints of dysphagia was evaluated at our outpatient clinic. His medical history included a right-sided pneumonia and endoscopic treatment of a Zenker's diverticulum. Endoscopy revealed an ulcerative adenocarcinoma of the esophagus at 28–34 cm from the incisors. Based on CT scans and endosonograpy, the tumor was staged as T3N1M0.

Operation

Six weeks after neoadjuvant chemoradiation (CROSS-scheme: weekly administration of Carboplatin® AUC = 2 en Paclitaxel® 50 mg/m^2 with concurrent 5 days weekly radiotherapy in fractions of 1.8 Gy, total 41,4 Gy [1]) the patient was admitted for open transthoracic esophagectomy with two-field lymphadenectomy followed by a right cervical gastric conduit anastomosis with the esophagus.

R. Gorter, M.D.
Pediatric Surgery, VU University Medical Center, Amsterdam, The Netherlands
e-mail: rr.gorter@vumc.nl

M.A. Cuesta, H.J. Bonjer (eds.), *Case Studies of Postoperative Complications after Digestive Surgery*, DOI 10.1007/978-3-319-01613-9_6,

Pathology

Radically resected T3N1 adenocarcinoma of the esophagus.

Postoperative Course: Identification and Treatment of the Complication

Postoperatively, the patient was admitted to the intensive care unit. On the chest radiograph a large pneumothorax was diagnosed on the right side and a second chest tube was inserted (Fig. 6.1). The second postoperative day, the patient was detubated, but during the following days, he became increasingly dyspnoic and oxygenation was poor. Because of aphony and stridor, the ENT doctor evaluated the vocal cords. Laryngoscopy showed bilateral vocal cord paralysis (Fig. 6.2). Because

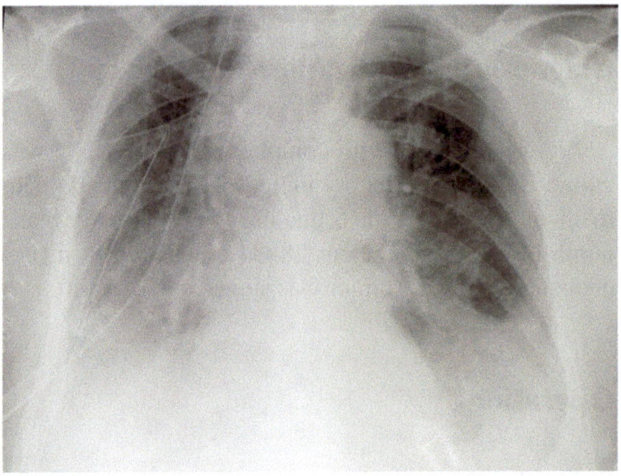

Fig. 6.1 Postoperative thorax X-ray

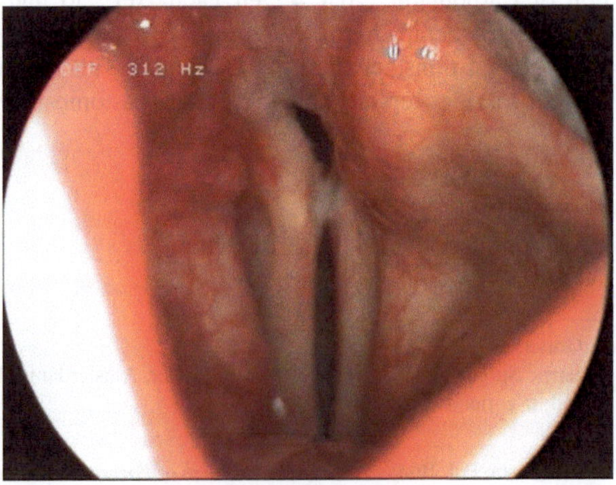

Fig. 6.2 Laryngoscopy showing vocal bilateral cord paralysis

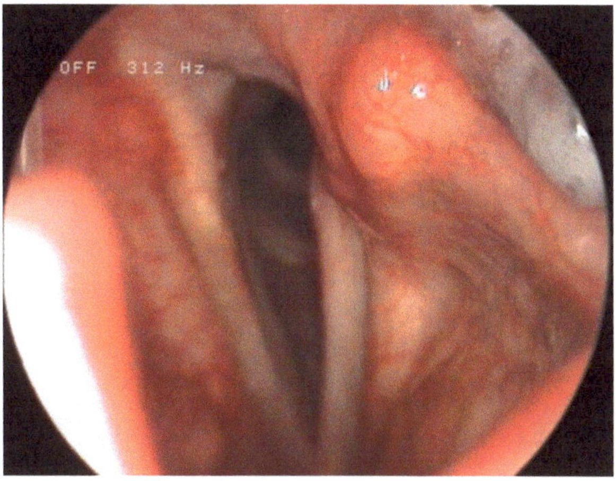

Fig. 6.3 Laryngoscopy after 6 months showing recovery of function of the right vocal cord

of the respiratory insufficiency and stridor, it was decided to perform a tracheostomy. On the 17th postoperative day, a bronchopneumonia was diagnosed for which intravenous antibiotics were started for 7 days. On the 19th postoperative day, it was decided to start oral feeding with the assistance of a logopedist. Aspiration was then noted clinically and the oral feeding was averted, whereas jejunostomy feeding was continued. Aspiration pneumonia developed again several days later and intravenous antibiotics were restarted. Revaluation of the vocal cord paralysis showed no signs of improvement. After discharge (1½ month after the initial surgery) the patient had not initiated oral intake and continued breathing through the tracheostomy. Intensive training with a speech language logopedist and progressive oral feeding started in an outpatient program. Six months after discharge, the patient was eating normally, and before a vocal cord plasty was planned, a new laryngoscopy showed recovery of the left vocal cord with normal spontaneous breathing (Fig. 6.3). After 2 months tracheotomy was retired without respiratory problems. He is still receiving speech therapy lessons to improve the quality of his voice.

Discussion

The recurrent laryngeal nerve (RLN) plays an essential role in the innervation of the intrinsic muscles of the larynx especially those responsible for movement of the vocal cords. Both uni- and bilateral lesions have been described with an incidence ranging between 15 and 80 % depending on the cervical dissection and extensiveness of the esophageal and lymph node dissection [1–3]. Most cases of unilateral RLN paralysis are seen after cervical oesophagogastrostomy. This patient developed bilateral RLN lesions after transthoracic oesophagectomy with right cervical anastomosis (Illustration 6.1). A cervical anastomosis is associated with a high incidence of RLN damage either temporarily or definitive [1–5]. The fact that a cervical anastomosis was performed on the right side may explain why the right RLN became damaged

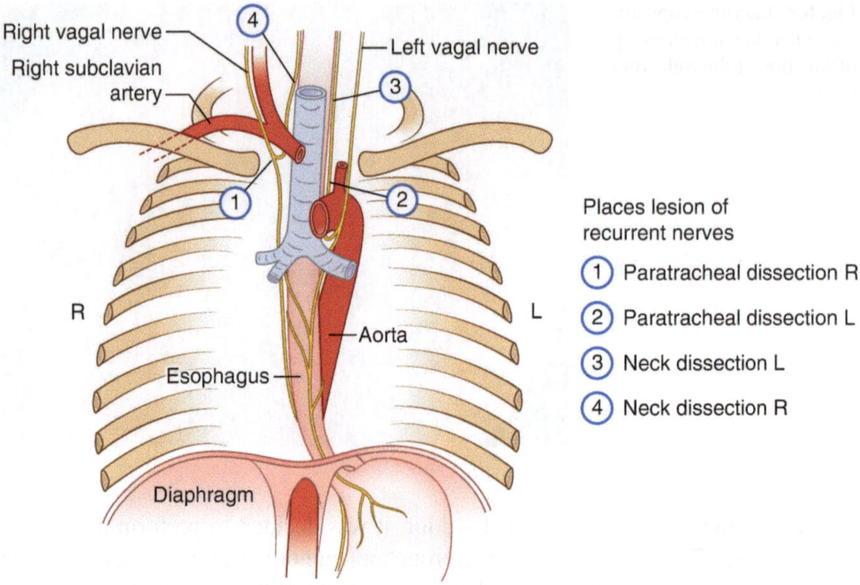

Illustration 6.1 Anatomy of the recurrent laryngeal nerve (RLN)

and possibly also the left RLN, since no paratracheal or aortopulmonary window lymphadenectomy was performed. Damage to the ipsilateral as well as the contralateral RLN is reported in 2 % of cases following transhiatal oesophageal resection [2]. Prevention of RLN lesion will include identification and eventually monitoring during cervical and high mediastinal lymph node dissection. Any atraumatic dissection and tractions will be avoided [4]. Symptoms associated with an unilateral lesion are hoarseness and infrequently stridor, while a bilateral lesion leads to aphony, swallowing dysfunctions and stridor with breathing difficulties causing significant secondary respiratory morbidity, prolonged hospital stay, and decreased quality of life [1–3]. The risk of developing postoperative pneumonia, due to decreased respiratory function, deficiency of the coughing mechanism, and aspiration, is significantly greater in patients suffering from postoperative RLN injury. Treatment in the acute phase depends on the severity of the symptoms. In most cases active physiotherapy and logopedy can offer satisfactory results, although in bilateral injury with paralysis in a median position, tracheostomy will be the only adequate treatment as described in this case. In a later stage several vocal cord procedures can be carried out for bilateral injury, in order to lateralize one or both vocal cords to improve the patency of the airways. Moreover, spontaneous recovery on one side is possible if only contusion of the nerve during operation. Both cordotomy and arytenoidectomy have been reported to have satisfactory results, although new techniques such as laryngeal pacing and botulinum toxin injection may be considered as therapeutical options in the near future [5].

References

1. Wright CD, Zeitels SM. Recurrent laryngeal nerve injuries after esophagectomy. Thorac Surg Clin. 2006;16:23–33.
2. Hulscher JB, van Sandick JW, Devriese PP, et al. Vocal cord paralysis after subtotal oesophagectomy. Br J Surg. 1999;86(12):1583–7.
3. Baba M, Natsugoe S, Shimada M, et al. Does hoarseness of voice from recurrent nerve paralysis after esophagectomy for carcinoma influence patient quality of life? J Am Coll Surg. 1999;188:231–6.
4. Gelpke H, Grieder F, Decurtins M, Cadosch D. World J Surg 2010;34:2379–82.
5. Rubin AD, Sataloff RT. Vocal fold paresis and paralysis. Otolaryngol Clin N Am. 2007;40:1109–31.

Chapter 7
Case on Trachea-gastric Conduit Fistula After Esophageal Resection

Koen Hartemink

Keywords Trachea fistula • Esophageal resection • Esophageal cancer

Diagnosis and Indication for Surgery

A 62-year-old male patient was referred to our hospital after esophageal resection performed in another hospital. His medical history revealed diabetes mellitus and an appendectomy. A few months before, an adenocarcinoma of the mid-esophagus had been found and the patient was treated by neoadjuvant chemo-radiotherapy according to the CROSS scheme (Carboplatin/Paclitaxel with concurrent radiotherapy in 23 fractions of 1.8 Gy). Restaging showed a reduction in size of the primary tumor without any signs of metastases and resection of the esophagus was planned.

Operation

A thoracolaparoscopic esophageal resection was done and a gastric conduit with an end-to-side cervical anastomosis was performed. The thoracoscopic phase was done in prone position during which the esophagus was resected and an en bloc carina lymphadenectomy was performed. Azygos vein was divided by means of Haemaloc clips®. Because the tumor was fixed to the right lung, a local resection of a pulmonary segment was done, after which a peroperative frozen section

K. Hartemink, M.D.
Intensive Care, Department of Surgery, VU University Medical Center, Amsterdam, The Netherlands
e-mail: k.hartemink@vumc.nl

M.A. Cuesta, H.J. Bonjer (eds.), *Case Studies of Postoperative Complications after Digestive Surgery*, DOI 10.1007/978-3-319-01613-9_7,

showed no tumor in the resection margin. The patient was turned in supine position for the abdominal phase of the operation in which a celiac trunk lymphadenectomy was done and the gastric conduit was created. Cervical incision and transection of the esophagus were done, followed by an end-to-side cervical anastomosis. A jejunostomy feeding tube was introduced for postoperative enteral feeding.

Pathology

Histopathological examination showed an adenocarcinoma with growth through the muscularis layer. One of nine lymph nodes showed a metastasis. Resection margins were free of tumor (pT3N1, R0 resection).

Postoperative Course: Identification and Treatment of the Complication

Postoperative recovery was uneventful and the patient was discharged from the hospital on the seventh postoperative day. One week after discharge from the hospital, the patient was readmitted because of pneumonia that was treated with antibiotics. Because of progressive complaints of dyspnoe, coughing, and persistence of the pneumonia, there was suspicion of a trachea-gastric conduit fistula. A fluoroscopic swallow study showed an anastomotic leakage of contrast (Fig. 7.1.a), and a CT-scan showed an infiltrate in the right lower lobe. An endoscopy showed partial dehiscence of the esophagogastric conduit anastomosis. Tracheobronchoscopy showed a defect (1 cm diameter) on the dorsal side of the proximal right main bronchus (Fig. 7.1b). The patient was transferred to our hospital for operative correction of the trachea-gastric conduit fistula.

At admission to our hospital, the patient was already intubated and mechanically ventilated, and after double intubation a right-sided thoracotomy was performed. A fistula was found between a semi-circular defect of the esophago-gastric conduit anastomosis and a defect on the dorsal side of the proximal right main bronchus (Fig. 7.2). Although the anastomosis was performed cervically, it had descended into the thorax. The esophagogastric conduit anastomosis was disconnected from the right bronchus, showing a t-shaped defect. The defect in the right main bronchus was closed with interrupted sutures (Fig. 7.3), and an intercostal muscle flap was used to reinforce the defect. After closure of the defect, the gastric conduit was re-anastomosed with the cervical esophagus (Fig. 7.4).

The postoperative course was initially uneventful. However, 2 weeks after reoperation, the patient developed respiratory failure due to vomiting and aspiration in both lungs, resulting in multiple organ failure and subsequent death.

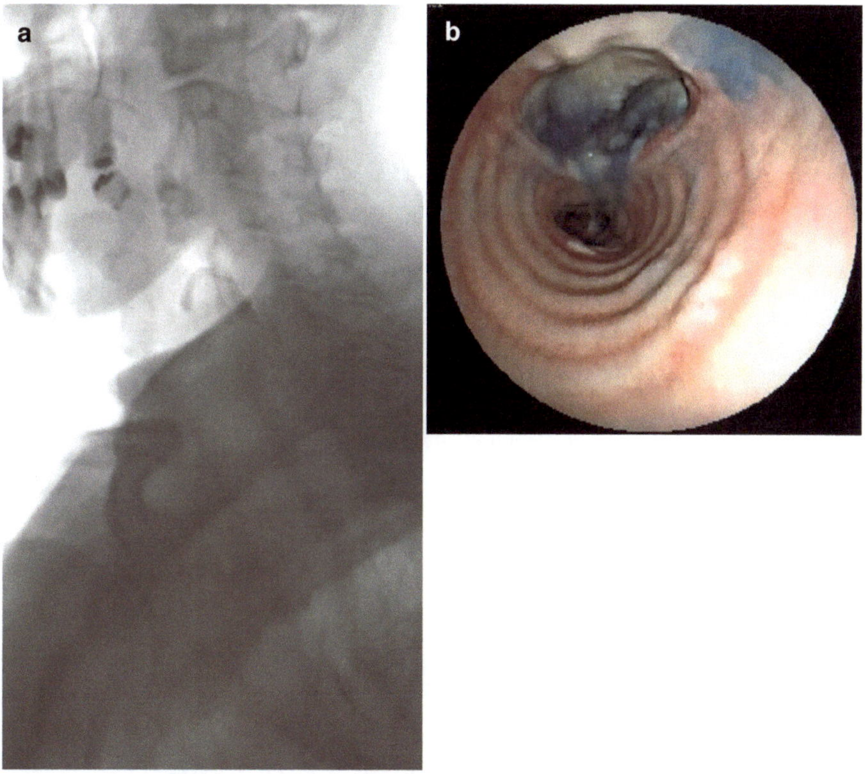

Fig. 7.1 Contrast swallow study shows leakage (*arrow*) (**a**) and tracheoscopy showing the fistula opening (**b**)

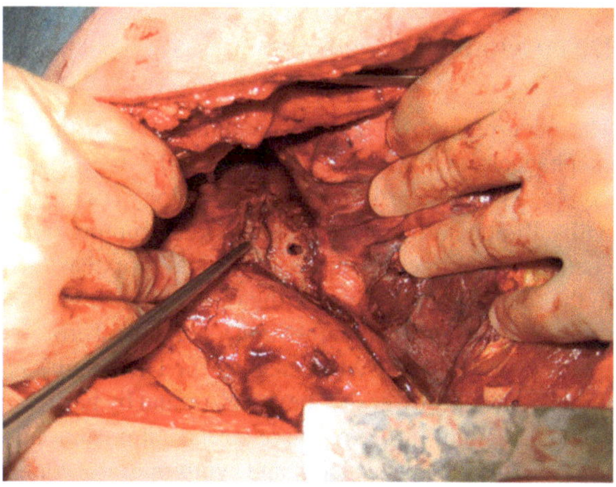

Fig. 7.2 Peroperative macroscopic picture showing a defect on the dorsal side of the proximal right main bronchus (*thin arrow*) and a defect in the gastric conduit (*thick arrow*)

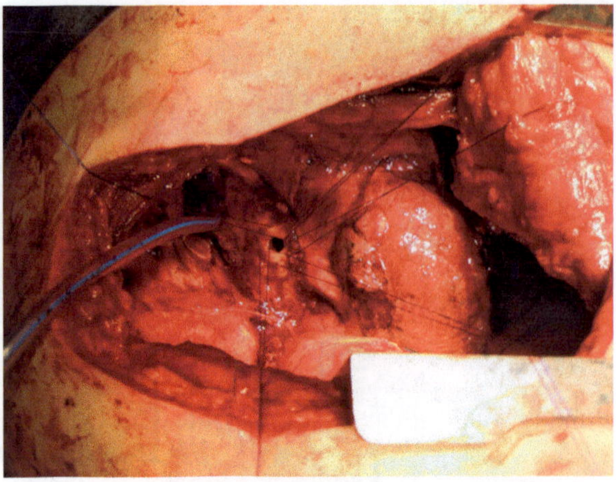

Fig. 7.3 Peroperative macroscopic picture showing the defect in the right main bronchus which was closed with interrupted sutures, and an intercostal muscle flap (not shown) was used to close the defect. A *gastric tube* in the cervical esophagus is seen

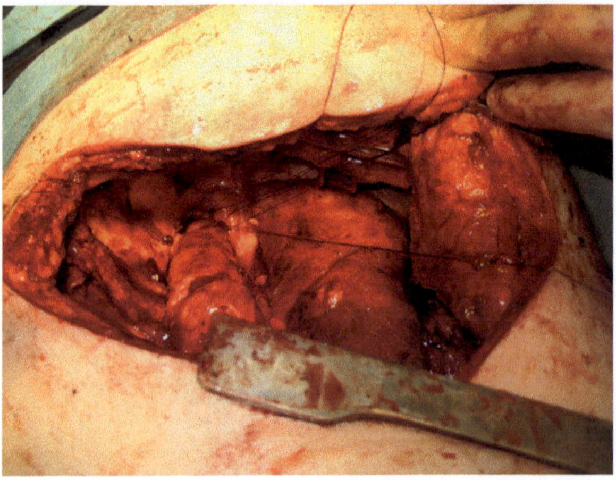

Fig. 7.4 Peroperative macroscopic picture showing the gastric conduit being re-anastomosed with the esophagus with interrupted sutures

Discussion

The occurrence of a gastric conduit fistula with trachea or bronchus following esophagectomy for cancer is very low (0.3–0.5 %) but is mostly a lethal complication [1, 2] The underlying pathophysiology consists of leakage of the anastomosis with subsequent mediastinal abscess and rupture into the posterior wall of the tracheobronchial tree, tracheal ischemia after extensive dissection, traumatic injuries to the trachea or bronchia during dissection, cuff-induced tracheal necrosis (during prolonged endotracheal intubation), or tracheal erosion by the gastric conduit staple line or clips [3, 4]. Yasuda et al. classified the fistulas in three types: caused by anastomotic leakage, by gastric necrosis, or/and by gastric ulcer [5]. Symptoms might be mild (coughing) or more severe (recurrent pneumonia or mediastinitis). Diagnosis is based on clinical suspicion and symptoms and confirmed by radiological contrast

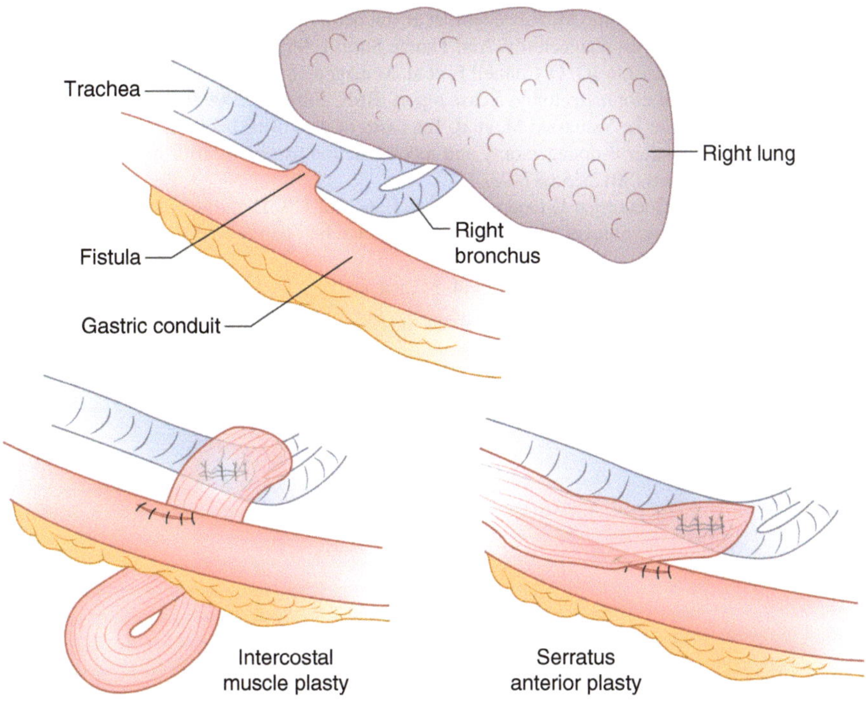

Illustration 7.1 Treatment of the tracheo-gastric conduit fistula by closure and muscle plasty

study and CT scan, esophagogastroscopy, and bronchoscopy [1] There are different possible management strategies (conservative, endoscopic, or surgical), and the approach depends on the patient's condition, site, and size of the fistula, the underlying cause, and the clinical presentation and severity of symptoms [4, 6] In patients having a very bad condition—locally and general—temporary treatment by means of stents may be an option to perform the definitive intervention at a better moment [7]. When conservative measures fail or the patient's condition worsens, a surgical approach becomes necessary. Surgical treatment consists of identification and dissection of the fistula, closure of the tracheal- and gastric-conduit defects with use of interposed vital tissue (pleural or pericardial tissue or a muscle-flap), and preservation if possible of the gastric conduit (Illustration 7.1) [1–6].

References

1. Nardella JE, Van Raemdonck D, Piessevaux H, et al. Gastro-tracheal fistula - unusual and life threatening complication after esophagectomy for cancer: a case report. J Cardiothorac Surg. 2009;4:69–71.
2. Kalmár K, Molnár TF, Morgan A, Horváth ÖP. Non-malignant tracheo-gastric fistula following esophagectomy for cancer. Eur J Cardiothoracic Surg. 2000;18:363–5.

3. Marty-Ané C-H, Prudhome M, Fabre J-M, et al. Tacheoesophagogastric anastomosis fistula: a rare complication of esophagectomy. Ann Thorac Surg. 1995;60:690–3.
4. Martin-Smith JD, Larkin JO, O'Connell F, et al. Management of gastro-bronchial fistula complicating a subtotal esophagectomy: a case report. BMC Surgery. 2009;9:20.
5. Yasuda T, Sugimura K, Yamasaki M, et al. Ten cases of gastro-tracheobronchial fistula: a serious complication after esophagectomy and reconstruction using posterior mediastinal gastric tube. Dis Esophagus. 2012;25:687–93.
6. Buskens CJ, Van Coevorden F, Obertop H, Van Lanschot JJB. Disturbed anastomotic healing after esophagectomy: a novel treatment of a benign tracheo-neo-esophageal fistula. Dig Surg. 2002;19:88–91.
7. Schweigert M, Dubecz A, Beron M, et al. Management of anastomotic leakage-induced tracheobronchial fistula following oesophagectomy: the role of endoscopic stent insertion. Eur J Cardiothorac Surg. 2012;41:74–80.

Chapter 8
Case on Herniation of the Stomach Into the Thorax After Laparoscopic Repair of a Type 3 Paraesophageal Hernia

Jelle P. Ruurda and Mark I. van Berge Henegouwen

Keywords Laparoscopic correction • Herniation • Paraesophageal hernia

Diagnosis and Indication for Surgery

A 65-year-old male presented at our outpatient clinic with progressive shortness of breath. Computed tomography of his chest demonstrated a type 3 paraesophageal hernia (Fig. 8.1a, b). Besides an umbilical hernia and an appendectomy and subsequent surgical repair of a cicatricial hernia at the site of appendectomy, he did not undergo previous abdominal surgery. His body mass index was 31 (186 cm, 107 kg).

Operation

At surgery, the completely intrathoracic stomach was laparoscopically repositioned into the abdomen. Hereafter, a tension-free cruraplasty could be performed with non-resorbable sutures, without the use of a mesh. The procedure was completed by a Toupet 270 degrees fundoplication.

J.P. Ruurda (✉)
Department of Surgery, University MC, Utrecht, The Netherlands
e-mail: j.p.ruurda@umcutrecht.nl

M.I. van B. Henegouwen
Department of Surgery, Academic Medical Center, Amsterdam, The Netherlands

M.A. Cuesta, H.J. Bonjer (eds.), *Case Studies of Postoperative Complications after Digestive Surgery*, DOI 10.1007/978-3-319-01613-9_8,

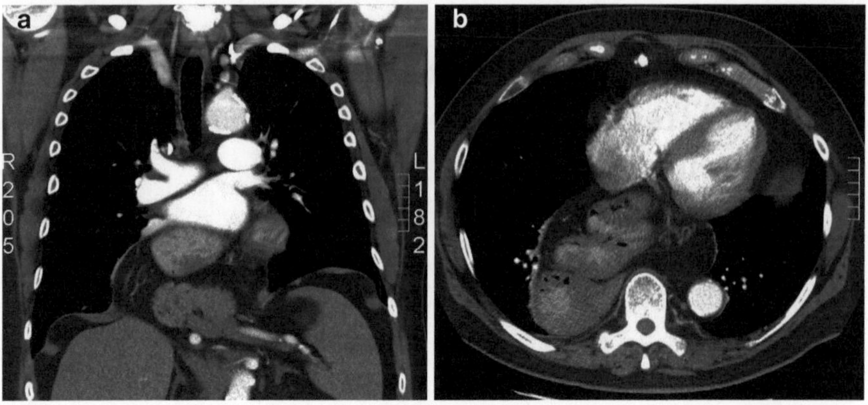

Fig. 8.1 (**a**, **b**) CT scan (sagital and transverse images) demonstrating a diaphragmatic hernia with an intrathoracic stomach and pancreas

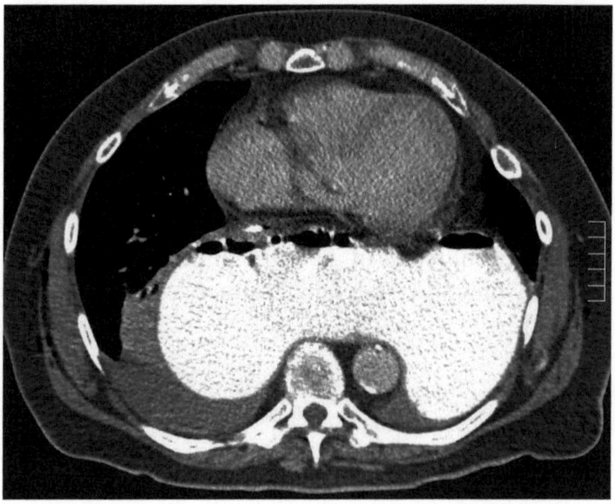

Fig. 8.2 CT scan on the third postoperative day, demonstrating re-herniation of the stomach into the thorax

Postoperative Course: Identification and Treatment of the Complication

Initially, recovery was uneventful and patient started on an oral diet at the first postoperative day. On the third postoperative day, his heart- and breathing frequency increased and his temperature went up to 38.5 °C. A CT scan demonstrated re-herniation of a huge dilated stomach into the thorax (Fig. 8.2) on which the patient was reoperated. In the short waiting time for surgery, the clinical condition of the patient deteriorated with a short period of cardiopulmonary resuscitation,

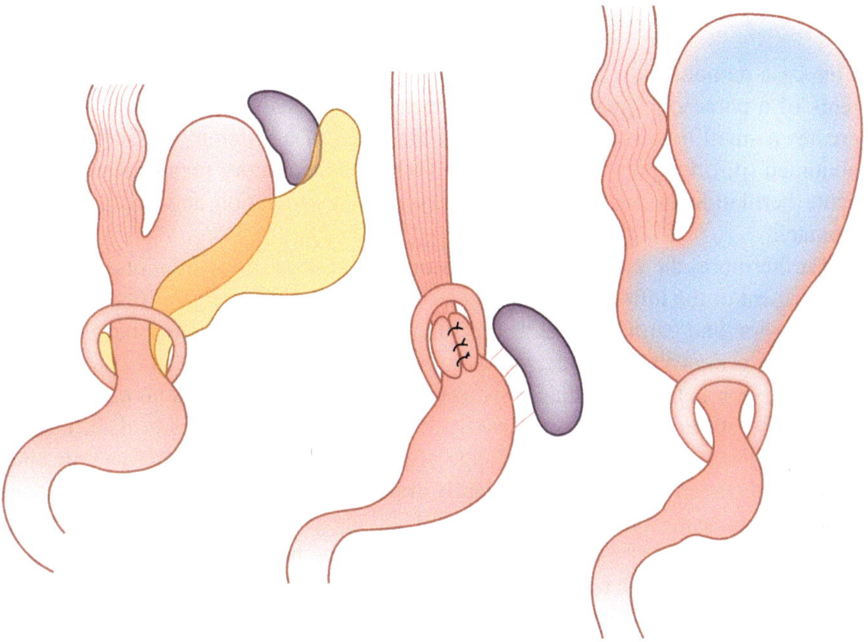

Illustration 8.1 Re-herniation of stomach after laparoscopic paraesophageal hernia repair. Acute operation by laparotomy, reposition of the stomach, and fixation

necessitating mechanical ventilation and hemodynamic support. Because of his deteriorated condition, an emergency laparotomy was performed.

At laparotomy, the stomach was found to have herniated through the 2–3 cm opening of an intact cruraplasty (Illustration 8.1). An important gastric dilatation of the strangulated stomach caused compression of lungs and heart, impairing cardiac inflow that caused the cardiopulmonary arrest. The stomach was opened and its contents immediately suctioned after which the clinical condition of the patient improved dramatically. The stomach could be repositioned into the abdomen after breakdown of the cruraplasty. It was found to be partly necrotic and damaged, necessitating resection of a part of the greater curvature.

The hiatus was reapproximated with non-resorbable sutures and a mesh. A fundoplication was not performed as the major part of the gastric fundus had been resected.

After surgery, the patient was admitted to the intensive care unit and needed hemodynamic and ventilatory support for another day. Further recovery was uneventful and the patient left the hospital on a normal diet 12 days after the laparotomy.

Discussion

This case demonstrates the important consequences of a re-herniation of the contents of a paraesophageal hernia after operation. A dehiscence of the hiatoplasty creates a small hole in the hiatus and in the event of a different pressure between abdomen (positive pressure) and thorax (negative inspiratory pressure) may cause acute herniation of the stomach with posterior strangulation and necrosis of the stomach.

Furthermore, the entrapment of the stomach, with gastric dilatation, will cause impairment of the inflow into the right atrium with cardiopulmonary instability and hypotension and cardiac arrest as a result. The mechanical situation may be compared to a pericard tamponade.

The lesson is that once diagnosis has been established, there is no time to wait. Very rapid surgical action is necessary in a clinically very quickly deteriorating patient. After fast opening and drainage of gastric contents, the hemodynamic situation of the patient will have dramatically improved and further resection and reconstruction can be performed. Prevention will include an adequate operative technique including resection of the sac, approximation of the hiatus and eventually gastropexy. The use of a mesh remains controversial and should only be used in the minority of cases in which the hiatus can not be approximated [1, 2].

References

1. Van der Peet DL, Klinkenberg Knol EC, Alonso Poza A, et al. Laparoscopic treatment of large paraesophageal hernias: both excision of the sac and gastropexy are imperative for adequate surgical treatment. Surg Endosc. 2000;14:1015–8.
2. Arafat FO, Teitelbaum EN, Hungness ES. Modern treatment of Paraesophageal hernia: preoperative evaluation and technique for laparoscopic repair. Surg Laparoscopic Endosc Percutan Tech. 2012;22:297–303.

Chapter 9
Case on Dysphagia After Laparoscopic Nissen Fundoplication

Miguel A. Cuesta and Donald L. van der Peet

Keywords Dysphagia • Gastroesophageal reflux disease • Nissen fundoplication

First Patient

Diagnosis and Indication for Surgery: Identification and Treatment of the Complication

A 47-year-old female patient was referred to our outpatient clinic for a second opinion due to persistent dysphagia incurred 4 months after a laparoscopic Nissen fundoplication. She could not pass bland or solid food and was fed enteral through a thin nasogastric tube in the duodenum. In the past she had undergone a laparoscopic sacrocolpopexy because of rectal prolapse. Indication for the fundoplication was a therapy resistant gastro-esophageal reflux disease (proton pump inhibitors).

The patient's condition was reasonably good, her weight was 64 kg (BMI of 25) and there were no other complaints such as pain, reflux esophagitis, or diarrhea. Moreover, her mental condition was good.

Her complaints were assessed by means of an X-swallow photo with marshmallows, esophagoscopy, and esophageal manometry. The swallow photo showed an incomplete passage to the stomach (Fig. 9.1a, b), and the manometry showed normal contractions of the esophageal body with a high and incomplete

M.A. Cuesta, M.D. (✉) • D.L. van der Peet
Department of Surgery, VU University Medical Center,
Amsterdam, The Netherlands
e-mail: ma.cuesta@vumc.nl

M.A. Cuesta, H.J. Bonjer (eds.), *Case Studies of Postoperative Complications after Digestive Surgery*, DOI 10.1007/978-3-319-01613-9_9,

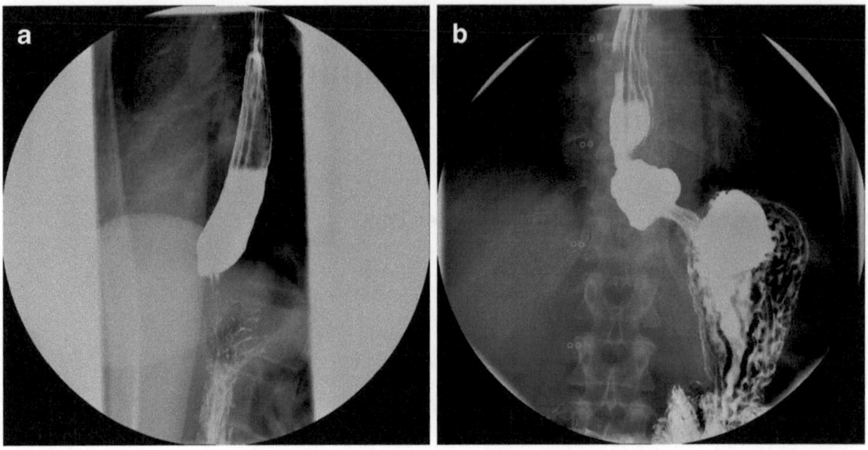

Fig. 9.1 (**a**, **b**) Swallow X-ray after Nissen fundoplication showing stenosis and telescopage of the esophagogastric junction

relaxation of the lower esophageal sphincter (LES) with a high pressure of 20 mmHg. On the esophagoscopy—distal of the Z-line—some gastric folds were visible before the wrap, indicating a misplaced wrap during the initial operation or some kind of herniation of the gastric fundus through the fundoplication.

It was clear that the previous fundoplication was the cause of the dysphagia and that motor dysfunction of the esophagus could be ruled out. A redo-procedure was indicated; to dismantle the 360° fundoplication, correct the position of the wrap, and convert the fundoplication in partial, Toupet like, 270° fundoplication.

Operation

This patient subsequently underwent laparoscopy and that showed a misplaced former fundoplication, created distally on the stomach. After undoing the wrap, a 270° fundoplication was performed at the correct place around the distal esophagus.

Postoperative Course

Postoperatively, the patient started with a bland diet at the second day. From then on, she gained weight and now is on a normal diet. During the last outpatient clinic visit, the patient again experienced reflux symptoms, the esophagoscopy showing reflux esophagitis. Medication with proton pump inhibitors has been initiated again with partial success.

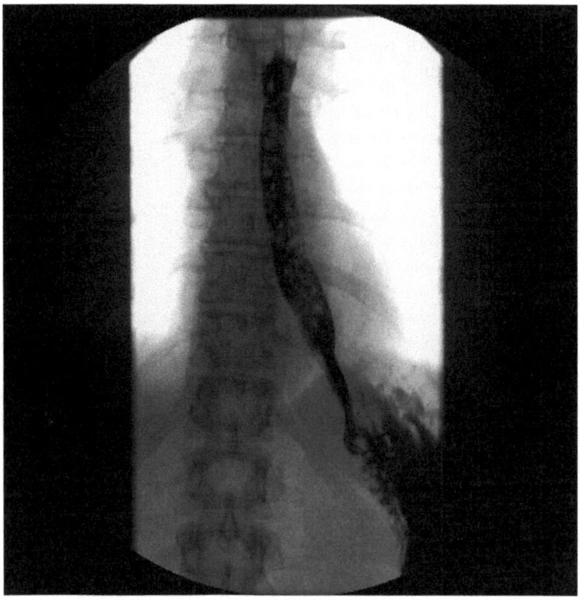

Fig. 9.2 Swallow X-ray showing no esophageal dilatation, but the passage of marshmallows is impaired

Second Patient

A 50-female-patient underwent a laparoscopic Nissen fundoplication because of a therapy-resistant reflux esophagitis. Previous to operation, the manometry showed insufficient contractions of the body of the esophagus with low pressures at the LES. Postoperative dysphagia was so important that patient had to be fed by a duodenal feeding tube. Swallow X-ray with marshmallows and manometry showed slow passage and almost no contractions of the esophagus (Fig. 9.2). A new operation was performed to take down the fundoplication showing no mechanical problems for the passage. Postoperatively, patient did not improve and continued with the enteral feeding and insufficient oral feeding. After many talks with patient and family, it was considered that the only surgical alternative was to perform a Roux-en-Y reconstruction with a small gastric pouch (Fig. 9.3). The operation was performed without complications, but after a long postoperative period of time in which all oral feeding possibilities have been tried and failed, a jejunostomy tube for feeding was definitively given in order to keep her weight stable. After 2 years, she is still having passage problems and oral feeding is not adequate. She has accepted the situation.

Discussion

Dysphagia is a normal early complaint after Nissen fundoplication, but will disappear after six weeks in the majority of patients. It will persist however in 5–10 % of patients. The most frequent complications are migration of the wrap, or wrap

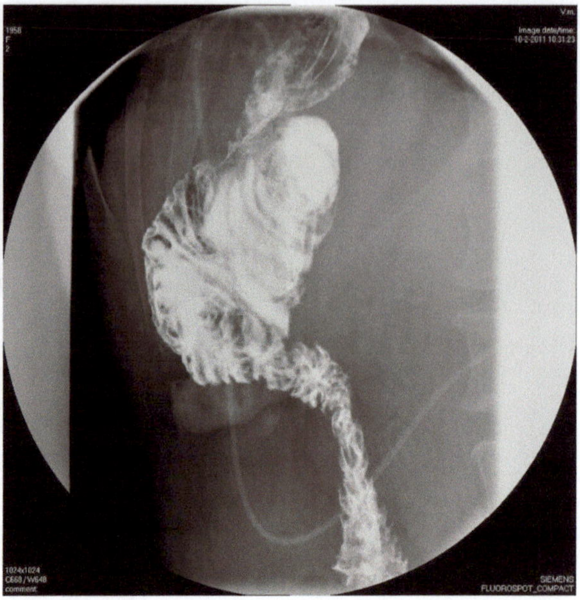

Fig. 9.3 Swallow X-ray showing the gastric pouch with the Roux-en-Y anastomosis

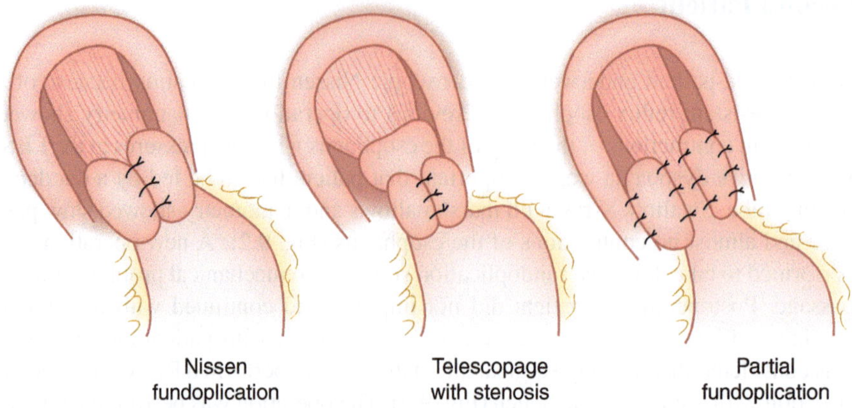

Illustration 9.1 Mid- and long-term postoperative dysphagia after fundoplication is a difficult problem to solve. If a mechanical problem is found, like a telescopage of esophagogastric junction, a reoperation should be performed. Switch to a partial fundoplication was performed in the first patient with normal manometry. If after different operations the patient cannot swallow and no mechanical obstruction can be found, conservative treatment and supplemental feeding should be given

fixed in the wrong place, like around the fundus; too tight fundoplication, or telescoping of the esophagogastric junction through the wrap; and torsion (Illustration 9.1). Another important cause is the postoperative dysphagia in those patients with esophageal contraction problems. The lesson of the first case is that the fundoplication should always be placed at the correct position around the distal esophagus.

Therefore, dissection of the distal esophagus is mandatory and at least 5 cm of distal esophagus should be placed intraabdominally. A partial—Toupet—fundoplication should have been performed, since postoperative dysphagia is significantly higher after Nissen fundoplication as compared to Toupet fundoplication [1], less reoperation rate and less belching problems. All grades of dysphagia are associated with an impaired quality of life. A wrap positioned in the wrong place or after telescoping of the esophagogastric junction will cause postoperative dysphagia and will not recover with conservative management or attempts of dilatations. A swallow X-ray is important to identify the problem. Correction will be done by relaparoscopy [2] or by laparotomy. Besides, questions will arise at reoperation whether to dismantle the fundoplication only or to switch the Nissen into a partial fundoplication. In our opinion, if the manometry of the body of the esophagus is normal, then a partial fundoplication will be the correct solution. If the manometry is not normal, no fundoplication should be performed, like in the second patient. Interesting is what to do with a patient with therapy-resistant esophagitis having abnormal esophageal contractions. Booth et al. performed a randomized trial [3] comparing whether Nissen or partial Toupet fundoplication would be preferable and whether preoperative esophageal manometry should be used to determine the degree of fundoplication performed. Preoperative esophageal manometry was used to stratify 127 patients with established gastro-esophageal reflux disease into effective (75 patients) and ineffective (52 patients) esophageal motility groups. Patients in each group were randomized to Nissen (64 patients) or Toupet (63 patients) fundoplication. Dysphagia of any degree (27 % versus 9 %); and chest pain on eating (22 % versus 5 %) were more prevalent at 1 year in the Nissen group, but there were no differences in postoperative symptoms between the effective and ineffective motility. They found that there is no reason to tailor the degree of fundoplication to preoperative esophageal manometry groups. No differences between partial and total fundoplication in impaired esophageal manometry is also found by others [4, 5]. In spite of this, there are a group of patients who are considered cripples after fundoplication and redo-procedures. Questions arise: (1) What is the cause of this problem, like in our second patient? and (2) Does surgery have a therapeutic value? Answering the first question is probably a combination of manometric problems, gastric emptying, and anatomical problems. Also, the role of vagal nerve(s) lesion may be important. Concerning the second question, Makris et al. studied the safety and efficacy of Roux-en-Y reconstruction, esophagojejunostomy (EJ), or gastrojejunostomy (GJ), for failed fundoplications [6]. Fourteen (64 %) patients had one, six (27 %) patients had two, and two (9 %) patients had three previous antireflux procedures. At a mean follow-up of 23 months, the average dysphagia score was 0.7 (range 0–2). The mean postoperative BMI was 25.4 compared to a preoperative BMI of 31.They concluded that RNY reconstruction with GJ or EJ for failed antireflux procedures may be considered a safe and valid surgical option in those difficult situations where a redo fundoplication is either non-feasible or expected to fail. Moreover, if after all these measures, the patient is still incapacitated to pass enough food orally, an alternative for supplementary feeding like a PEG should be done.

References

1. Broeders JA, Mauritz FA, Ahmed Ali U, et al. Systematic review and meta-analysis of laparoscopic Nissen versus Toupet fundoplication for gastro-esophageal reflux disease. Br J Surg. 2010;97:1318–30.
2. Awais O, Luketich JD, Schuchert MJ, et al. Reoperative antireflux surgery for failed fundoplication: an analysis of outcomes in 275 patients. Ann Thorac Surg. 2011;92:1083–9.
3. Booth MI, Stratford J, Jones L, et al. Randomized clinical trial of laparoscopic total (Nissen) versus posterior partial (Toupet) fundoplication for gastro-oesophageal reflux disease based on preoperative oesophageal manometry. Br J Surg. 2009;95:57–63.
4. Pizza F, Rossetti G, Del Genio G, et al. Influence of esophageal motility on the outcome of laparoscopic Total fundoplication. Dis Esophagus. 2008;21:78–85.
5. Chrysos E, Tsiaoussis J, Zoras OJ, et al. Laparoscopic surgery for gastroesophageal reflux disease patients with impaired esophageal peristalsis: total or partial fundoplication? J Am Coll Surg. 2003;197:8–15.
6. Makris KI, Lee T, Mittal SK. Roux-en-Y reconstruction for failed fundoplication. J Gastrointest Surg. 2009;13:2226–32.

Chapter 10
Case on Iatrogenic Esophageal Perforation

Miguel A. Cuesta and Donald L. van der Peet

Keywords Esophageal perforation • Iatrogenic perforation • Empyema • Mediastinitis • Stent

Diagnosis and Indication for Surgery: Identification and Treatment of the Complication

A 62-year-old male patient had been operated on by a cardiac surgeon because of a mitral stenosis. The valve had been replaced through a sternotomy. Postoperatively, the patient was admitted to the intensive care department, and there he developed a respiratory infection with respiratory insufficiency. The patient was treated by mechanical ventilation and antibiotics. After a period of 4 weeks, he still could not be disconnected from the mechanical ventilator and in order to rule out an insufficiency of the new implanted valve, a cardiac trans-esophageal ultrasound was performed. The valve was found to work correctly, but the patient's low-grade sepsis persisted, which impeded weaning him from mechanical ventilation. Moreover, he developed an acute renal insufficiency requiring hemodialysis. The CT scan showed mediastinitis with free air in the mediastinum and a suspicion of a right thoracic empyema (Figs. 10.1 and 10.2). To rule out an esophageal perforation, an esophagoscopy was performed showing an esophageal perforation at 30 cm of incisors line. The clinical condition of the patient was considered too unstable for surgery and he was treated primarily by a stent and thoracic drainage (Fig. 10.3). The septic condition persisted and 5 days later, a mediastinal abscess, located in the right superior and mid

M.A. Cuesta, M.D. (✉) • D.L. van der Peet
Department of Surgery, VU University Medical Center,
Amsterdam, The Netherlands
e-mail: ma.cuesta@vumc.nl

M.A. Cuesta, H.J. Bonjer (eds.), *Case Studies of Postoperative Complications after Digestive Surgery*, DOI 10.1007/978-3-319-01613-9_10,

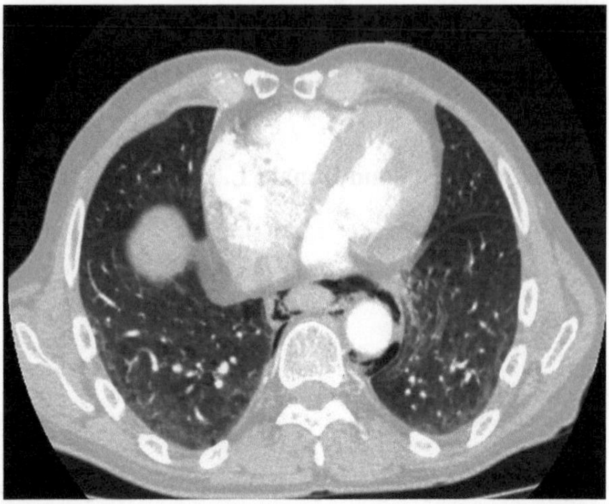

Fig. 10.1 Mediastinitis by esophageal perforation

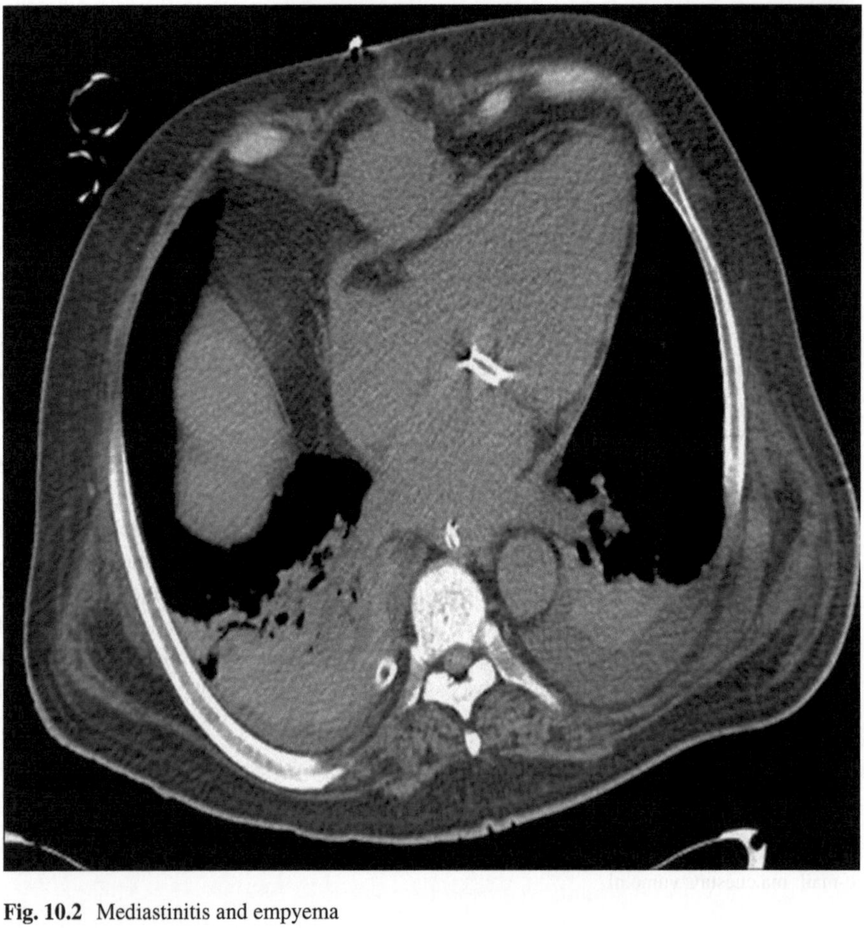

Fig. 10.2 Mediastinitis and empyema

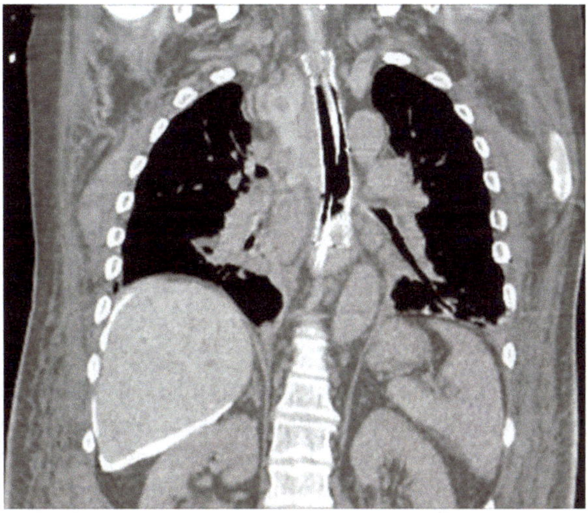

Fig 10.3 Stent placed in the esophagus

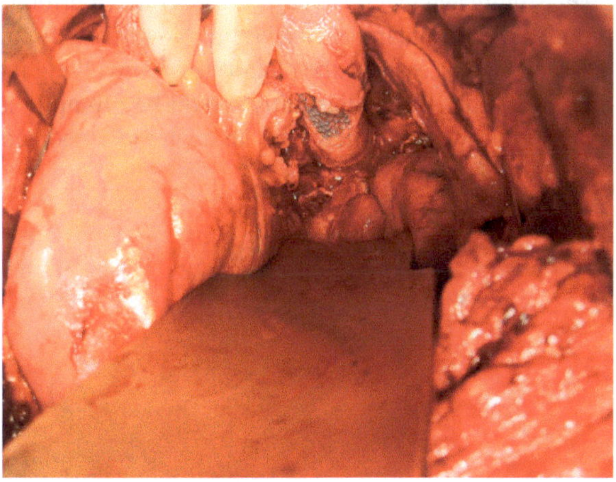

Fig. 10.4 Defect of the esophagus showing the stent

mediastinum, was drained through a right cervical incision. The patient's clinical condition did not improve and after much deliberation a decision was taken to perform a right explorative thoracotomy to drain the empyema and fix the perforation.

Operation

A large esophageal perforation was seen at operation including destruction of at least five cm of the mid-esophagus (Fig. 10.4). An esophageal resection was performed, a gastric conduit created, and anastomosed at cervical level. In addition, decortication of the right lung was performed and the thorax drained.

Postoperative Course

After 3 weeks of mechanical ventilation via a tracheotomy, the patient's condition finally improved so he could be retired from mechanical ventilation. Also the renal function recovered. His clinical situation was restored after a long period of rehabilitation.

Discussion

Following a trans-esophageal ultrasound, this patient's iatrogenic esophageal perforation was first treated with a stent (Illustration 10.1a). Even with a critically ill patient, stent treatment for a longer existing perforation combined with mediastinitis and thoracic empyema is not an optimal treatment option. It should be preserved for acute perforations with intact mediastinal pleura without contamination of the mediastinum and pleural cavity [1–3]. A direct perforation of the esophagus through the mediastinal pleura or a delay in diagnosis will contribute to disruption of the mediastinal abscess into the pleural cavity involving the formation of an empyema. The empyema and mediastinitis should be promptly and adequately drained. The only option for this patient was an explorative thoracotomy on the right side with treatment of the perforation.

a

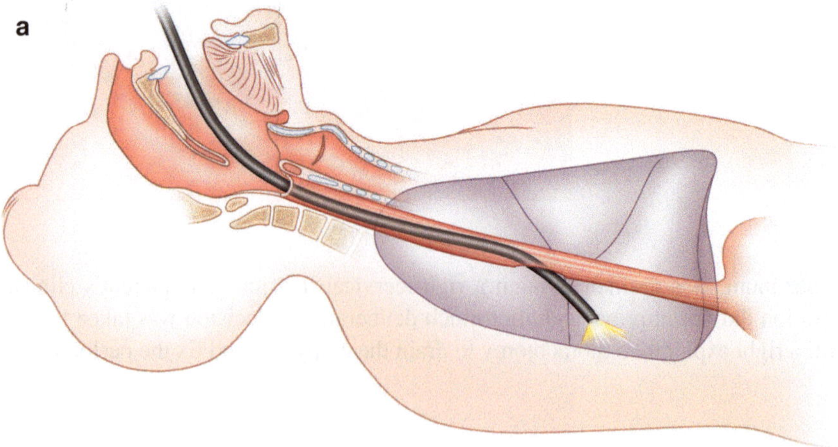

Illustration 10.1 (**a**) Iatrogenic esophageal perforation. (**b**) Two possibilities, (a) esophageal perforation with intact mediastinal pleura may be treated by stent placement and (b) patient with esophageal perforation with empyema treated by a right thoracotomy, lung decortication, closure of the perforation, and muscular flap

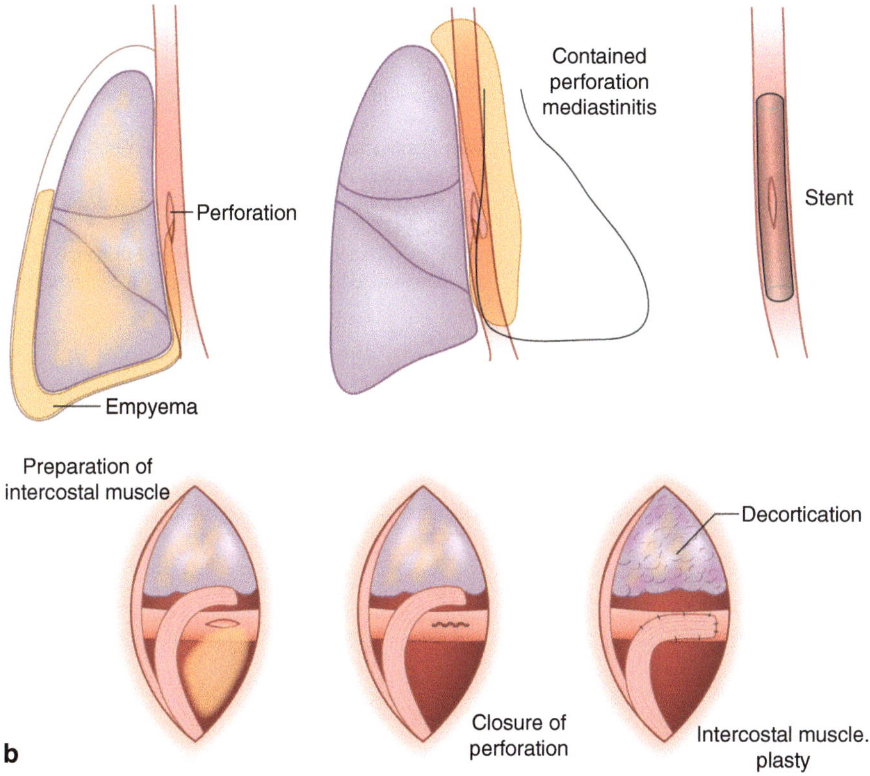

Illustration 10.1 (continued)

Yet, the question may be: How to manage an iatrogenic esophageal perforation? In case of a small perforation with intact pleura and no empyema (contained rupture), a stent could be sufficient with eventually a drainage of the medistinitis, but close observation remains important. In case of an "open" perforation with empyema, the perforation should be closed primarily, in two layers, with some kind of muscular flap or fundoplication if the perforation is distal. The empyema should be treated by decortication of the lung and drainage (Illustration 10.1b). Important factor here is adequately draining the place of the closed perforation. There is also an option for thoracoscopic exploration with adequate debridement and drainage [4]. If the leakage reappears, the drain should be maintained for a long period of time in order to have a controlled fistula. The option to drain the empyema percutaneously and to cover the perforation by means of a stent is not optimal. In the patient here presented, having a large perforation and necrosis of the esophagus around the stent, the only treatment option should have been an esophageal resection with the formation of a gastric conduit anastomosis in the neck.

References

1. Pla V, Cuesta MA, van den Broek WT. Treatment of thoracic esophageal perforations. Cir Esp. 2005;77:327–31.
2. Freeman RK, Ascioti AJ. Esophageal stent placement for the treatment of perforation, fistula or anastomotic leak. Semin Thorac Cardiovasc Surg. 2011;23:154–8.
3. Ryom P, Ravn JB, Schmidt S, et al. Aetiology, treatment and mortality after oesophageal perforation in Denmark. Dan Med Bull. 2011;58:A4267.
4. Haveman JW, Nieuwenhuijs VB, Kobold JP, et al. Adequate debridement and drainage of the mediastinum using open thoracotomy or video assisted thoracoscopic surgery for Boerhaave's syndrome. Surg Endosc. 2011;25:2492–7.

Chapter 11
Case on Peritonitis After Unrecognized Perforation Following Heller Myotomy and Dor Fundoplication for Achalasia

Miguel A. Cuesta and Donald L. van der Peet

Keywords Peritonitis • Perforation • Heller myotomy • Dor fundoplication • Achalasia

Diagnosis and Indication for Surgery

A 16-year-old boy presented with dysphagia for solid food and weight loss of 5 kg during the final year of his secondary education.

Diagnosis revealed achalasia, as based on the manometry findings involving hypoactivity of the contractions and no relaxation of the lower esophageal sphincter (LES). In another hospital, the patient had been dilated twice without improvement and now he was referred to our center for a laparoscopic Heller myotomy.

Operation

During the laparoscopic intervention, it was difficult to develop the plane between the muscular layer of the esophagus and the mucosa. It seemed that two different planes were developing. Two small iatrogenic perforations were made and were closed with 4-0 stitches. Myotomy was performed adequately, on 6 cm of the distal esophagus and on 2 cm of the proximal stomach. Across the defect an

M.A. Cuesta, M.D. (✉) • D.L. van der Peet
Department of Surgery, VU University Medical Center, Amsterdam, The Netherlands
e-mail: ma.cuesta@vumc.nl; dl.vdpeet@vumc.nl

M.A. Cuesta, H.J. Bonjer (eds.), *Case Studies of Postoperative Complications after Digestive Surgery*, DOI 10.1007/978-3-319-01613-9_11,

anterior Dor fundoplication (180°) was created without mobilizing the short gastric vessels.

Postoperative Course: Identification and Treatment of the Complication

The second day after operation the patient could ingest some bland liquids; on the third day he developed fever and upper abdominal pain. A CT scan with oral contrast was performed, and leakage of contrast was found at the distal esophagus (Fig. 11.1a, b) A laparoscopic exploration was performed. Leakage of gastric content was seen in the upper abdomen, and after removal of the stitches of the Dor plasty, a 3-cm long perforation was seen at the distal part of the mucosa (Illustration 11.1). This extended perforation was possibly caused by necrosis of the mucosa. The perforation was carefully closed again with a 5.0 PDS continuous suture, and a Dor plasty was created to cover the defect. The abdomen was drained and patient received a central line for feeding. He recovered in a week time. A new control by swallow X-ray showed a normal passage and no leakage.

Discussion

This patient possessed an unusual complication. Boeckstaens et al. have published recently a randomized study of a "total of 201 patients randomly assigned to pneumatic dilation (95 patients) or laparoscopic Heller myotomy (LHM) (106)" [1]. The

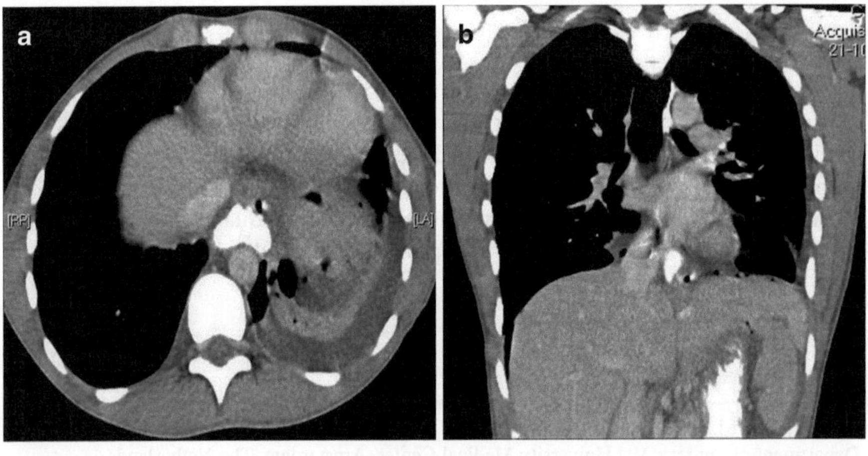

Fig. 11.1 (**a**) CT scan showing leakage of contrast at the myotomy site. (**b**) CT scan with leakage of contrast

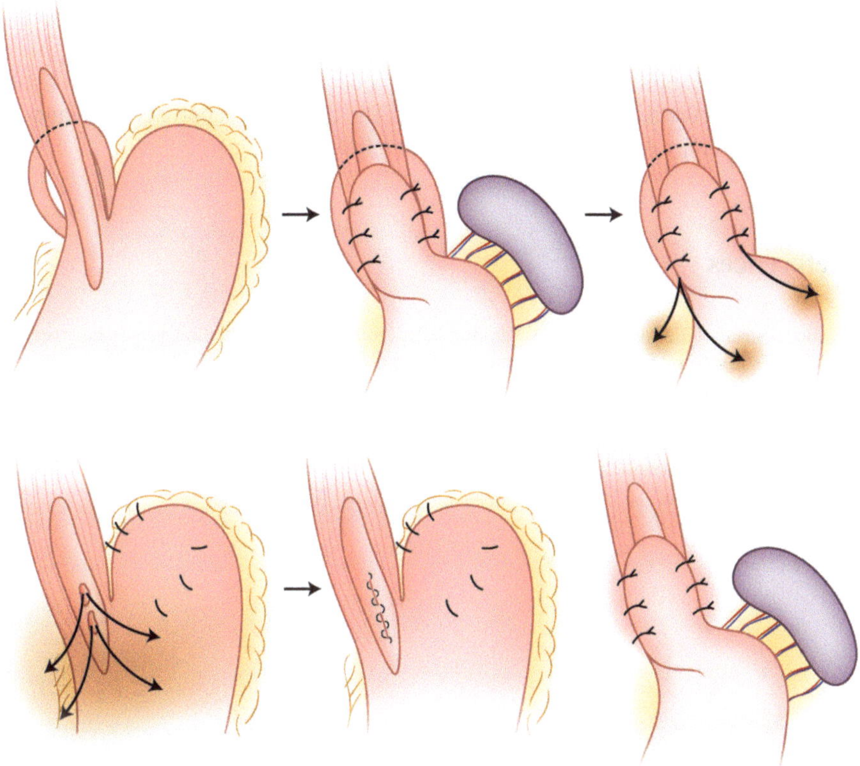

Illustration 11.1 Heller's myotomy with Dor fundoplication as treatment of idiopathic achalasia. Postoperative leakage with peritonitis. Laparoscopically approached: Dor fundoplication was dismantled, mucosa perforation seen, and closed by running suture. Dor fundoplication was added

therapeutic success with pneumatic dilation with the random group was 90 % after 1 year of follow-up and 86 % after 2 years as compared with a rate of the group with LHM of 93 % after 1 year and 90 % after 2 years. Perforation of the esophagus occurred in 4 % of the patients during pneumatic dilation, whereas mucosal tears occurred in 12 % during LHM. There were no postoperative perforations in this series. Zaninotto et al. published the outcome of a study of 400 patients treated for achalasia by means of Heller myotomy and Dor fundoplication, and they determined conversion and morbidity rates of 1.5 % and 1.9 %, respectively, whereas the mortality was 0 % [2]. Moreover, Lan Wang and You Ming Li reviewed 16 papers on the outcomes of surgical treatment of recurrent achalasia and complications involved. "The most common intraoperative complication was gastrointestinal perforation, including gastric and esophageal perforation in 1.5–20 % of patients.

Besides, some patients experienced pneumothorax (1.9–6.7 %). Early postoperative complications included pulmonary complications (1.3–4 %). Some patients experienced persistent and severe chest pain, which prolonged the time to hospital discharge" [3].

The possibility of complications must never be discounted. Difficulties in finding the plane during the dissection and tears of the mucosa can be regarded as the causes for the complication of the patient here. It is possible that dissection in the wrong plane induced the ischemia and perforation. The aggressive approach by diagnosis and relaparoscopy eventually solved the complication.

References

1. Boeckstaens GE, Annese V, des Varannes SB, et al. Pneumatic dilation versus laparoscopic Heller's myotomy for idiopathic achalasia. N Engl J Med. 2011;364:1807–16.
2. Zaninotto G, Constantini M, Rizzetto C, et al. Four hundred laparoscopic myotomies for esophageal achalasia: a single centre experience. Ann Surg. 2008;248:986–93.
3. Wang L, Li YM. Recurrent achalasia treated with Heller myotomy: A review of the literature. World J Gastroenterol. 2009;14:7122–26.

Chapter 12
Case on Esophagojejunostomy Leakage Following Extended Total Gastrectomy

Jose L. Garcia Sabrido and Wenceslao Vasquez Jimenez

Keywords Esophagojejunostomy • Gastrectomy • Gastric cancer • Leakage • Stent • Lymphadenectomy

First Patient

Diagnosis and Indication for Surgery

In view is a 55-year-old female patient, without a previous medical history, who had an ulcerated lesion of 3 cm at the lesser curvature of the stomach. The biopsy was positive for poorly differentiated adenocarcinoma and signet ring cells. The tumor was staged by means of CT scan and endoscopic ultrasonography as T3N + M0. The patient was treated by neo-adjuvant systemic chemotherapy according to the MAGIC protocol scheme (three cycles of epirubicin, cisplatin, and fluorouracil) [1].

Operation

After three cycles of chemotherapy, and after an interval of 6 weeks, the patient underwent open surgery. A total gastrectomy with lymphadenectomy type D2 resection with splenic preservation was performed. The reconstruction consisted of an end-to-side esophagojejunostomy carried out with a 21-mm circular stapler. The Roux-en-Y loop was 60 cm (Fig. 12.1). Two Jackson-Pratt drains were placed in the right and left subdiaphragmatic spaces at the esophagojejunal anastomosis.

J.L.G. Sabrido, M.D. (✉) • W.V. Jimenez, M.D., Ph.D.
Department of Surgery, Gregorio Marañon Hospital, Madrid, Spain
e-mail: jlgsabrido@gmail.com, jlgsabrido@ciriii.hggm.es

M.A. Cuesta, H.J. Bonjer (eds.), *Case Studies of Postoperative Complications after Digestive Surgery*, DOI 10.1007/978-3-319-01613-9_12,

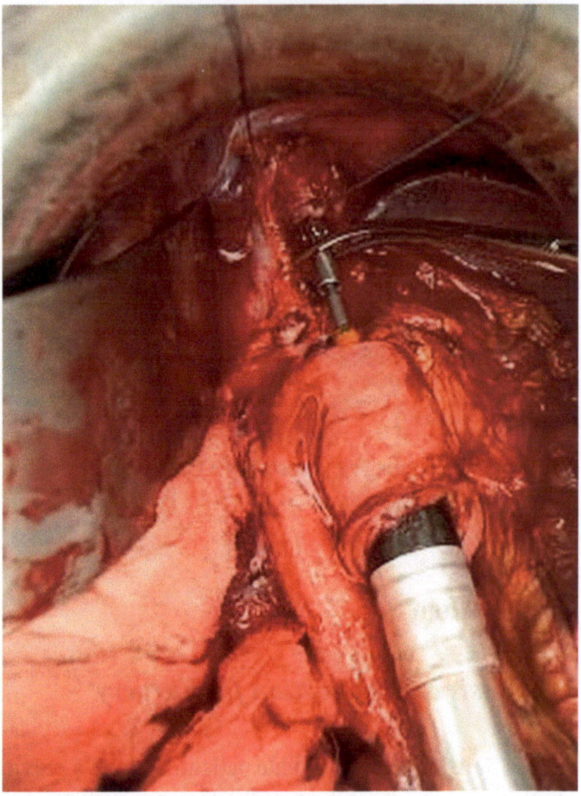

Fig. 12.1 End-to-side esophagojejunostomy anastomosis by means of circular stapler

Pathology

The pathological stage was pT3N1M0.

Postoperative Course: Identification and Treatment of the Complication

On the 6th postoperative day, after taking oral liquids, the patient achieved fever, pain in the upper left abdomen, and an increase in the amount of left drain volume, which was opalescent, with an amylase level of 800 UI/L. White cell count showed leukocytosis of 20,000 with left deviation of 95 %.

First a swallow X-ray (Fig. 12.2) and after a CT scan with double contrast showed leakage at the level of the esophagojejunal anastomosis with a perianastomotic fluid collection of 4 cm in diameter, communicating with the left drain.

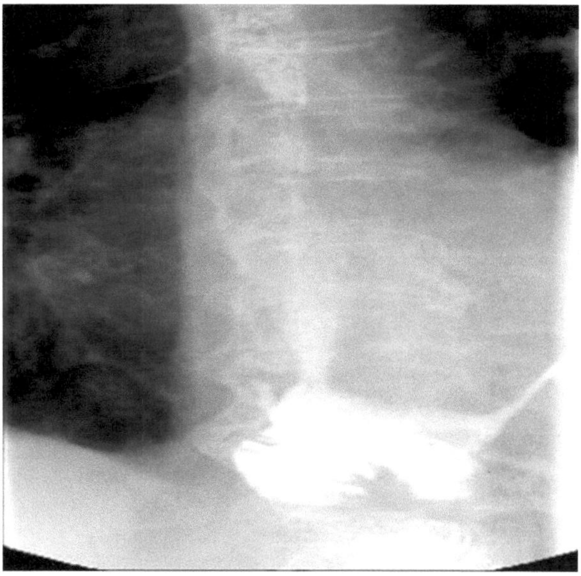

Fig. 12.2 Leakage of contrast from the esophagojejunostomy

Oral intake was stopped, and administration of IV fluids and iv broad spectrum antibiotics was initiated. At the 8th postoperative day, the patient improved; however, the volume of the drainage remained high (approximately, 500 mL/day). An expandable endoprosthesis was then inserted at the level of the esophagojejunostomy that immediately sealed the anastomotic leakage (Illustration 12.1, Fig. 12.3).

The patient continued to evolve favorably; oral ingestion started again at the 12th postoperative day. The patient was discharged on the 18th postoperative day. She was scheduled to complete her adjuvant systemic chemotherapy.

Second Patient

Diagnosis and Indication for Surgery

A 69-year-old man diagnosed with a proximal gastric adenocarcinoma was found elsewhere unresectable at explorative laparotomy because of lymph nodes metastases along the celiac trunk. The tumor seemed attached to the aorta at the level of the hiatus, and the surgeon preferred not to resect the tumor at this stage. The patient was referred to our hospital and treated by neoadjuvant chemotherapy (MAGIC protocol scheme [1]), three sessions, and at the new CT scan, it appeared that the tumor had regressed and could be resected.

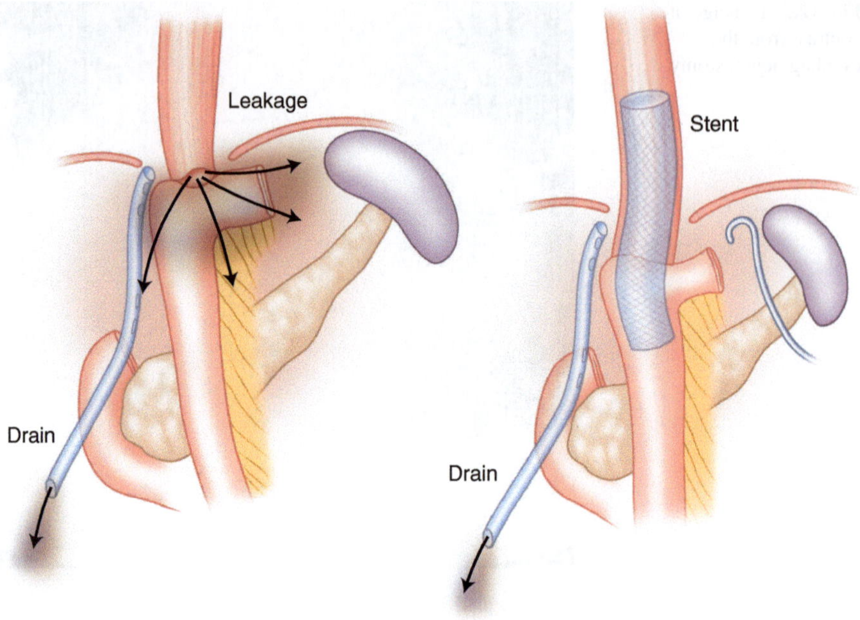

Illustration 12.1 Leakage of the esophagojejunostomy is showed with perianastomotic leakage. Stent is placed by esophagoscopy and the abscess has been drained percutaneously. If there is general peritonitis, like in the second patient, a laparotomy should be done with rinsing of the abdomen, stent at the anastomosis, and drains

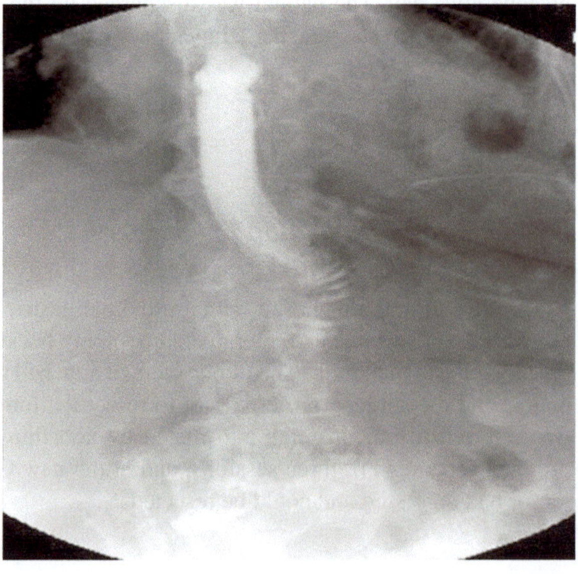

Fig. 12.3 Control of the leakage of the esophagojejunostomy with the placement of an endoprosthesis

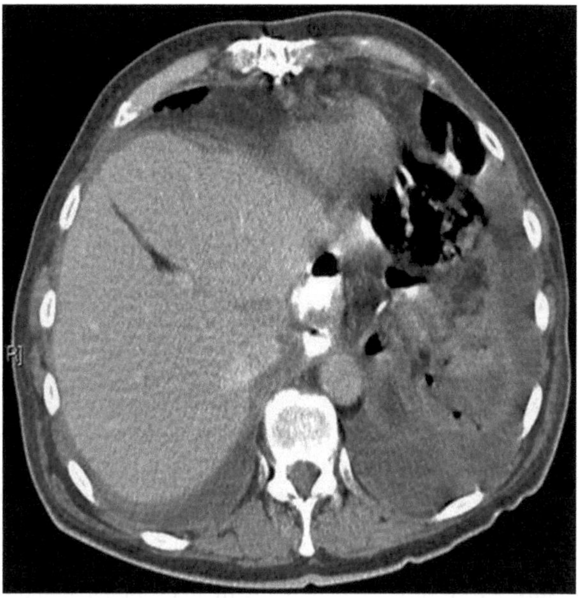

Fig. 12.4 CT scan of anastomotic leakage of esophagojejunostomy with general peritonitis

Operation

A new laparotomy showed that a total gastrectomy could be performed, extended to the distal 7 cm of the esophagus, splenectomy, and lymphadenectomy of the celiac trunk. An esophagojejunostomy was performed transhiatally with a Roux-en-Y long loop through the transverse mesocolon in an end-to-side fashion (circular stapler 25 mm).

Pathology

The pathological study showed an adenocarcinoma pT3N1M0, radical resected with a resection margin of 1 cm, and metastases in 3 of the 15 studied lymph nodes.

Postoperative Course: Identification and Treatment of the Complication

The postoperative course was complicated, at day 8 by a leakage of the esophagojejunostomy, necessitating an exploratory laparotomy. An abscess was found around of the anastomosis in the upper abdomen and lower mediastinum, but a clear anastomotic leakage could not be identified. Drains were left at the mediastinum and hiatus area, draining pus. Five days later a CT scan (Fig. 12.4) was performed because of continuing sepsis and clinical deterioration showing multiple abscesses around the anastomosis. A new relaparotomy showed a leakage at the anastomosis and a stent was placed by esophagoscopy at the level of the anastomosis after draining the abscesses and rinsing the abdomen. Leakage was no longer seen following this procedure, and patient could be taken off the mechanical ventilation. Finally, the patient was discharged. Four years later, the patient developed a local recurrence around the anastomosis well responding to chemotherapy. He is now 1 year after detection of the recurrent disease and doing well.

Discussion

Esophago-jejunostomy leakage is a much-feared postoperative complication, occurring in 4–27 % of cases after total gastrectomy and being associated with a mortality of 60 %. Moreover, 30–50 % of patients with leakage of an esophago-jejunal anastomosis will later develop a stenosis at that level [2].

Factors involved in the prevention include: (a) optimization of the nutritional status before surgery, patients with an esophageal and gastric cancer usually have a poor oral intake, and enteral nutrition should be given through a nasojejunal tube; (b) a perfect surgical technique, distal esophageal margins should be well perfused and free of cancer by intra-operative frozen-section evaluation [3, 4]. The jejunal loop to be anastomosed needs to have enough length and a good perfusion. The best way to reach the esophagus, without any tension of the jejunal loop, is the transmesocolic route. The esophago-jejunal Roux-Y anastomosis is usually performed in an end-to-side fashion by means of a 25-mm circular stapler. Placement of a drain does not diminish the incidence of anastomotic leak, but may decrease the immediate clinical impact of such a complication and may allow the possibility of a less invasive treatment such as the placement of a stent [5]. Diagnosis of this complication is based on clinical signs, usually between the seventh and tenth postoperative day; the use of a CT scan of thorax and abdomen with double contrast will provide sufficient information about the anastomotic leakage and the presence of peri-anastomotic abscesses, mediastinitis, or general peritonitis and the use of the gastroscopy in those cases without a clear diagnosis after clinical and radiological evaluation, or in a case whereby the possibility of treatment by means of a stent is being considered. In most of the cases during endoscopic evaluation, a stent should be placed.

Concerning the treatment, patient should be admitted to Intensive Care or Medium Care. Resuscitation measures are very important to achieve an optimal circulation and urinary flow; a broad-spectrum IV antibiotics should, according to protocol, be started immediately after diagnosis and an adequate control of anastomotic leakage: (1) In case a hemodynamically unstable patient is in critical septic condition despite resuscitation measures, the patient should be operated on urgently, including either closure of the distal esophageal stump plus cervical esophagostomy and jejunostomy for feeding or esophago-jejunal dismantling and placement of drains in the distal esophagus and in the jejunum and (2) In case of a hemodynamically stable patient, time is available to perform a quick study of anastomotic leakage. If the leakage is <30 % of the circumference, treatment may be conservative, including: sepsis control, adequate local drainage of fluid-collections, stent placement, and enteral feeding by microtube through the anastomosis or TPN [6, 7]. If the leakage is >30 %, then the esophago-jejunostomy should be dismantled and adequately drained [8]. A reconstruction may be performed 6–12 weeks later in order to redo the anastomosis.

References

1. Cunningham D, Allum WH, Stenning SP, et al. Perioperative chemotherapy versus surgery alone for resectable gastroesophageal cancer. N Engl J Med. 2006;355:11–20.
2. Garcia Sabrido JL, Vasquez Jimenez W. How to prevent, early diagnose, and treat major postoperative complications after gastric surgery. In: Cuesta MA, Bonjer HJ, editors. Treatment of complications after digestive surgery, chapter 9. London: Springer; 2013.
3. Deguchi Y, Fukagawa T, Morita S. Identification of risk factors for esophagojejunal anastomotic leakage after gastric surgery. World J Surg. 2012;36(7):1617–22.
4. Kight CE. Nutrition considerations in esophagectomy patients. Nutr Clin Pract. 2008;23:521–8.
5. Takeyoshi I, Ohwada S, Ogawa T, et al. Esophageal anastomosis following gastrectomy for gastric cancer: comparison of hand-sewn and stapling technique. Hepatogastroenterology. 2000;47:1026–9.
6. Dai YY, Gretschel S, Dudeck O, et al. Treatment of oesophageal anastomotic leaks by temporary stenting with self-expanding plastic stents. Br J Surg. 2009;96:887–91.
7. Blackmon SH, Santora R, Schwarz P, et al. Utility of removable esophageal covered self-expanding metal stents for leak and fistula management. Ann Thorac Surg. 2010;89:931–6.
8. Lang H, Piso P, Stukenborg C, et al. Management and results of proximal anastomotic leaks in a series of 1114 total gastrectomies for gastric carcinoma. Eur J Surg Oncol. 2000;26:168–71.

Chapter 13
Case on Leakage of the Duodenal Stump Following Gastrectomy

Jose L. Garcia Sabrido and Wenceslao Vasquez Jimenez

Keywords Gastrectomy • Antrectomy • Vagotomy • Gastrojejunostomy • Pyloric obstruction • Peptic stenosis • Duodenal leakage

Diagnosis and Indication for Surgery

In view is a 60-year-old male patient with a long-standing history of a peptic ulcer, treated with ranitidine, proton pump inhibitors, and eradication of Helicobacter pylori with antibiotics. He had been referred to the emergency room due to an obstruction of the upper gastrointestinal tract lasting several days. He had been vomiting after meals for 3 weeks, resulting in a 7 kg weight loss.

After clinical assessment, an abdominal CT scan showed a gastric dilatation. The follow-up gastroscopy revealed a stenosis of the duodenal bulb due to severe antro-duodenal fibrosis. The biopsies were compatible with a chronic inflammation without signs of cancer.

Diagnosis was a pyloric obstruction due to peptic stenosis.

Operation

A laparoscopic antrectomy, truncular vagotomy, and gastrojejunostomy by means of Roux-en-Y reconstruction was performed.

Two vacuum drainages (Jackson-Pratt) were placed: one at the duodenal stump and another close to the gastric stump.

J.L.G. Sabrido, M.D. (✉) • W.V. Jimenez, M.D., Ph.D.
Department of Surgery, Gregorio Marañon Hospital, Madrid, Spain
e-mail: jlgsabrido@gmail.com, jlgsabrido@ciriii.hggm.es

M.A. Cuesta, H.J. Bonjer (eds.), *Case Studies of Postoperative Complications after Digestive Surgery*, DOI 10.1007/978-3-319-01613-9_13,

Pathology

The pathologic evaluation showed an antral peptic ulcer with intense antro-duodenal inflammatory response, without malignant disease.

Postoperative Course: Identification and Treatment of the Complication

The postoperative course was favorable until the fourth day. Biliary fluid was then seen in the duodenal stump drain having an initial production of 400 mL/24 h. The patient complained of abdominal pain, but he was hemodinamically stable without signs of sepsis. The performed abdominal CT scan revealed abundant intra-abdominal fluid and pneumoperitoneum.

A laparoscopic surgical exploration was then performed. This located a free biliary collection in the abdominal cavity and fibrin depositions, but its origin could not be determined. Conversion to laparotomy followed, in which a diffuse biliary peritonitis and dehiscence of the duodenal stump was seen. After aspiration and washing of the cavity, a terminal duodenostomy was performed by means of a 22F Foley catheter, using a purse string suture, and placing an omental patch around the closure. The suture was tested with an instillation of 50 mL of saline into the catheter. The Foley catheter was exteriorized through the right upper abdomen (Figs. 13.1 and 13.2, Illustration 13.1). In addition, a Jackson-Pratt vacuum drainage was placed close to the duodenal stump. The postoperative evolution was good, with

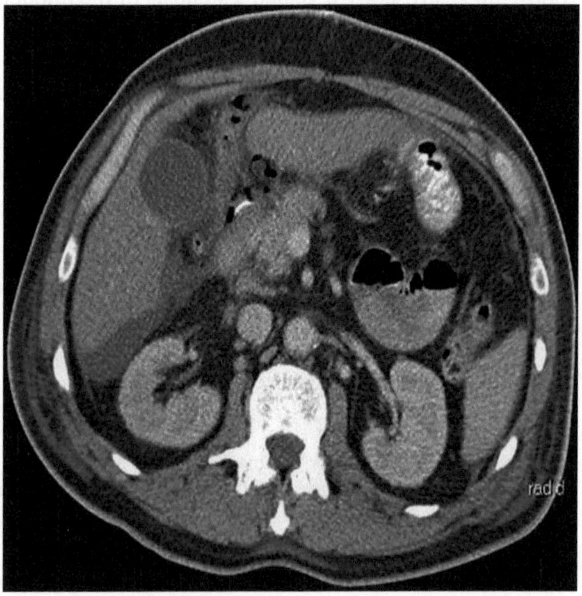

Fig. 13.1 Leakage of the duodenal stump with subhepatic fluid collection and air

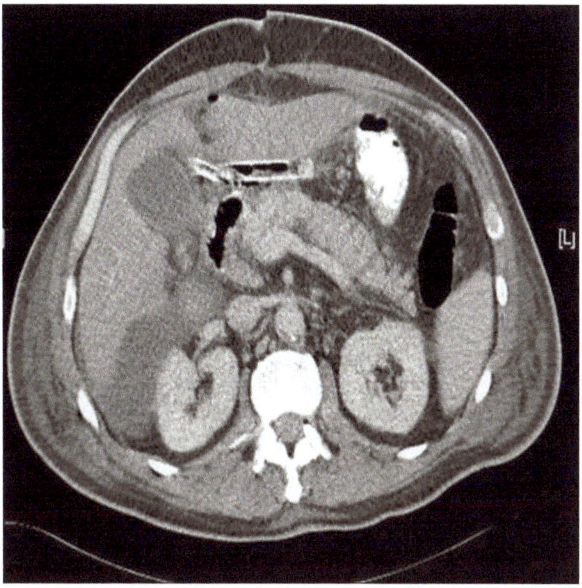

Fig. 13.2 After operative drainage and treatment of the leakage of the duodenal stump (Foley's catheter and drain)

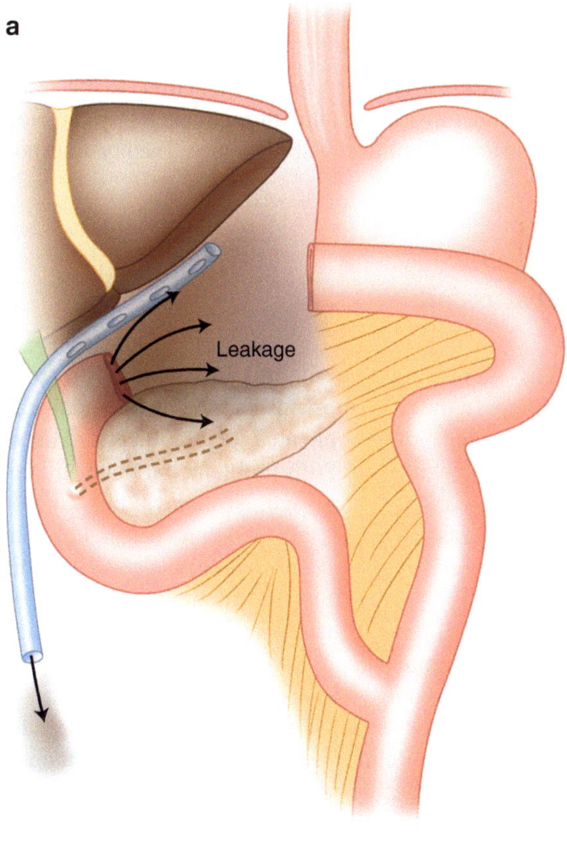

Illustration 13.1 (**a**, **b**) Surgical treatment of duodenal leakage after gastrectomy included a duodenostomy for control of the leakage, wrapping of the omentum, abdominal rinsing, and abdominal drainage

Illustration 13.1
(continued)

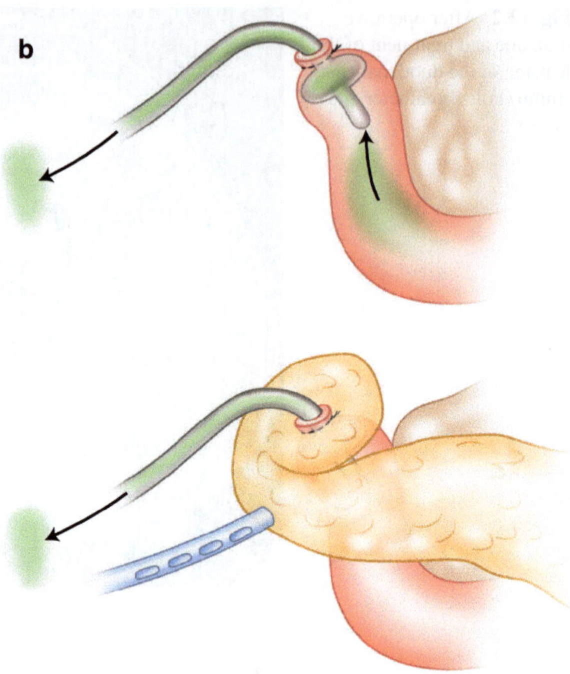

progressive decrease of drain production. At the 24th postoperative day radiological control with gastrographin through the Foley catheter did not show any leakage; the catheter was removed subsequently. Twenty-four hours later, the vacuum drainage also was retired.

Discussion

The main cause of peritonitis following gastrectomy is the leakage of duodenal stump. In the past, surgeons learned how to deal with a difficult duodenum during the surgery of complicated peptic ulcers. Many ingenious ways have been described to deal with this problem, but none will completely prevent a significant incidence of stump leakage. Nowadays, this kind of surgery is incidental. While treating gastric cancer, the duodenum has no inflammation, fibrosis, or cancer. The patient, here described, shows how to deal with a difficult duodenal stump during treatment of a complicated duodenal ulcer, in order to prevent the leakage. Moreover, invasive gastric cancer is generally treated by neoadjuvant chemotherapy, and immunosuppression may increase the rate of duodenal stump leakage after gastrectomy [1].

The closure of the duodenal stump has to be safe; it is usually performed with linear stapler. Reinforcement of the stump by sutures is not recommended, because the duodenal wall is thick but weak. In those cases where the stump closure is considered unsafe, a lateral duodenotomy is recommended; this creates duodenal decompression, which can also be achieved with the placement of a nasogastric/transjejunal tube up to the end of the duodenal stump. Lateral duodenotomy implies the introduction of a Foley-like tube through a purse string suture, being exteriorized and sealed by wrapping omentum around it. The lateral duodenotomy will emerge through the upper-right abdominal wall, above the level of the duodenum, to assure adequate drainage [2, 3]. The tube should remain for 3 or 4 weeks before removal, in order to assure a good canalized fistula and thereby reducing the possibility of a peritoneal leakage. Adequate use of the external drains left in subhepatic area is also important.

In the infrequent case of gastrectomy used because of a complicated peptic ulcer, we specify two manoeuvres that are useful for the closure of a difficult stump: the Nissen closure is performed in those cases with a difficult to manage duodenum in which the duodenal stump is closed by means of separated stitches of the anterior wall of the duodenum with the fibrotic posterior wall plus omentoplasty, or the Finsterer-Bancroft-Plenk closure is a good alternative to the Nissen closure. It consists of three steps: the division of the antrum 6-cm from the pylorus, keeping its irrigation from the pyloric and gastroepiploic arteries; the mucosa cuff being resected following the submucous layer up to the pylorus, which is closed with stitches that take the pyloric muscular layer, and to attach the anterior and posterior antrum walls with stitches and a second continuous suture layer.

This complication occurs postoperatively rather early, usually between the fourth and seventh postoperative days. The most important signs and symptoms are fever, abdominal pain, tachycardia, and (if a drain is still in situ) the presence of biliary and duodenal leakage through it.

At physical exploration, the patient may appear as septic, hemodynamically unstable, dyspnoic, and the abdomen may show signs of distension and peritonitis. Patient should then be admitted to the Medium Care or Intensive Care department for initial resuscitation.

The CT scan of the abdomen with double contrast will show not only the duodenal leakage but also signs of local or general peritonitis, such as free air and fluid collections.

The leakage of the duodenal stump appears in 1–3 % of gastric resections. Nowadays, the mortality associated with this complication is, due to improvements in postoperative critical care, between 0 and 12 %.

Initial resuscitation by fluid reposition and adequate antibiotic treatment is important followed in the majority of cases by relaparotomy. The most commonly used technique is the terminal duodenotomy. A 22 or a 24 French, Petzer or Foley catheter is introduced through the duodenal leakage at the stump and a purse string is made with nonabsorbable material. This procedure can be complemented with wrapping and fixation of the major omentum around the suture (Wu technique), which contributes to closing it [2, 3]. A Penrose and a sump drain are left subhepatic and in the Morrison pouch. A temporary gastrostomy for suction and a jejunostomy for feeding are created. Abdomen should be rinsed and drained. Skin should be left open.

The only option for conservative approach will be the situation in which the duodenal leakage is fistulized and drained totally through a drain. Moreover, the patient should be hemodynamically stable and no intra-abdominal collections are allowed to be present on the CT scan. But also in this situation, if the flow is persistent and higher than 500 mL/24 h (high-flow bilio-pancreatic fistula), then surgical exploration could be indicated. In this case, the high flow may be associated with distal obstruction (afferent loop syndrome) or the presence of local abscess.

Total parenteral nutrition (TPN) through a central venous access should be initiated early after reoperation because these patients have an increased catabolism and do not get enteral food for several days.

The use of octreotide or somatostatin analogues (e.g., Lanreotide®) has demonstrated the efficacy of decreasing the fistula production during the first week; however, its share in the closure of the fistula is still controversial.

References

1. Garcia Sabrido JL, Vasquez JW. How to prevent, early diagnose, and treat major postoperative complications after gastric surgery. In: Cuesta MA, Bonjer HJ, editors. Treatment of complications after digestive surgery, chapter 9. London: Springer; 2013.
2. Tsuei BJ, Schwartz RW. Management of the difficult duodenum. Curr Surg. 2004;61:166–71.
3. Isik B, Yilmaz S, Kirimlioglu V, et al. A life-saving but inadequately discussed procedure: tube duodenostomy. Known and unknown aspects. World J Surg. 2007;31:1616–24.

Chapter 14
Case on Re-bleeding After Repair of Bleeding Duodenal Ulcer

Jose L. Garcia Sabrido and Wenceslao Vasquez Jimenez

Keywords Duodenal ulcer • Hematemesis • Melena • Gastroscopy • Duodenotomy • Peptic ulcer • Peptic ulcer bleeding

Diagnosis and Indication for Surgery

In view is a 35-year-old male patient, evaluated in the emergency room with hematemesis and melena. The patient possessed a history of smoking, a duodenal ulcer treated irregularly with proton pump inhibitors (PPIs), and a positive *Helicobacter pylori* breathing test with irregular treatment. He was also taking Diclophenac® 75 mg orally for 2 days due to a traumatic lesion of the right leg. At examination, the patient was in shock with signs of hypoperfusion, with a blood pressure of 90/40 mmHg and a heart rate of 110/min.

Two peripheral intravenous 14F lines were placed in his upper limbs. The hemoglobin was 7 g/dL, platelets were 350,000, and coagulation times in normal range. Two packed cell blood concentrates were transfused.

Gastroscopy summarily showed an ulcer of 2.5 cm in the posterior side of the first portion of the duodenum, classified as Forrest IIb (bleeding with visible vessel) (Fig. 14.1). Adrenaline was infiltrated together with contact diathermia therapy and the bleeding stopped. The patient was admitted to the ICU and received 80 mg Omeprazol® intravenously as a bolus and as a continuous perfusion afterwards. The *Helicobacter pylori* test was positive.

Four hours after the first procedure, the patient complained about abdominal pain, hematemesis, and hypotension. A second endoscopic procedure was

J.L.G. Sabrido, M.D. (✉) • W.V. Jimenez, M.D., Ph.D.
Department of Surgery, Gregorio Marañon Hospital, Madrid, Spain
e-mail: jlgsabrido@gmail.com, jlgsabrido@ciriii.hggm.es

M.A. Cuesta, H.J. Bonjer (eds.), *Case Studies of Postoperative Complications after Digestive Surgery*, DOI 10.1007/978-3-319-01613-9_14,

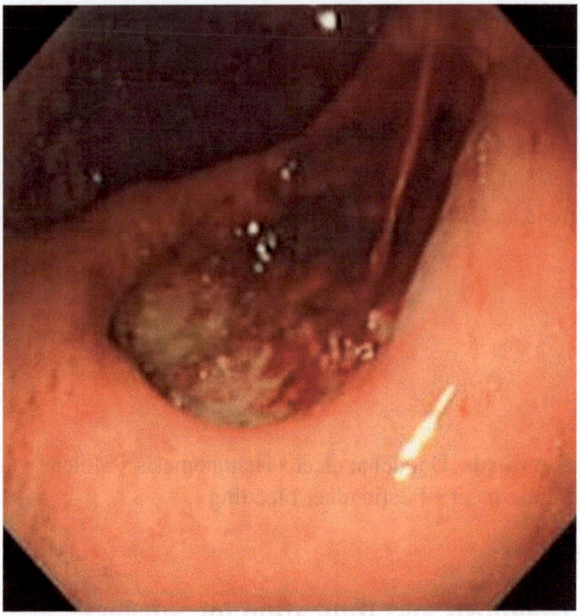

Fig. 14.1 Gastroscopy showing a bleeding postpyloric ulcer at the posterior side

performed with evidence of active bleeding in the ulcer; the bleeding could not be controlled with adrenaline and clips.

Operation

Due to his hemodynamic instability and failure of the endoscopic treatment, surgery was indicated. A medial laparotomy was done, followed by a Kocher maneuver, a longitudinal duodenostomy at the level of the pylorus, and identification of the ulcer. Hemostatic sutures were placed in the four quadrants of the ulcer with Prolene 3/0®. The bleeding was controlled. Peroperatively, the patient remained hypotensive, requiring inotropes and transfusion of eight packed cell units. The duodenotomy was closed in one layer with PDS 4/0. A nasogastric tube was placed in the antrum, and he was readmitted to the ICU.

Postoperative Course

Twenty-four hours after surgery, hematemesis and hypotension recurred with a hemoglobin of 7 g/dL. Blood and clots were removed by flushing saline through the nasogastric tube. A new gastroscopy showed a recurrent ulcer bleeding; so again clips were placed and bleeding partially became controlled. Additionally, an

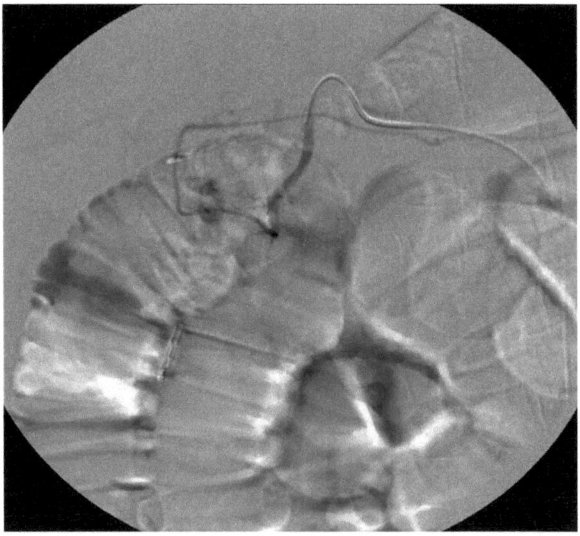

Fig. 14.2 Celiac trunk angiography shows active bleeding (blush) at the gastroduodenal artery after surgery

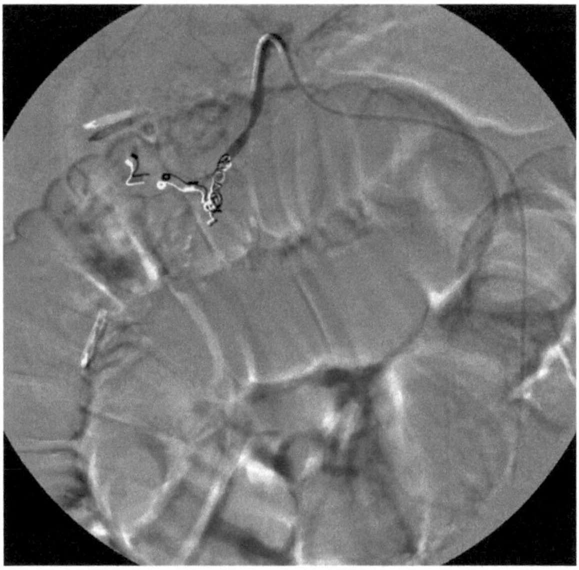

Fig. 14.3 Selective embolization of gastroduodenal artery by means of coils

angiography was performed, showing a bleeding from the gastroduodenal artery with a blush (Fig. 14.2) and consequently an embolization with coils was performed (Fig. 14.3).

The patient evolved favorably leading to discharge at the 8th postoperative day with *Helicobacter pylori* eradication therapy for 2 weeks. A second *Helicobacter pylori* breath test was negative.

Illustration 14.1 (**a**, **b**)
Selective angiography and coiling of the gastroduodenal artery

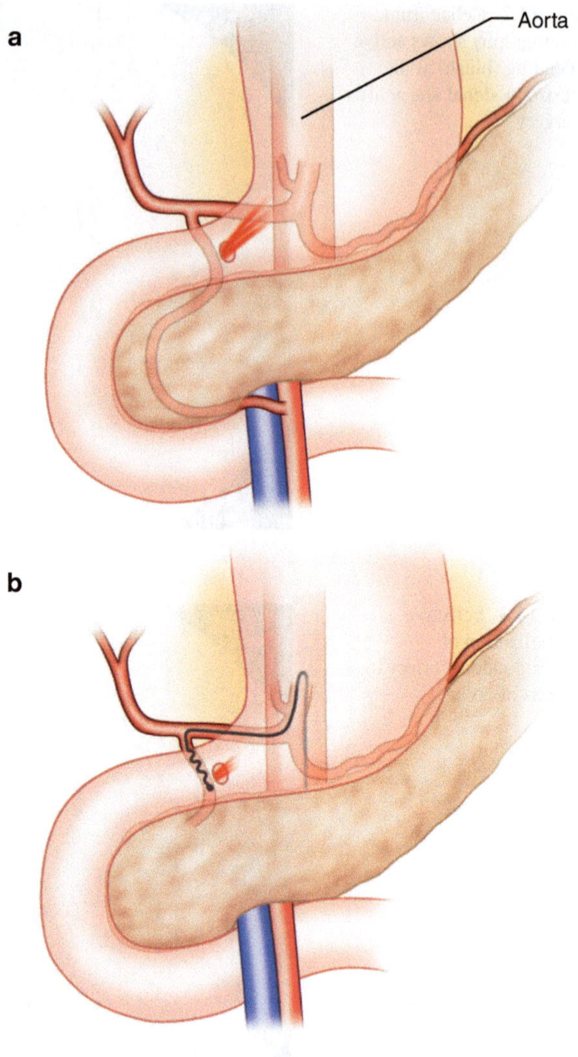

Discussion

Acute bleeding is the most common complication of peptic ulcer disease and its mortality lies between 5 and 10 %. Endoscopic treatment solves bleeding in the majority of patients; however 5–10 % of patients have re-bleeding and require surgery or embolization (Illustration 14.1a, b). After surgery, the risk of re-bleeding is about 4 %. The factors that increase the risk of re-bleeding are: an ulcer larger than 2 cm, localized in the lesser curvature or posterior side of the duodenal bulb, and hypovolemic shock.

Chapter 15
Case on Stenosis of a Side-to-Side Gastrojejunostomy After a Laparoscopic Subtotal Gastrectomy

Alfredo Alonso Poza and Francisco Nevarez Noboa

Keywords Stenosis • Gastrojejunostomy • Lymphadenectomy • Gastric cancer • Laparoscopic gastrectomy

Diagnosis and Indication for Surgery

We view a 65-year-old male patient, known for having hypertension and Diabetes mellitus type II, who had a stroke 3 years ago with left hemiparesia, and now he is studied because of anemia. Through gastroscopy he was diagnosed having a gastric adenocarcinoma in the antrum. Dissemination study by CT scan showed no metastatic disease. The tumor was staged as T3N1M0.

Operation

A subtotal laparoscopic gastrectomy with a D2 lymphadenectomy and spleen preservation was performed. A stapled side-to-side Roux-en-Y anastomosis in the greater curvature was performed with closure of the insertion of de endostapler by means of another mechanical stapler.

Postoperative Course and Identification of the Complication

On the 5th postoperative day, a transit X-ray was performed for control showing a slow passage of the contrast with gastric remnant dilatation, but no leakage (Fig. 15.1).

A.A. Poza, M.D., Ph.D. (✉) • F.N. Noboa, M.D.
Department of Surgery, Hospital del Sureste, Madrid, Spain
e-mail: alfredo.alonsop@salud.madrid.org

M.A. Cuesta, H.J. Bonjer (eds.), *Case Studies of Postoperative Complications after Digestive Surgery*, DOI 10.1007/978-3-319-01613-9_15,

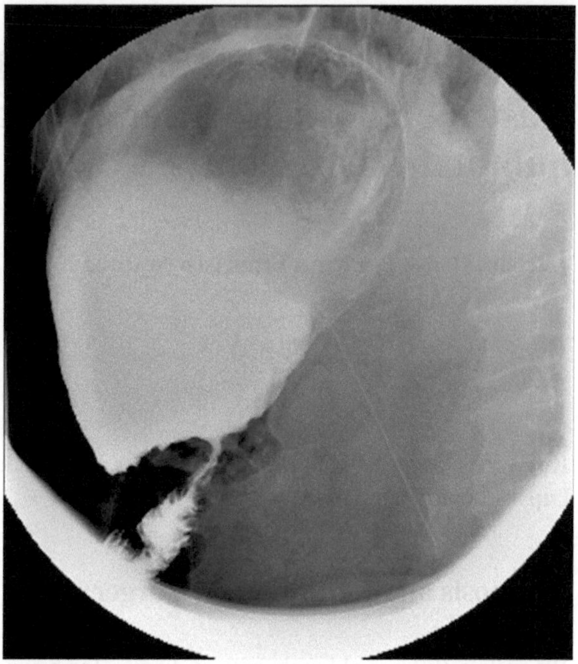

Fig. 15.1 Stenosis gastrojejunostomy

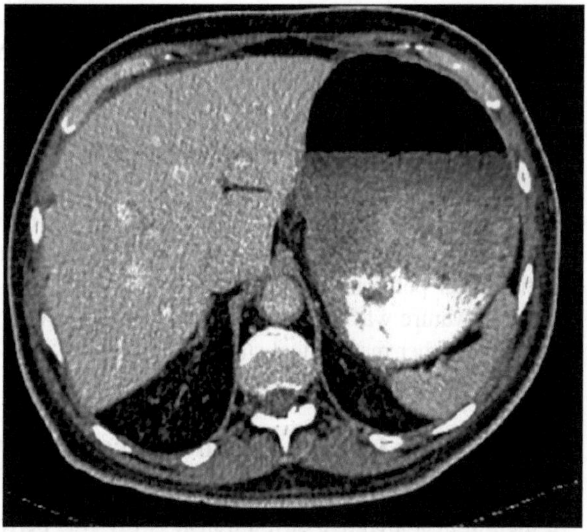

Fig. 15.2 CT scan showing the gastric dilatation

Patient, taking a semisolid diet, was discharged at the 10th postoperative day. He was readmitted on the 14th postoperative day with upper left quadrant pain and experiencing vomiting. A CT scan with oral contrast was performed showing a marked dilatation of the gastric remnant with significant stenosis of the anastomosis (Fig. 15.2 and Illustration 15.1a, b).

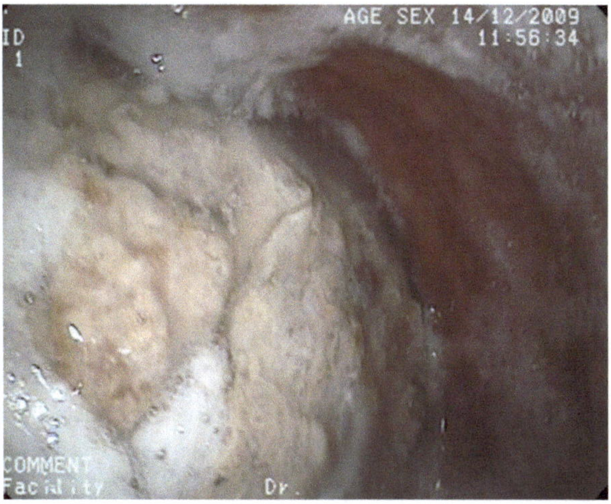

Fig. 15.3 Gastroscopy showing the bezoar

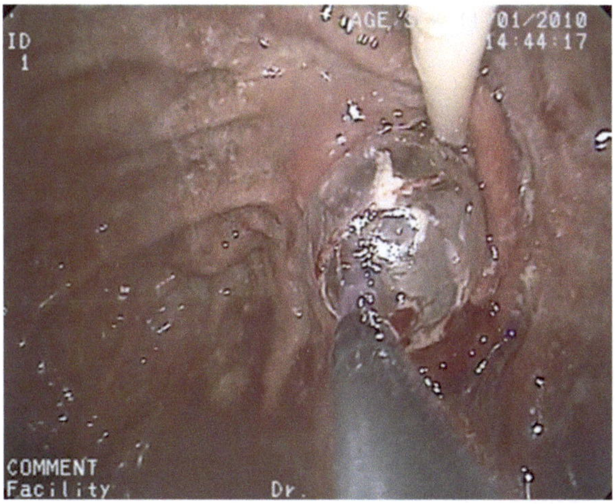

Fig. 15.4 First balloon dilatation up to 13 mm

Patient was treated with total parenteral nutrition (TPN) and nasogastric tube for gastric decompression.

It was proposed to dilate the stenosed anastomosis. However, at the first attempt a large bezoar was found at the gastrojejunostomy (Fig. 15.3).

Conservative medical treatment was established with pancreatic enzymes in order to dissolve the bezoar. During the second gastroscopy, the anastomosis could be visualized and dilated by means of a balloon up to 1.3 cm (Fig. 15.4). An enteral feeding tube could be introduced through the stenosis. TPN was replaced by enteral feeding (Fig. 15.4).

During the 4th balloon dilatation, a 3, 5-cm dilatation could be achieved (Fig. 15.5a).

Six months postoperatively, a new gastroscopy showed an adequate patency of the gastrojejunostomy and a normal CT scan (Fig. 15.5b).

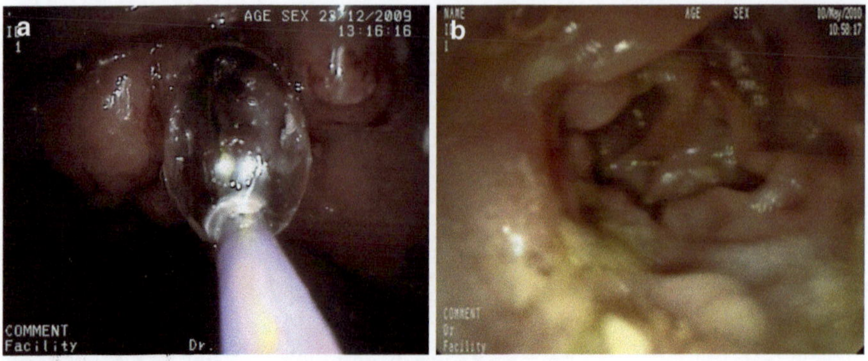

Fig. 15.5 (**a**) Dilatation up to 35 mm. (**b**) Patent gastrojejunostomy at 6 months postoperatively

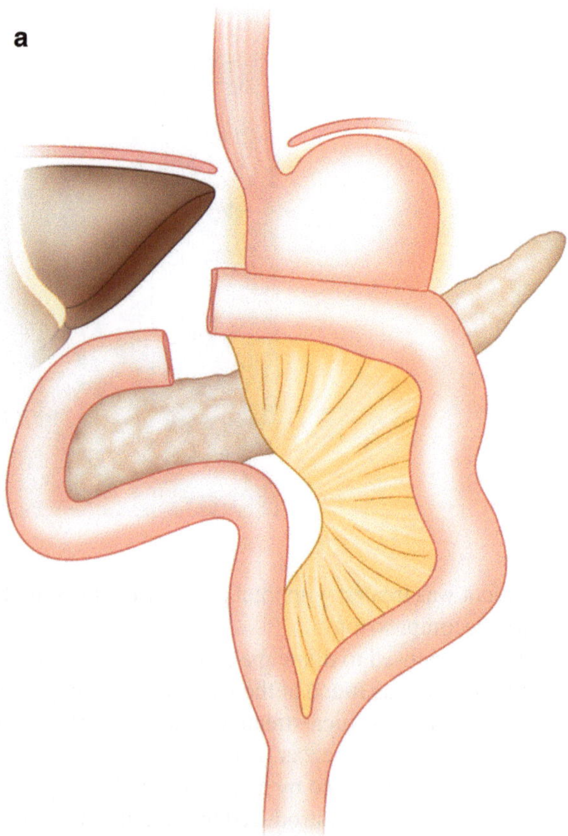

Illustration 15.1 (**a, b**) After partial gastrectomy, stenosis can be found at the gastrojejunostomy or at the efferent loop of the anastomosis. Once stenosis is diagnosed, patient should be treated by nasogastric tube and TPN. A dilatation program should be scheduled by progressive balloon dilatation. If an enteral feeding tube can be passed through the stenosed anastomosis, enteral feeding can replace the TPN

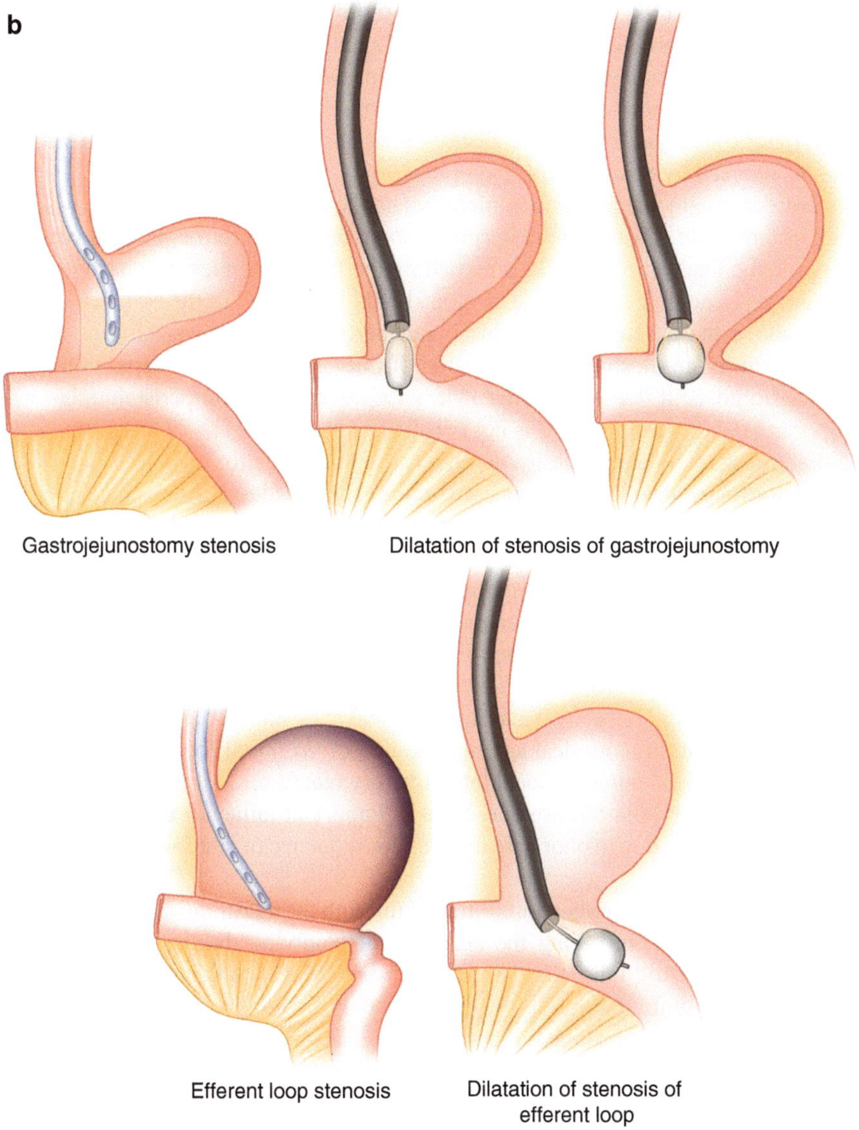

Illustration 15.1 (continued)

Discussion

Gastric-outlet obstruction and intestinal obstruction are relatively frequently occurring complications after gastrectomy. Five percent of all gastrectomies are complicated with stenosis/obstruction of any anastomoses.

The main cause of the obstruction is an area of inflammatory adhesions adjacent to the anastomosis, probably as consequence of small suture-line leakages and bleeding. Clearly, these complications are preventable. Moreover, functional paralysis of the stomach, common in patients after long-standing gastric dilatation as resulting from pyloric stenosis, may mimic gastric-outlet obstruction. Gastric peristalsis may also be reduced by postoperative hypopotasemia.

There are many mechanical problems related to the gastro-jejunostomy, whether ante or retrocolic. Gastric outlet occurs in about 5 % of all retrocolic anastomoses. A retrocolic anastomosis can be stenosed by the transverse mesocolon. In order to prevent this, the defect in the mesocolon should be sutured to the stomach at least 2-cm above the anastomosis. If this is not performed, the mesocolon may slide down resulting in mechanical obstruction of one or both jejunal loops. In making the anastomosis, it does not matter if it is isoperistaltic or antiperistaltic, but it is important that the anastomosis is not twisted or obstructed [1].

Following a total gastrectomy, another cause of obstruction may become the torsion of the long loop of the jejunum used for the esophago-jejunostomy. Furthermore, if antecolic anastomosis is performed, an internal hernia between the loop and colon may be the cause of obstruction.

Benign stenosis after esophago-jejunostomy occurs in 26–42 % of patients, which is of significant influence on the nutritional status and quality of life. Despite the technical and postoperative improvements, the incidence of benign stenosis has not changed in the last 15 years.

Stenosis is associated with anastomotic leakages and cardiovascular disease. Stenosis after anastomotic leakage may be due to (a) initial local ischemia manifested as a leakage and/or (b) local inflammatory reaction.

Also, cardiovascular disease may have an important influence on the anastomosis healing process due to poor irrigation, as consequence of atherosclerosis or a low cardiac output.

Diagnosis of this complication. If transit through the anastomosis is impaired for longer than 5 days, involving the necessity of emptying the gastric remnant by means of nasogastric tube, then diagnostic assessment is indicated by means of a CT scan using oral contrast. It will help not only for diagnosing the level of the obstruction but also for ruling out abscesses or leakages that should be treated first. Stenosis may be found at the level of the esophago-jejunostomy, the gastro-jejunostomy, or after a Billroth II anastomosis at the afferent or efferent loop. Gastroscopy is the next step in order to assess the stenosis/obstruction and to evaluate the possibility for dilatation therapy. If possible, progressive balloon dilatation done in several sessions will be the treatment of choice [1].

Decompression of the stomach is the initial step, along with adequate feeding by means of intestinal feeding tube introduced by the gastroscopist distal of the stenosis or by TPN.

Treatment depends on the diagnosis. If abscesses are present, these must first be drained percutaneously before the dilatation program can be started. If there is only stenosis, a dilatation program will be scheduled. Dilatation by means of a balloon will frequently lead to optimal results. Currently, most of literature is based on balloon dilatation for stenosis of anastomosis after gastric bypass for morbid obesity showing that dilatation is safe and efficient to solve the problem [1, 2].

If dilatation is not possible or obstruction is complete because of a technical problem, such as internal hernia or torsion, then reoperation will need to be planned.

References

1. Garcia Sabrido JL, Vasquez JW. How to prevent, early diagnose, and treat major postoperative complications after gastric surgery. In: Cuesta MA, Bonjer HJ, editors. Treatment of complications after digestive surgery, chapter 9. London: Springer; 2013.
2. Ukleja A, Afonso BB, Pimentel R, et al. Outcome of endoscopic balloon dilation of strictures after laparoscopic gastric bypass. Surg Endosc. 2008;22:1746–50.

Chapter 16
Case on Leakage After Closure of a Duodenal Perforation

Jose L Garcia Sabrido and Wenceslao Vasquez Jimenez

Keywords Duodenal perforation • Arthrosis • Laparoscopy • Omentoplasty • Duodenal ulcer • Perforation closure

Diagnosis and Indication for Surgery

We behold a 78-year-old male patient with a history of arthrosis and a chronic use of oral NSAID's and opiates. He had been evaluated at the emergency room because of abdominal pain lasting 72 h. At examination, the patient was hypotensive with a good reaction to fluid therapy. Clinical examination showed signs of generalized peritonitis, being confirmed by CT scan with abundant intra-abdominal fluid collections, submesocolic pneumoperitoneum, and air bubbles at the level of the hepatoduodenal ligament. The history was compatible with a perforated duodenal ulcer secondary to NSAID's use, and subsequently a diagnostic laparoscopy was performed.

Operation

A generalized peritonitis with a perforation larger than 1 cm at the level of the duodenal bulb was found. After abdominal lavage, the perforation was closed with sutures and an omentoplasty was added. Moreover, the subhepatic space was drained.

J.L.G. Sabrido, M.D. (✉) • W.V. Jimenez, M.D., Ph.D.
Department of Surgery, Gregorio Marañon Hospital, Madrid, Spain
e-mail: jlgsabrido@gmail.com, jlgsabrido@ciriii.hggm.es

M.A. Cuesta, H.J. Bonjer (eds.), *Case Studies of Postoperative Complications after Digestive Surgery*, DOI 10.1007/978-3-319-01613-9_16,

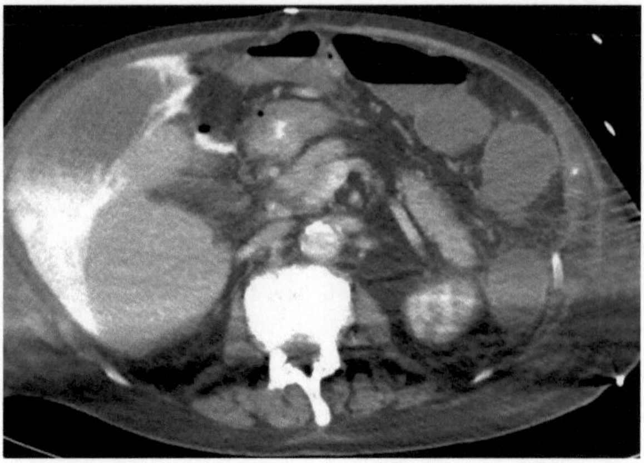

Fig. 16.1 Leakage of the duodenum following closure of a perforation

Postoperative Course: Identification and Treatment of the Complication

At the fifth postoperative day, the patient had severe abdominal pain with a tachycardia and hypotension. The complete blood count showed 23,000 leucocytes, 98 % of them segmented, a hemoglobin of 14 g/dL, and mild coagulation alterations. The abdominal CT scan with oral contrast (gastrographin) showed leakage of contrast at the duodenal level (Fig. 16.1).

A supra-umbilical laparotomy found a dehiscence of the primary suture with an important generalized peritonitis. The antrum of the stomach and the duodenal bulb were resected with use of a stapler, and both the gastric and duodenal stump staple lines were reinforced with PDS continuous sutures. A reconstruction by means of a Roux-Y gastrojejunostomy was performed. The patient recovered slowly on the Intensive Care Unit and could start with oral feeding and medication progressively after 3 weeks.

Discussion

Perforated duodenal ulcers (Illustration 16.1) that cover more than 1/3 of the circumference are not suitable to primary suture reparation due to the high risk of leakage. Moreover the first choice is the horizontal closure and omentum plasty with adequate use of drains. Gastric resection will be used only exceptionally. Perforations equal or shorter than 1/3 of the circumference are suitable for primary suture and omentoplasty.

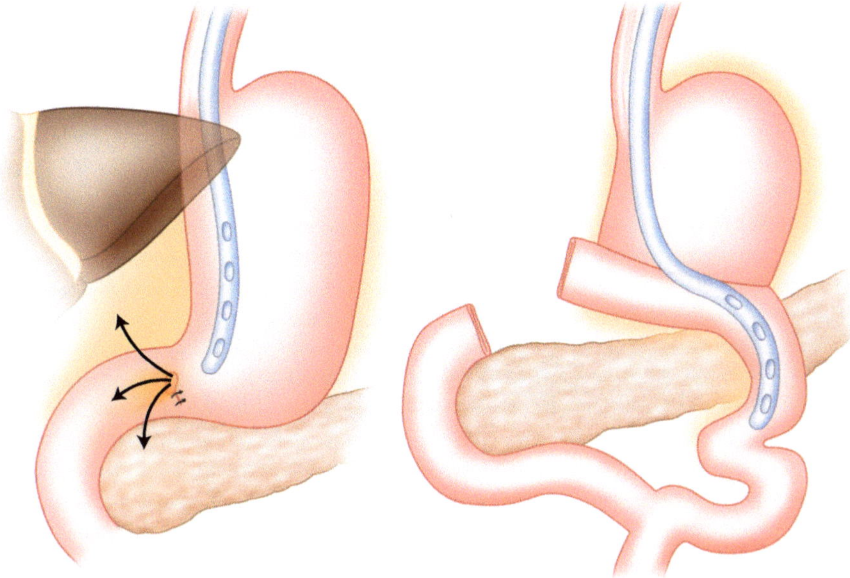

Illustration 16.1 Perforated duodenal ulcers that cover more than 1/3 of the circumference are not suitable to primary suture reparation due to the high risk of leakage. Perforations equal or shorter than 1/3 of the circumference are suitable for primary suture and omentoplasty. In the case of leakage a partial gastrectomy should be done with a Roux-en-Y anastomosis and adequate drainage

Chapter 17
Case on Leakage After Closure of a Perforated Duodenal Diverticulum

Ramon Gorter and J. Wolter Oosterhuis

Keywords Perforation • Duodenal diverticulum • Peritonitis • Laparoscopy • Papilla of Vater

Diagnosis and Indication for Surgery

In view is a 76-year-old female patient, who presented at our cardiac care unit because of acute distress, dyspnoe, and chest pain. Her medical history included arterial hypertension, hypercholesterolemia, a cholecystectomy, hysterectomy, and a diaphragmatic hernia. On physical examination, she was acutely ill, her blood pressure was 100/60 mm Hg, her pulse 80 beats/min, without fever. Her abdomen was painful with signs of generalized peritonitis. Laboratory findings were normal except for a mild leukocytosis of 13.4×10^9/L. The electrocardiogram did not show any sign of acute ischemia. A CT scan with double contrast revealed free fluid and air in the retroperitoneal space as well as in the right upper quadrant. The diagnosis of a perforation of a hollow organ—probably a duodenal ulcer—was made, and a laparoscopic exploration was proposed.

Operation

Diagnostic laparoscopy revealed intra-abdominal and retroperitoneal biliary fluid. Due to the reduced visibility, conversion to a laparotomy was performed, showing a

R. Gorter, M.D. (✉)
Pediatric Surgery, VU University Medical Center, Amsterdam, The Netherlands
e-mail: rr.gorter@vumc.nl

J.W. Oosterhuis
Department of Surgery,VU University Medical Center, Amsterdam, The Netherlands

M.A. Cuesta, H.J. Bonjer (eds.), *Case Studies of Postoperative Complications after Digestive Surgery*, DOI 10.1007/978-3-319-01613-9_17,

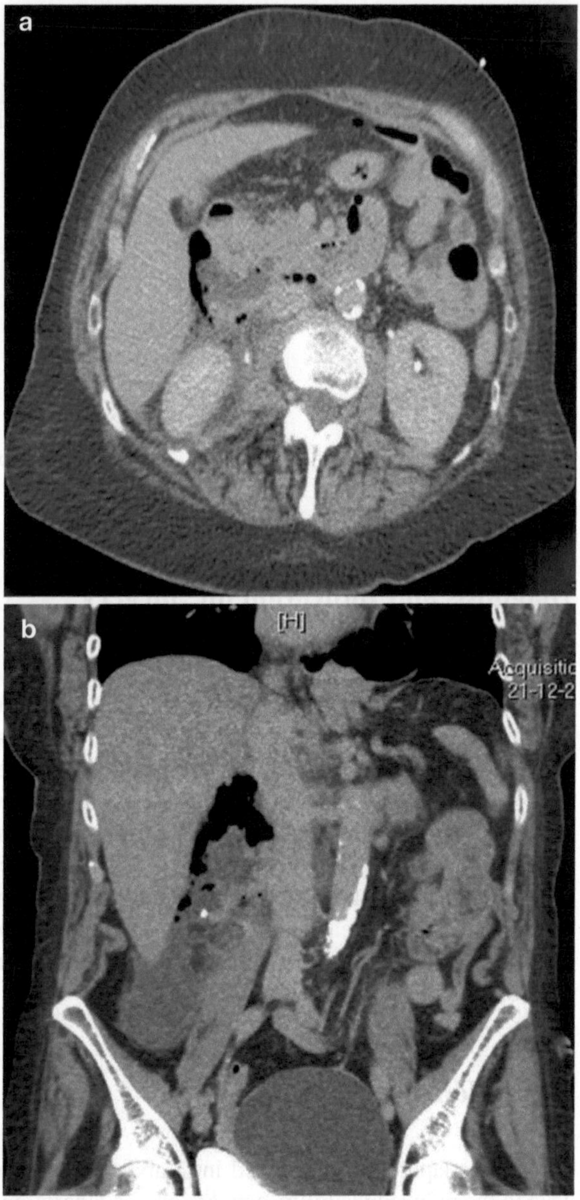

Fig. 17.1 (**a**) CT showing duodenal perforation. (**b**) CT scan showing duodenal perforation

perforated duodenal diverticulum of the descending part of the duodenum (Fig. 17.1a, b). The diverticulum was resected using a GIA® stapler; the suture line was inverted and closed by means of a purse string suture (Illustration 17.1a). To control the possible damage of the papilla of Vater, a T-drain was placed in the common bile duct and the retroperitoneal space was drained.

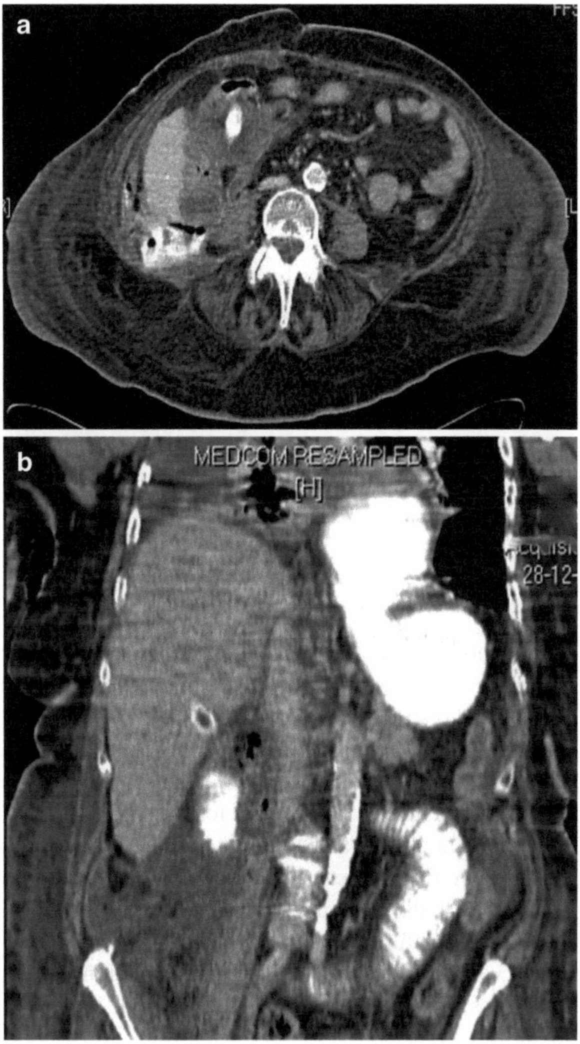

Fig. 17.2 (**a**, **b**) CT scan showing paracolic abscess

Postoperative Course: Identification and Treatment of the Complication

On the Intensive Care Unit (ICU) she was treated for septic shock, with mechanical ventilation, fluid resuscitation, inotropes, and intravenously applied broad-spectrum antibiotics. After 3 days, mechanical ventilation was terminated, but on the seventh postoperative day her clinical condition deteriorated. She had abdominal pain and the surgical drain produced intestinal contents. She experienced a tachycardia of 117 beats/min with a normal blood pressure and fever of 39.2 °C. A CT scan showed important free fluid and air in the retroperitoneal space around the duodenum extending to the right paracolic space (Fig. 17.2a, b). This fluid was drained

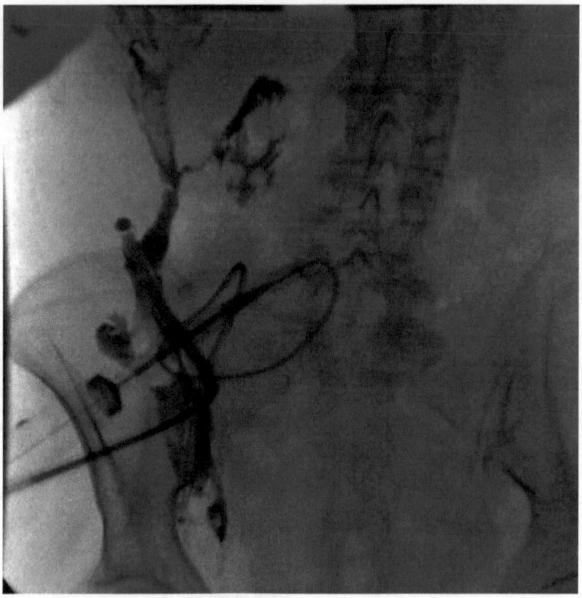

Fig. 17.3 Fistulogram showing the fistula's tracks

percutaneously, revealing a mixture of bile and bowel contents. After drainage, the patient entered a severe septic shock, and a relaparotomy was performed.

At the reoperation, two defects in the duodenal suture line were detected and sutured. Additionally, necrosis around the head of the pancreas was removed. Furthermore, the T-drain seemed to be dislocated, hence it was replaced. After extensive lavage, two drains were left, one right paracolic and one at the level of the duodenum, and she was admitted to the ICU. Cultures of the intra-abdominal fluid revealed an *Enterococcus faecalis*. Patient recovered from the septic situation, and on the 7th day after the second operation, she was discharged from the ICU and admitted to the surgical ward.

She was treated with total parenteral nutrition, a nasogastric tube, and intravenous antibiotics. Her condition improved and oral feeding was started on her 10th postoperative day.

After the second operation, she had seven episodes of high fever and right abdominal pain. After exclusion of pneumonia or urinary tract infection, a CT scan with double contrast showed one or two abscesses located at the right paracolic space in communication with the duodenum. Analysis of the drained fluid revealed organic fibers and an amylase of 30.000 U/L. A contrast medium administered through the drains showed persistent leakage of the duodenal defect and an extensive fistula complex in the retroperitoneal space (Fig. 17.3, Illustration 17.1b). New and old drains were draining pus and intestinal contents up to the 18th postoperative day when the drains were progressively mobilized and finally removed. After a visit to the hairdressing saloon and normal oral intake she could be discharged. On the outpatient policlinic, she was doing well and she was dismissed from surveillance.

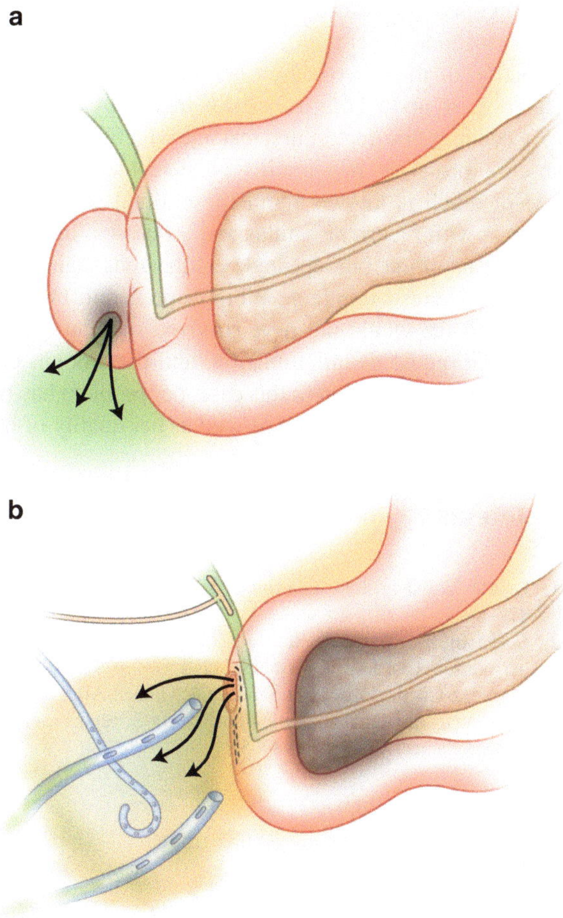

Illustration 17.1 (**a, b**) Perforation of a duodenal diverticulum should be treated by resection after papilla of Vater control. Leakages should be treated by percutaneous drainage

Discussion

Leakage after closure of a perforated duodenal diverticulum is a rare but serious complication. In literature not much is known about its optimal treatment strategy.

Duodenal diverticula are common with an estimated incidence between 5 and 22 % [1, 2]. They are usually located at the second part of the duodenum at the mesenteric or pancreatic border [3]. Most are asymptomatic, although in about 5 % of cases, complications occur such as bleeding, inflammation, or even perforation (with a mortality rate up to 30 %) [1–3]. As the location is in the second part of the duodenum, perforation usually leads to leakage of duodenal contents in the retroperitoneal and peritoneal spaces, leading to abscess formation or generalized peritonitis and sepsis. Due to its rarity, there are no equivocal guidelines concerning the initial management. Several authors consider nonoperative management (parenteral feeding, percutaneous drainage of abscesses, and intravenous antibiotics) in stable and non-septic patients as the treatment strategy of choice although in literature, the resection of the diverticulum is still considered to be the golden standard [1–3]. However, in up to 41 % of patients treated by diverticulectomy such complications may occur as bile duct injury, leakage with fistula formation (20 %), intra-abdominal abscess formation, pancreatitis, persistent leakage, and sepsis [2, 3].

Not much is known about the optimal treatment strategy in especially those patients with recurrent fistulas and abscesses. In our patient in view, a reoperation was not an option, but repeated percutaneous drainages were performed. In her case, an extensive resection (e.g., Whipple procedure) was one of the considered options. However, she would not have survived such an operation due to her poor clinical condition, grade of inflammation, and the amount of affected tissue. Although it meant a long admission in this case, her problem has been solved; her condition has now significantly improved as well as her quality of life.

References

1. Duarte B, Nagy KK, Cintron J. Perforated duodenal diverticulum. Br J Surg. 1992;79: 877–81.
2. Bergman S, Koumanis J, Stein LA, et al. Duodenal diverticulum with retroperitoneal perforation. Can J Surg. 2005;48:332–4.
3. Martinez-Cecilia D, Arjano-Sanchez A, Gomez-Alvarez M, et al. Conservative management of perforated duodenal diverticulum: a case report and review of the literature. World J Gastroenterol. 2008;14:1949–51.

Chapter 18
Case on An Acute Complication of the Wilkie Syndrome

Miguel A. Cuesta and Donald L. van der Peet

Keywords Wilkie syndrome • Complications • Peritonitis • Pneumatosis

Diagnosis and Indication for Surgery

We now regard a 16-year-old female patient, a high school student without previous complaints, who suddenly became ill, experiencing abdominal pain and vomiting. The general practitioner observed her at home under an initial diagnosis of gastroenteritis. After 3 days, the complaints worsened and the patient was referred to our surgical department. She appeared to be dehydrated, had a fever of 38.7 °C, tachycardia, and she displayed a poor general aspect. Physical examination of the abdomen showed upper abdominal pain with signs of local peritonitis. The laboratory results showed a leukocytosis of 21,000/L and a CRP of 180 mg/L were found. A CT scan with oral and IV contrast was performed. A gastric dilatation with pneumatosis in the stomach wall was found with dilatation of duodenum and possible compression of the horizontal part of the duodenum (Fig. 18.1). Differential diagnosis was made between annular pancreas and duodenal web.

Operation

At emergency laparotomy, a clear compression of the horizontal part of duodenum by the superior mesenteric vessels against the spine was seen. Moreover, gastric dilatation with necrosis of the fundus was found (Fig 18.2).

M.A. Cuesta, M.D. (✉) • D.L. van der Peet
Department of Surgery, VU University Medical Center, Amsterdam, The Netherlands
e-mail: ma.cuesta@vumc.nl; dl.vdpeet@vumc.nl

M.A. Cuesta, H.J. Bonjer (eds.), *Case Studies of Postoperative Complications after Digestive Surgery*, DOI 10.1007/978-3-319-01613-9_18,

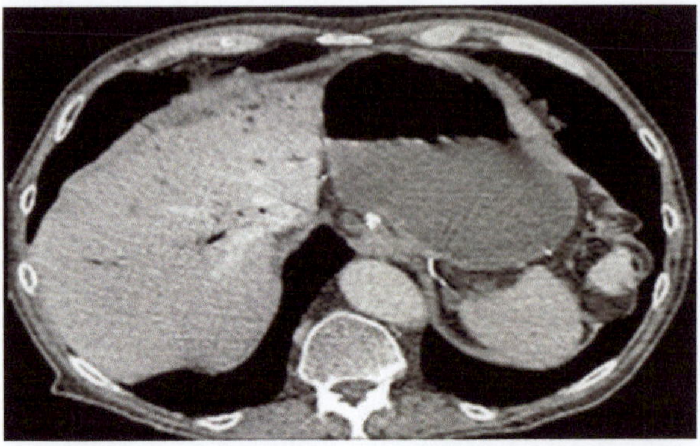

Fig. 18.1 CT scan showing gastric dilatation and pneumatosis. Gas in the portal veins

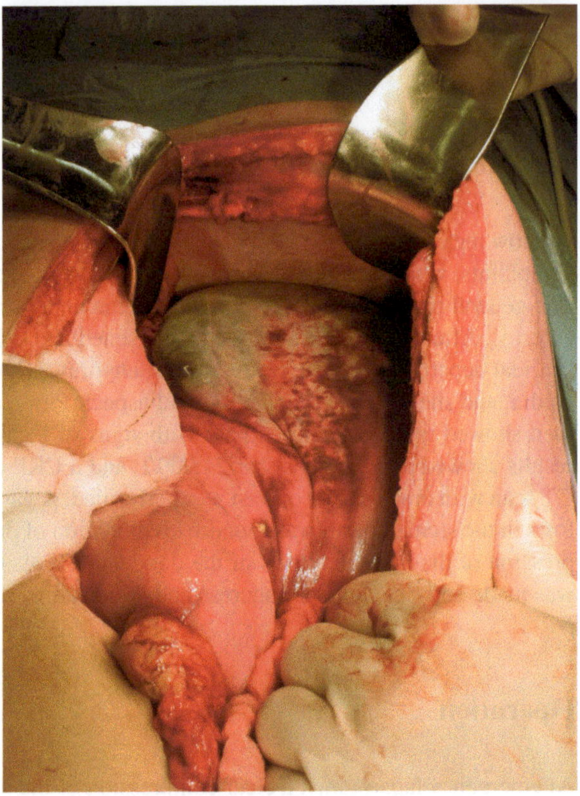

Fig. 18.2 Aspect of the operation, stomach is dilated and the greater curvature is necrotic

A resection of the necrotic part of the gastric fundus along the greater curvature was performed by means of staplers and a running suture over it. Moreover, to treat the cause, a side-to-side duodenojejunostomy was performed in two layers (Fig. 18.3).

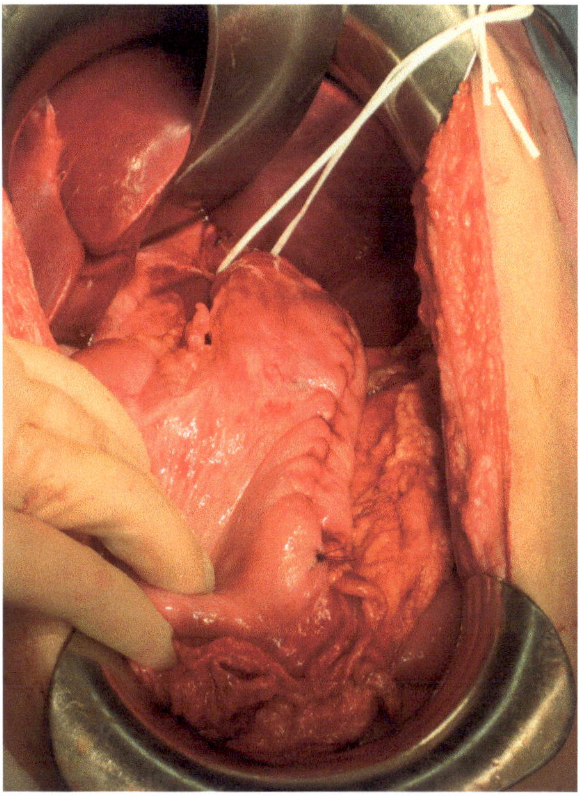

Fig. 18.3 After resection of the greater curvature and duodenojejnunostomy

Postoperative Course

Postoperatively, the patient recovered very quickly and could initiate oral feeding progressively from the 3rd day on. At day 7 she went home and after a period of 4 weeks she could reinitiate her daily activities and studies.

Discussion

Wilkie's syndrome is a rare cause of duodenal passage problems. It is produced by compression of the superior mesenteric artery on the horizontal duodenal part. Chronic complaints are typical with dilatation of the duodenum and stomach. Acute complication is very rare and in this young patient led to gastric dilatation and necrosis of the greater curvature.

Chapter 19
Case on Distal Duodenal Perforation After Double Balloon Endoscopy (DBE)

Marijn Poelman and Chris J.J. Mulder

Keywords Perforation • Double balloon endoscopy (DBE) • Celiac sprue • Laparotomy • Proximal jejunum

Diagnosis and Indication for Surgery: Identification of the Complication

A 56-year-old female patient, known for having celiac sprue since 7 years, was admitted at the surgical ward of a hospital because of vomiting and weight loss. The CT scan with double contrast revealed a stenosis in the duodenojejunal junction (Fig. 19.1). A gastroscopy done up to the distal part of the duodenum showed no anomalies, and in order to investigate the distal part and jejunum, a double balloon endoscopy (DBE) was performed (Illustration 19.1a). Here, a tumor was seen and localized in the horizontal part of the duodenum. Biopsies were taken for histological examination. The patient developed progressive abdominal pain after the procedure and on the X-ray of the abdomen free air was observed. A CT scan showed signs of a perforation (Fig. 19.2) with pneumoperitoneum and free fluid at the level of the tumor in the ligament of Treitz and patient was operated on.

M. Poelman, M.D.
Department of Surgery, VU University Medical Center, Amsterdam, The Netherlands
e-mail: mm.poelman@vumc.nl

C.J.J. Mulder
Department of Gastroenterology, VU University Medical Center, Amsterdam, The Netherlands
e-mail: cjmulder@vumc.nl

M.A. Cuesta, H.J. Bonjer (eds.), *Case Studies of Postoperative Complications after Digestive Surgery*, DOI 10.1007/978-3-319-01613-9_19,

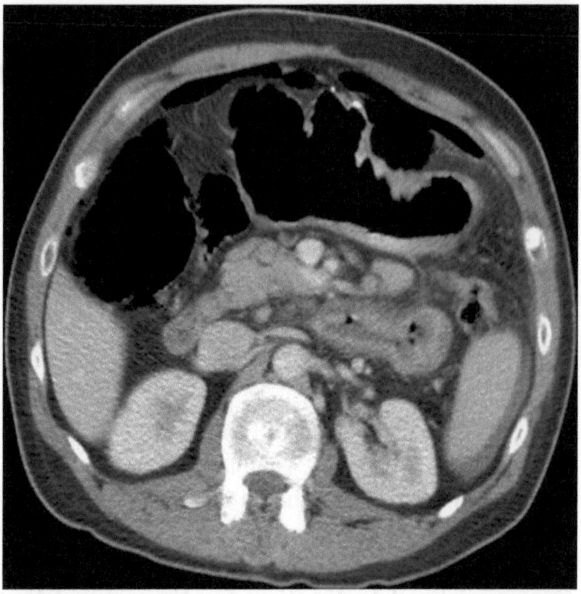

Fig. 19.1 Thickness with stenosis at horizontal part of the duodenum (tumor) with intraabdominal free air

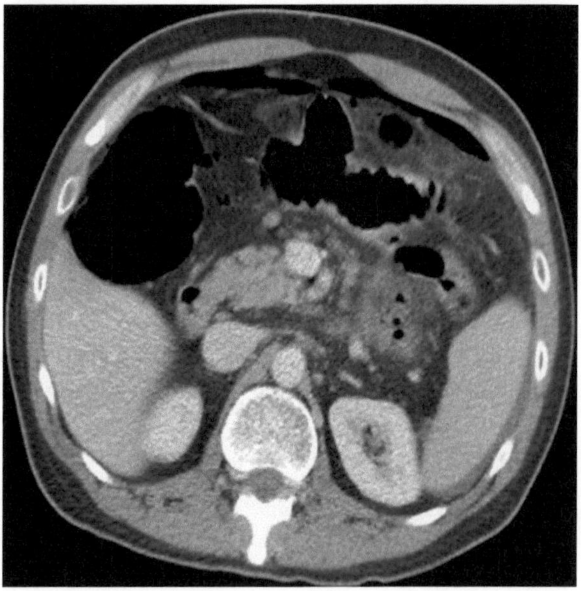

Fig. 19.2 Perforation with pneumoperitoneum and free air and fluid collection at the level of Treitz ligament

Illustration 19.1 (**a**) Double balloon endoscopy. Perforation as complication. (**b**) Resection of tumor after perforation

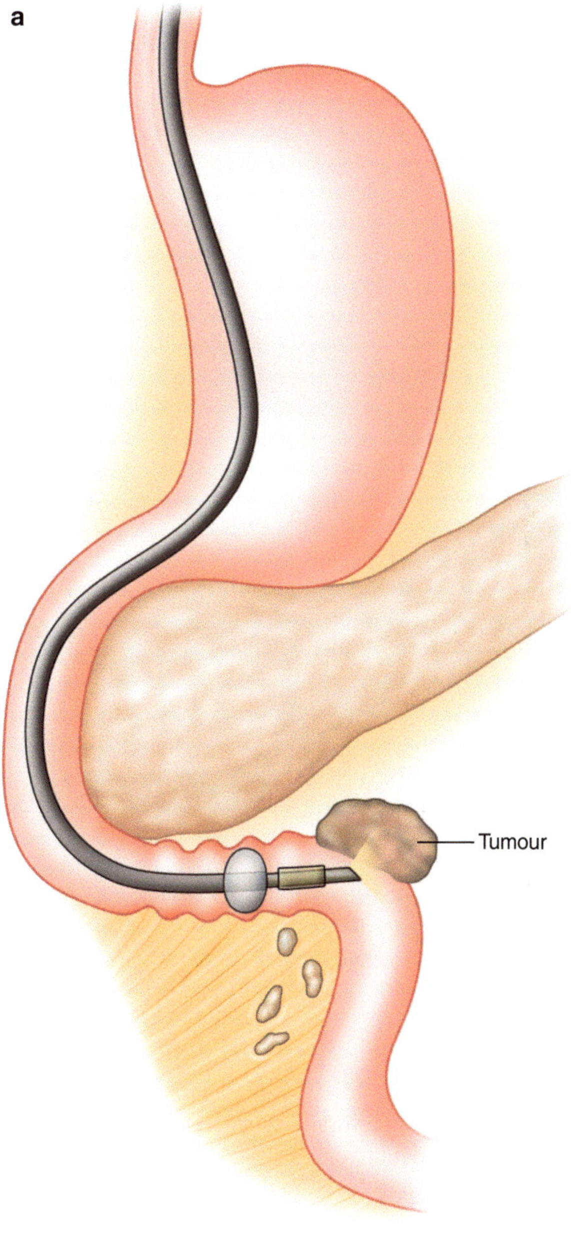

b

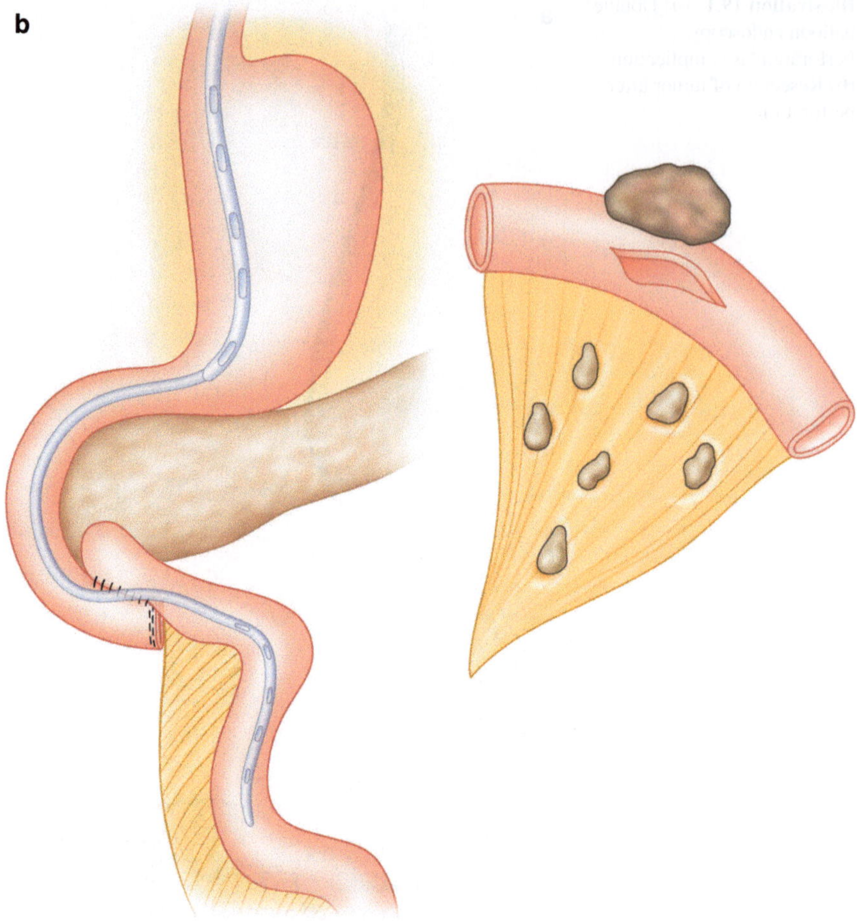

Illustration 19.1 (continued)

Operation

At laparotomy a perforation was seen in the tumor localized at the junction between the distal duodenum and the proximal jejunum. The tumor was 4 cm, and enlarged lymph nodes were found in the mesentery at the level of ligament of Treitz. A radical resection was performed followed by an end-to-side anastomosis between the descending part of the duodenum and the proximal jejunum (Illustration 19.1b).

Pathology

Pathological examination demonstrated a B-cell lymphoma, radically resected.

Patient recovered.

Discussion

Xin et al. [1] performed a systematic review about the indications and complications of the diagnostic double balloon endoscopy after a 10-year experience of its application. A total of 66 articles involving 12,823 procedures were included. Suspected mid-GI bleeding (MGIB) was the most common indication (62.5 %), followed by symptoms/signs only (7.9 %), small-bowel obstruction (5.8 %), and Crohn's disease (5.8 %). Inflammatory lesions (37.6 %) and vascular lesions (65.9 %) were the most common findings, respectively. The pooled total enteroscopy rate was 44.0 % by combined or antegrade-only approach. The pooled minor and major complication rates were 9.1 and 0.72 %, respectively. They concluded that the detectability and complication risk of diagnostic DBE are acceptable.

Reference

1. Xin L, Liao Z, Jiang YP, Li ZS. Indications, detectability, positive findings, total enteroscopy, and complications of diagnostic double-balloon endoscopy: a systematic review of data over the first decade of use. Gastrointest Endosc. 2011;74:563–70.

Chapter 20
Case on Duodenal Leakage After Resection of an Insulinoma of the Head of the Pancreas

Miguel A. Cuesta and Donald L. van der Peet

Keywords Duodenal leakage • Insulinoma • Pancreas • Laparoscopic enucleation • Pancreatic leakage

Diagnosis and Indication for Surgery

In our focus is a 48-year-old male patient, who, after series of collapses, was diagnosed with an insulinoma of 3 cm in the head of the pancreas. The tumor was visible on the MRI scan (Fig. 20.1).

Operation

The patient underwent a laparoscopic enucleation after laparoscopic ultrasonography. A distance of 3–4 mm with the pancreatic duct could be seen. After performing a Kocher maneuver, the tumor was excised. In the pancreas opening no leakage of pancreatic fluid was observed, leaving a drain at the level of the pancreas.

Postoperative Course: Identification and Treatment of the Complication

Postoperatively, the patient experienced abdominal pain and the amylase level in the drain was high (20,000 U/ml), suggesting the existence of a pancreatic leakage. A CT scan confirmed some leakage from the pancreas with a fluid collection

M.A. Cuesta, M.D. (✉) • D.L. van der Peet
Department of Surgery, VU University Medical Center, Amsterdam, The Netherlands
e-mail: ma.cuesta@vumc.nl; dl.vdpeet@vumc.nl

M.A. Cuesta, H.J. Bonjer (eds.), *Case Studies of Postoperative Complications after Digestive Surgery*, DOI 10.1007/978-3-319-01613-9_20,

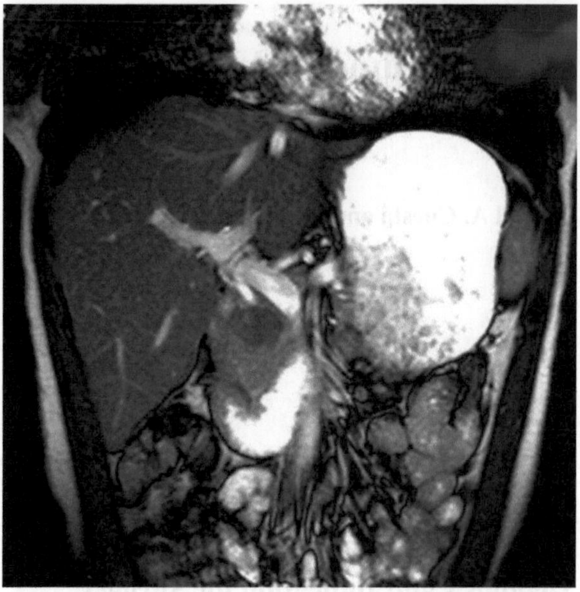

Fig. 20.1 MRI, insulinoma in head of the pancreas

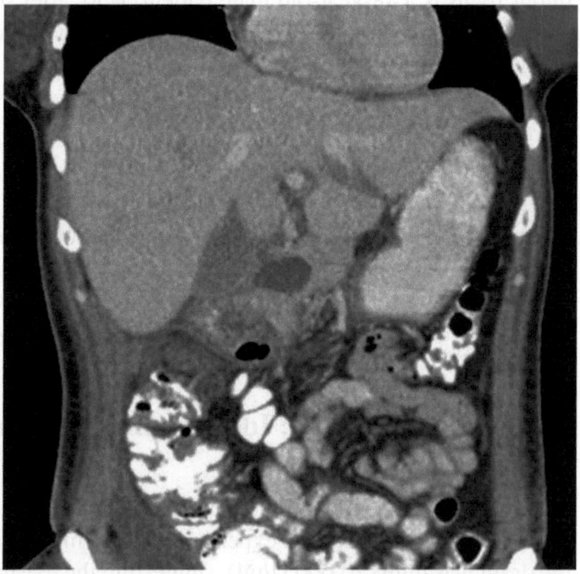

Fig. 20.2 CT scan showing local leakage of pancreas

around the duodenum (Fig. 20.2) (Illustration 20.1a). The location of the drain in the middle of the collection was considered good. On the 10th postoperative day, the patient became hemodynamically unstable, with decreasing Hemoglobin levels. On the performed CT more fluids and clots were visible in the abdomen, and

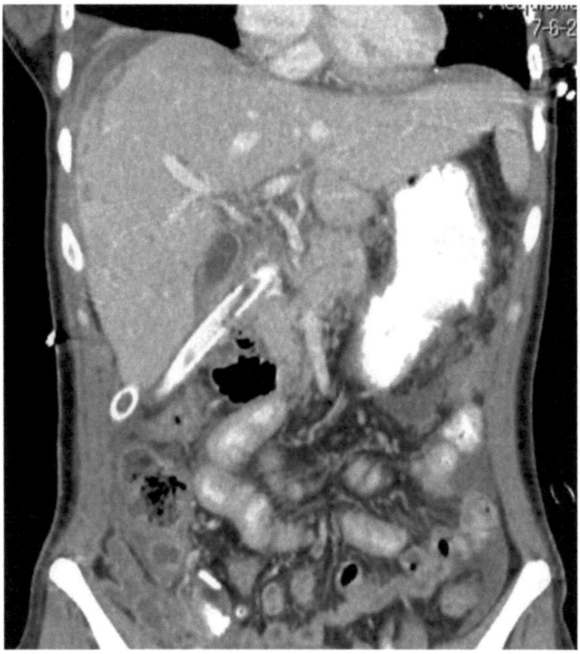

Fig. 20.3 Duodenal leakage direct to the drain

on the CT angiography a blush was found around the head of the pancreas, but it could not be coiled. Liver perfusion was considered irregular. An explorative laparotomy through a subcostal incision was done. A bleeding caused by some small vessels around the junction between pancreatic head and the common bile duct was found and fixed with stitches. Moreover, the aspect of the duodenal wall was considered fragile and inflamed. The patient recovered, but on the 7th postoperative day intestinal contents came through the drain. The CT scan with contrast showed a duodenal fistula of the descending part of the duodenum (Fig. 20.3) with adequate drainage and no intra-abdominal collections. The patient was treated by total parenteral nutrition (TPN) and after 7 days drain production decreased and then ceased. The patient could reinitiate oral feeding. After 3 weeks, she acquired a feeling of gastric fullness and started vomiting. A new CT scan with oral contrast showed an important stenosis of the descending part of the duodenum with a gastric dilatation. Nasogastric tubing and TPN was given. Deliberation by the multidisciplinary group considered two possibilities for treating the stenosis, endoscopic dilatation or surgery.

Considering the risk of perforation, the first option was adopted. After four balloon dilatations, passage (2.5 cm) was considered sufficient; oral feeding could be initiated and this was well tolerated (Illustration 20.1b).

One year after operation, the patient has been doing well; her weight is optimal and there are no signs of recurrence of the insulinoma.

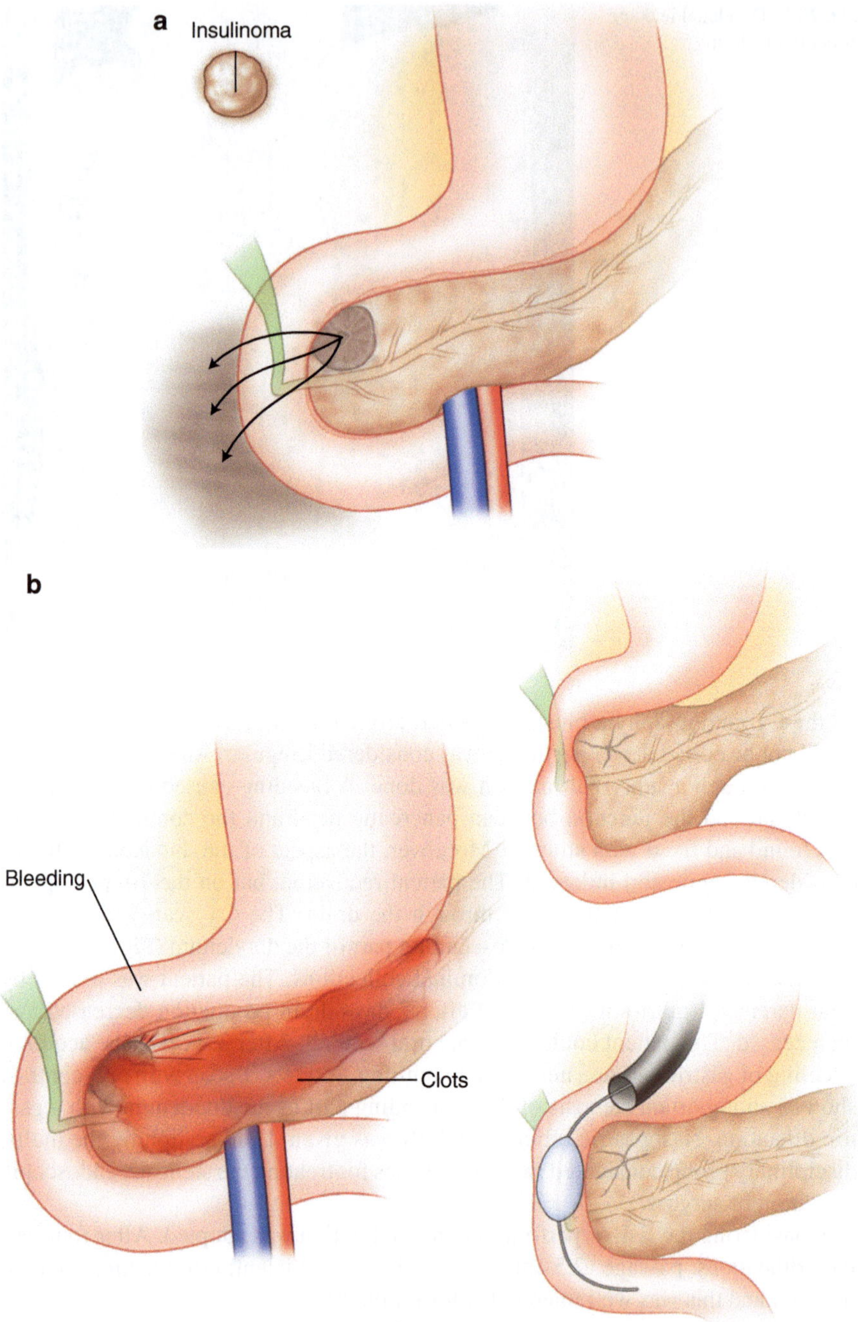

Illustration 20.1 (**a**, **b**) Benign insulinomas of the pancreas should be operated laparoscopically. Small tumors or preoperative unidentified tumors will be localized by visual inspection and laparoscopic ultrasonography. After enucleation, the most frequent complication is the pancreatic fistula. Drainage should be maintained until no production of the fistula. If suspicion that the main pancreatic duct (PD) is the cause of the fistula, the PD should drained by ERCP

Discussion

In our department Berends et al. described ten patients treated laparoscopically because of insulinoma of the pancreas [1]. There were localized all over the pancreas with a maximal size of 3 cm. Laparoscopic ultrasonography was used to localize properly the insulinoma during the operation. Six tumors could be excised laparoscopically, four patients being converted to laparotomy. Five complications were observed: two after laparoscopy (two pancreatic fistulas, one treated by drainage and the other by drainage, ERCP, and drain in the pancreatic duct) and three after laparotomy (pancreatic collection around the duodenum treated by percutaneous drainage, and two paralytic ileus, one of them treated by laparotomy, finding no obstruction). All patients recovered from the hypoglycemia.

Reference

1. Berends FJ, Cuesta MA, Kazemier G, et al. Laparoscopic detection and resection of insulinomas. Surgery. 2000;128:386–91.

Chapter 21
Case on Postoperative Intraluminal Bleeding Following a Gastric Bypass

Jose L. Garcia Sabrido and Wenceslao Vasquez Jimenez

Keywords Intraluminal bleeding • Gastric bypass • Morbid obesity • Dyslipidemia

Diagnosis and Indication for Surgery

We regard a 34-year-old female patient, BMI 45 kg/m^2, with a history of hypertension and dyslipidemia, and scheduled for a laparoscopic gastric bypass. Gastroscopy did not show abnormalities, and abdominal ultrasound showed severe hepatic steatosis.

Eight hours before surgery she received thromboembolic prophylaxis with subcutaneous 5,000 UI heparin.

Operation

The laparoscopic gastric bypass was performed with a long-loop Roux-Y technique; the feeding loop measured 100 cm and the jejunojejunostomy was performed at 45 cm from the ligament of Treitz, antecolic, with a side-to-side anastomosis, by means of an endoscopic linear stapler 60 mm/3.5 mm. The gastric reservoir had a volume of approximately 30 mL and was created using two shots of an endostapler 60 mm/3.5 mm. The closure of the gastro-jejunostomy was done by a continuous suture with Vycril 3/0®, followed by a serosa layer stitches with silk 3/0. Two vacuum laminate drains were placed close to the gastro-jejunostomy and gastric remnant. The procedure was evaluated as routine with no technical difficulties.

J.L.G. Sabrido, M.D. (✉) • W.V. Jimenez, M.D., Ph.D.
Department of Surgery, Gregorio Marañón Hospital, Madrid, Spain
e-mail: jlgsabrido@gmail.com, jlgsabrido@ciriii.hggm.es

M.A. Cuesta, H.J. Bonjer (eds.), *Case Studies of Postoperative Complications after Digestive Surgery*, DOI 10.1007/978-3-319-01613-9_21,

Postoperative Course: Identification and Treatment of the Complication

During the intraoperative period, a nasogastric tube was placed and then withdrawn 12 h later. Postoperative analgesia included NSAID's (Dextroprofen 50 mg) alternating with Acetaminophen 1 g, thereby achieving good pain control.

The patient had a good oral tolerance to clear fluids in the first hours after the procedure. Twenty-four hours following the operation, the patient developed hematemesis, tachycardia, mild hypotension, and a decreased hemoglobin (7 g/dL).

Summarily, a gastroscopy was performed showing an intraluminal bleeding at the level of the stapled gastrojejunostomy. The bleeding was treated with diathermia and a hemostatic clip. Following this procedure, the patient quickly recovered without further complications.

Discussion

The incidence of bleeding following gastric bypass is between 0.9 and 4.4 %, and it seems that bleeding is more frequent after laparoscopic than open bypass [1]. In a laparoscopic bypass, the most likely places for intraluminal bleeding are the gastrojejunostomy and the jejunojejunostomy (Illustration 21.1), and for intraperitoneal bleeding, the suture line of the gastric remnant and the trocar openings (Figs. 21.1, 21.2, and 21.3). Postoperative bleeding after gastric bypass should be diagnosed by means of gastroscopy. If a bleeding is seen at the gastrojejunostomy, it should be treated by diathermia or clips. If patient is steadily bleeding from other source or hemodynamically unstable, CT angiography may be helpful to establish the cause. Otherwise explorative laparotomy should be done [2, 3].

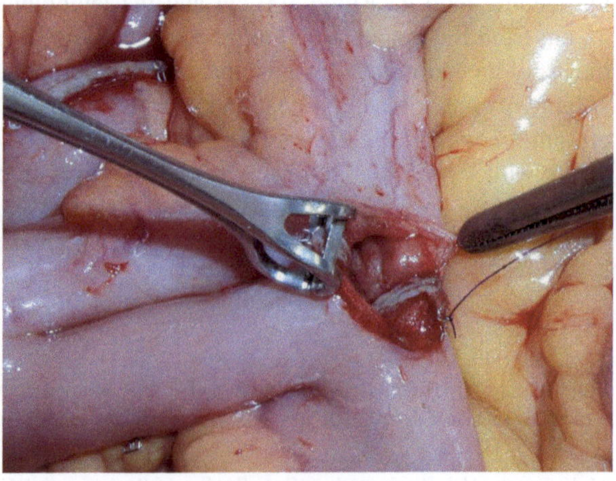

Fig. 21.1 Review of the suture line with stapler after jejunojejunostomy

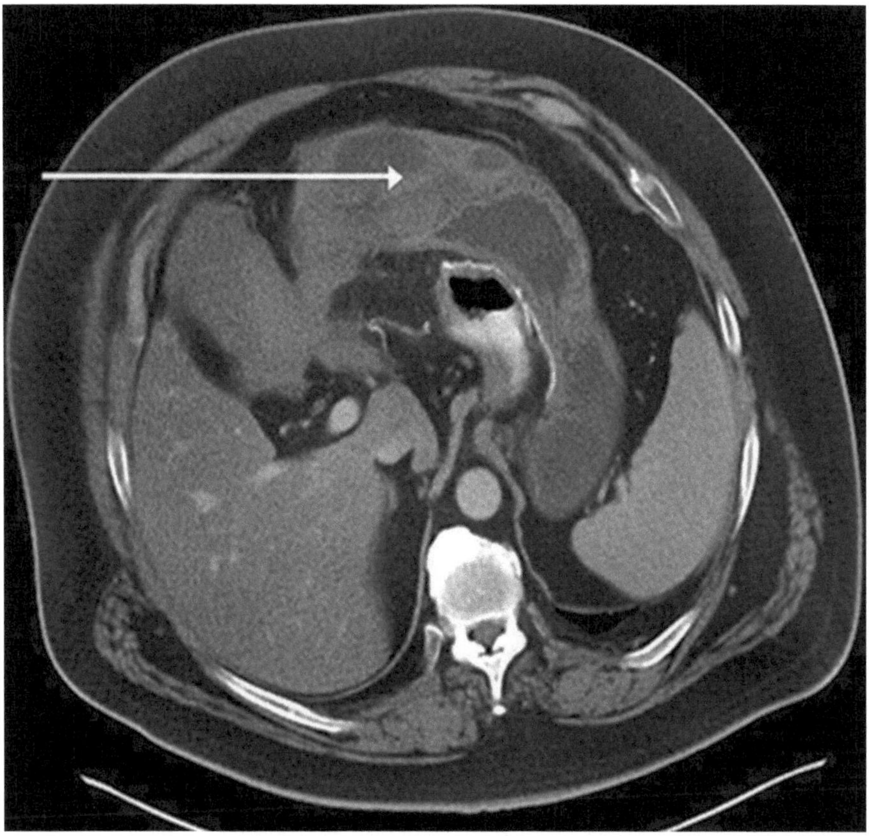

Fig. 21.2 *Arrow* showing intra-abdominal hematoma at the level of the suture line of the gastric remnant

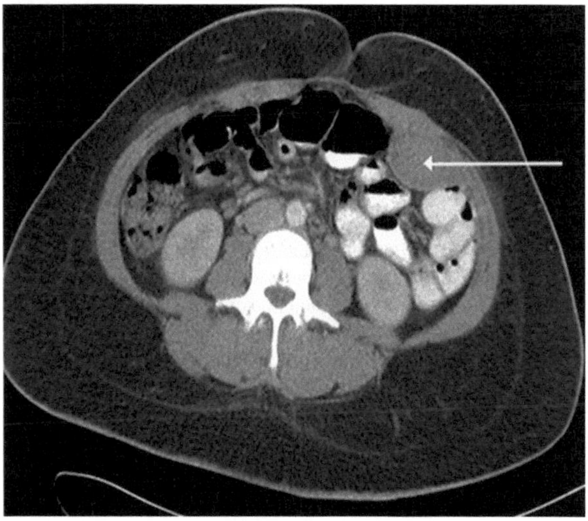

Fig. 21.3 *Arrow* showing hematoma of the abdominal wall associated with the trocar entrance

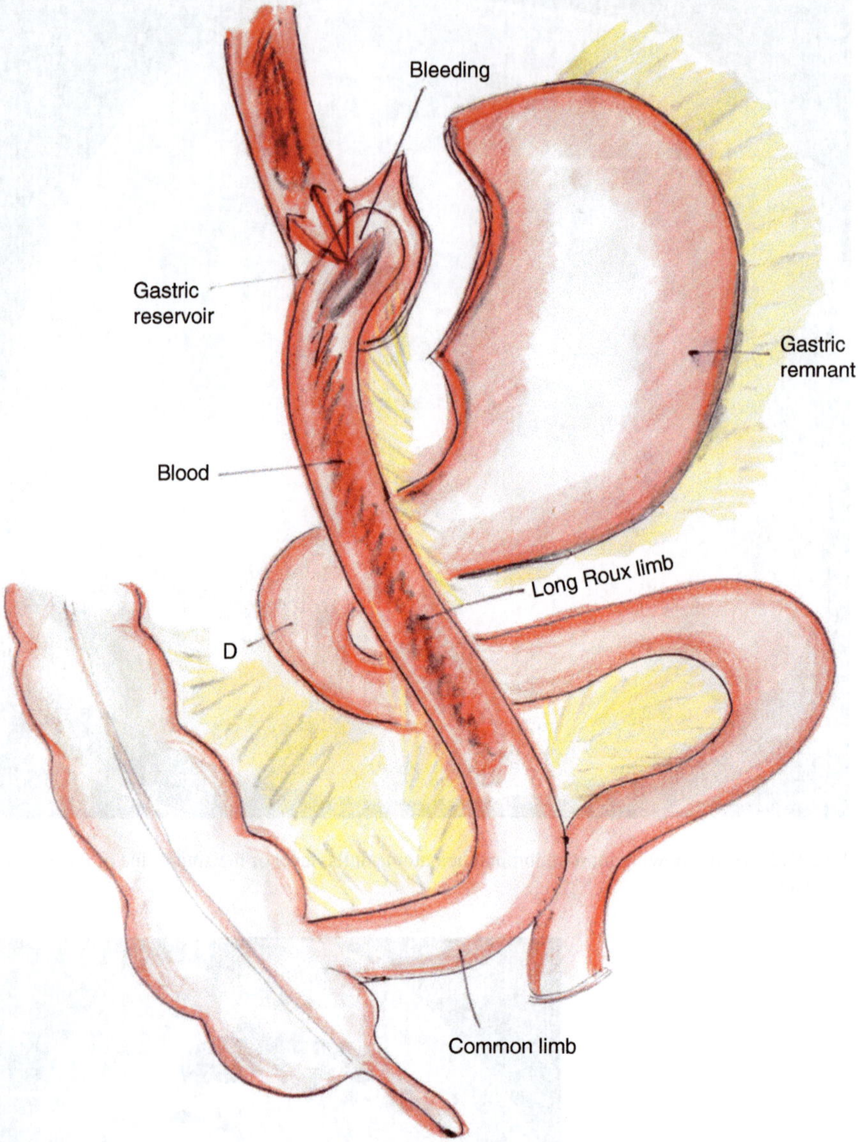

Illustration 21.1 Potential places for intraluminal bleeding after gastric bypass. Postoperative bleeding after gastric bypass because obesity should be diagnosed by means of gastroscopy. If a bleeding is seen at the gastrojejunostomy it should be treated by diathermia or clips. If patient is steadily bleeding from other source or hemodynamically unstable, CT angiography may be helpful to establish the cause. Otherwise explorative laparotomy should be done

References

1. Mehran A, Szomstein S, Zundel N, Rosenthal R. Management of acute bleeding after laparoscopic Roux-en-Y gastric bypass. Obes Surg. 2003;13:842–7.
2. Nguyen NT, Rivers R, Wolfe BM. Early gastrointestinal hemorrhage after laparoscopic gastric bypass. Obes Surg. 2003;13:62–5.
3. Jamil LH, Krause KR, Chengelis DL, et al. Endoscopic management of early upper gastrointestinal hemorrhage following laparoscopic Roux-en-Y gastric bypass. Am J Gastroenterol. 2008;103:86–91.

Chapter 22
Case on Complication of Sleeve Gastrectomy

Ignace M.C. Janssen and Frits J. Berends

Keywords Leakage • Laparoscopy • Gastric bypass • Morbid obesity • Adjustable gastric band • Sleeve gastrectomy

Diagnosis and Indication for Surgery

A 36-year old woman had received an adjustable gastric band 7 years earlier, but the band had been removed because of infection. Her BMI was 40.

Operation

Six months later a sleeve gastrectomy was performed because of weight regain. This procedure commenced laparoscopically but had to be converted to open surgery due to firm adhesions between the liver and the stomach.

Postoperative Course: Identification and Treatment of the Complication

Three days postoperatively gastrointestinal contents were noted in the drain. The patient had little abdominal complaints and only a slightly elevated CRP. A covered stent was inserted on day 5. However, the leak was in the top of the sleeve,

I.M.C. Janssen, M.D. (✉) • F.J. Berends, M.D.
Department of Surgery, Rijnstate,
Arnhem, The Netherlands
e-mail: ijanssen@alysis.nl; fberends@alysis.nl

M.A. Cuesta, H.J. Bonjer (eds.), *Case Studies of Postoperative Complications after Digestive Surgery*, DOI 10.1007/978-3-319-01613-9_22,

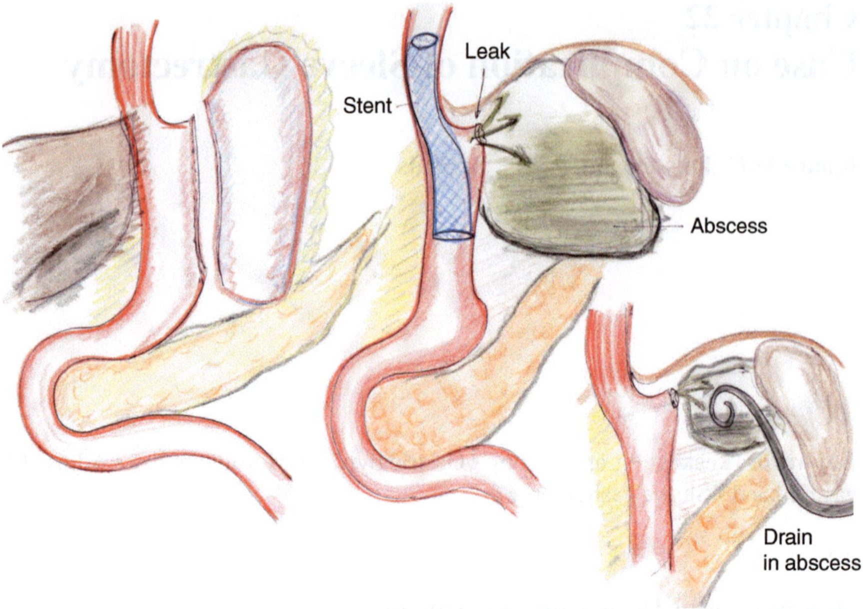

Illustration 22.1 If there is leakage after sleeve gastrectomy, the abdomen should be drained and the leakage covered by a stent. If fistula develops, a reoperation should be performed by conversion the sleeve gastrectomy in a gastric bypass

where it was created too wide, so that the leak was not well covered and a fistula persisted. She developed a septic profile, and a CT scan showed a peri-splenic abscess. The abscess was drained percutaneously and a naso-jejunal tube was placed (Illustration 22.1). She recovered well but a gastrocutaneous fistula persisted after removal of the drain. The general condition of the patient strongly improved in a couple of weeks and she agreed to another operation. During explorative laparotomy it was found that there was enough fundus left to safely close the proximal stomach and resect the part with the fistula. The sleeve was then converted to a gastric bypass. The postoperative period was uneventful.

Discussion

Sleeve gastrectomy is a surgical weight-loss procedure in which the stomach is reduced to about 25 % of its original size, by surgical removal of a large portion of the stomach, following the major curve [1]. The open edges are then attached together (often with surgical staples) to form a sleeve or tube with a banana shape. The procedure permanently reduces the size of the stomach. The procedure is performed laparoscopically and is not reversible. Sleeve gastrectomy (also called gastric sleeve) is usually performed on extremely obese patients, with a body mass index of 40 or more, where the risk of performing a gastric bypass or duodenal switch procedure may be too large. A two-stage procedure is performed: the first is a sleeve gastrectomy, and the second is a conversion into a gastric bypass or duodenal switch. Patients usually lose a large quantity of their excess weight after the sleeve gastrectomy procedure alone. If weight loss ceases the second step is performed. For patients that are obese but not extremely obese, sleeve gastrectomy alone is a suitable operation with low risks. The sleeve gastrectomy currently is acceptable weight loss surgery option for obese patients as a single procedure. Compared to other bariatric procedures, perioperative risk of LSG appears to be relatively low even in patients considered "high risk." The overall reported mortality rate for LSG is 0.3 %. Complication rates range from 0 to 29 % (average 11.2 %) in literature. Major complications after LSG are: staple line leakage 0–5.5 % and internal bleeding 0–14.5 % [2].

Staple line leakage—Staple line leakage after LSG typically arises in the first days after surgery. Symptoms are similar as in leakage after RYGB with tachycardia, abdominal pain, leukocytosis, and fever. Diagnosis of a leak is made via contrast (gastrografin) swallow or abdominal computed tomography (CT) scan. When a drain is present, ingestion of methylene blue (5 mL in 250 mL of water) can provide clear evidence of a leak. Patients can be treated depending on the onset or detection of the leak. This divides the management of leaks as to whether they were early (1–3 days) or late and whether or not sepsis is present.

Early leak—In a patient with an early leak, the patient should be taken back to the operating room for a laparoscopic or open washout and placement of drains. An attempt can be made to repair the hole in the sleeve through suturing the hole, closure with an omental patch, or insertion of a T-tube through the defect [3, 4]. Intravenous antibiotics are administered. Endoscopic insertion of a nasogastric or nasojejunal tube can be considered especially when closing the leak has failed. A feeding jejunostomy is a more patient friendly alternative.

References

1. Berends FJ, Janssen IMC. Prevention and treatment of complications after Bariatric Surgery. In: Cuesta MA, Bonjer HJ, editors. Treatment of complications after digestive surgery, chapter 10. London: Springer; 2013.
2. Shi X, Karmali S, Sharma AM, Birch DW. A review of laparoscopic sleeve gastrectomy for morbid obesity. Obes Surg. 2010;20:1171–7.
3. Tan JT, Kayawasam S, Wijeratne T, Chandratna HS. Diagnosis and management of gastric leaks after sleeve gastrectomy for morbid obesity. Obes Surg. 2010;20:403–9.
4. Court I, Wilson A, Benotti P, et al. T-tube gastrostomy is a novel approach for distal staple line disruption after sleeve gastrectomy for morbid obesity: case report and review of the literature. Surgery. 2009;145:106–13.

Chapter 23
Case on Leakage of Gastric Bypass

Ignace M.C. Janssen and Frits J. Berends

Keywords Leakage • Gastric bypass • Morbid obesity • Peritonitis

Diagnosis and Indication for Surgery

A 45-year old man presented with a BMI of 55 without serious comorbidity.

Operation

He received a laparoscopic Roux-en-Y gastric bypass. No drains were placed.

Postoperative Course: Identification and Treatment of the Complication

On Postoperative day 1, there was a slight fever and his pulse was 105 bpm. There was an abdominal tenderness that was attributed to the surgery the day before. No further action was undertaken. On postoperative day 2, the patient complained of abdominal pain. His pulse remained 105 bpm. Blood examination revealed a leukocytosis and elevated CRP. Upper gastrointestinal radiograph series did not show any

I.M.C. Janssen, M.D. (✉) • F.J. Berends, M.D.
Department of Surgery,
Rijnstate, Arnhem, The Netherlands
e-mail: ijanssen@alysis.nl; fberends@alysis.nl

M.A. Cuesta, H.J. Bonjer (eds.), *Case Studies of Postoperative Complications after Digestive Surgery*, DOI 10.1007/978-3-319-01613-9_23,

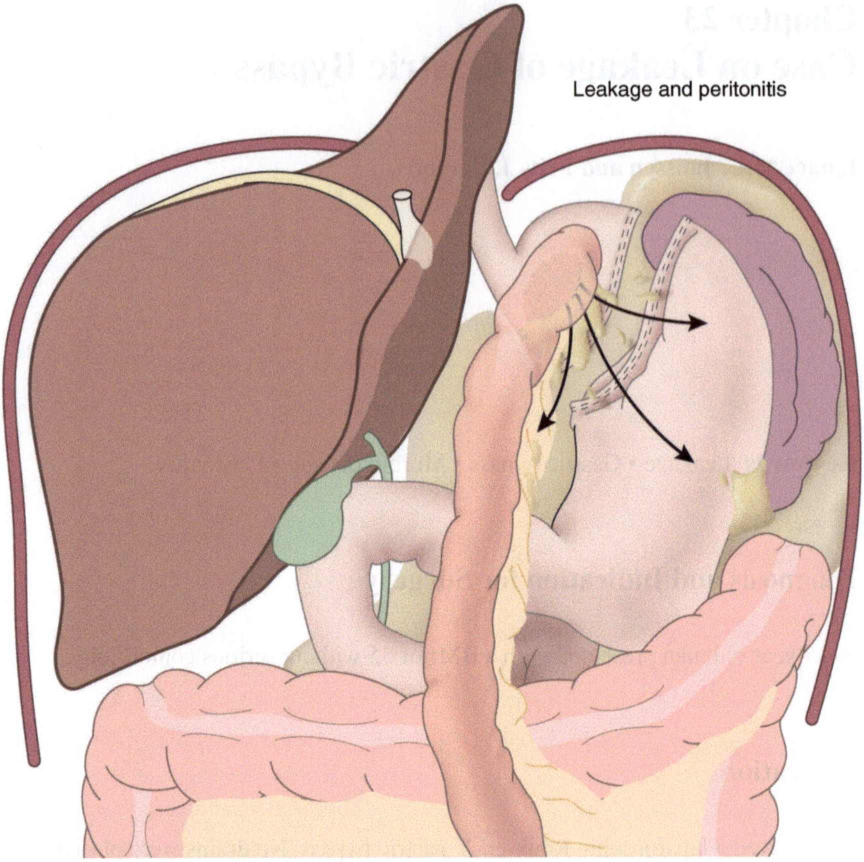

Illustration 23.1 After confirmation of leakage of the gastrojejunostomy of a gastric bypass, abdomen should be rinsed and adequately drained

leakage. Intravenous antibiotics were started and the patient was instructed to abstain from food and drink. The next day the patient developed a slight tachypnoea. Furthermore, his situation was unchanged. On the 5th postoperative day the patient collapsed but recovered soon. Shortly thereafter he developed a full-blown septic profile and a serious dyspnea. He was transported to the intensive care and was intubated and mechanical ventilated. Emergency CT scan now revealed a contrast leak from the gastrointestinal junction (Illustration 23.1). Urgent surgery confirmed a leak in the gastrointestinal anastomosis and a generalized peritonitis. The abdomen was drained and rinsed. The patient remained 4 weeks on the intensive care unit. In that period, he was operated on three times for abdominal sepsis and ended with an open abdomen and a large abdominal wall hernia. He needed prolonged mechanical ventilation because of additional acute respiratory distress syndrome.

He also developed polyneuropathy hampering later remobilization. After a total hospital stay of 4 months he was discharged to a clinic for further revalidation.

Discussion

A Roux-Y Gastric Bypass (RYGB) consists of a small gastric pouch and a Roux-en-Y reconstruction of the jejunum, creating an alimentary limb of 75–200 cm that is attached to the pouch and a biliopancreatic limb of about 50 cm [1].

Most leaks in weight-loss surgery arise from the gastrointestinal anastomosis after gastric bypass surgery. Reported incidence can be as high as 6 %. However, leaks also occur at the staple line of the excluded stomach or of the gastric tube in sleeve gastrectomy. Finally, accidental damage of small intestine or colon by laparoscopic instruments can happen outside the view of the camera.

There is no sure way to prevent a gastrointestinal leakage. Many surgeons evaluate the integrity of the GI anastomosis by testing it with methylene blue dye or through insufflations of air through the gastric tube while the anastomosis is submerged in saline. When no bubbles are seen, there is no apparent leak. Also reinforcement techniques are used for staple lines to prevent leakage, such as fibrin glue, buttressing materials, and over sewing. However, these measures add to the operative costs while there is little evidence that they can prevent leakage.

Leaving wound drains near to the gastrointestinal anastomosis obviously cannot prevent leakage but may help to detect a leak early. Furthermore, having a drain in place can be very helpful in case of a leak because it is an essential part of the treatment and it may prevent needing a reoperation [1].

Symptoms of leak can be very discrete and sometimes merely consist of tachycardia or abdominal tenderness. Other symptoms include fever, tachypnea, and leukocytosis. Especially tachycardia >100 BPM and respiratory distress are the most sensitive physical signs for postoperative leak. CRP is elevated after all operative procedures and discrete elevations are therefore not very reliable. When reconvalescense after surgery is out of the ordinary, a leak must be suspected. As physical examination in the obese patient is mostly of limited value, further diagnostics can be considered [2]. Barium swallow or computed tomography can radiographically demonstrate a leak; however, a (false) negative result does not rule out the possibility of leak. Reported sensitivity and specificity of CT scan for GI leakage can be very high, even up to 100 % in some reports.

As the mortality rate after GI leakage can be as high as 15 %, it is mandatory to treat the leak as soon as possible. Therefore, it is questionable if the effort of additional diagnostic procedures should be undertaken at all. Urgent surgical intervention is probably the best response when a leak is suspected. Most often a laparoscopic approach at reoperation after initial laparoscopic weightloss surgery is feasible.

References

1. Berends FJ, Janssen IMC. Prevention and treatment of complications after bariatric surgery. In: Cuesta MA, Bonjer HJ, editors. Treatment of complications after digestive surgery, chapter 10. London: Springer; 2013.
2. Hamilton EC, Sims TL, Hamilton TT, et al. Clinical predictors of leak after laparoscopic Roux-en-Y gastric bypass for morbid obesity. Surg Endosc. 2003;17:679–84.

Chapter 24
Case on Complication of Adjustable Gastric Band Converted in a Gastric Bypass

Ignace M.C. Janssen and Frits J. Berends

Keywords Gastric band • Gastric bypass • Morbid obesity • Adjustable band • Laparoscopy • Dysphagia

Diagnosis and Indication for Surgery

A 27-year-old female presented with a BMI of 37 and additional hypertension.

Operation

She received a laparoscopic adjustable band.

Postoperative Course: Identification and Treatment of the Complication

She successfully lost weight until a BMI of 29. The band was inflated several times to ensure enough restriction and progressive weight loss. Although she was very content with her weight loss there was a distinct dysphagia. Bread and meat was impossible for her to swallow and after a few years she had adapted to a diet consisting mainly of fluids and mashed food. Once in a while she vomited. Upper

I.M.C. Janssen, M.D. (✉) • F.J. Berends, M.D.
Department of Surgery, Rijnstate,
Arnhem, The Netherlands
e-mail: ijanssen@alysis.nl; fberends@alysis.nl

M.A. Cuesta, H.J. Bonjer (eds.), *Case Studies of Postoperative Complications after Digestive Surgery*, DOI 10.1007/978-3-319-01613-9_24,

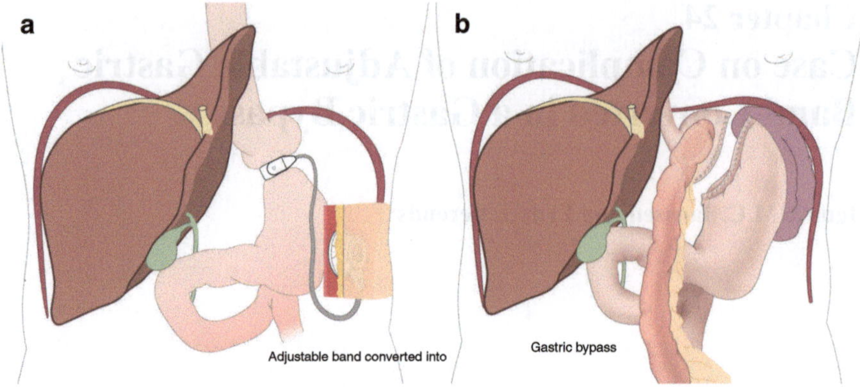

Illustration 24.1 (**a, b**) Complications of the gastric band with dilatation of the gastric pouch and the esophagus should be converted to gastric bypass

gastrointestinal contrast series demonstrated a very tight band, a pouch, and esophageal dilatation. The band was deflated slightly. As a result intake improved, but her weight increased with 5 BMI points. Control contrast series demonstrated a decrease in pouch diameter. The patient was referred to lifestyle training again to regain weight loss, but instead she gained another 3 BMI points. On reinflating the band her vomiting and dysphagia returned immediately. The patient was operated and the band was laparoscopically removed and converted to a gastric bypass (Illustration 24.1). Her recovery was uneventful and in the following year her BMI dropped again to 27 kg/m^2.

Discussion

Adjustable gastric banding is one of the most frequently performed bariatric operations in morbidly obese patients. Laparoscopic adjustable gastric banding (LAGB) is a safe and effective method of weight loss and reduction of comorbidities associated with obesity. Despite its good safety profile compared with Roux-en-Y gastric bypass, patients with LAGB can manifest unique complications that are distinctive to the LAGB and need a special assessment and treatment. The most common complications are: Pouch enlargement, band slip, band erosion, esophageal dilatation, reflux, port rotation, port-site infection, and breakage of the tubing [1].

In the assessment of a patient with a LAGB, one should make an upper gastrointestinal radiograph series. The band is placed just below the gastroesophageal junction. The pouch in the first year is hardly visible but will extend to a size of appropriately 50–80 mL. The right position of the band is seen on the radiography if it has an angle of approximately 45° toward the left shoulder.

Band slip and pouch dilatation—The most important cause of slippage is an increased pressure in the pouch due to vomiting. In a lot of cases overfilling is the real cause. Most patients feel that they have the best support of the band if they can hardly eat. They will ask for filling of the band if they don't lose weight. Prevention of overfilling is prevention of pouch dilatation and helps to get a good long-term result. The patient with a band slippage and obstruction usually presents with dysphagia, vomiting, regurgitation, and food intolerance. The diagnosis is easily made by an upper gastrointestinal series. Complications related to band slip include gastric perforation, necrosis of the slipped stomach (type-V prolapse), upper gastrointestinal bleeding, and aspiration pneumonia.

Pouch enlargement or prolapse is diagnosed when dilation of the proximal gastric pouch is present with or without change in the angle of the band on an upper abdominal radiograph and in the absence of signs of obstruction. The lower esophagus may or may not be dilated. Pouch enlargement is also a pressure-related phenomenon that may be surgically induced by band over inflation or overeating with vomiting, resulting in high pressure in the pouch. Primary placement of the band with too much fundus above the band gives a high risk of pouch dilatation. Symptoms of pouch enlargement can be: lack of satiety, heartburn, regurgitation, and occasional chest pain. The diagnosis is made with an upper gastrointestinal series [1].

Band slip and pouch dilatation can be classified depending on the part of the body of the stomach that moves though the band or on the dilatation of the stomach or placement of the band [1].

Incidence of slippage varies in literature. O'Brien and Dixon reported 25 % of band slip in their first 500 patients using the perigastric approach (accessing the right crus perigastrically) and only 4.8 % of slippage in the last 600 patients with the pars flaccida technique (accessing the right crus through the pars flaccida) [2, 3]. Other published literature reports an incidence of slip of 1–22 %.

Since the amount of tissue of the stomach in the band is bigger at the body of the stomach than at the angle of His (normal band position), obstruction of the gastrointestinal tract can occur when the band slips. Band slip can be posterior or anterior, depending on whether the anterior or posterior region of the stomach herniates through the band. In all patients with obstructive complaints and pain not responding to emptying of the band, a gastroscopy is mandatory to rule out gastric ischemia or necrosis. These conditions require an immediate surgical intervention.

Laparoscopic removal or repositioning of the band is the preferred method of treatment for both slippage and pouch dilatation. In patients who were successful in losing weight with the gastric band repositioning can be considered. If the patient did not experience significant weightloss, removing the band and creating a gastric bypass in one or two tempi is the preferred option. In situations of substantial prolapse where reduction is not possible or when evidence of intra abdominal infection is present, the most prudent management is removal of the gastric band.

References

1. Berends FJ, Janssen IMC. Prevention and treatment of complications after bariatric surgery. In: Cuesta MA, Bonjer HJ, editors. Treatment of complications after digestive surgery, chapter 10. London: Springer; 2013.
2. Eid I, Birch DW, Sharma AM, et al. Complications associated with adjustable gastric banding for morbid obesity: a surgeon's guides. Can J Surg. 2011;54:61–6.
3. O'Brien PE, Dixon JB. Weight loss and early and late complications – the international experience. Am J Surg. 2002;184:42S–5.

Chapter 25
Case on Problems with Laparoscopic Adjustable Gastric Band: Erosion and Migration

Ignace M.C. Janssen and Frits J. Berends

Keywords Gastric band • Laparoscopy • Morbid obesity • Band erosion • Adjustable gastric band • Band migration

First Patient

Operation, Identification and Treatment of the Complication

Three weeks after receiving a laparoscopic adjustable gastric band, a 42-year-old woman returned to the hospital with an infection of the wound where the port connected to the band's tubing was placed. The patient was initially treated with antibiotics; however, after a few days the wound spontaneously opened and a collection of pus leaked out. At the bottom of the wound the port and tubing were visible. The patient was reoperated and the port was removed. The tubing was cut, filled with antibiotics, and pushed back into the abdominal cavity. Three months later the patient had not lost any weight. She could eat normally, but complained of abdominal discomfort. Blood examination demonstrated elevated CRP and leukocytosis. Gastroscopy revealed a band that had eroded into the stomach and was visible for one-third of the circumference. It was suggested to the patient to remove the band laparoscopically but she insisted on being referred to another hospital where the band was removed gastroscopically (Fig. 25.1 and Illustration 25.1a). Three months later a biliopancreatic diversion was done from which she recovered uneventfully. After 1 year she had an excess weight loss of 90 %.

I.M.C. Janssen, M.D. (✉) • F.J. Berends, M.D.
Department of Surgery, Rijnstate, Arnhem, The Netherlands
e-mail: ijanssen@alysis.nl; fberends@alysis.nl

M.A. Cuesta, H.J. Bonjer (eds.), *Case Studies of Postoperative Complications after Digestive Surgery*, DOI 10.1007/978-3-319-01613-9_25,

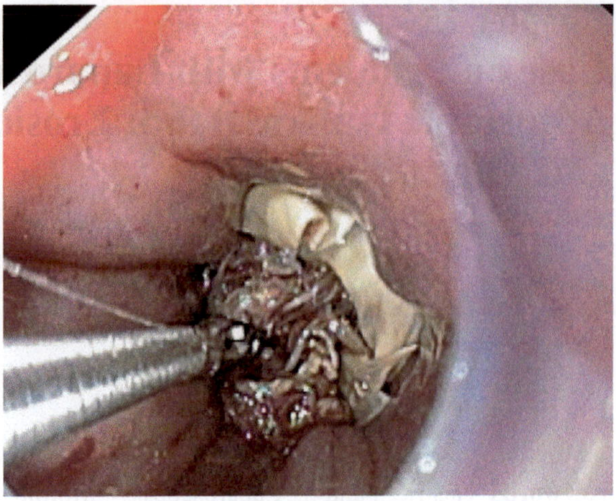

Fig. 25.1 Erosion of the band in distal esophagus. Attempt to removal by endoscopy

Second Patient

Diagnosis and Indication for Surgery

A 42-year-old woman had been operated 3 years previously because of obesity, having a BMI of 35. A laparoscopic gastric band was then performed without technical problems. In the course of the following year, the patient had importantly reduced her weight until she gained a BMI of 26. She was happy with the outcome of the operation. Three years later and now 3 months before the referral to us, she began to have extra difficulties with passing food. She felt that something had changed as she had lost an additional four kg. At gastroscopy it was observed that the connection tube has migrated in distal direction. The CT scan showed that the band was fixed in the first loop of jejunum and a kind of fixed triangle was formed between the band, connection tube, and the port (Figs. 25.2 and 25.3).

Operation

At operation, after cutting the connection tube first the port was taken out. Then by laparoscopy we could see the tube and the inflammatory reaction around the proximal part of the stomach. The duodenum and proximal part of jejunum were localized, but it was impossible to see in which part of these the band was fixed. Through a small subcostal incision and a pyloroplasty the band that was fixed between duodenum and jejunum could be taken out. After this, pyloroplasty was closed in horizontal direction and the incision closed after leaving a drain (Illustration 25.1b). Postoperative course went uneventful.

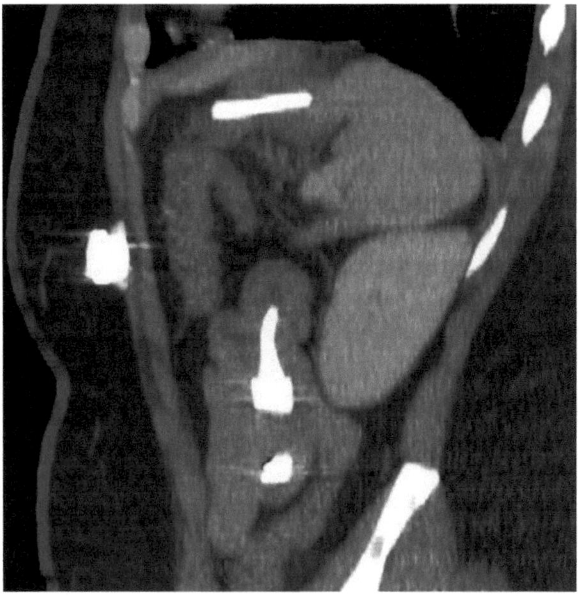

Fig. 25.2 CT scan, migration after erosion of the gastric band up to the first part of jejunum

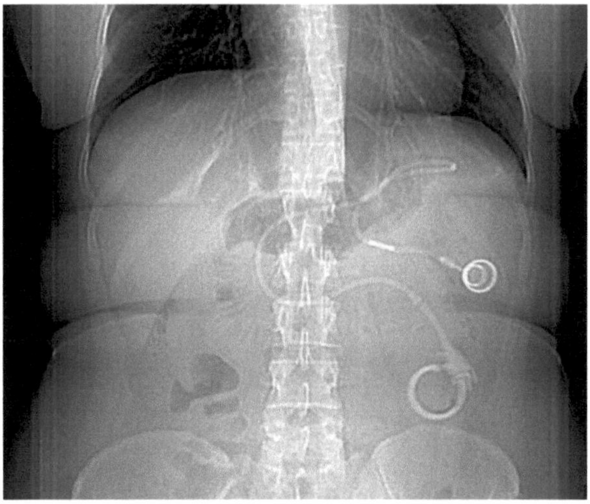

Fig. 25.3 Plain X-ray showing the migration

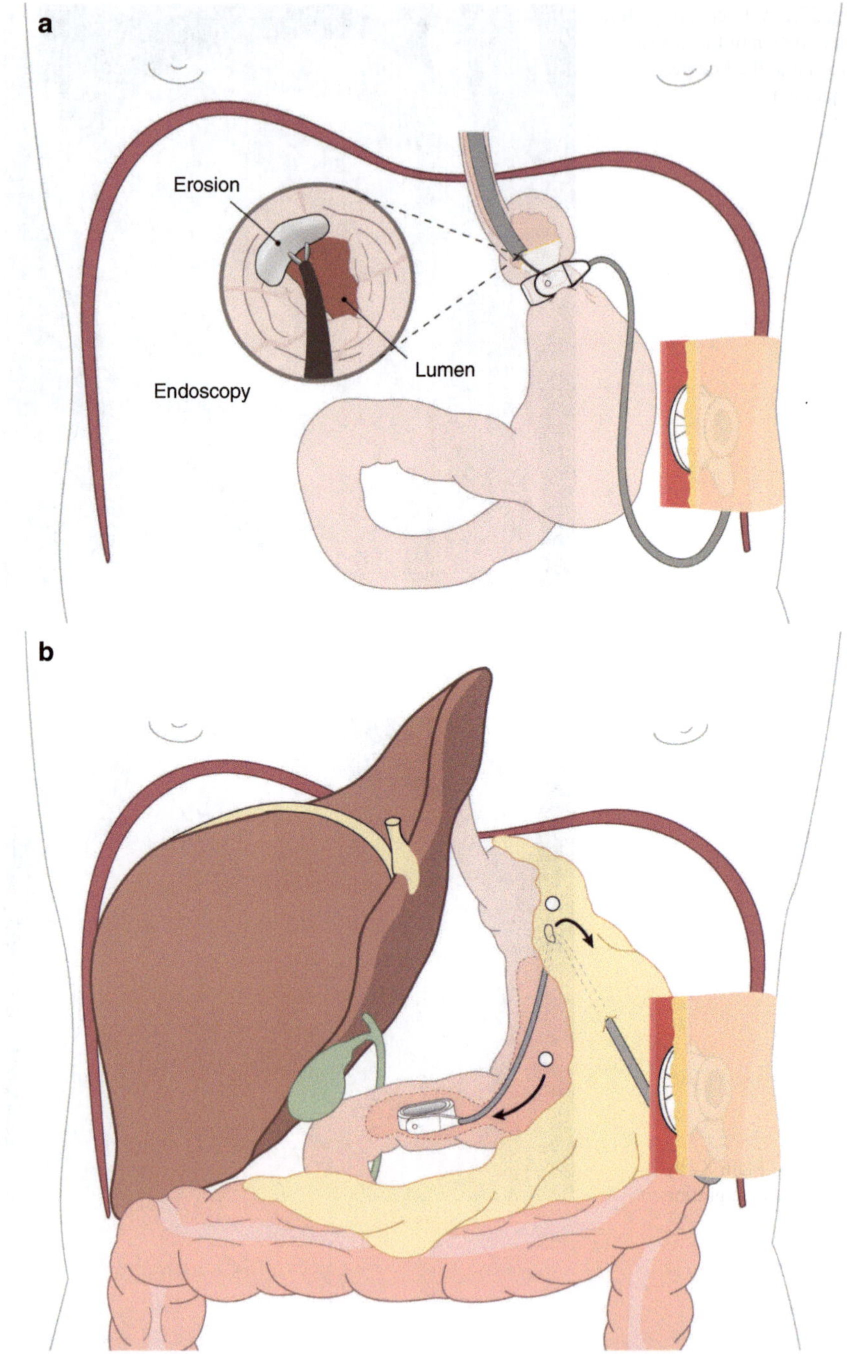

Illustration 25.1 (**a**) Adjustable gastric band showing erosion on the proximal stomach. Gastric band was removed by gastroscopy using a gastric band cutter. (**b**) Adjustable gastric band showing first erosion through gastric wall and then migrating until the duodeno-jejunal junction. Removed by pyloroplasty

Discussion

Band erosion—Band erosion is an uncommon complication of LAGB. The band gradually erodes through the stomach wall into the gastric lumen. The reported incidence is around 1 %, with an estimated prevalence varying from 0 to 11 % [1, 2]. Band erosion may be the result of gastric-wall injury during band placement or tight anterior fixation.

A high index of suspicion is required for diagnosis of band erosion as most patients are asymptomatic. When symptomatic, complaints related to erosion include loss of restriction, nonspecific epigastric pain, gastrointestinal bleeding, intra-abdominal abscesses, or port-site infection. The diagnosis is often made at the time of gastroscopy.

The recommended treatment is complete removal of the eroded gastric band, gastroscopically and laparoscopically or via laparotomy. Removing a band that has eroded into the stomach can be difficult owing to the extensive inflammatory response around the proximal stomach and left lobe of the liver. This is the rationale for a gastroscopic approach: With the scope a thin metal wire is positioned around the band. The two ends of the wire are brought through a thin flexible shaft which is gently brought down through the esophagus to the band. The wires are pulled with force against the flexible shaft thus cutting through the silicone band. From the outside, the port must be surgically removed and the tubing cut. After this, the band can be removed orally, most of the times. This procedure can only be performed when the band is well visible within the stomach [1–3].

Because of the difficult direct laparoscopic approach, transgastric techniques have been proposed to facilitate band removal. Using distal transgastric ports, the band can be removed with a combined laparoscopic/endoscopic approach. It is surgically easier to operate and close a gastrotomy in normal gastric tissue than near an eroded band. In the case of acute gastric perforation, laparotomy with wide drainage is necessary.

Port-site infection—Port-site infections can be classified as early and late. Early infections will manifest with the cardinal signs of erythema, swelling, and pain. These infections typically occur in the immediate postoperative period. These infections with cellulitis alone may be treated with oral antibiotics. If the response is inadequate, then intravenous antibiotic use is warranted. When the infection does not respond to intravenous antibiotics and is limited to the port, the port can be removed and the tubing knotted and left inside the abdomen. A new port may be placed when all signs of infection are gone. The tubing can be connected with laparoscopic guidance.

Late port site infections are often caused by band erosion with ascending infection. This usually manifests several months after surgery and can be associated with loss of restriction. Gastroscopy must be done to confirm the diagnosis of band erosion. In each case of erosion, removal of the band is necessary.

Tube breakage—Breakage or damage of the tube typically refers to leakage of the tubing leading into the port or a place where there is a metal connector. To prevent leakage from the port, the use of a standard coring needle is strongly discouraged, and only Huber (noncoring) needles should be used to access the port. If port access is difficult or if the tubing connected to the port is at risk of perforation, then band adjustment under fluoroscopy is advised. Tube breakage usually manifests as a slow leak with the loss of the injected fluid volume on aspiration and the absence of restriction. It can be difficult to identify the leak site, but local exploration of the port site can confirm the diagnosis.

Leakage from the intra-abdominal tubing is more difficult to diagnose. Injection of dilute nonionic iodinated contrast into the port under fluoroscopy can help to identify the site of the leak. Another approach is to inject diluted methylene blue into the port under direct laparoscopic visualization of the tubing and the band. Port, tubing, or band replacement is usually necessary depending on the site of the leakage and type of band used [1].

References

1. Berends FJ, Janssen IMC. Prevention and treatment of complications after bariatric surgery. In: Cuesta MA, Bonjer HJ, editors. Treatment of complications after digestive surgery, chapter 10. London: Springer; 2013.
2. Abu-Abeid S, Szold A. Laparoscopic management of Lap-Band erosion. Obes Surg. 2001;11:87–9.
3. El-Hayek K, Timratana P, Brethauser SA, Chand B. Complete endoscopic/transgastric retrieval of eroded gastric band: description of a novel technique and review of the literature. Surg Endosc. 2013;27:2974–9.

Chapter 26
Case on Jaundice and Hepatic Failure After Major Hepatic Resection

Miguel A. Cuesta

Keywords Jaundice • Hepatic failure • Hepatic resection • Rectal cancer • Liver insufficiency • Liver metastases • RFA • Liver cyst

First Patient

Diagnosis and Indication for Surgery

A 75-year-old male patient was operated at the end of 2009 because of proximal rectal cancer, stage III, by means of low anterior resection.

Six months later, a CT scan revealed two liver metastases on segments 1 and 2 of the liver.

Patient was proposed to be treated by resection of segments 2 and 3 and radiofrequency (RFA) of the lesion located on segment 1.

Operation

Through a subcostal incision, after inspection and US, five metastases were found, the two known ones and another three between 8 and 15 mm: one in segment 4a, another in 4b, and the last in segment 8. An attempt was made to resect segment 1, but because

M.A. Cuesta, M.D.
Department of Surgery, VU University Medical Center,
Amsterdam, The Netherlands
e-mail: ma.cuesta@vumc.nl

M.A. Cuesta, H.J. Bonjer (eds.), *Case Studies of Postoperative Complications after Digestive Surgery*, DOI 10.1007/978-3-319-01613-9_26,

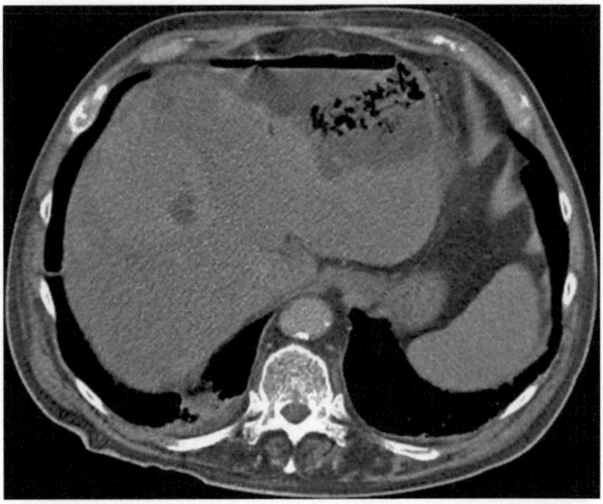

Fig. 26.1 Liver abscess at the surface of segments 2 and 3 resection

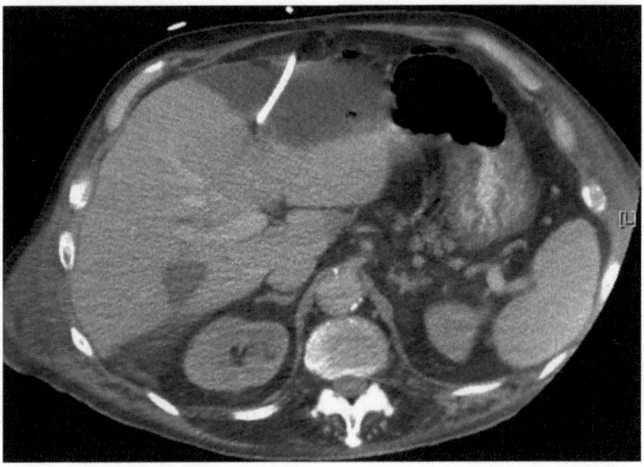

Fig. 26.2 Percutaneously drained liver abscess

of fixation to the hilar plate, RFA was performed, but also used to treat the lesions located in segments 4a and 4b and 8. Moreover, segments 2 and 3 were resected.

Postoperative Course: Identification of the Complication

Operation had no complications and the patient could be discharged at sixth postoperative day. After 3 months, he was again admitted to the hospital because of high fever and upper abdominal pain. On the CT scan, an abscess was found at the level of the resection being drained percutaneously (Figs. 26.1 and 26.2). New admissions followed with new abscesses, not only in the resection area but also in rest of the liver. Progressive hepatic failure developed with hypoalbuminemia, altered coagulation, and edema. Finally, the patient died.

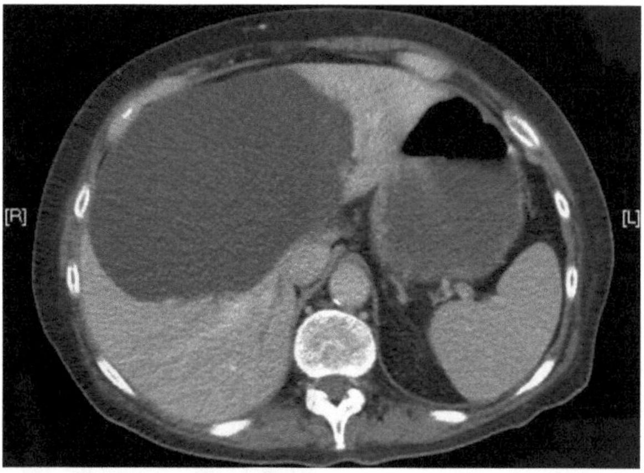

Fig. 26.3 Liver cyst

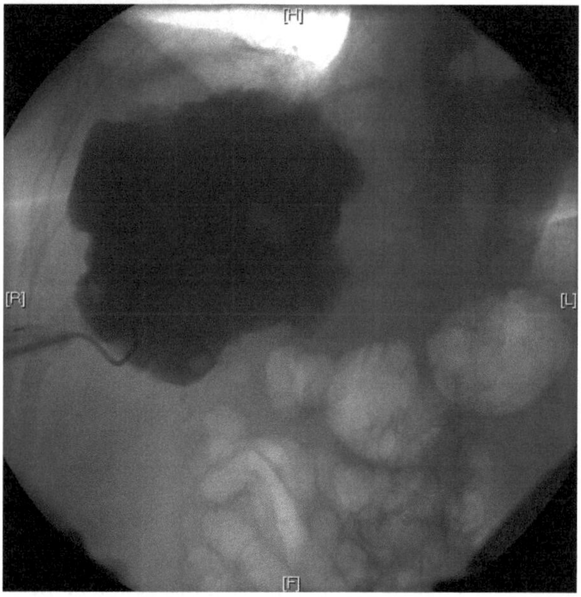

Fig. 26.4 Liver cyst treated by alcohol injection

Second Patient

Diagnosis and Indication for Surgery

A 65-year-old female patient already known having a huge liver cyst and being conservatively treated was admitted from another hospital with mechanical complaints of the upper digestive tract, as caused by a cyst of 25 cm found by CT scan (Fig. 26.3). An open cholecystectomy had been performed 7 years before. It was decided to treat the cyst by alcohol injection, and the treatment was considered successful (Fig. 26.4). Patient was readmitted 3 weeks later with a distended abdomen

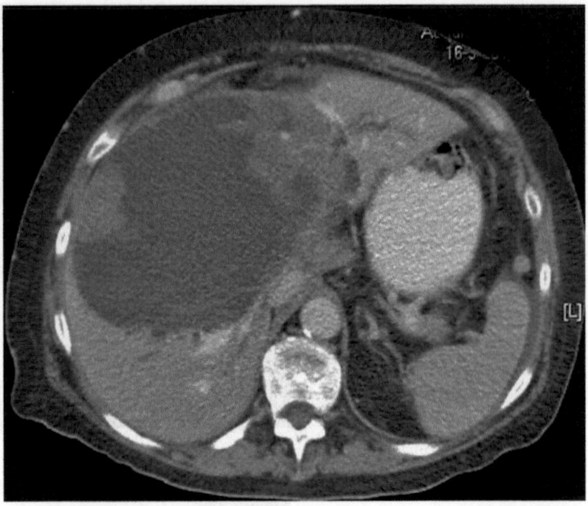

Fig. 26.5 Liver cyst showing clots inside and compression of the vena cava

and two edematous legs and decreased hemoglobin rate. On CT scan and duplex study, the cyst appeared unchanged in size, but showing clots inside as sign of bleeding. An important compression of the retrohepatic vena cava was found to produce an inferior vena cava syndrome (Fig. 26.5). Moreover, the patient had a low albumin and coagulation disorders as caused by a liver insufficiency. After correction of the coagulation disorders by vitamin K and plasma factors, a decision was taken to perform a partial cystectomy of the cyst in order to decrease the pressure on the vena cava, to decompress the liver parenchyma, and to diminish the mechanical complaints.

Operation

A subcostal incision was performed, and a partial cystectomy performed after drainage by puncture. Hereafter a brown fluid with some necrosis was drained, a possible effect of alcohol therapy. Inspection of the cyst was done, vena cava inferior and hilar elements appeared visible and not covered by cyst wall tissue. After deroofing, the wall of the cyst was sent to pathology for study. Omentum plasty was performed in the cyst. Patient recovered very quickly, edema disappeared, and she was discharged at the ninth postoperative day.

Discussion

Liver insufficiency is characterized by a deficit in factors produced by the liver such as albumin, coagulation factors, and glucose metabolism or eliminated by the liver like ammonia. Decrease of these functions determine the clinic of the patients such as progressive jaundice, ascites and peripheral edema, coagulation problems and encephalopathy (excessive nitrogen load and ammonia) [1].

Reference

1. Rahbari NN, Garden OJ, Padbury R, et al. Posthepatectomy liver failure: a definition and grading by the international study group of liver surgery (ISGLS). Surgery. 2011;149:713–24.

Chapter 27
Case on Biliary Leakage and Abscess After Liver Resection

Suzanne S. Gisbertz

Keywords Biliary leakage • Abscess • Liver resection • Hemicolectomy • Adenocarcinoma

Diagnosis and Indication for Surgery

A 66-year-old lady underwent a right hemicolectomy in 2008 because of an adenocarcinoma stage T3N0M0.

One year later, three liver metastases were found on the CT scan: in segments 5, 6, and 4b (Fig. 27.1). She was treated with neoadjuvant chemotherapy in the form of Xeloda®, in three cycles. A very important response of the metastases was observed on the CT scan. Six weeks later, she underwent a liver resection of the above segments 5, 6, and 4b.

Postoperative Course: Identification and Treatment of the Complication

Her postoperative period was complicated by a high-production bile leakage along the drain (Fig. 27.2). The subhepatic collection was treated by a percutaneous drain and in order to decrease the flow, an ERCP and a papillotomy with stent placement were performed (Fig. 27.3 and Illustration 27.1). Leakage decreased significantly and finally the drains could be retired. One month later, a deep wound abscess was

S.S. Gisbertz, M.D.
Department of Surgery,
Academic Medical Centre,
Amsterdam, The Netherlands
e-mail: s.gisbertz@antoniusziekenhuis.nl

M.A. Cuesta, H.J. Bonjer (eds.), *Case Studies of Postoperative Complications after Digestive Surgery*, DOI 10.1007/978-3-319-01613-9_27,

Fig. 27.1 Liver metastases

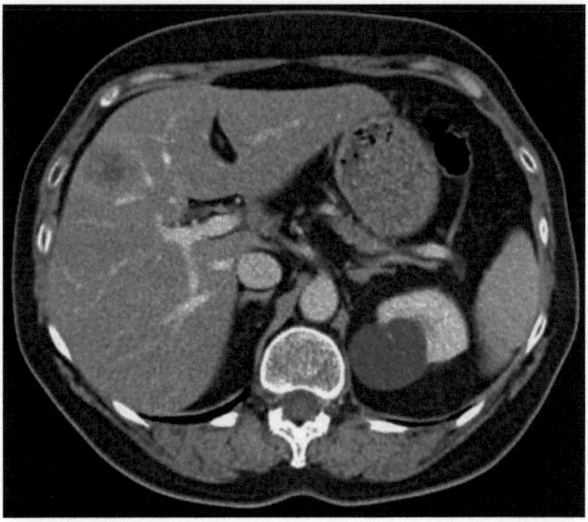

Fig. 27.2 Leakage of bile

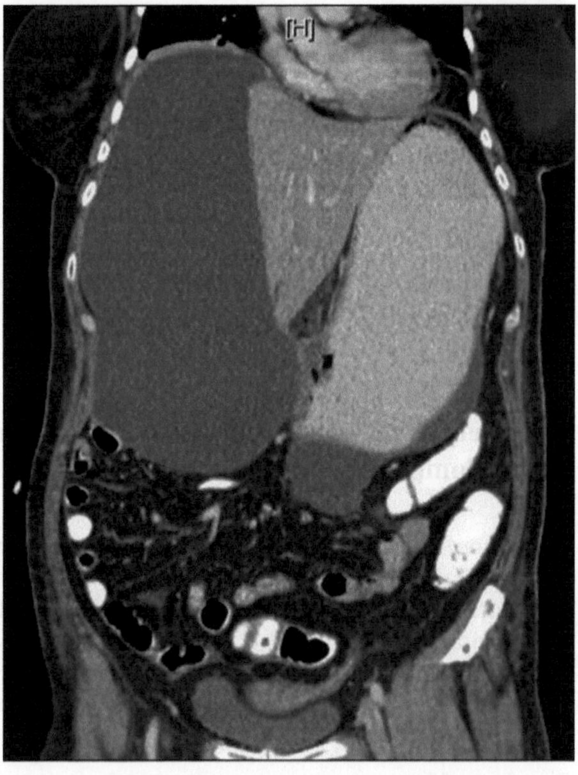

drained. Four months after operation, she was admitted again to the hospital because of abdominal pain and high fever. On the CT scan, an abscess was found at the place of the liver resection and it was drained percutaneously (Fig. 27.4). Moreover,

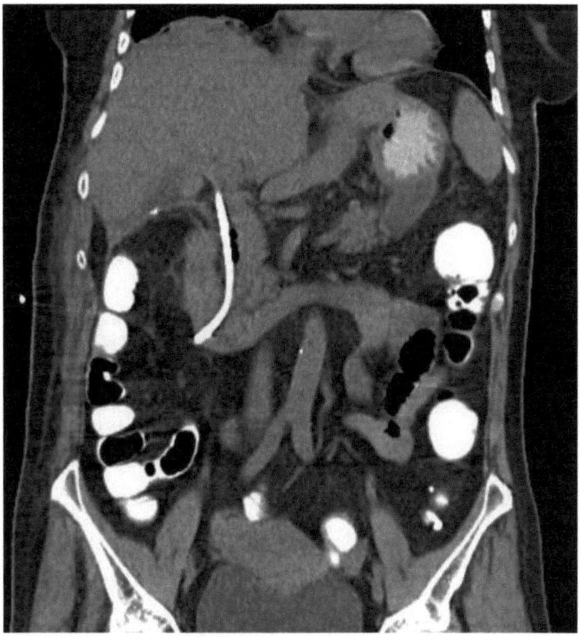

Fig. 27.3 Percutaneously drainage and endoprosthesis

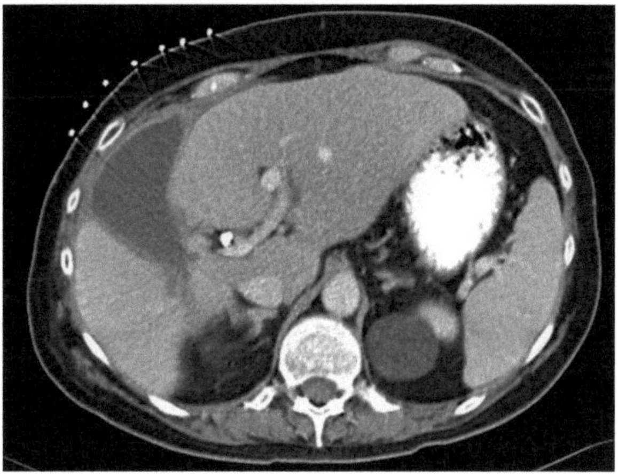

Fig. 27.4 Recurrent liver abscess

thinking that the biliary stent was occluded, this was removed by a new ERCP. In the period of 3 months after, the patient was admitted twice because of recurrence of the abscess, being subsequently drained. Ten months postoperatively, a recurrence of two metastases was seen on the control CT scan (Fig. 27.5). On the Oncology Multidisciplinary Commission, the second-line chemotherapy, Irinotecan®, was proposed. During the two cycles, she reacted with fever, and on the CT scan again a small abscess was diagnosed in the liver, including pulmonary metastases. In spite of drainage of the abscess and chemotherapy, the pulmonary metastases showed to be progressive. The patient decided to stop treatment.

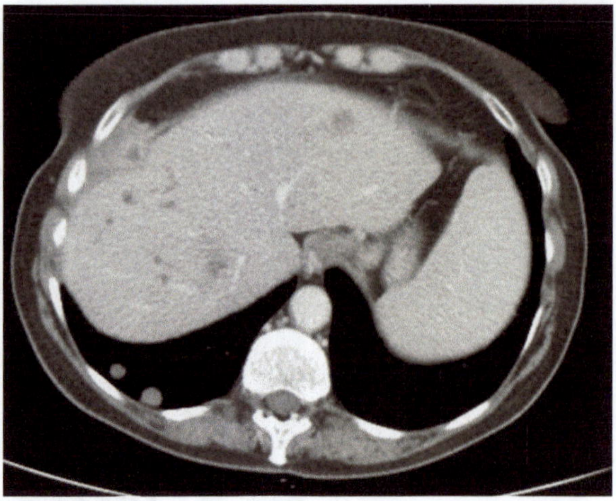

Fig. 27.5 Recurrent metastases

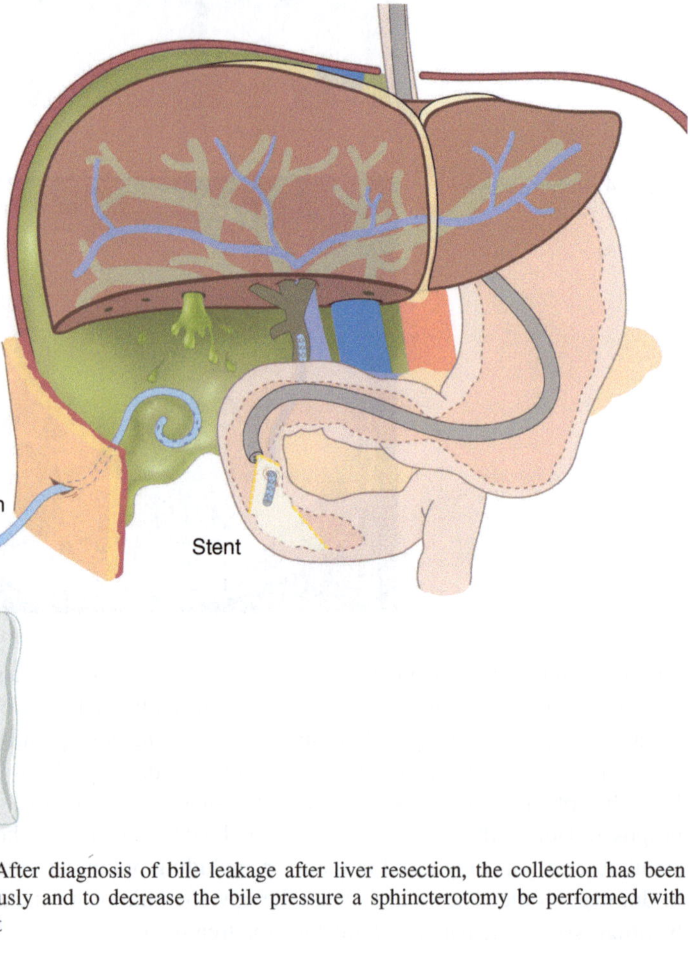

Illustration 27.1 After diagnosis of bile leakage after liver resection, the collection has been drained percutaneously and to decrease the bile pressure a sphincterotomy be performed with placement of a stent

Discussion

Biliary complications are the most common and potentially serious complications and can appear postoperatively as fistulas and/or bile collections, as a diffuse bile peritonitis, or as a sepsis due to the existence of segments with poor bile drainage [1].

Biliary fistulas were recently classified in three grades [2]: grade A biliary fistula has little or no clinical impact on the patient; the fistula is controlled by drainage, the drainage volume decreases daily, and bile drainage lasts less than 1 week. Grade B biliary fistula causes a change in the patient's clinical situation and treatment, requiring additional radiological or endoscopic approaches, the hospital stay is lengthened, or it is a grade A fistula with more than 1 week's hospital stay. Grade C biliary fistula requires laparotomy for treatment, and occasionally a clinical situation of sepsis or multisystemic failure occurs. Hospital stay is very prolonged, and patients may have secondary complications (e.g., wall abscesses).

Prevention is implemented by performing a systematic intraoperative cholangiography (IOC) in the case of hemihepatectomies or extended LRs. When a hepatectomy is finished, the bile duct must also be explored by IOC or by injecting serum through the cystic duct to identify minor biliary leaks on the liver surface. Segments that have become ischemic during the liver resection should be excised.

Treatment. Injury to a principal hepatic duct must be treated with an HJ reconstruction. If a segment is left poorly drained, it must be excised to avoid secondary infectious complications or the biliary radicle sutured if it is of little importance.

If it appears as a biliary fistula through the drain, which does not close conservatively, we must identify the origin by performing a cholangiography through the drain or an ERCP, which allows a papillotomy to be performed, and also insert a nasobiliary drain or an endoscopic plastic prosthesis. If endoscopic treatment fails, the next step is surgical treatment. If it appears as an infected perihepatic collection, detected by CT, a radiological drain must be inserted and if a high volume of drainage is maintained it should be treated as a biliary fistula.

Infected collections. Favoring factors include liver resections with biliodigestive anastomoses, patients with previous chemotherapy, the application of intraoperative radiofrequency, and immunodepressed patients [3].

In the presence of fever, leukocytosis, and increased CRP, we must indicate an emergency abdominal CT. If there are clinical data of sepsis or air inside the collection, the collection must be drained radiologically as an emergency procedure. On rare occasions these collections are not resolved with radiological treatment and surgical treatment is necessary. In selected cases with less than 38 °C fever, no leukocytosis, and no hemodynamic repercussion, antibiotic treatment can be started under clinical, analytical, and serial-CT guidance [1].

References

1. Parrilla Paricio P, Robles Campos R, Sanchez BF. Prevention and treatment of major complications of liver surgery. In: Cuesta MA, Bonjer HJ, editors. Treatment of complications after digestive surgery, chapter 11. London: Springer; 2013.

2. Koch M, Garden OJ, Padbury R, et al. Bile leakage after hepatobiliary and pancreatic surgery: a definition and grading of severity by the International Study Group of Liver Surgery. Surgery. 2011;149:680–8.
3. Zimmitti G, Roses RE, Andreou A, et al. Greater complexity of liver surgery is not associated with an increased incidence of liver-related complications except for bile leak: an experience with 2,628 consecutive resections. J Gastrointest Surg. 2013;17:57–64.

Chapter 28
Case on A Patient with Biliary Strictures in One-Half of the Liver After Liver Transplantation

Geert Kazemier and Herold J. Metselaar

Keywords Biliary strictures • Liver transplantation • Hepatocellular carcinoma • Steatohepatitis • Liver cirrhosis

Diagnosis and Indication for Surgery

A 57-year-old male patient with end-stage liver disease because of nonalcoholic steatohepatitis-induced liver cirrhosis and three hepatocellular carcinomas smaller than 2 cm each was placed on the waiting list for liver transplantation. His medical history revealed no other abnormalities, apart from the liver disease. Physical examination showed a patient in good clinical condition with slight jaundice. He was depended on diuretic medication to control ascites. Severity of cirrhosis was considered Child-Pugh B and his Model for End-Stage Liver disease score was 17. CT scanning showed no signs of metastatic disease, and portal vein, hepatic artery, hepatic veins, and inferior vena cava were patent.

Liver Transplantation

After a waiting time of 5 months, a blood type compatible liver from a 51-year-old brain dead, heart beating donor became available. The donation pocedure was uneventful. Explorative laparotomy in the recipient through a J-shaped incision

G. Kazemier, M.D. ✉
Department of Surgery, VU University Medical Center, Amsterdam, The Netherlands
e-mail: g.kazemier@vumc.nl

H.J. Metselaar
Department of Gastroenterology, Erasmus Medical Center, Rotterdam, The Netherlands

M.A. Cuesta, H.J. Bonjer (eds.), *Case Studies of Postoperative Complications after Digestive Surgery*, DOI 10.1007/978-3-319-01613-9_28,

revealed no evidence for tumor spread outside the liver and removal of the diseased liver was straightforward. The liver graft was reperfused after the side-to-side cavo-cavostomy and portal venous anastomosis were performed. Cold-ischaemia time was 510 min and warm ischemia time was 23 min. The arterial anastomosis was performed after reperfusion and took 19 min to complete. An end-to-end biliary anastomosis was performed without the use of a T-tube to restore bile flow. The estimated total blood loss was 2,300 mL and no blood transfusions were administered. Intra- and direct postoperative Doppler color ultrasonography showed intact arterial, portal, and hepatic venous blood flow. However, on the first postoperative day, turbulent flow was noticed in several right portal vein branches during routine Doppler ultrasonography. Arterial flow and flow in the left portal vein and hepatic veins were normal.

Postoperative Course

Postoperatively, liver function was recovering quickly with peak transaminases of 400 IU/L Therefore, surgical intervention was deemed unnecessary. Ultrasound imaging on the following days showed persistent turbulent flow in the right portal vein branches but normal flow patterns in all other vessels. Postoperative recovery was complicated by a wound infection which was treated by draining the wound and the patient was discharged on the 24th postoperative day. Immunosuppressive therapy consisted of tacrolimus and low-dose prednisone.

Follow-Up and Second Operation

During the following months, the patient suffered from recurrent attacks of cholangitis with high fever, bilirubin levels up to 150 μmol/L, and positive blood cultures with Gram-positive and Gram-negative bacteria. On subsequent endoscopic retrograde cholangiopancreatographic interventions (ERCPs), multiple strictures in the right posterior, and inferior branches of the biliary tree were diagnosed, while bile ducts in the left half of the liver and the biliary anastomosis remained unaffected (Fig. 28.1). Portal venous flow was uncompromised in the left half of the liver, but portal flow to the right hemiliver was diminished due to thrombosis of portal braches in the right anterior and posterior liver. All other vascular structures were unaffected. Several endoscopic procedures of dilatation and stenting of different biliary stenosis in the right hemiliver were only temporarily successful. Additional treatment with ursodeoxycholic acid did not resolve symptoms.

Eventually, 15 months after transplantation, a right hemihepatectomy was performed (Illustration 28.1). This operation was cumbersome due to extensive adhesions of the right hemi liver and difficulty to identify and control hilar structures. The postoperative course was complicated by a wound infection, which was treated by draining the wound and biliary leakage from the stump of the right bile duct resolved by draining the biloma percutaneously and subsequent endoscopic

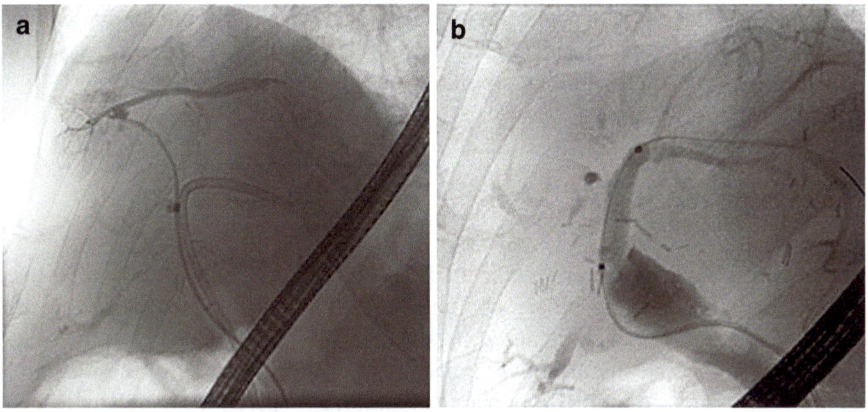

Fig. 28.1 ERCP images showing abnormal bile ducts on the right side of the liver (**a**) and normal bile ducts in the left hemi-liver (**b**)

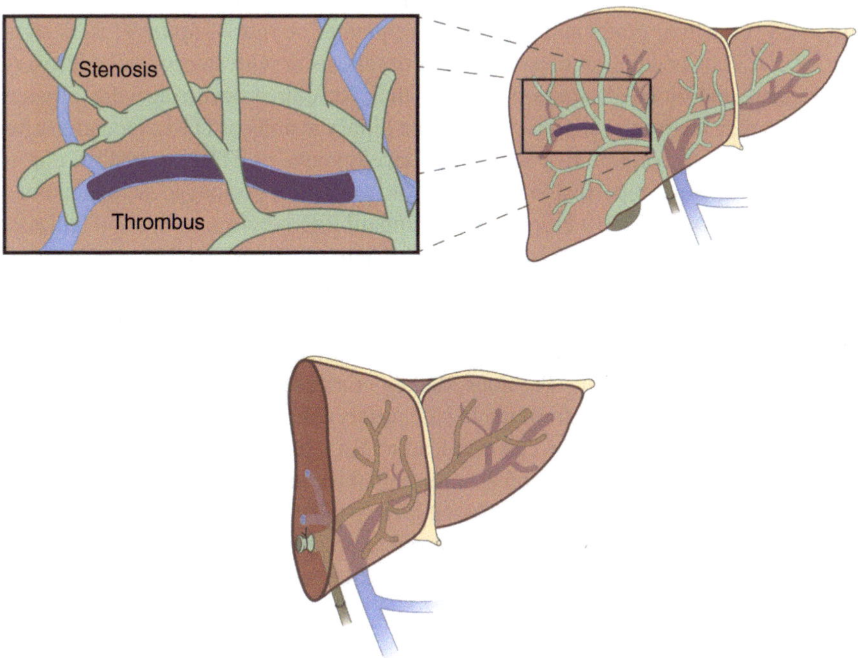

Illustration 28.1 After liver transplantation, right posterior and inferior branches of the biliary tree were stenosed causing recurrence cholangitis. Moreover portal branches of the right anterior and posterior liver were thrombosed. Decision was taken to perform a right hemihepatectomy

stenting. Patient was discharged from the hospital on the 20th day. Histopathological examination of the removed right hemiliver revealed extensive damage and irregularity of the biliary epithelium, ductopenia in the majority of portal tracts, intact arterial and hepatic venous circulation, and extensive circulatory impairment and thrombosis of the portal venous system. The patient recovered from the surgery and is currently asymptomatic with slightly elevated bilirubin levels, but otherwise normal liver function on low-dose tacrolimus immunosuppressive monotherapy.

Discussion

Biliary complications form a significant cause of morbidity and mortality after liver transplantation [1]. Early biliary complications, either leakage or stenosis at the anastomotic site, are usually caused by surgical failure and typically occur in the first days postoperatively after liver transplantation. The majority of these complications can be treated by ERCP or percutaneously; a reoperation is rarely indicated. Biliary complications occurring later after transplantation are mostly due to biliary strictures not at the anastomotic site. Those non-anastomotic strictures (NAS) are often diffusely present but sometimes affect predominantly one or more segments or one liver half. They represent a considerable cause of graft loss as they can affect up to 25 % of liver grafts and lead to retransplantation rate of up to 50 % in some series. NAS can occur after hepatic artery thrombosis or with an open hepatic artery. Both share radiological similarities, and, thus, strictures occurring with a patent hepatic artery are often called ischemic-type biliary lesions or ITBL. Donation after cardiac death is a major risk factor for development of ITBL, probably due to increased ischemia–reperfusion injury in those grafts [2]. Prolonged ischemia times, bile salt toxicity, and AB0 blood type incompatibility between donor and recipient have also been recognized as risk factors [3]. There is increasing interest in impaired biliary microcirculation as a possible cause of ITBL [4] and urokinase treatment of the graft has been shown to prevent its development [5]. Intra-and extrahepatic bile ducts have a unique anatomic feature in that they are provided with blood by a peribiliary capillary plexus. Previous studies concluded that this plexus is exclusively provided with blood from the hepatic artery. Recent studies showed however that impairment in portal flow can also lead to NAS [6] and that the contribution of portal venous microvascular blood flow through the bile duct is 40 % [7]. Particularly after liver transplantation, when the blood flow to the intrahepatic bile ducts through the gastroduodenal artery is no longer possible because of complete transection of the hepatoduodenal ligament this can become clinically important, as is illustrated in the described patient.

References

1. Pascher A, Neuhaus P. Bile duct complications after liver transplantation. Transpl Int. 2005;18:627–42.
2. Dubbeld J, Hoekstra H, Farid W, et al. Similar liver transplantation survival with selected cardiac death donors and brain death donors. Br J Surg. 2010;97:744–53.
3. Heidenhain C, Pratschke J, Puh G, et al. Incidence of and risk factors for ischemic-type biliary lesions following orthotopic liver transplantation. Trans Int. 2009;23:14–22.
4. Ren J, Lu MD, Zheng RQ, et al. Evaluation of the microcirculatory disturbance of biliary ischemia after liver transplantation with contrast-enhanced ultrasound. Liver Transpl. 2009;15:1703–8.
5. Lang R, He Q, Jin ZK, et al. Urokinase perfusion prevents intrahepatic ischemic-type biliary lesion in donor livers. World J Gastroenterol. 2009;15:3538–41.
6. Farid WRR, De Jonge J, Slieker JC, et al. The importance of portal venous blood flow in ischemic-type biliary lesions after liver transplantation. Am J Transplant. 2011;11(4):857–62.
7. Slieker JC, Farid WR, van Eijck CH, et al. Significant contribution of the portal vein to blood flow through the common bile duct. Ann Surg. 2012;255:523–7.

Chapter 29
Case on Patient with a Stenosis of the Cavocavostomy After Liver Transplantation

Geert Kazemier and Herold J. Metselaar

Keywords Cavocavostomy • Liver transplantation • Crigler–Najjar syndrome • Complications • Budd Chiari syndrome

Diagnosis and Indication for Surgery

A 21-year-old girl suffering from Crigler–Najjar syndrome type I was successfully treated with light therapy until her 18th life year. Due to therapy-resistant progressive hyperbulirubinaemia patient was evaluated for a liver transplantation. There were no signs of liver cirrhosis and the MELD score was 19. Her height was 157 cm and her weight 72 kg. CT scanning of the liver and surrounding vascular structures including the vena cava showed no abnormalities.

Liver Transplantation

After 1 year on the waiting list, a blood group identical liver from a brain dead, heart-beating donor was offered and accepted. The donor was 54-year-old and weight of 80 kg. and a length of 175 cm. The donation procedure was uneventful. During the transplantation, the liver graft was reperfused after the side-to-side cavocavostomy and portal venous anastomosis were performed. The side-to-side cavocavostomy was difficult to perform because of size difference between the graft

G. Kazemier, M.D. ✉
Department of Surgery, VU University Medical Center, Amsterdam, The Netherlands
e-mail: g.kazemier@vumc.nl

H.J. Metselaar
Department of Gastroenterology, Erasmus Medical Center, Rotterdam, The Netherlands

M.A. Cuesta, H.J. Bonjer (eds.), *Case Studies of Postoperative Complications after Digestive Surgery*, DOI 10.1007/978-3-319-01613-9_29,

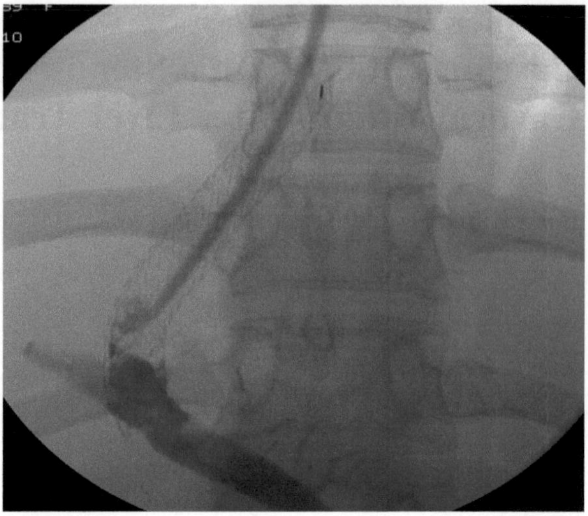

Fig. 29.1 In a combined percutaneous, trans-hepatic, and transjugular approach, a 10 mm covered stent was placed from the main portal vein into the recipient vena cava, creating adequate portal outflow directly into the vena cava

and the abdominal cavity of the recipient. Cold-ischaemia time was 415 min and warm ischaemia time was 44 min. The arterial anastomosis was performed after reperfusion. An end-to-end biliary anastomosis was performed without the use of a T-tube to restore bile flow. The estimated total blood loss was 1,300 mL and no blood transfusions were administered. Intra-operative Doppler color ultrasonography showed intact arterial, portal, and hepatic venous blood flow.

Directly postoperatively, transaminases raised considerable to 5,700 IU/L, probably because of the large for size graft. Transaminases lowered in the following days to values below 500 IU/L and the liver function recovered quickly with an INR of 1.1 at day 3 after transplantation. Immunosuppressive therapy consisted of basiliximab, tacrolimus, and low-dose prednisone. Routine Doppler ultrasonography direct postoperatively showed normal signals in all vascular structures of the transplant and a triphasic flow in the hepatic veins, despite a narrow cavocavostomy. At 1 week after transplantation the flow in the hepatic veins was monophasic. One week later the flow was absent and patient developed an acute Budd–Chiari syndrome. Triphasic, contrast enhances CT scan suggested torsion of the cavocavostomy. In a combined percutaneous, trans-hepatic, and transjugular approach, a 10 mm covered stent was placed from the main portal vein into the recipient vena cava, creating adequate portal outflow directly into the vena cava (Fig. 29.1). After this procedure, the liver function improved rapidly and patient was discharged 50 days after the liver transplantation without coumarines or platelet aggregation suppression.

Discussion

Hepatic venous outflow complications after liver transplantation are rare [1]. Particularly after introduction of the side-to-side cavocavostomy as gold standard for venous reconstruction during liver transplantation of whole organs at our institution more than 10 years ago, only once did occlusion of the left and middle hepatic

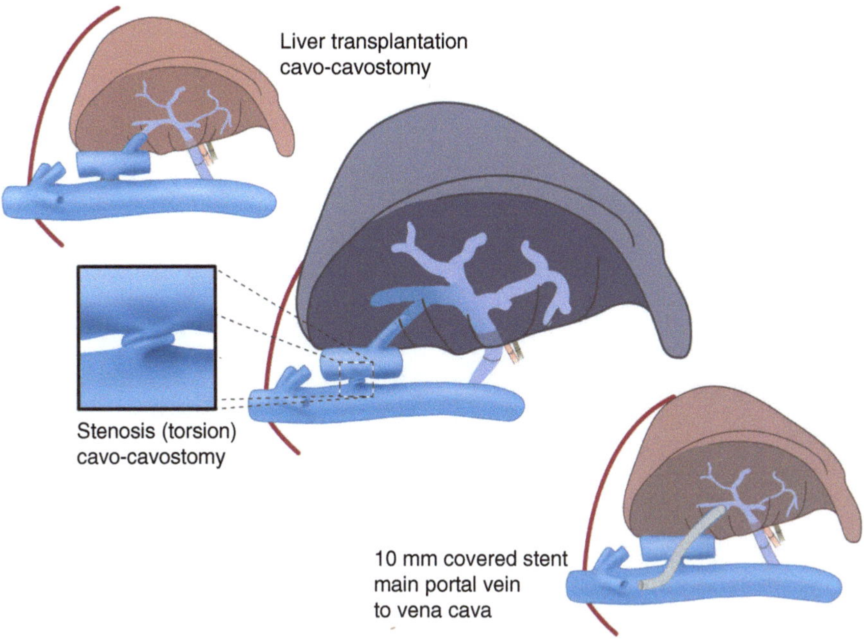

Illustration 29.1 After liver transplantation with a cavocavostomy. The side-to-side cavocavostomy was difficult to perform because of size difference between the graft and the abdominal cavity of the recipient. Patient developed an acute Budd–Chiari syndrome probably by a torsion of the cavo-cavostomy. In a combined percutaneous, trans-hepatic, and transjugular approach, a 10 mm covered stent was placed from the main portal vein into the recipient vena cava, creating adequate portal outflow directly into the vena cava

vein due to technical failure lead to partial venous congestion of part of the graft, but not to graft loss. Other centers report comparable low incidences of venous outflow complications with side-to-side cavocavostomy [2]. When venous outflow obstructions after liver transplantation develop however, symptoms can vary from mild ascites to acute failure of the graft. Especially if the latter is the case, a prompt intervention is mandatory. Surgical correction of the venous outflow can be very challenging because the liver will be congested, and swollen, and consequently very fragile, hampering easy handling particularly of the most dorsally located anastomosis: the site-to-site cavocavostomy. Percutaneous correction of the stenosis via placement of a covered stent as in a transjugular portosystemic shunt or TIPSS procedure in cirrhotic patients is the preferred technique in those patients as is shown in this case (Illustration 29.1).

References

1. Darcy MD. Management of venous outflow complications after liver transplantation. Tech Vasc Interv Radiol. 2003;10:240–5.
2. Navarro F, Le Moine MC, Fabre JM, et al. Specific vascular complications of orthotopic liver transplantation with preservation of the retrohepatic vena cava: review of 1361 cases. Transplantation. 1999;68:646–50.

Chapter 30
Case on CBD Lesion During Laparoscopic Cholecystectomy

Oliver R.C. Busch, Klaske A.C. Booij, Dirk J. Gouma, and Thomas M. van Gulik

Keywords Common bile duct • CBD lesion • Laparoscopic cholecystectomy • Symptomatic cholecystolithiasis • Bile duct injury

Diagnosis and Indication for Surgery

A 71-year-old female patient underwent a laparoscopic cholecystectomy because of symptomatic cholecystolithiasis.

Operation Description, Identification, and Treatment of Complication

During operation, the surgeon noticed a bile duct injury, possibly a complete transection of the common bile duct (CBD). The surgeon contacted our center for advice from the operating room. We recommended to leave a catheter in the proximal part of the divided bile duct and the patient was referred to our center. One day after operation the patient arrived in our hospital. Cholangiography using the catheter which was left in the bile duct showed a normal intrahepatic biliary anatomy, no absence of any segmental bile duct. Furthermore, a proximal CBD without a connection with the distal CBD was seen (Fig. 30.1). Based upon these findings, patient was suspected of having a type D bile duct injury. The patient was in a good condition without signs of abdominal sepsis. Therefore, a direct reconstruction was performed 2 days after initial operation. The hepatoduodenal ligament was explored by

O.R.C. Busch, M.D., Ph.D. (✉) • K.A.C. Booij • D.J. Gouma • T.M. van Gulik
Department of Surgery, Academic Medical Center, Amsterdam, The Netherlands
e-mail: o.r.busch@amc.uva.nl

M.A. Cuesta, H.J. Bonjer (eds.), *Case Studies of Postoperative Complications after Digestive Surgery*, DOI 10.1007/978-3-319-01613-9_30,

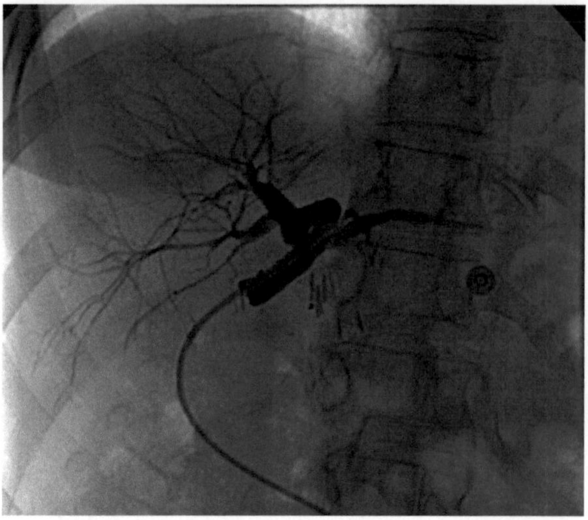

Fig. 30.1 Cholangiography by a drain in the proximal CBD which shows a complete transection of the CBD

a subcostal incision. Besides a complete divided CBD a complete transection of the right hepatic artery was seen. At first, a venous reconstruction of the right hepatic artery was performed. Secondly, a bile duct reconstruction was done by using a Roux-en-Y hepaticojejunostomy (Illustration 30.1). The patient had an uncomplicated postoperative course and left the hospital on day 7. One year after reconstruction, patient did not have any complaints.

Discussion

The most devastating complication after cholecystectomy is Bile Duct Injury (BDI), with a reported incidence of 0–1.5 %. The key issue in the management of BDI is prevention. Prevention is only adequate with the awareness of pre- and intraoperative risk factors, the use of CVS, experience in performing cholecystectomy and knowledge of the different escape strategies in the case of a difficult cholecystectomy. BDI can be diagnosed either peroperatively or in the direct or late postoperative phase. In case BDI occurs, the severity of the injury should be classified thoroughly before a proper treatment can be chosen. The treatment of BDI should be performed by a multidisciplinary team and only if sufficient experience in dealing with this complication is present. If not, the patients should be referred to a tertiary center. Even after an objectively excellent outcome of treatment, the reported QoL is still reduced [1].

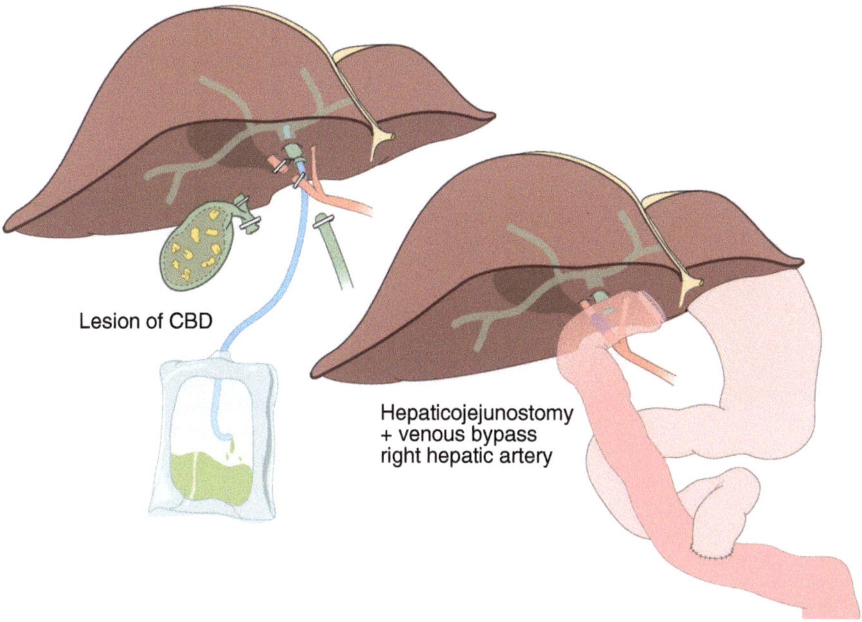

Illustration 30.1 After diagnosing a complete transection of the CBD by laparoscopic cholecystectomy, it was recommended to leave a catheter in the proximal part of the divided bile duct and to transfer the patient to a specialized center. At operation, first, a venous reconstruction of the right hepatic artery was performed and, second, a bile duct reconstruction was done by means of a Roux-en-Y hepaticojejunostomy

Reference

1. Booij KAC, Gouma DJ, van Gulik TM, Busch ORC. Prevention and treatment of major complications after cholecystectomy. In Cuesta MA and HJ Bonjer, editors. Treatment of complications after Digestive Surgery. Chapter 12 a. Springer, London 2013.

Chapter 31
Case on CBD Lesion During Laparoscopic Cholecystectomy

Oliver R.C. Busch, Klaske A.C. Booij, Dirk J. Gouma, and Thomas M. van Gulik

Keywords CBD lesion • Laparoscopic cholecystectomy • Cholecystolithiasis • Hepaticojejunostomy • Balloon angioplasty

Diagnosis, Indication for Surgery and Operation

A 30-year-old female patient had complaints of cholecystolithiasis and therefore a laparoscopic cholecystectomy was performed.

Postoperative Course: Identification and Treatment of Complication

Because of jaundice a week after operation, an ERCP was performed which demonstrated a complete transection of the CBD. Therefore, a hepaticojejunostomy was created which was complicated by fever, acute respiratory distress syndrome, and sepsis requiring intensive care treatment. Because of persistent fever and jaundice, patient was referred to our clinic. Computer tomography (CT) of the abdomen showed dilated intrahepatic bile ducts of the posterior segments, suggesting that a segmental bile duct was not connected to the hepaticojejunostomy (Fig. 31.1). Drainage of the right hepatic ducts was established by a percutaneous transhepatic

O.R.C. Busch, M.D., Ph.D. (✉) • K.A.C. Booij • D.J. Gouma • T.M. van Gulik
Department of Surgery, Academic Medical Center,
Amsterdam, The Netherlands
e-mail: o.r.busch@amc.uva.nl

M.A. Cuesta, H.J. Bonjer (eds.), *Case Studies of Postoperative Complications after Digestive Surgery*, DOI 10.1007/978-3-319-01613-9_31,

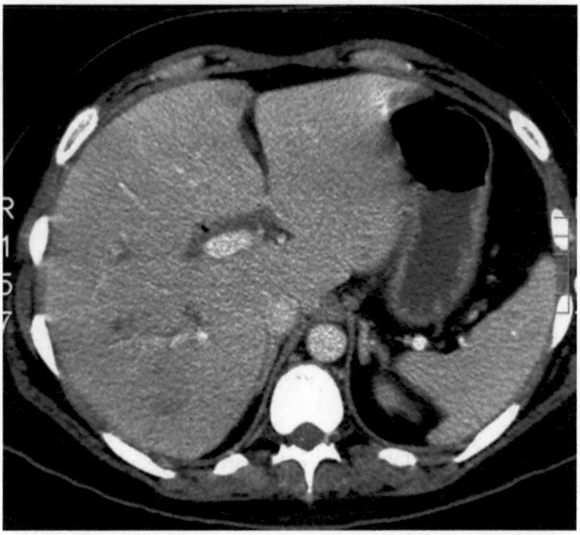

Fig. 31.1 Computer tomography of the abdomen revealed dilated bile ducts of the posterior segments of the right liver

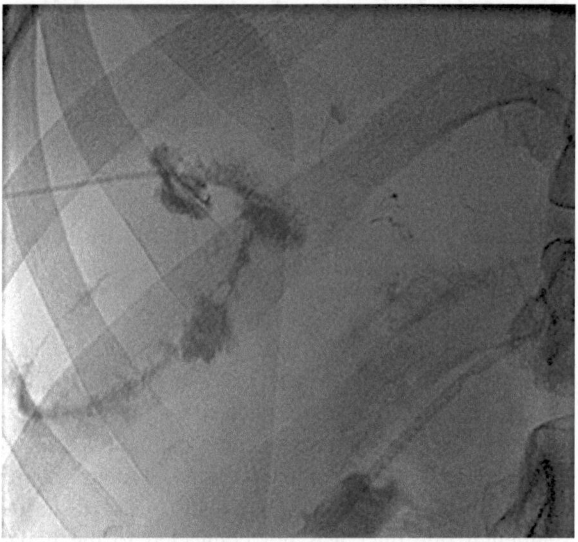

Fig. 31.2 PTC demonstrated leakage of the segmental bile ducts which were not included in the hepaticojejunostomy

cholangiography (PTC) catheter (Fig. 31.2). Further analysis by magnetic resonance cholangiopancreatiocography (MRCP) revealed that the bile ducts of segments VI and VII were not drained by the hepaticojejunostomy. Six months after initial operation, a new hepaticojejunostomy was constructed (Illustration 31.1). The

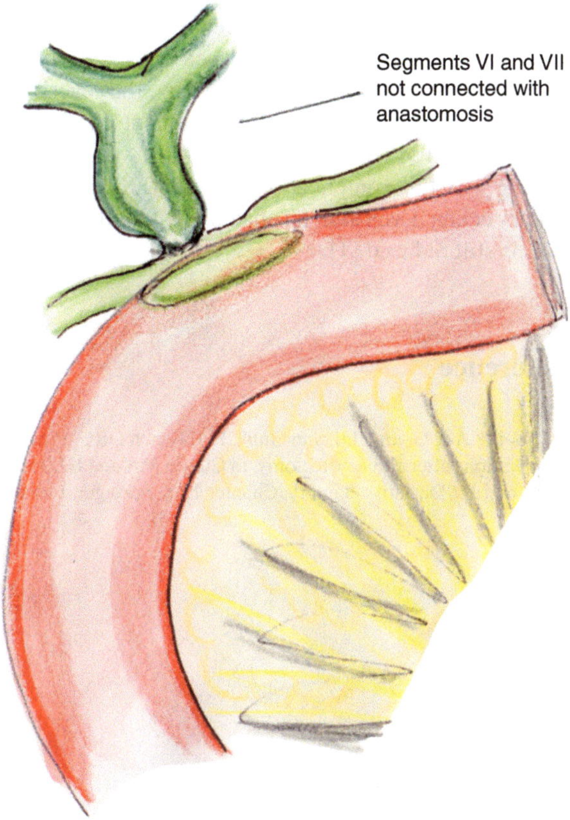

Illustration 31.1 A hepaticojejunostomy was performed because of transection of the CBD during laparoscopic cholecystectomy. Because of persistent fever and jaundice a CT scan of the abdomen showed dilated intrahepatic bile ducts of the posterior segments, suggesting that a segmental bile duct was not connected to the hepaticojejunostomy. After drainage by PTC, further analysis by MRCP revealed that the bile ducts of segments VI and VII were not drained by the hepaticojejunostomy. Six months after initial operation, a new hepatico-jejunostomy was performed

postoperative course was uneventful. Currently, 8 years after hepaticojejunostomy, patient was treated twice because of stenotic complaints of the anastomosis requiring PTC and balloon angioplasty.

Discussion

The most devastating complication after cholecystectomy is Bile Duct Injury (BDI), with a reported incidence of 0–1.5 %. The key issue in the management of BDI is prevention. Prevention is only adequate with the awareness of pre- and intraoperative risk factors, the use of CVS, experience in performing cholecystectomy and knowledge of the different escape strategies in the case of a difficult cholecystectomy. BDI can be diagnosed either peroperatively or in the direct or late postoperative phase. In case BDI occurs, the severity of the injury should be classified thoroughly before a proper treatment can be chosen. The treatment of BDI should be performed by a multidisciplinary team and only if sufficient experience in dealing with this complication is present. If not, the patients should be referred to a tertiary center. Even after an objectively excellent outcome of treatment, the reported QoL is still reduced [1].

Reference

1. Booij KAC, Gouma DJ, van Gulik TM, Busch ORC. Prevention and treatment of major complications after cholecystectomy. In Cuesta MA and HJ Bonjer, editors. Treatment of complications after Digestive Surgery. Chapter 12 a. Springer, London 2013.

Chapter 32
Case on Hepatic Abscess After Double Lesion (CBD and Right Hepatic Artery) During Cholecystectomy

Miguel A. Cuesta

Keywords Hepatic abscess • Double lesion • Right hepatic artery • Cholecystectomy • Conversion • Cholelithiasis

Identification and Treatment of Complication

A 56-year-old female patient was transferred to our unit because of biliary leakage after a converted laparoscopic cholecystectomy had been performed in another hospital. It was her fifth postoperative day; patient had a productive drain of more than 700 cc bile per day, she was treated with broad spectrum antibiotics, and had a gastric tube for enteral feeding. She was not jaundiced, had fever, and a deep wound infection had already been drained. A complete blood examination, a CT scan of the thorax and abdomen, and ERCP were performed (Fig. 32.1). A proximal and complete lesion of the hepatic duct was seen (type D BDI) with an insufficiently drained subhepatic collection. Along with this, a decrease of arterial circulation of the hepatic right segments was also observed. A PTC drain was placed to properly drain the collection.

Patient was treated conservatively during 2 weeks in order to improve her general condition and to treat the wound sepsis. After a postoperative period of 6 weeks she was reoperated.

M.A. Cuesta, M.D.
Department of Surgery, VU University Medical Center, Amsterdam, The Netherlands
e-mail: ma.cuesta@vumc.nl

M.A. Cuesta, H.J. Bonjer (eds.), *Case Studies of Postoperative Complications after Digestive Surgery*, DOI 10.1007/978-3-319-01613-9_32,

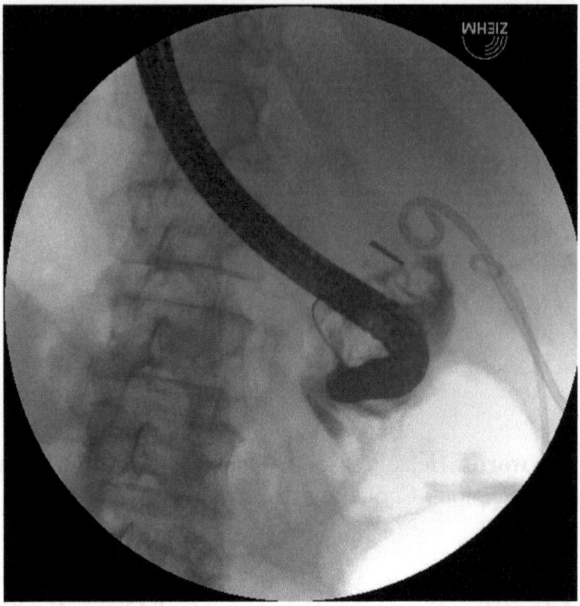

Fig. 32.1 ERCP showing the complete CBD lesion

Operation

A bilio-digestive anastomosis by means of a Roux-en-Y loop was performed (Illustration 32.1).

Postoperative Course

Postoperatively, she had a small biliary leakage through the drain, being treated conservatively. Splints and percutaneous drain were removed 6 weeks after operation once cholangiography showed that the anastomosis was patent and had no leaks. She did postoperatively quite well, but a significant depression required her to follow psychological support.

Eighteen months later she was acutely admitted to the Intensive Care Unit because of septic shock caused by a right hepatic abscess. On the CT scan it became clear that the right segments of the liver were atrophic and progressively replaced by a big abscess (Fig. 32.2). Patient was mechanically ventilated with high PEEP, the liver abscess drained twice percutaneously (Illustration 32.1), and she received iv broad spectrum antibiotics (Fig. 32.3). Slowly she could be retired from mechanical ventilation and after a recovery period of 5 weeks she could be admitted to a revalidation center. Since then, she is controlled at an outpatient polyclinic. Remarkably, she has only general complaints and an adequate liver function. On CT scan a hypertrophic left lobe and atrophic right segments without signs of portal

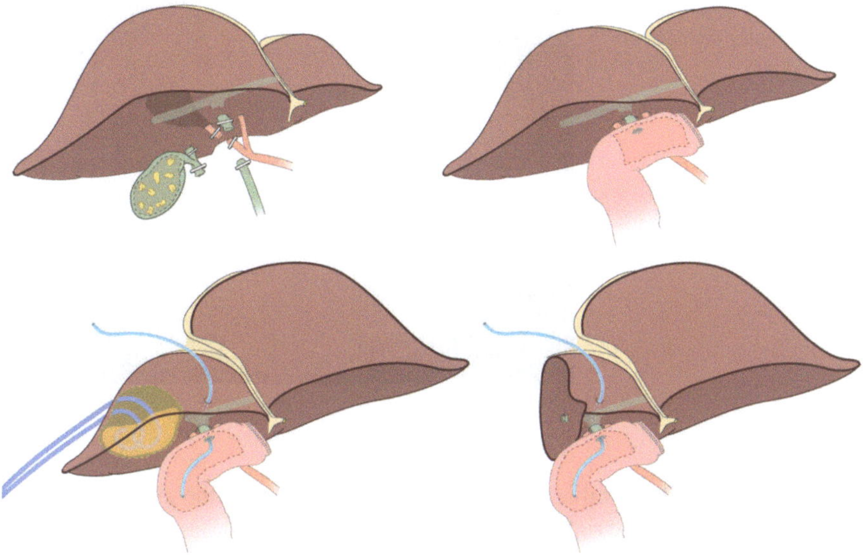

Illustration 32.1 During conversion to open cholecystectomy an unrecognized lesion was performed of the CBD. It was identified as a type D BDI. A hepaticojejunostomy was performed. One-half year later she was admitted because of liver abscesses in the relative atrophic right lobe of the liver with hypertrophic left lobe, and signs of a lesion of the right hepatic artery. Conservatively treated by drainage she recovered. In case of recurrence, a right hepatectomy should be done

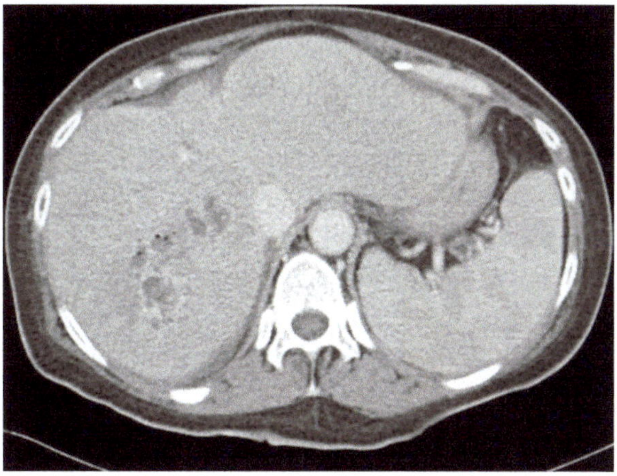

Fig. 32.2 CT scan. Atrophic right liver lobe with abscesses

Fig. 32.3 CT scan guided percutaneously drainage of the abscesses

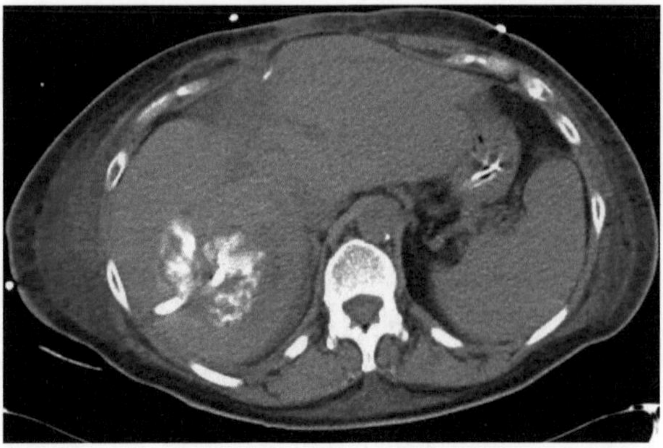

hypertension or dilated biliary system are seen. In the event the abscess recurs, a resection of the atrophic right lobe will need to be considered.

Discussion

The most devastating complication after cholecystectomy is Bile Duct Injury (BDI), with a reported incidence of 0–1.5 %. The key issue in the management of BDI is prevention. Prevention is only adequate with the awareness of pre- and intraoperative risk factors, the use of CVS, experience in performing cholecystectomy and knowledge of the different escape strategies in the case of a difficult cholecystectomy. BDI can be diagnosed either peroperatively or in the direct or late postoperative phase. In case BDI occurs, the severity of the injury should be classified thoroughly before a proper treatment can be chosen. The treatment of BDI should be performed by a multidisciplinary team and only if sufficient experience in dealing with this complication is present. If not, the patients should be referred to a tertiary center. Even after an objectively excellent outcome of treatment, the reported QoL is still reduced [1].

Reference

1. Booij KAC, Gouma DJ, van Gulik TM, Busch ORC. Prevention and treatment of major complications after cholecystectomy. In Cuesta MA and HJ Bonjer, editors. Treatment of complications after Digestive Surgery. Chapter 12 a. Springer, London 2013.

Chapter 33
Case on Unrecognized CBD Stones After Laparoscopic Cholecystectomy

Akash M. Metha

Keywords CBD stones • Laparoscopic cholecystectomy • Anorexia • Biliary leakage • Acute cholecystitis

First Patient

Diagnosis and Indication for Surgery

A 35-year-old female patient, with no previous history, was presented to the Emergency Department because of progressive upper-right abdominal pain since 5 days. Patient experienced nausea and anorexia. On physical examination, the upper-right quadrant of the abdomen was tender, though there were no local signs of peritonitis. A leukocytosis of 8.9×10^9/L and a C-reactive protein of 132 mg/L were found. Hepatic tests were all within the normal range. Abdominal ultrasonography showed an acute cholecystitis with gallstones. Intrahepatic bile ducts were mildly dilated, without dilatation of the common bile duct (CBD). Patient was admitted and it was decided to perform a laparoscopic cholecystectomy.

Operation Description

During laparoscopy, a severely inflamed gallbladder was visualized; and due to severe edema of the wall, the critical view of safety of the Hilar structures could

A.M. Metha, M.D.
Department of Surgery, VU University Medical Center,
Amsterdam, The Netherlands
e-mail: a.metha@nki.nl

M.A. Cuesta, H.J. Bonjer (eds.), *Case Studies of Postoperative Complications after Digestive Surgery*, DOI 10.1007/978-3-319-01613-9_33,

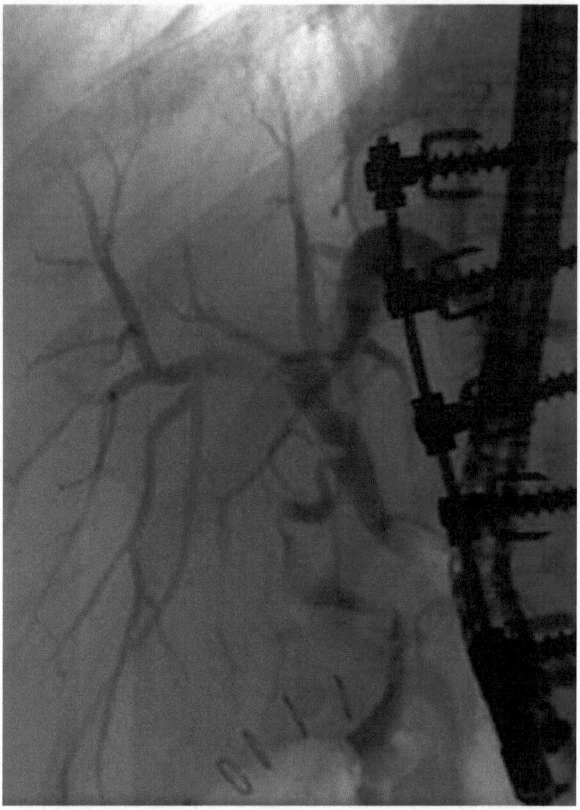

Fig. 33.1 CBD stone and leakage of the cystic duct by ERCP after laparoscopic cholecystetomy

not be obtained properly. Therefore, the procedure was converted to an open cholecystectomy through a subcostal incision. A standard retrograde cholecystectomy was performed.

Postoperative Course: Identification and Treatment of Complication

At third postoperative day, she experienced increasing abdominal pain and leakage of bile-like liquid from the subcostal wound. Biochemical analysis demonstrated elevated level of alkaline phosphatase. Abdominal CT scan showed intraperitoneal fluid collections in all quadrants, and on the ERCP, a leakage was seen from the stump of the cystic duct with an occluding bile stone in the CBD (Fig. 33.1). A sphincterotomy was performed and an endoluminal stent was placed covering the defect of the cystic duct. The same day, percutaneous ultrasonography-guided drainage of the intra-abdominal bile collection was performed. After an intravenous antibiotic treatment for 1 week, the patient was discharged with the percutaneous drain still in place. Ten days later, the drain could be removed without any complications. Six weeks after the initial ERCP, the procedure was repeated by removing the stent and visualizing the biliary ducts. Cystic duct leakage had ceased, there were no strictures of the common bile duct, and no CBD stones could be identified. The patient was discharged from further follow up.

Second Patient

Diagnosis and Indication for Surgery

A 38-year-old female patient with no significant comorbidity presented to the outpatient clinic with episodic upper right quadrant abdominal pain, provoked by ingestion of fatty food. Ultrasonography showed gallstones with normal CBD. Biochemical analysis showed hepatic tests within normal ranges.

Operation Description

An elective laparoscopic cholecystectomy was performed; critical view of safety of the Hilar structures was properly obtained and the procedure went well, except for the fact that a total of six endoscopic clips had to be applied to the cystic duct, which was of an exceptionally large size.

Postoperative Course: Identification and Treatment of Complication

The postoperative course was unremarkable and the patient could be discharged the next day. However, approximately 2 weeks later, she presented again to the Emergency Department with ongoing right-upper quadrant pain, similar to the attacks she had experienced prior to the cholecystectomy. Moreover, her feces had become progressively lighter, while the urine had become darker. Liver function tests were as follows: bilirubin 91 μmol/L, with elevated alkaline phosphatase of 271 U/L, being lipase and amylase levels normal. Abdominal ultrasonography showed dilatation of the common bile duct and intrahepatic bile ducts without any evident CBD stones. Emergency ERCP demonstrated bile stones in the CBD (Fig. 33.2); hence, a sphincterotomy was performed, followed by extraction of the stones. The next day, the patient could be discharged. Outpatient follow-up

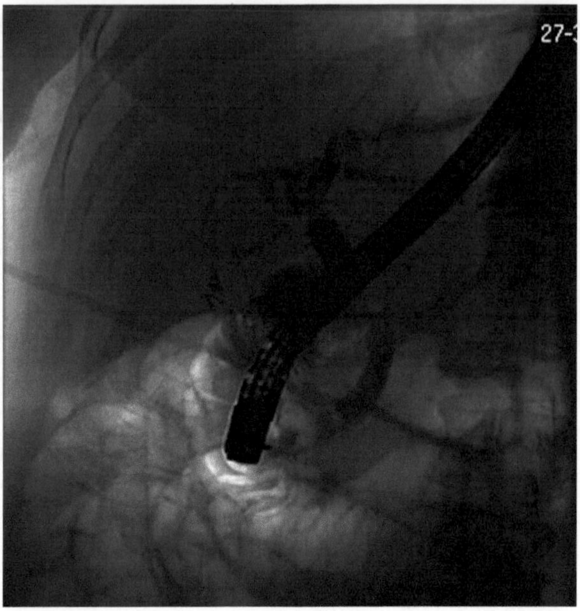

Fig. 33.2 CBD stone by ERCP after laparoscopic cholecystectomy

demonstrated normalization of the hepatic tests abnormalities with simultaneous decrease of the abdominal pain. Approximately 2 months after the initial operation, the patient was discharged from further follow up.

Discussion

The first patient exhibited signs of biliary leakage 3 days after a cholecystectomy due to acute cholecystitis. During ERCP, leakage from the cystic duct (type A BDI) was demonstrated in conjunction with a CBD stone. Although biochemical analysis and abdominal ultrasound had been performed preoperatively, no signs were found suggesting the presence of a CBD stone. Various studies advocate the routine use of intra-operative cholangiography to detect unknown CBD stones. Notable is a lack of conclusive evidence that performing this procedure in all patients undergoing cholecystectomy is either feasible or efficient, whereas the incidence of CBD stones in patients with uncomplicated symptomatic cholecystolithiasis without signs of biliary obstruction is relatively low. However, intra-operative cholangiography is associated with few complications and, given experienced hands, will not lead to significantly longer operating times. Especially in patients at risk for biliary injury (e.g., acute cholecystitis) and in case of conversion from a laparoscopic to an open procedure, cholangiography may be routinely used to visualize biliary anatomy and to minimize the risk of postoperative complications by the timely detection of CBD stones. If CBD stones are found during laparoscopic cholangiography, various options are available for removal: flushing of the CBD after intravenous administration of glucagon, intra-operative transcystic, or through choledochotomy, the retrieval of stones followed by choledochoscopy. Another possibility is to perform an ERCP immediately postoperatively. In the first patient, performing intra-operative cholangiography during this complicated cholecystectomy would have led to earlier detection of the CBD stone, which could have been removed either perioperatively or immediately postoperatively, thereby possibly preventing the biliary leakage.

The second patient underwent an elective laparoscopic cholecystectomy because of gallstones; neither hepatic function tests nor ultrasonography demonstrated any signs indicative of CBD stones. However, ERCP performed due to ongoing complaints and elevated cholestasis parameters approximately 2 weeks postoperatively demonstrated two CBD stones that were subsequently extracted. Though intra-operative cholangiography would probably have identified the CBD stones, the pre-operative and intra-operative case history yields no signs or symptoms, which lead to a higher, a priori chance of a positive cholangiography. The presence of a wide cystic duct during operation is the explanation for passage of stones from the gallbladder to the CBD. Importantly, if after laparoscopic cholecystectomy a patient repeats the same colic pain resembling the previous complaints, the presence of CBD stones always has to be excluded.

In conclusion, the existence of CBD stones is frequently a cause of complications after cholecystectomy. Primarily, the incidence of preoperative history, liver function tests, and ultrasound should together form the basis for further decision making regarding preoperative MRCP. In cases of complications during cholecystectomy, intra-operative cholangiography may be a valuable tool to assess biliary anatomy and minimize the risk of CBD-stone related complications. However, routine use of this technique is probably not warranted.

Chapter 34
Case on Recurrence of Acute Gallstone Pancreatitis: When to Perform a Cholecystectomy?

Marijn Poelman

Keywords Gallstone pancreatitis • Acute pancreatitis • Laparoscopic cholecystectomy • Endoscopic retrograde cholangio-pancreatography • Papillotomy

Timing of laparoscopic cholecystectomy for acute gallstone pancreatitis is a current matter of interest. Must the operation be performed during the same admission in the event the mild acute pancreatitis has disappeared? Or must it be done after a period of 6 weeks once the patient has completely recovered? Taking the second option frequently means a longer period of time entailing risks for recurrence of the acute pancreatitis and other risks. Currently, a randomized study regarding this controversy is being performed in the Netherlands, named the PONCHO trial.

Patient

Diagnosis and Indication for Surgery

A 28-year-old nurse came to the emergency unit with heavy pain in the upper abdomen. Three months earlier, she had been admitted because of a mild acute gallstone pancreatitis. Because of her training period as nurse, she then had refused to be operated on by laparoscopic cholecystectomy. At the First Aid examination, she appeared ill. Elevated serum bilirubin, amylase, and lipase were found. An ultrasound showed again small gallstones, a light dilated CBD, and a mildly swollen pancreas. A gallstone acute

M. Poelman, M.D.
Department of Surgery, VU University Medical Center, Amsterdam, The Netherlands
e-mail: mm.poelman@vumc.nl

M.A. Cuesta, H.J. Bonjer (eds.), *Case Studies of Postoperative Complications after Digestive Surgery*, DOI 10.1007/978-3-319-01613-9_34,

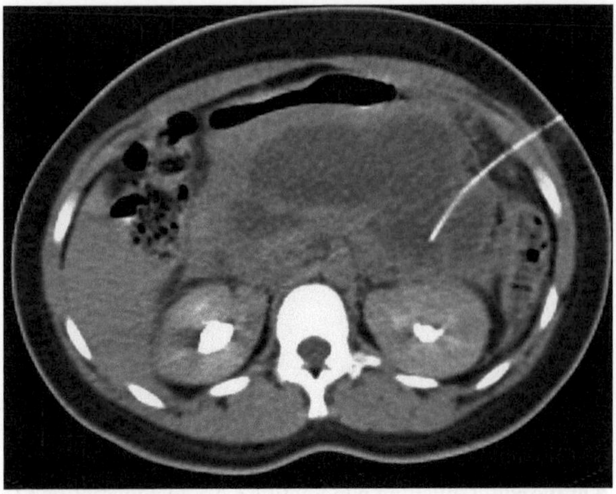

Fig. 34.1 Necrotizing acute pancreatitis, abscess percutaneously drained

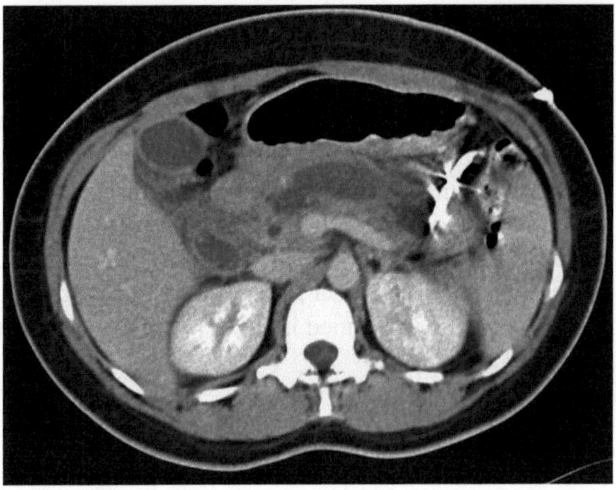

Fig. 34.2 Clear improvement after drainage

pancreatitis was diagnosed. Because of her fever and a Ranson score of 4, a CT-scan of the abdomen was performed, showing a necrotizing acute peripancreatitis.

An ERCP was not performed because there were no signs of obstruction of the CBD. Clinically, the patient had periods of ups and down, yet after 3 weeks she developed intermittent fever. A mass was palpated in the epigastric area. A new CT-scan was performed and a pancreatic abscess was diagnosed (Fig. 34.1) with suspected gas imaging. Decision was taken for a radiological drainage of the collection and treatment with iv antibiotics was started. She recovered well and a CT-scan was repeated a week later (Fig. 34.2) to evaluate the size of the fluid collection, showing an important reduction. A culture of the fluid proved sterile. The production by the drain ceased and it was removed. She was discharged shortly after and was referred to the surgical outpatient clinic for planning a laparoscopic cholecystectomy.

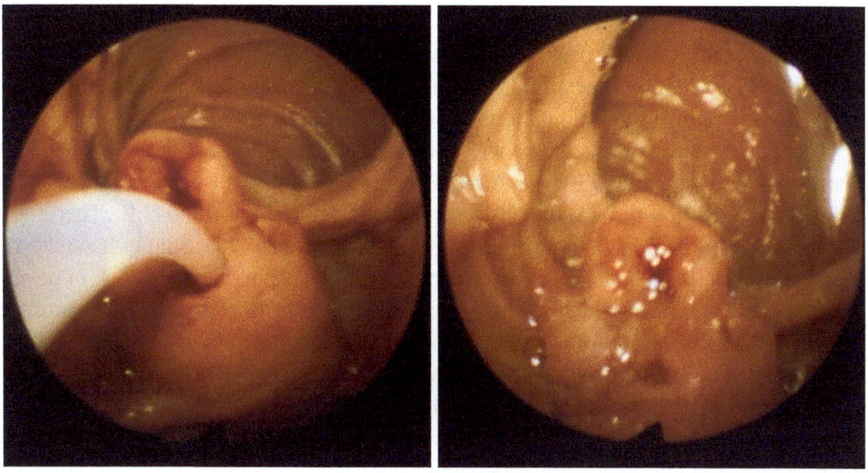

Fig. 34.3 Sphincterotomy by ERCP

Unfortunately, she returned 3 days after discharge because of pain in the upper abdomen. No mass was palpated in the upper abdomen, but serum bilirubin, amylase, and lipase had been elevated again and an ultrasound showed an edematous acute pancreatitis without pseudocyst and an obstructive gallstone in the CBD with dilatation. An endoscopic retrograde cholangio-pancreatography (ERCP) and papillotomy were performed, the gallstone being extracted from the CBD (Fig. 34.3). A new CT-scan showed no new fluid collections. The recurrent pancreatitis turned out to be mild and she recovered well within a week.

Surgery was performed 3 weeks after the second discharge. An uncomplicated laparoscopic cholecystectomy was performed.

Discussion

Acute biliary pancreatitis can be distinguished as mild (Ranson score < 3) or as severe pancreatitis. The recurrence rate of acute gallstone pancreatitis is known to be as high as 60 % when treated conservatively without cholecystectomy [1–3]. Mildly acute gallstone pancreatitis is treated conservatively; usually in the event the patient has recovered in a couple of days and the amylase rate in serum has normalized, then the gallbladder can be taken out by laparoscopy. Only in the case of stones in the CBD with obstruction parameters, an ERCP and sphincterotomy will be indicated before cholecystectomy [4, 5].

The timing of surgery is different for both groups. A recent RCT shows that patients with mild pancreatitis can be treated safely with a cholecystectomy within 48 h [2]. This treatment approach demonstrated a shorter length of hospital stay and did not show an increase in complication rate. Currently in the Netherlands, the PONCHO trial is being performed, in which the timing of the cholecystectomy serves as the pertaining question: Must the cholecystectomy be done very early during the same admission or must it be postponed for 6 weeks? [6].

In case of necrotizing acute pancreatitis, no evidence is available on how to treat these patients. An early, ERCP and papillotomy in the case of CBD obstruction, is advised for lowering the risk of gallstone pancreatitis recurrence to 0–2 %. Therefore, the timing of the cholecystectomy in this situation is more flexible. Studies have shown that patients with encountered gallstones pancreatitis have an increased risk of developing biliary complications, such as acute cholecystitis, CBD stones, and recurrence acute pancreatitis, and therefore in that situation cholecystectomy is indicated [3].

The timing of the cholecystectomy after severe pancreatitis depends on the clinical course. In case of fluid collections, it is usually postponed and executed after radiological drainage. In case of operative interventions for these collections, cholecystectomy can be done simultaneously.

In the case at hand, one could argue that at the first admission of this patient, a laparoscopic cholecystectomy should have been performed. That seems obvious! During her second stay, no indication was found for ERCP and patient was adequately treated. The question rose again when to remove the gallbladder. Acute pancreatitis recurred shortly after the patient was dismissed. An ERCP and sphincterotomy were performed and a delayed cholecystectomy done. Since the third episode of pancreatitis was mild, one can argue that a cholecystectomy within 48 h after the onset of symptoms should have been performed in order to reduce the chance for a new and unpredictable recurrence.

References

1. Wilson CT, de Moya MA. Cholecystectomy for acute gallstone pancreatitis: early vs delayed approach. Scan J Surg. 2010;99:81–5.
2. Aboulian A, Chan T, Yaghoubian A, et al. Early cholecystectomy safely decreases hospital stay in patients with mild gallstone pancreatitis: a randomized prospective study. Ann Surg. 2010; 251:615–9.
3. Ito K, Whang EE. Timing of cholecystectomy for biliary pancreatitis: do the data support current guidelines? J Gastrointest Surg. 2008;12:2164–70.
4. Van Geenen AJM, van der Peet DL, Mulder CJJ, et al. Recurrent acute biliary pancreatitis: the protective role of cholecystectomy and endoscopic sphincterotomy. Surg Endosc. 2009;23: 950–6.
5. Lee JK, Ryu JK, Park JK, et al. Role of endoscopic sphincterotomy and cholecystectomy in acute biliary pancreatitis. Hepatogastroenterology. 2008;55:1981–5.
6. Bouwense SA, Besselink MG, van Brunschot S, et al. Pancreatitis of biliary origin, optimal timing of cholecystectomy (PONCHO trial): study protocol for a randomized controlled trial. Trials. 2012;26:13–225.

Chapter 35
Case on Complicated Retained Stones in the Common Bile Duct After Multiple Sphincterotomies by ERCP

Gwen M.P. Diepenhorst

Keywords Retained stones • Common bile duct • Sphincterotomy • ERCP • CBD stone

First Patient

Diagnosis and Indication for Surgery

Our first patient is a 55-year-old female presenting with a biliary pancreatitis. Because of dilated CBD with stones, an ERCP and sphincterotomy were performed. One stone could not removed, and the gastroenterologist left two stents behind. This procedure was complicated by a post-ERCP acute pancreatitis. Patient refused surgical exploration of the CBD and cholecystectomy, and 1 year later, because of fever the stent was found occluded and consequently replaced.

A MRCP demonstrated recurrent stones in the common bile duct (CBD) and after a new attempt to remove the stones by new sphincterotomy, this was unsuccessful and finally patient agreed to undergo a classic open cholecystectomy with CBD exploration.

Operative Description

Through a subcostal incision, cholecystectomy and exploration of the CBD were performed, being multiple stones removed from the CBD, and a T-tube was placed.

G.M.P. Diepenhorst
Department of Surgery, VU University Medical Center, Amsterdan, The Netherlands
e-mail: g.diepenhorst@vumc.nl

M.A. Cuesta, H.J. Bonjer (eds.), *Case Studies of Postoperative Complications after Digestive Surgery*, DOI 10.1007/978-3-319-01613-9_35,

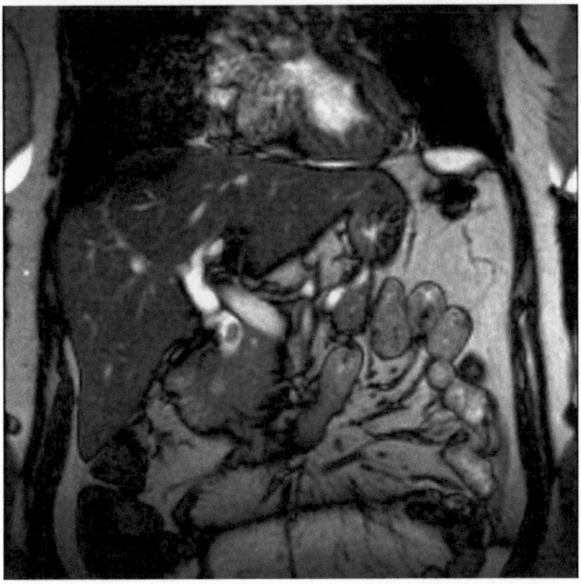

Fig. 35.1 MRCP showing recurrence CBD stone

Subsequent cholangiography demonstrated adequate patency of the CBD and no stones.

Postoperative Course: Identification and Treatment of Complication

Due to postoperative intermittent fever, the patient was treated with broad spectrum antibiotics. Histological evaluation of the gallbladder showed no signs of malignancy. The patient was discharged from the hospital in good condition, having the T-tube removed at the outpatient clinic. One year later, however, biliary colics recurred with high fever and recurring CBD stones could be demonstrated on MRCP (Fig. 35.1).

Despite repeated ERCPs with sphincterotomy and placement of stents, biliary symptoms persist. Six months later, the patient—still refusing a new operation—developed a new acute cholangitis due to an occluded stent, followed by stent replacement. The patient could then be convinced about the necessity of a new operation, and a new operative exploration of the CBD was performed during which multiple large stones were extracted. We decided to perform a bilio-digestive anastomosis consisting of a choledochoduodenotomy in an end-to-side fashion. Postoperatively, she developed abdominal pain with fever and a septic profile. Subsequent CT scan demonstrated free intra-abdominal fluid with signs of a general peritonitis. During relaparotomy a purulent peritonitis was found as well as a partial necrotic omentum. The necrotic omentum was resected and the abdominal cavity rinsed thoroughly. Postoperatively, the patient became increasingly septic, and a new CT scan demonstrated multiple fluid collections in Douglas' pouch, subhepatic right, and in the retroperitoneum. The next day, a relaparotomy was performed due to clinical deterioration.

Peroperatively, leakage was found because of the choledochoduodenostomy, and a T-tube was placed through the anastomosis, the abdominal cavity was rinsed, and new drains placed. Post-operatively, subphrenic fluid collections developed, which were treated by percutaneous drainage. In addition, the patient developed a pancreatic fistula, with an average production of 500 cc/day being conservatively treated with somatostatine and total parenteral nutrition (TPN). Despite these measures the patient showed progressive clinical deterioration and at the 6th postoperative day, feces appeared through the subcostal incision. A new surgical intervention was performed, in which a fecal peritonitis was found caused by a colon perforation at the level of hepatic flexure. The perforated segment was resected and a deviating colostomy created. The wound was closed by means of a Vycril mesh. Patient was again admitted to the intensive care department, mechanically ventilated, and broad spectrum antibiotics and TPN administered. She developed pneumonia as well as a wound infection, treated by VAC therapy. She improved clinically and could be transferred from the intensive care to the medium care. Six weeks after the last operation, she could leave the hospital in a reasonable condition for a revalidation center. Pancreatic fistula closed some weeks later. Two years later, understandably, the patient still refused a new operation to close the colostomy and for repair of cicatricial hernia.

Second Patient

Diagnosis and Indication for Surgery

Our second patient is a 73-year-old man presenting with complaints of diarrhea, abdominal bloating, and fever. Medical history included a Billroth-II resection for benign ulcer, COPD, and an elaborate cardiac history consisting of paroxysmal atrial fibrillation and myocardial infarction. Laboratory study showed an acute phase reaction with an elevated white blood cell count and cholestasis. An abdominal ultrasound depicted diffuse gallbladder wall thickening, characteristic of an acute cholecystitis with an impacted obstructing stone in the neck of the gallbladder.

Operation Description

After consideration of the patient's general medical condition, percutaneous transhepatic gallbladder drainage was considered to be the initial treatment of choice.

Fig. 35.2 MRCP showing recurrence CBD stone

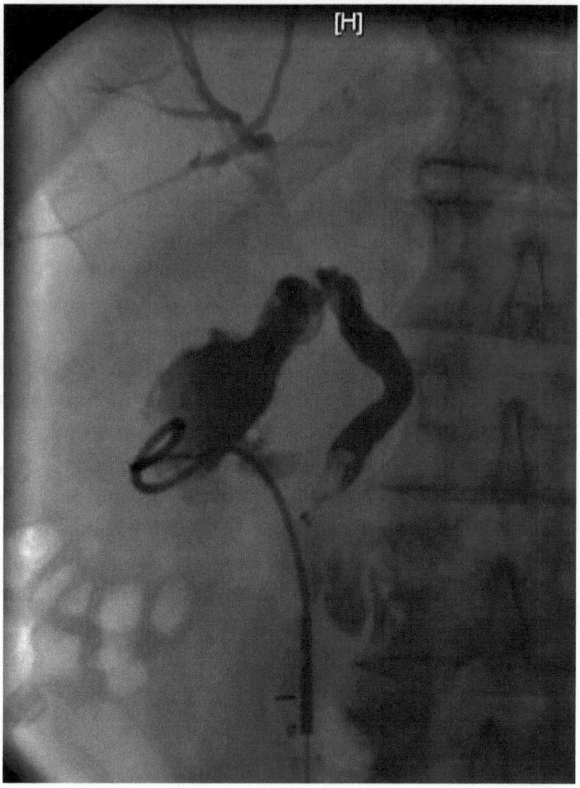

Ultrasound-guided drainage yielded 30 cc of pus and the drain was left in place. After the procedure, ultrasound and posteriorly cholangiography showed no signs of leakage and the following days the drain production decreased. The patient was discharged in good clinical condition with the drain in place and an elective laparoscopic cholecystectomy planned. Before operation, a new cholangiography in the outpatient setting demonstrated a stone in the distal CBD with slightly dilated intrahepatic bile ducts. However, outflow of contrast to the CBD, intra-hepatic bile ducts, as well as to the duodenum appeared to be adequate. In addition, imaging showed a limited amount of contrast leakage, possibly alongside the course of the drain (Fig. 35.2). The patient was readmitted to hospital and an attempted removal of the residual CBD stone by ERCP was undertaken, unsuccessful in part due to technical limitations after the BII resection.

Consequently, an open cholecystectomy with CBD exploration and intraoperative cholangiography was performed. Peroperative cholangiography after removal of the gallbladder demonstrated the presence of a fixed stone in the distal CBD. After a Kocher maneuver an open exploration of the CBD allowed removal of a single stone and placement of a T-drain. During exploration, it seemed that the space between instruments and posterior aspect of the pancreas was very thin. During intraoperative cholangioscopy, a perforation proximal of the papilla vater on

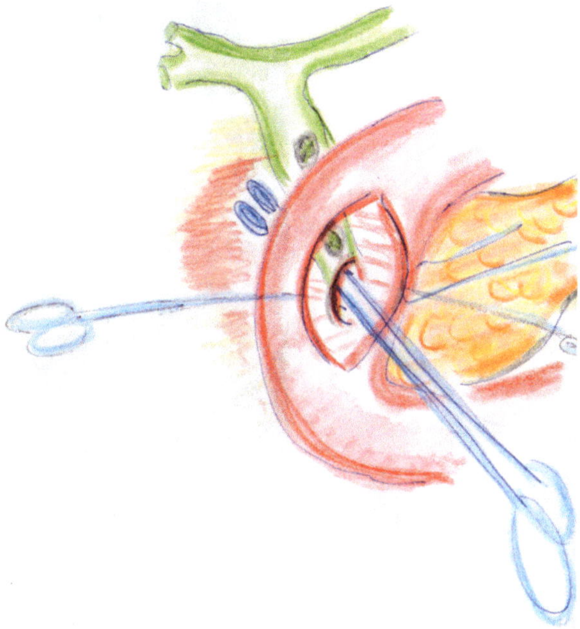

Illustration 35.1 In patients who underwent multiple ERCPs and sphincterotomies, an open CBD exploration will be high risk operation for complications. Perforation at the level of the papilla is of difficult treatment. In the first patient a choledochoduodenostomy was the treatment of choice and in the second a Whipple procedure

the posterior side was identified. Multiple attempts, first by performing a bilio-digestive anastomosis, and second, stenting the perforation, were unsuccessful (Illustration 35.1). Therefore, a Whipple procedure was considered as only option and consequently performed. Postoperative histological examination of the specimen demonstrated signs of a chronic pancreatitis without signs of malignancy.

Postoperative Course: Identification and Treatment of Complication

At day 10, patient demonstrated septic clinical deterioration with fecal and biliary drain production and subsequently a relaparotomy was performed (Fig. 35.3). At operation, fecal contamination was found coming from a necrotic segment of the transverse colon near the hepatic flexure, being resected and anastomosed. Furthermore, the hepatico-jejunostomy showed a limited amount of anastomotic leakage, being the right subhepatic space drained.

Postoperatively, bile leakage continued so that a PTC drain was placed. Hospital stay was further complicated by development of pneumonia as well as pleural fluid collections on both sides. Gradually, the patient improved clinically with an expectant policy, antibiotic treatment, and enteral nutrition. Percutaneous drain production decreased and could be removed several weeks later. Finally, the patient was discharged from the hospital with the PTC catheter in place. A month later a

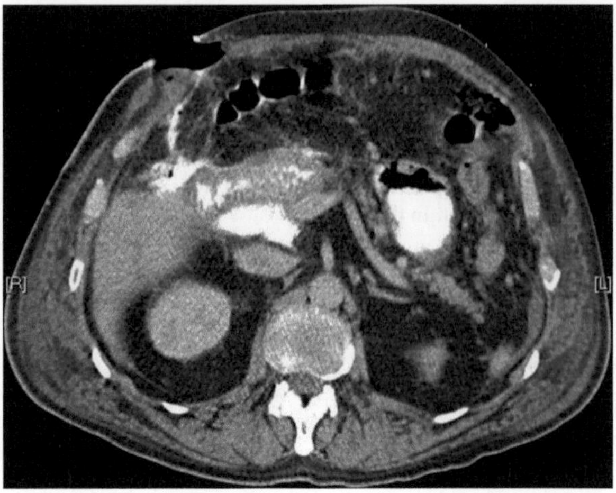

Fig. 35.3 CT scan showing contrast leakage following Whipple

transhepatic cholangiography demonstrated adequate contrast flow through the hepatico-jejunostomy without signs of leakage after which the PTC stent was initially closed off and finally removed. On the outpatient clinic, the patient complained about the loss of an incisive tooth, probably occurred during intubation. Orthodontist costs were reimbursed. Patient is doing well.

Discussion

In these two cases, retained stones in the CBD after multiple sphincterotomies lead to elaborate clinical complications. Retained CBD stones remain a challenging problem, and if controversy exists regarding ideal management, it is the opinion of the surgeon that patient should be operated on.

Since the 1980s, ERCP followed by sphincterotomy has become the most widely used method for imaging and treating CBD stones [1]. Magnetic resonance cholangiopancreatography (MRCP) serves as a noninvasive and sensitive test for detection of bile duct stones, but it is relatively expensive and provides no option for therapy. Repeated endoscopic stone extraction by ERCP is an accepted treatment modality and avoids surgery. However, this technique will only provide temporary relief from primary duct stones and repeated endoscopic treatment will be required. In a prospective study in patients undergoing repeated endoscopic stone extractions, the mean number of endoscopies carried out per patient was 7.3 and failure to completely clear the duct occurred in 36.4 % of all endoscopies [2]. Current options in management of CBD and gallbladder stones are open cholecystectomy and CBD exploration; laparoscopic cholecystectomy and laparoscopic CBD exploration (LCBDE); endoscopic sphincterotomy (ES) and subsequent laparoscopic cholecystectomy; or laparoscopic cholecystectomy followed by ES [3].

A number of studies have directly compared endoscopic and surgical interventions in management of CBD stones. Four randomized trials have compared open surgery and ES for the treatment of CBD stones, reporting a high success rate for both procedures (90–95 %) without a significant difference in morbidity and mortality but a longer hospital stay after surgery [4]. A trial comparing ES and surgery in patients with severe cholangitis showed less morbidity (34 % vs. 66 %) and less mortality (10 % vs. 32 %) associated with ES [5].

A number of trials have compared laparoscopic CBD exploration with ES as treatment for CBD stones. One of these randomized studies shows laparoscopic cholecystectomy plus laparoscopic CBD exploration and endoscopic retrograde cholangiopancreatography sphincterotomy plus laparoscopic cholecystectomy to be equivalent in effectiveness and cost, with shorter hospital stay after laparoscopic CBD exploration. Other trials confirm these findings, demonstrating laparoscopic CBD exploration and ES to be effective intervention strategies in detection and removal of CBD stones, without significant differences in complication or mortality rates with a shorter hospital stay in the laparoscopic approach to CBD exploration [6].

In summary, there is still an indication for open surgery if ES fails or if stones cannot be removed endoscopically. As alternative for ERCP, laparoscopic CBD exploration should be preferred for fit patients (ASA I and II).

ES should be the management of choice for patients with severe cholangitis.

These two patients had gallstones and CBD stones. Traditional treatment will consist of open or laparoscopic cholecystectomy and CBD exploration. As alternative for surgical CBD exploration, ERCP and papillotomy has been developed in many countries as first choice treatment, in order to clear the CBD stones before laparoscopic cholecystectomy. Questions arises, how many attempts should a gastroenterologist perform in the event the first treatment is not successful and if the use of a stent should be considered safe to assure the free pass of bile through the papilla. In elderly patients, the stent may be considered as alternative for operation. From the surgical point of view, it seems logical to perform ERCP and papillotomy, one or two times, and, if not successful, to indicate a cholecystectomy and CBD exploration. In the first case, seven ERCPs with four sphincterotomies were performed, and in the second case, four ERCPs and one sphincterotomy.

It is imaginable that repeated papillotomies may cause covered perforation of the papil and may alter the wall between papilla and posterior aspect of pancreas. This problem may explain the complication in these two cases, the pancreas leakage in the first patient, and the perforation—in spite of proper technique—near the papilla in the second. The other complication as found in both cases of the hepatic flexure perforation of the colon may be attributed to a technical complication during surgery, which should have been avoided.

References

1. Barwood NT, Valinsky LJ, Hobbs MS, et al. Changing methods of imaging the common bile duct in the laparoscopic cholecystectomy era in Western Australia: implications for surgical practice. Ann Surg. 2002;235:41–50.
2. Kohn GP, Hassen AS, Banting SW, et al. Endoscopic management of recurrent primary bile duct stones. ANZ J Surg. 2008;78:579–82.
3. Gouma DJ, Terpstra OT. Gallstone disease – surgical aspects. In: van Lanschot JJB, Gouma DJ, Jansen PLM, Jones EA, Pinedo HM, Schouten WR, et al., editors. Integrated medical and surgical gastroenterology. Houten: Bohn Stafleu Van Loghum; 2004. p. 158–66.
4. Targarona EM, Ayuso RM, Bordas JM, et al. Randomised trial of endoscopic sphincterotomy with gallbladder left in situ versus open surgery for common bileduct calculi in high-risk patients. Lancet. 1996;347:926–9.
5. Lai EC, Mok FP, Tan ES, et al. Endoscopic biliary drainage for severe acute cholangitis. N Engl J Med. 1992;326:1582–6.
6. Cuschieri A, Lezoche E, Morino M, et al. E.A.E.S. multicenter prospective randomized trial comparing two-stage vs single-stage management of patients with gallstone disease and ductal calculi. Surg Endosc. 1999;13:952–7.

Chapter 36
Case on Complications After ERCP and Sphincterotomy

Miguel A. Cuesta

Keywords Papilla Vater perforation • ERCP • Sphincterotomy • Necrotizing acute pancreatitis • Multiple organ failure (MOF)

First Patient

ERCP and Papillotomy and Acute Necrotizing Pancreatitis

Diagnosis and Indication for Surgery

A 29-year-old obese female patient known with immunosuppressive disease underwent elsewhere an ERCP because of a suspicion for having CBD stones with colics and alteration of liver enzymes. As consequence of the ERCP without papillotomy, she developed in the course of 2 days a necrotizing acute pancreatitis (CT scan confirmed) with multiple organ failure (MOF). Patient was intubated and ventilated with a high PEEP of 14, and acute dialysis became necessary because of the acute renal insufficiency. Due to her obesity (BMI 47), ventilation was becoming difficult and on a new CT scan important volumes of fluids were seen in the abdomen (Fig. 36.1) and clinically an abdominal compartment syndrome was diagnosed.

M.A. Cuesta, M.D.
Department of Surgery, VU University Medical Center, Amsterdam, The Netherlands
e-mail: ma.cuesta@vumc.nl

M.A. Cuesta, H.J. Bonjer (eds.), *Case Studies of Postoperative Complications after Digestive Surgery*, DOI 10.1007/978-3-319-01613-9_36,

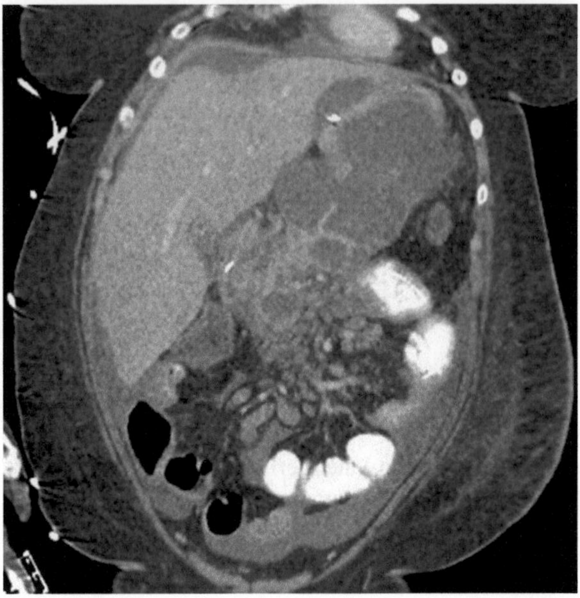

Fig. 36.1 CT scan showing acute necrotizing pancreatitis and huge fluid collection

Operation

Consequently, surgeon performed a long transversal upper abdomen laparotomy in order to decompress the abdomen and there a huge fluid collection was drained. Abdomen was left open and temporarily closed by means of a double Vicryl® mesh.

Postoperative Course: Identification and Treatment of Complication

The next day feces appeared under the mesh, inspection revealed that the leakage came from the colon, and a reoperation was planned. At relaparotomy, an opening was found in the transverse colon near the splenic flexure. Her upper abdomen was changed as a plastron, and surgeon closed the colon distal of perforation by staples and after dissection of the transverse mesentery, the surgeon could create a colostomy at the middle-right abdomen. Two drains were left, one along the colon and the other in the pancreatic area. Abdomen was rinsed and closed temporarily by means of a VAC system. On CT scan a retrogastric abscess was diagnosed and percutaneously drained (Fig. 36.2). Colostomy remained vital and productive and wound started to granulate. Ventilation was difficult and a tracheotomy was given. At the same time, the patient's clinical condition improved, her renal function recovered, and she could be extubated. Eight weeks after her admission to the Intensive Care Unit, patient could go to a revalidation center. She did not wish the

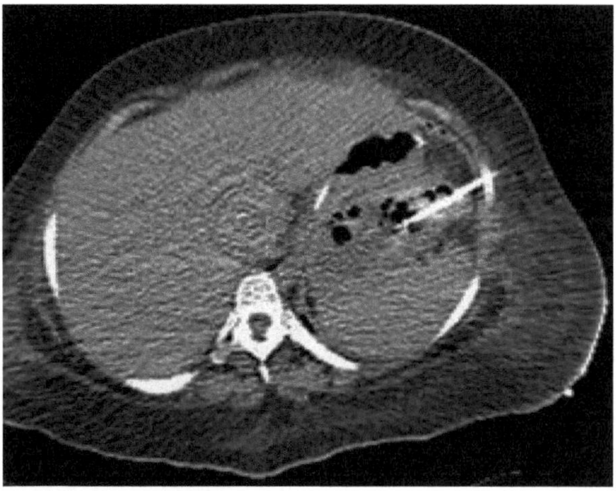

Fig. 36.2 CT scan showing a retrogastric abscess, being percutaneously drained

VAC system for this period, which was feasible because the wound was smaller with healthy granulating bottom. Local care by Polimem® was applied to the surface of the wound.

After a period of revalidation and having gained a BMI of 35 a year later, she underwent a new operation to close the wound and the colostomy.

Second Patient

ERCP and Sphincterotomy and Papilla of Vater Perforation

Diagnosis and Indication for ERCP

A 64-year-old man underwent an ERCP and endoscopic papillary with large balloon dilatation because of cholelithiasis and CBD stone in the CBD. He had had colics for 2 years and if not jaundiced cholestasis had been observed in the lab study. At the ERCP a stone was removed through sphincterotomy by balloon and Dormia catheter. Post-ERCP, patient had high fever and abdominal pain.

Postoperative Course: Identification and Treatment of Complication

The day after, a CT scan revealed retroperitoneal emphysema with fluid collection as sign of papilla of vater perforation (Fig. 36.3). The patient was treated by broad spectrum antibiotics, nasogastric tube, and total parenteral nutrition (TPN). After

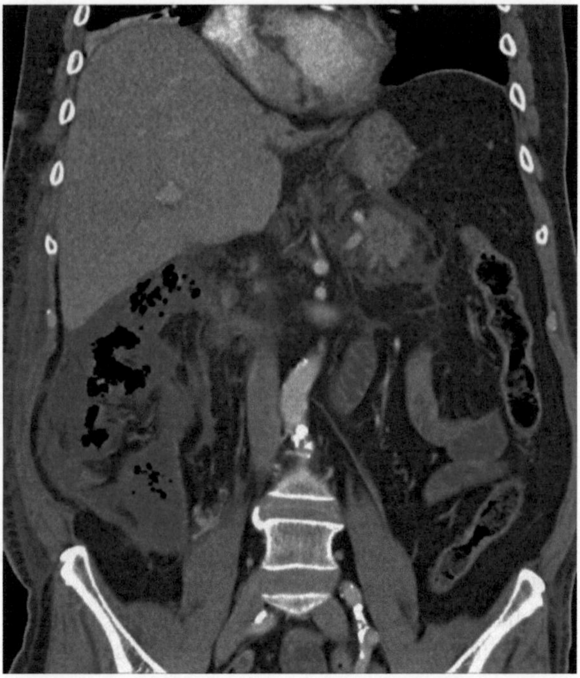

Fig. 36.3 CT scan, retroperitoneal emphysema, and abscess

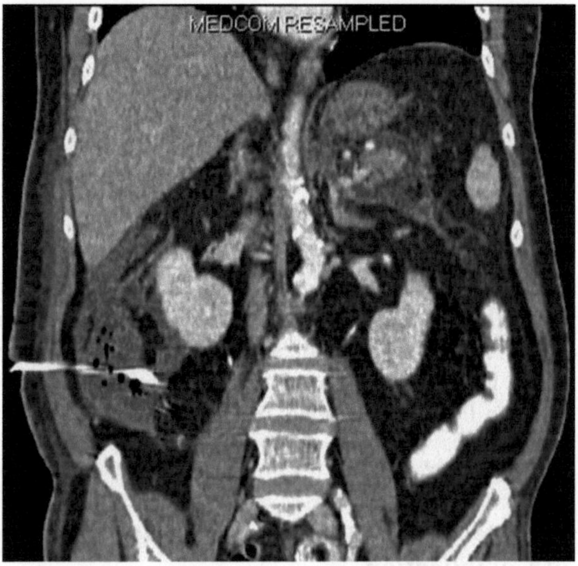

Fig. 36.4 CT scan showing retroperitoneal abscess percutaneously drained

referral, a new CT scan showed retroperitoneal abscess, being drained by CT-guided percutaneous drainage (Fig. 36.4). Slowly the condition of the patient improved and after 2 weeks the drain could be removed (Illustration 36.1). He was scheduled to undergo a laparoscopic cholecystectomy.

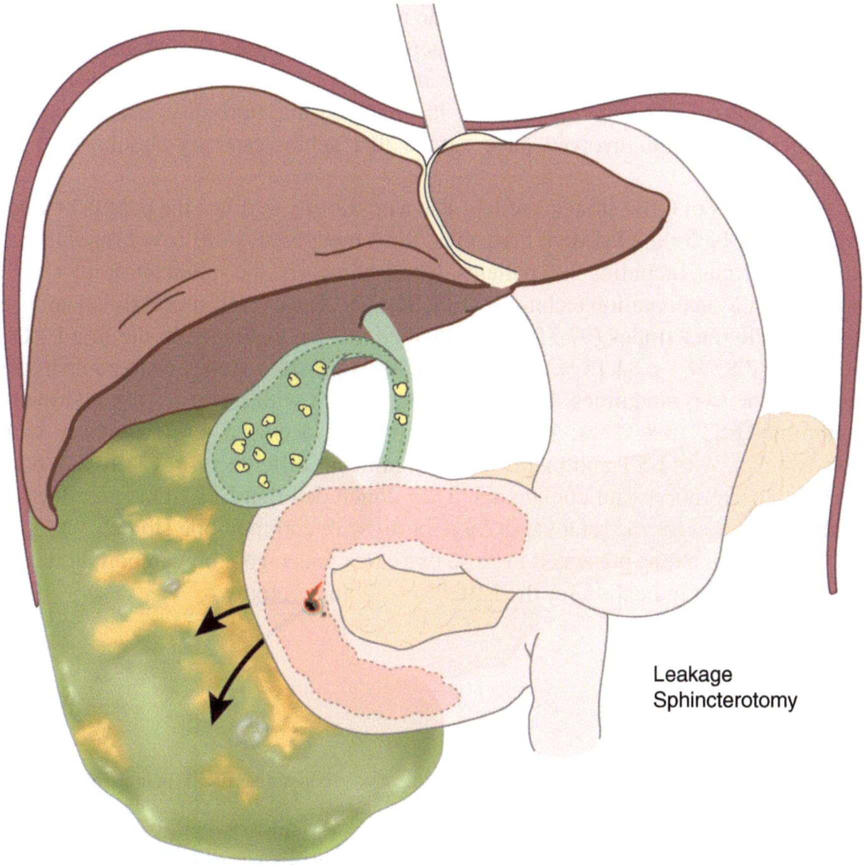

Illustration 36.1 After perforation of papilla of vater by sphincterotomy, this will be percutaneously drained

Discussion

Originally, the ERCP had been designed and used to assess the biliary duct, but subsequently the possibility arose to intervene the papilla of vater by means of sphincterotomy. A review of 119 patients who underwent an ERCP with or without sphincterotomy in our department was carried out in a period when papillotomy was extensively used for assessment of jaundice, acute pancreatitis, and for CBD stones [1]. The study showed a high positive predictive value (over 85 %) for the presence of CBD stones in patients with acute cholangitis, persistent obstructive jaundice or in the acute phase of gallstone pancreatitis. The complication rate of ERCP with sphincterotomy was 14 % with a mortality rate of 2 %. These results argued for more selective use of preoperative ERCP to be used only for patients with acute cholangitis, persistent jaundice or acute gallstone pancreatitis.

Complications, such as perforation with retroperitoneal abscesses, bleeding, and acute pancreatitis, were found to be frequent. Evidence-based studies and the introduction of MRCP has since decreased the numbers of unnecessary ERCP, especially in normal-size CBD and consequently has reduced the morbidity. Indications are stricter now and all involved have agreed that sphincterotomy should be done selectively.

In the cases of CBD stones, there is also a possibility to dilate the papilla of vater by means of balloon dilatation. Feng et al. did a meta-analysis of seven randomized controlled trials, including 790 patients, which compared the sphincterotomy (EST) with the balloon dilatation technique (EPLBD) [2]. The overall successful clearance rates of bile duct stones (97.35 % vs. 96.35 %), stone clearance in the first ERCP session (87.87 % vs. 84.15 %), and removal of large-sized stones were comparable between the two modalities. EPLBD was associated with fewer overall complications than EST (5.8 % vs. 13.1 %). Hemorrhage occurred less frequently with EPLBD than with EST and there was no significant difference in post-ERCP pancreatitis, perforation, and cholangitis. They concluded that EPLBD is an effective and safe method for the removal of large or difficult common bile stones.

The complications presented in these two cases underscore how important it is to establish a good indication for the ERCP and sphincterotomy.

References

1. Rijna H, Borgstein PJ, Meuwissen SG, et al. Selective preoperative ERCP in laparoscopic biliary surgery. Br J Surg. 1995;82:1130–3.
2. Feng Y, Zhu H, Chen X, et al. Comparison of endoscopic papillary large balloon dilatation and endoscopic sphincterotomy for retrieval of choledocholithiasis: a meta-analysis of randomized controlled trials. J Gastroenterol. 2012;47:655–63.

Chapter 37
Case on Lost Stones in Abdomen After Laparoscopic Cholecystectomy

Miguel A. Cuesta

Keywords Lost Stones • Subphrenic abscess • Umbilical abscess • Laparoscopic cholecystectomy

First Patient

Diagnosis and Indication for Surgery

A 44-year-old male patient was admitted in the hospital with the diagnosis of acute cholecystitis, and a laparoscopic intervention was planned.

Operation

During intervention and after suction of the bile, stones fell into the abdominal cavity, being taken out in a bag as much as possible (Illustration 37.1). Moreover, the cystic duct was wide and had to be stapled.

M.A. Cuesta, M.D.
Department of Surgery, VU University Medical Center, Amsterdam, The Netherlands
e-mail: ma.cuesta@vumc.nl

M.A. Cuesta, H.J. Bonjer (eds.), *Case Studies of Postoperative Complications after Digestive Surgery*, DOI 10.1007/978-3-319-01613-9_37,

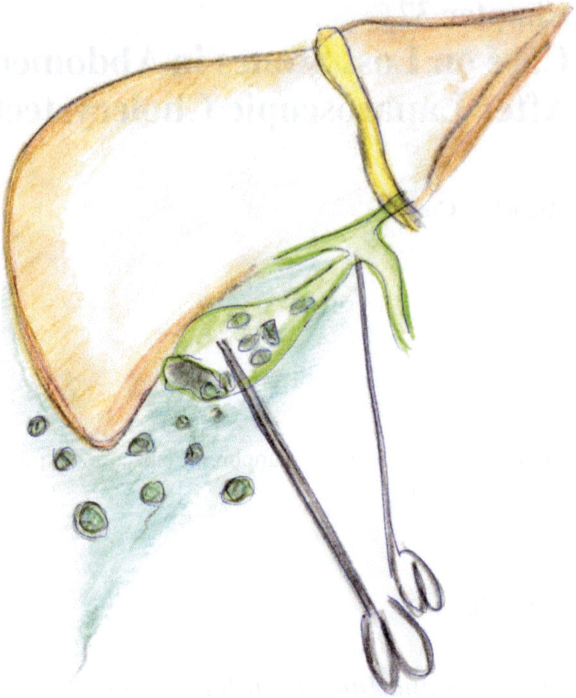

Illustration 37.1 Lost stones during cholecystectomy should be removed completely. Otherwise, the morbidity caused is very high

Postoperative Course: Identification and Treatment of the Complication

Patient did well postoperatively but 3 weeks after operation he had fever and abdominal pain in the right upper abdomen and flank. Readmission followed and differential diagnosis was made regarding problems with the integrity of CBD or retained stones. A US showed some dilatation of the CBD, and on the ERCP no stones were detected, and neither lesion of the CBD was seen. Because of persistent fever and pain, a CT scan was performed, and here a subphrenic collection with gas and structures alike stones were seen in the subphrenic and subhepatic areas (Figs. 37.1 and 37.2). A new laparoscopic exploration was performed in which pus was drained from both spaces and some stones were removed. After operation patient persisted having pain and fever; he was impeded in going back to work as machinist at a construction company. A new CT scan showed that the subfrenic abscess had not disappeared and on its posterior aspect there was at least one retained stone. Moreover, stones were seen in two other locations, that is, in the gallbladder region and probably in the pouch of Morrison. In the meantime, patient walked stooped due to flank pain, and a new laparoscopic intervention was proposed with a high chance for conversion.

Conversion to laparotomy was necessary because the subhepatic region was not accessible, being both abscesses drained and different stones removed. Recovery

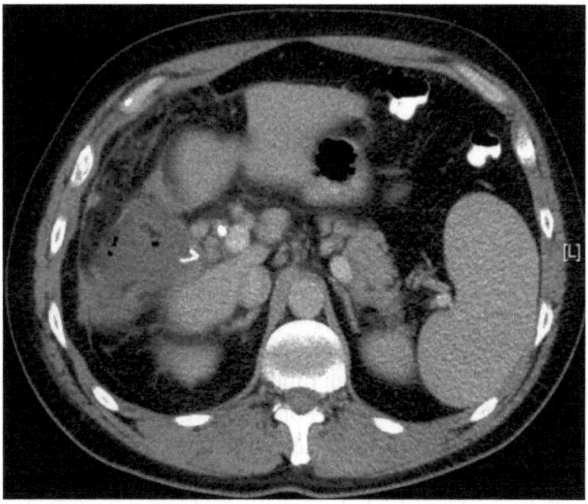

Fig. 37.1 CT scan showing subhepatic lost stones in an abscess

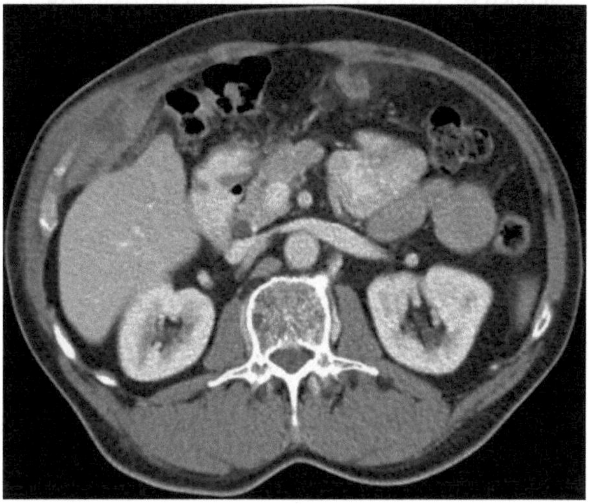

Fig. 37.2 CT scan, lost stones in the lateral subfrenic space

for the patient took another 6 months. After active physiotherapy and much patience, patient finally reinitiated his work as machinist.

Second Patient

Diagnosis and Indication for Surgery

A 34-year-old female patient was operated electively because of gallstones by a laparoscopic cholecystectomy. During operation an important leakage of small and large stones as well as bile into the abdomen occurred. Moreover, a bleeding coming from the gallbladder bed was difficult to control.

Postoperative Course: Identification and Treatment of the Complication

While patient initially recovered and was discharged, yet after a period of several weeks she returned with pain in the right abdomen. On the US and the CT scan no problems were detected and the surgeon tried to convince her that everything was satisfactory . In the mean time, she was referred to the urologist because of an infection of the urinary tract. For the next 2 years, the patient continued to experience chronic complaints and was not able to return to her previous occupation at a kindergarten. After some referrals for pain to outpatient clinic and physiotherapist, she subsequently visited the gynecologist for pain in her lower abdomen. She was examined by US for a possible cyst in the right ovary. By US and vaginal examination, a right ovary cyst with solid contents was diagnosed and patient was proposed to undergo another intervention by laparoscopy with possible conversion to laparotomy. Hereafter, inflammation was found around her right ovary fixed to the bladder and proved difficult to mobilize. The gynecologist converted the operation to a Pfannenstiel incision and at the location between the right adnexa of the uterus and the bladder; several old gallstones were found and removed. The right ovary was found normal and left untouched.

Third Patient

Postoperative Course: Identification and Treatment of the Complication

After undergoing an elective laparoscopic cholecystectomy in which some leakage of bile and stones occurred, a 67-year-old patient recovered and was discharged. After a period of 2 months, the umbilical scar became red and inflamed and the surgeon drained it under local anesthesia. The wound then closed and patient felt well for some time. Six months later, the patient was readmitted because of recurrent umbilical abscess. A CT scan was performed revealing a large abscess with a large stone of about 2 cm (Fig. 37.3). No other stones or fluid collection were visible in the rest of abdomen. Under anesthesia the scar was opened, and the pus and stone removed. Wound again was closed by secondary intention and the patient recovered definitely.

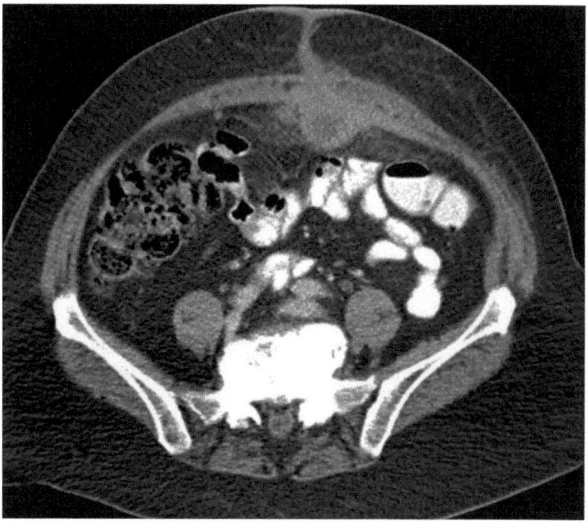

Fig. 37.3 CT scan, subumbilical abscess, and stone

Discussion

The lessons regarding these three patients are, first, that during laparoscopic (or open) cholecystectomy all lost stones in the abdomen should be removed. Second, that in case of recurrence of complaints in the upper and right abdomen a CT scan should be done [1]. The found stones should be located and removed. Spilled stones located in the pouch of Morrison are difficult to find. Finally, if the patient has problems with the spine while standing or walking, a lengthy physiotherapy should be initiated in order to ensure the patient is able to return to an active life.

Reference

1. Loffeld RJ. The consequences of lost gallstones during laparoscopic cholecystectomy. Neth J Med. 2006;64:364–6.

Chapter 38
Case on Late Stenosis of Biliodigestive Anastomosis with Cholangitis (After Laparoscopic Cholecystectomy)

Miguel A. Cuesta and Chris J.J. Mulder

Keywords Balloon dilatation • Gallstones • Biliodigestive anastomosis • Cholangitis • Laparoscopic cholecystectomy

Diagnosis and Indication for Surgery

A 32-year-old female patient, residing in another country, was referred to our department by the gastroenterologist because of a complete stop in her common hepatic duct.

Nine months before she had been operated on for symptomatic gallstones by means of a laparoscopic cholecystectomy.

During laparoscopy, the surgeon diagnosed a CBD lesion and converted the operation to subcostal laparotomy. His description of the operation reads that "a total division of the CBD was seen, and after mobilization of the proximal CBD and Kocher manoeuvre, an end-to-end anastomosis was performed with drainage of the CBD by means of a T-tube." Patient recovered well and the T-tube was removed 2 months later after certainty that there was no stenosis or dilatation and a good passage to duodenum. After a normal period of 6 months, the patient returned with complaints and was admitted to the department of Gastroenterology because of obstructive jaundice. On CT scan and ERCP a complete stop was seen in the CBD at the level of hepatic duct (Fig. 38.1), so the patient was drained by means of a PTC

M.A. Cuesta, M.D. (✉)
Department of Surgery, VU University Medical Center, Amsterdam, The Netherlands
e-mail: ma.cuesta@vumc.nl

C.J.J. Mulder
Department of Gastroenterology, VU University Medical Center, Amsterdam, The Netherlands

M.A. Cuesta, H.J. Bonjer (eds.), *Case Studies of Postoperative Complications after Digestive Surgery*, DOI 10.1007/978-3-319-01613-9_38,

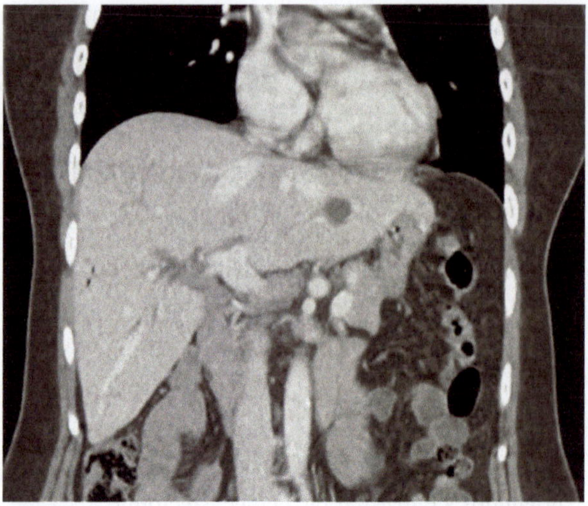

Fig. 38.1 CT scan, stop in the CBD with intrahepatic duct dilatation

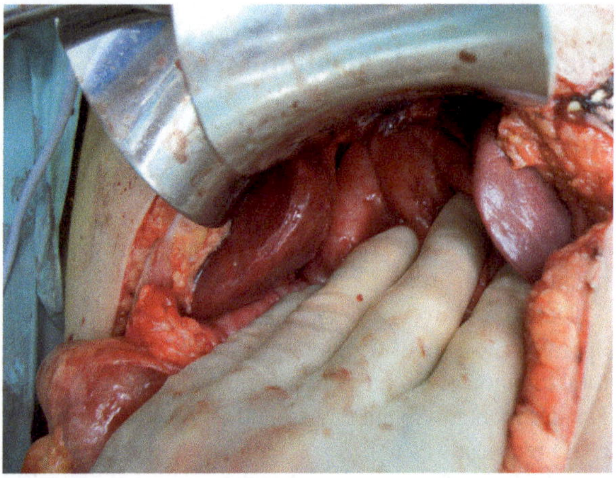

Fig. 38.2 Operation view hepaticojejunostomy

drain introduced through the left hepatic duct, and an operation was planned for reconstruction.

Operation

At operation, done through a subcostal incision, a biliodigestive anastomosis with a Roux-en-Y anastomosis was performed (Fig. 38.2, and Illustration 38.1). Patient did postoperatively well and could go home with the PTC drain after 10 days. Six weeks later, a cholangiography showed a good patent anastomosis and the PTC drain was removed.

Postoperative Course: Identification and Treatment of Complication

Eighteen months later she was again readmitted because of periods of acute cholangitis probably caused by stenosis of the bilio-digestive anastomosis. She was treated initially with iv Antibioticss. On the PTC, a stenosis of anastomosis was found (Fig. 38.3), which was consequently dilated by means of a balloon (Fig. 38.4a and Illustration 38.1) with success. Patient is currently under control at the outpatient clinic.

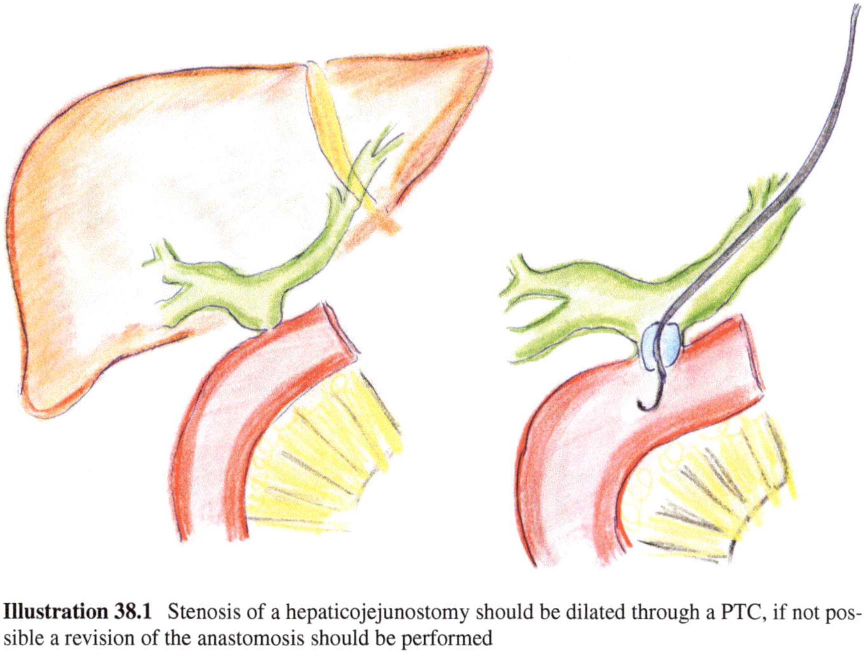

Illustration 38.1 Stenosis of a hepaticojejunostomy should be dilated through a PTC, if not possible a revision of the anastomosis should be performed

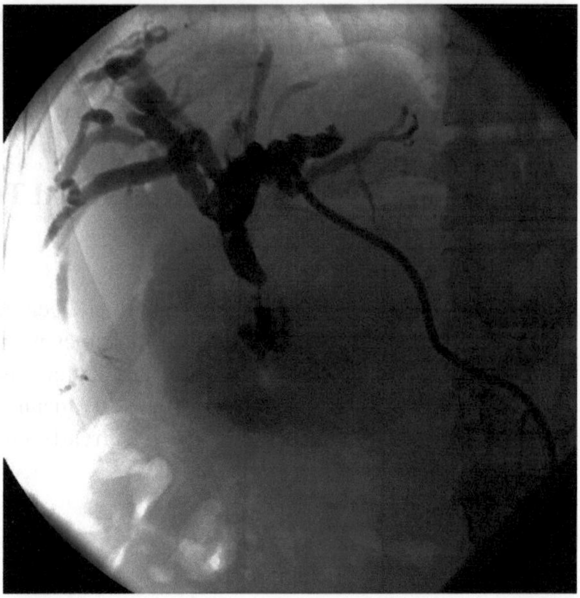

Fig. 38.3 PTC showing stenosis hepaticojejunostomy

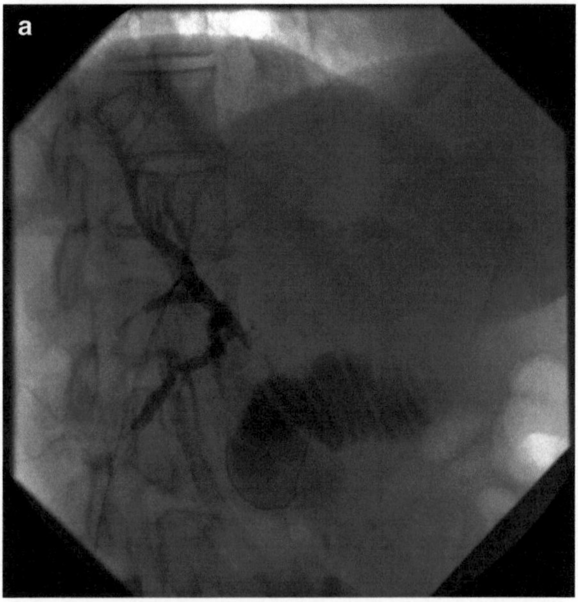

Fig. 38.4 (**a**) contrast X-ray stenosis common hepatic duct, (**b**) PTC balloon dilatation

Fig. 38.4 (continued)

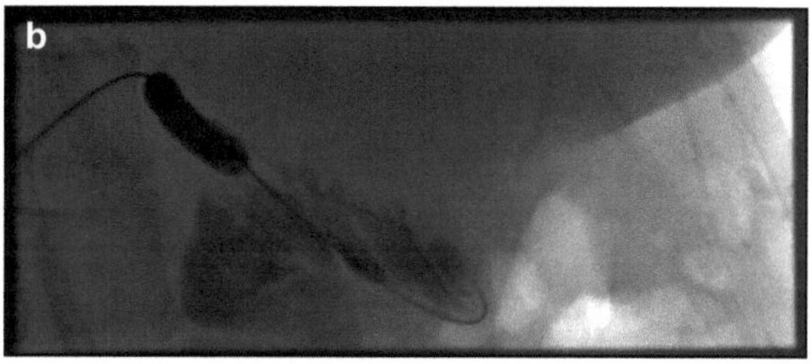

Discussion

Roux-en-Y biliodigestive anastomosis is the most common method to treat surgically the consequences of Bile Duct Injuries (BDI) (see Chaps. 30–32) [1, 2]. In the case of stenosis of the anastomosis with jaundice or cholangitis, the patency of the anastomosis must be restored. The problem of this complication is the difficulty to reach the anastomosis by gastric route. Therefore, the percutaneous and more recently the use of Double Balloon Endoscopy (DBE) routes are important to solve the stricture. The first choice for treatment will be the percutaneous dilatation [3, 4]. Nevertheless this treatment has a 27 % of restenosis in 30 months of follow-up. Creation of transgastric or jejunal routes to intervene repeatedly the anastomosis is also a procedure that will help the access [5]. Another nonsurgical alternative is the use of DBE to reach the anastomosis and proceed to dilate and stent the anastomosis [4]. If these procedures are not successful, redo surgery will be performed. Stenosis is known to relapse frequently after the creation of a new anastomosis.

References

1. Booij KAC, Gouma DJ, van Gulik TM, Busch ORC. Prevention and treatment of major complications after cholecystectomy. In: Cuesta MA, Bonjer HJ, editors. Treatment of complications after digestive surgery, chapter 12. London: Springer; 2013.
2. Costamagna G, Shah SK, Tringali A. Current management of postoperative complications and benign biliary strictures. Gastrointest Endosc Clin N Am. 2003;13:635–48.
3. Vos PM, van Beek EJ, Smits NJ, et al. Percutaneous balloon dilatation for benign hepaticojejunostomy strictures. Abdom Imaging. 2000;25:134–8.
4. Parlak E, Cicek B, Disibeyaz S, et al. Endoscopic retrograde cholangiography by DBE in patients with Roux-en-Y hepaticojejunostomy. Surg Endosc. 2010;24:466–70.
5. Parlak E, Disibeyaz S, Oztas E, et al. Endoscopic treatment of biliary disorders in patients with Roux-en-Y hepaticojejunostomy via a permanent access loop. Endoscopy. 2011;43:73–6.

Chapter 39
Case on Complication After Surgical Treatment of a Klatskin Tumor

Oliver R.C. Busch and Miguel A. Cuesta

Keywords Klatskin tumor • Cholangiocarcinoma • Liver resection • Bile leakage • Hemihepatectomy • Cholangitis

First Patient

Diagnosis and Indication for Surgery

A 61-year-old male patient presented with jaundice which was caused by a hilar cholangiocarcinoma. Preoperative staging revealed a Bismuth–Corlette classification type III a (Illustration 39.1a), and biliary drainage was achieved by percutaneous transhepatic cholangiography (PTC) catheter for both left and right hemiliver. After diagnostic laparoscopy and neoadjuvant short course radiotherapy a liver resection was performed.

Operation

During surgical exploration, no distant metastases were encountered and a central liver resection, including segments I, IV, V, and VIII was performed with a hepaticojejunostomy for drainage of the segmental bile duct of segment II/III and VI/VII

O.R.C. Busch, M.D., Ph.D. (✉)
Department of Surgery, Academic Medical Center, Amsterdam, The Netherlands
e-mail: o.r.busch@amc.uva.nl

M.A. Cuesta, M.D.
Department of Surgery, VU University Medical Center, Amsterdam, The Netherlands
e-mail: ma.cuesta@vumc.nl

M.A. Cuesta, H.J. Bonjer (eds.), *Case Studies of Postoperative Complications after Digestive Surgery*, DOI 10.1007/978-3-319-01613-9_39,

a

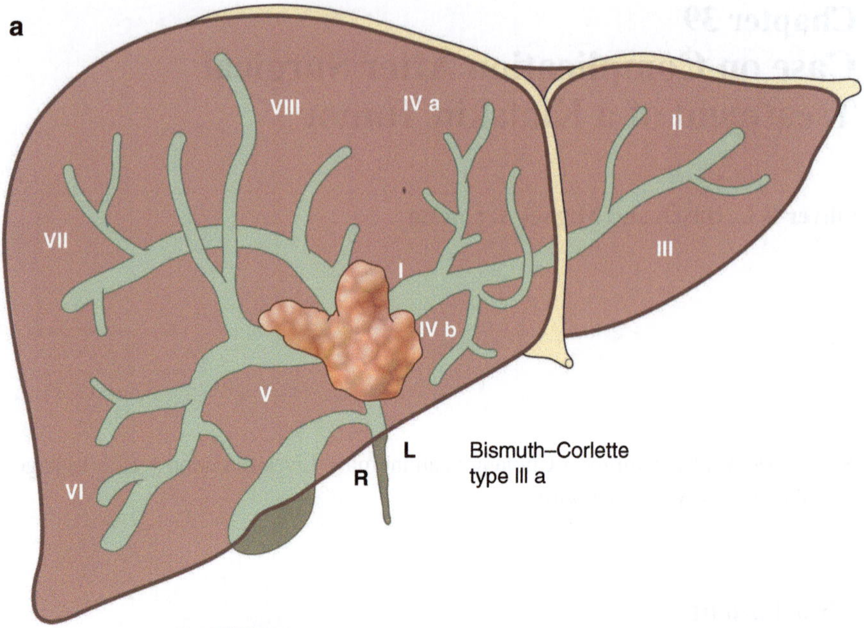

b

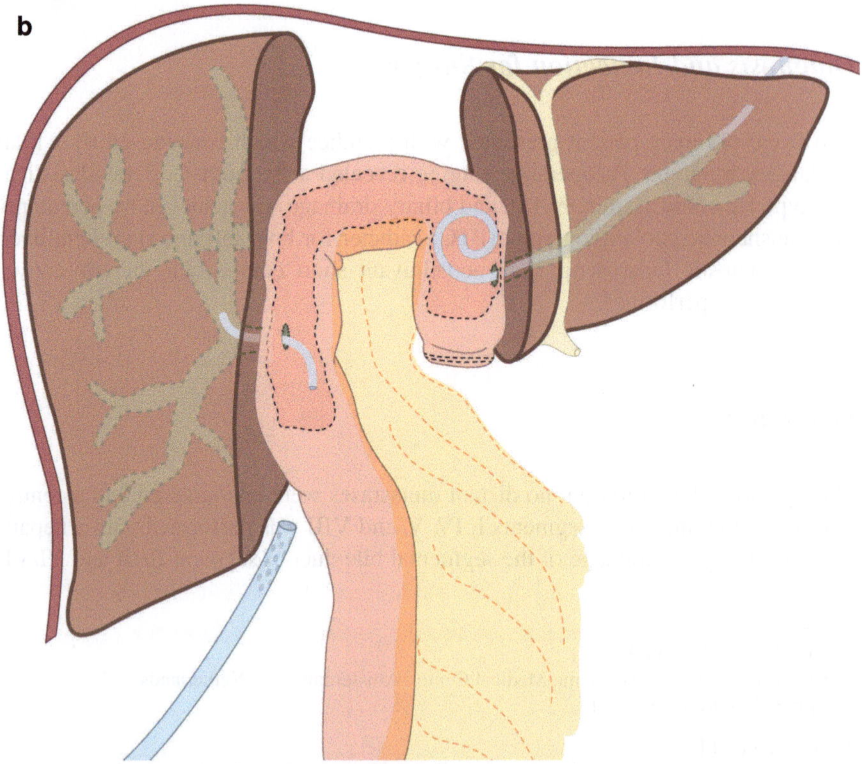

Illustration 39.1 (**a**) Corlette–Bismuth tumor type III a. (**b, c**) Resection of the Klatskin tumor Bismuth–Corlette type III a in the first patient with the leakage of the right hepaticojejunostomy, being fixed and drained

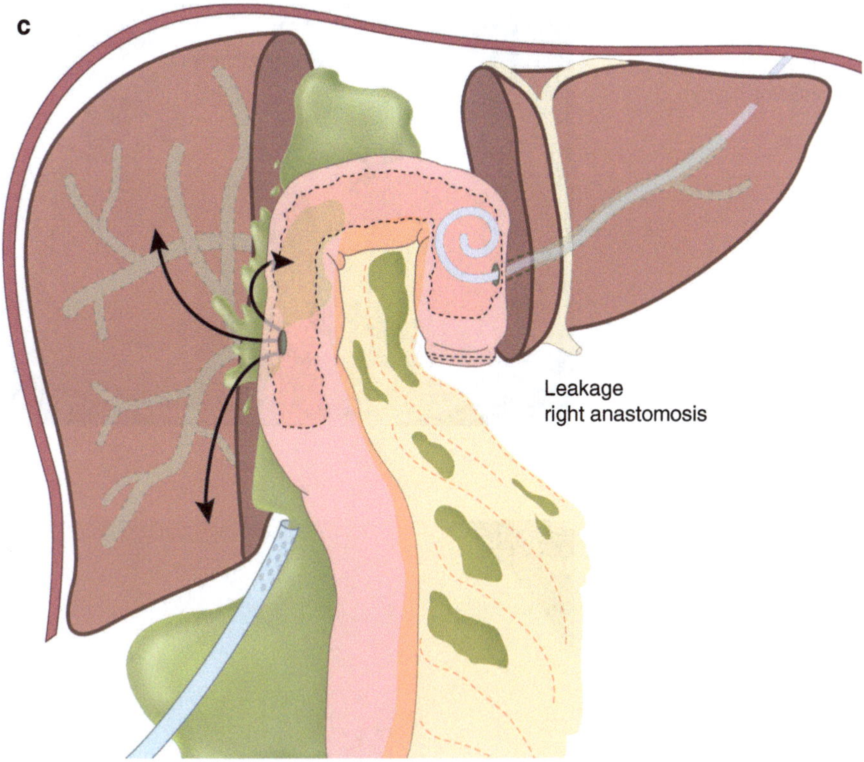

Illustration 39.1 (continued)

(Illustration 39.1b). The PTC catheter in the segmental duct II/III was placed across the left hepaticojejunostomy.

Postoperative Course: Identification and Treatment of the Complication

Three days after operation, the clinical condition of the patient deteriorated resulting in a septic shock requiring resuscitation on the intensive care unit. CT of the abdomen (Fig. 39.1) showed a partial infarction of the right hemiliver with normal arterial and portal blood flow. Furthermore, fluid and air were visualized in the resection cavity. Based upon these findings and the clinical condition, a relaparotomy was mandatory. During surgical exploration a leakage was found of the right hepaticojejunostomy which was sutured across a silastic catheter. After 2 days, patient returned to the general ward. Twelve days after initial operation, the abdominal catheter produced 300 ml a day. Visualization of the different bile duct catheters revealed no leakage of the hepaticojejunostomy (Fig. 39.2) but still some bile

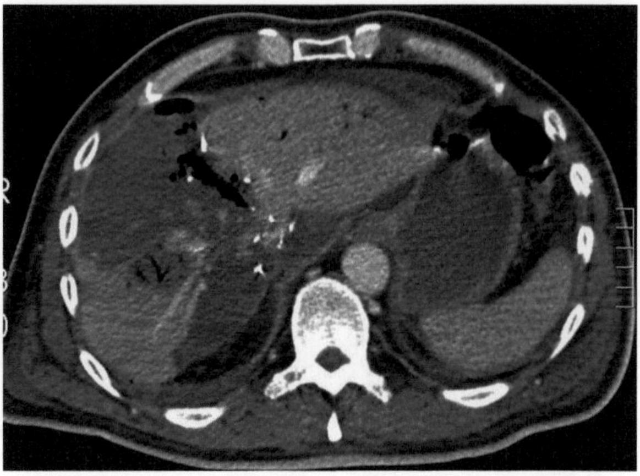

Fig. 39.1 CT showed partial infarction of the right hemiliver and fluid and air in the resection cavity

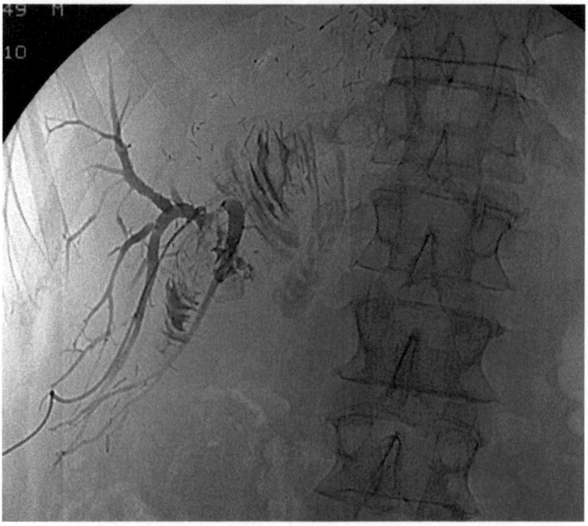

Fig. 39.2 PTC demonstrated sufficient hepaticojejunostomy of the segmental bile ducts VI and VII

leakage from the remnants of segment IV and VIII into the resection cavity was seen (Fig. 39.3). Therefore, a new PTC catheter was placed to decompress this segmental bile duct (Illustration 39.1c). Twenty-one days after resection the patient was discharged from hospital and several drains were removed 3 months after operation. Histological examination revealed a complete resection of a cholangiocarcinoma without lymph node metastases.

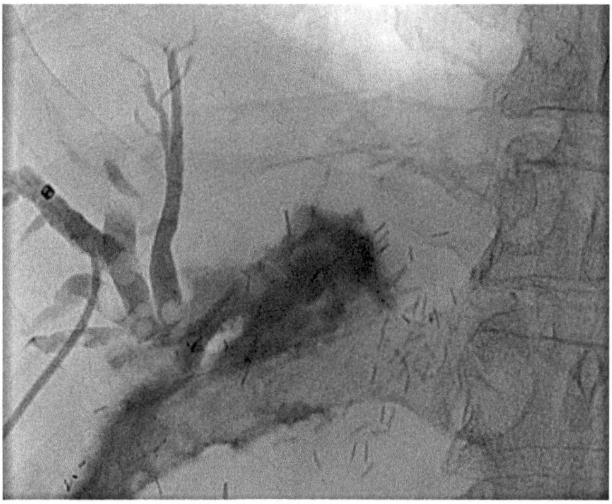

Fig. 39.3 PTC showed dilatation of the bile ducts of remnants of segment IV and VIII leakage into the resection cavity

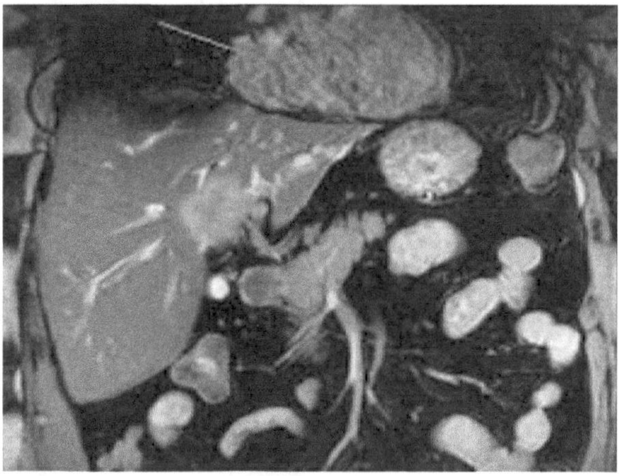

Fig. 39.4 MRCP showing mass Klatskin tumor with dilatation left system

Second Patient

Diagnosis and Indication for Operation

A 58-year-old metal worker was diagnosed having a mass forming Klatskin tumor found during study because of silent obstructive jaundice and 10 kg weight loss. His bilirubin was 275 mmol/l and he was treated initially by a PTC drain. A MRCP was done showing a tumor of 4 cm at the hepatic bifurcation with dilatation of the left system (Fig. 39.4). Dissemination study showed no distance metastases and he was proposed to undergo a laparotomy.

Operation

During operation a tumor of 4 cm located on the left hepatic duct was dissected and an extended left hemihepatectomy was performed (segments 1–5 and 8), with anastomosis of the posterior branch to the common hepatic duct.

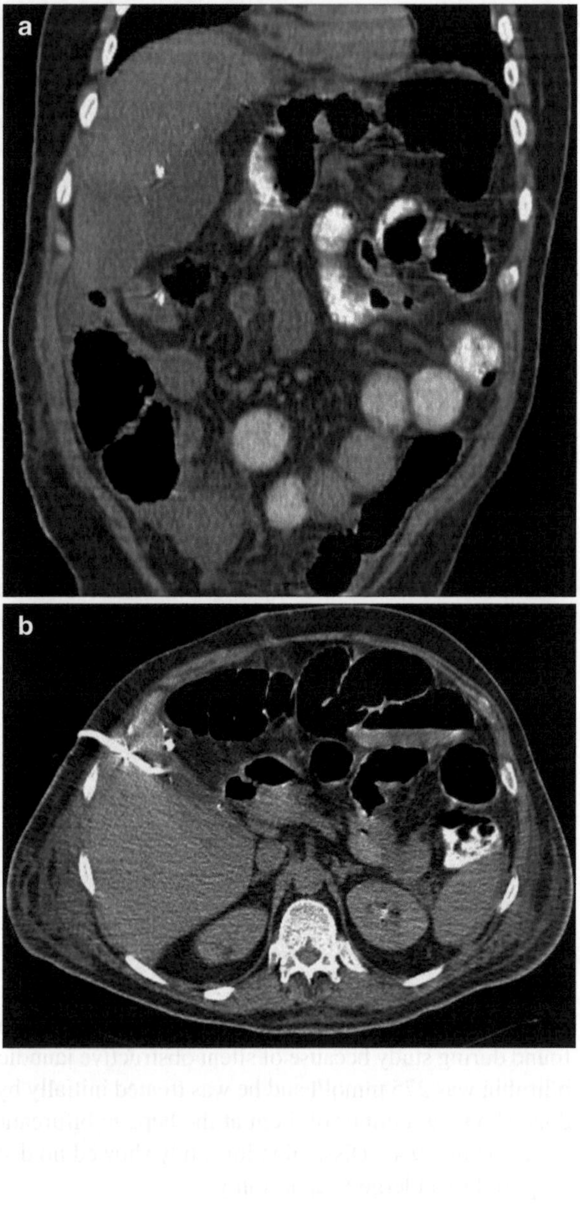

Fig. 39.5 (**a**) CT scan revealing subfrenic and paracolic abscess. (**b**) Abscess drained

Pathology

Mass forming cholangiocarcinoma, 6 cm, radical resected, with important perineural and intraneural growth. Obstructive cholangitis.

Postoperative Course: Identification and Treatment of the Complication

From the beginning bile leakage was seen in the drain. Patient was doing well and conservative treatment was established. In the fifth day he developed fever and shivering. Under diagnosis of acute cholangitis or intra-abdominal abscess, a CT scan revealed an abscess on the hepatic surface and paracolic space right (Fig. 39.5a). A percutaneous drainage was performed (Fig. 39.5b) An ERCP with stenting was done without decreasing the bile production. Situation became stable, but one week later patient developed again high fever and abdominal pain. Patient was admitted to the Medium Care ward and a new CT scan revealed a new abscess, being percutaneously drained. Drain produced 600-800 per day but stools color was normal. Patient was well and stable and went home with the drain. After two weeks, production decreased progressively and the drain could be retired.

Chapter 40
Case on Postoperative Bleeding After Whipple Procedure

Miguel A. Cuesta and Suzanne S. Gisbertz

Keywords Whipple procedure • Peutz Jegher syndrome • Intraabdominal bleeding

First Patient

Postoperative Intraluminal Bleeding Diagnosis and Indication for Surgery

A 40-year-old male patient was sent to the emergency department because of obstructive jaundice and abdominal pain. The US and CT scan with double contrast revealed a possible stone in the papilla of Vater with intrahepatic biliary duct dilatation (Fig. 40.1); consequently, an ERCP was proposed. On the ERCP, a polyp mass was found at duodenum, and a stent was introduced through papilla for bile drainage (Fig. 40.2). Biopsies were taken. Moreover, multiple small polyps were seen in the stomach. The possibility of a familial polyposis coli was considered but not confirmed by family history. Post ERCP, the patient developed progressive abdominal pain in the whole abdomen with signs of intestinal obstruction. On the CT scan, an invagination of a big polyp in the small bowel was seen and the patient was operated on. On operation, multiple polyps were palpated in the small bowel and colon. The invaginated part of ileum was resected and a primary side-to-side anastomosis was done. Diagnosis was established as Peutz Jegher syndrome.

M.A. Cuesta, M.D. (✉)
Department of Surgery, VU University Medical Center, Amsterdam, The Netherlands
e-mail: ma.cuesta@vumc.nl

S.S. Gisbertz, M.D.
Department of Surgery, Academic Medical Center, Amsterdam, The Netherlands
e-mail: s.gisbertz@antoniusziekenhuis.nl

M.A. Cuesta, H.J. Bonjer (eds.), *Case Studies of Postoperative Complications after Digestive Surgery*, DOI 10.1007/978-3-319-01613-9_40,

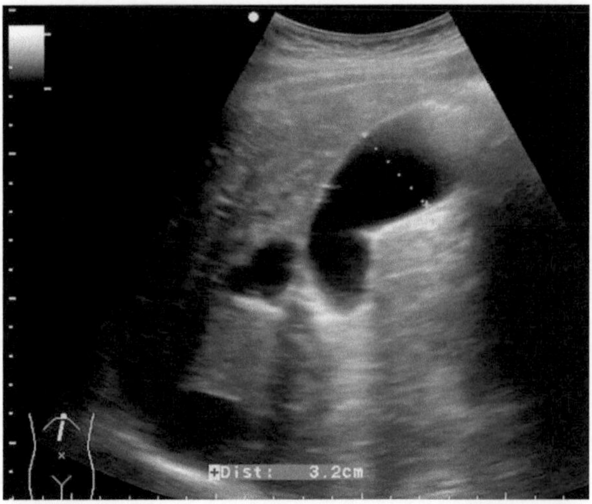

Fig. 40.1 US showing a dilated CBD of 2 cm

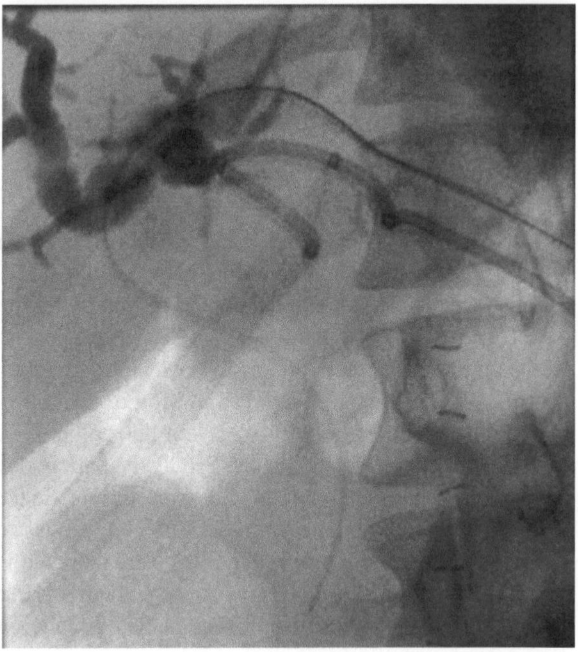

Fig. 40.2 ERCP and sphincterotomy, stop distal CBD, placement of a stent

Operation

CT scan and MRI enteroclysis showed a huge polypoid mass in duodenum and in the small bowel and colon (Figs. 40.3 and 40.4). Policy was executed as treating the multiple polyps in steps, starting with the duodenum. Two attempts were undertaken for resecting the huge polyps by duodenoscopy, but this was considered

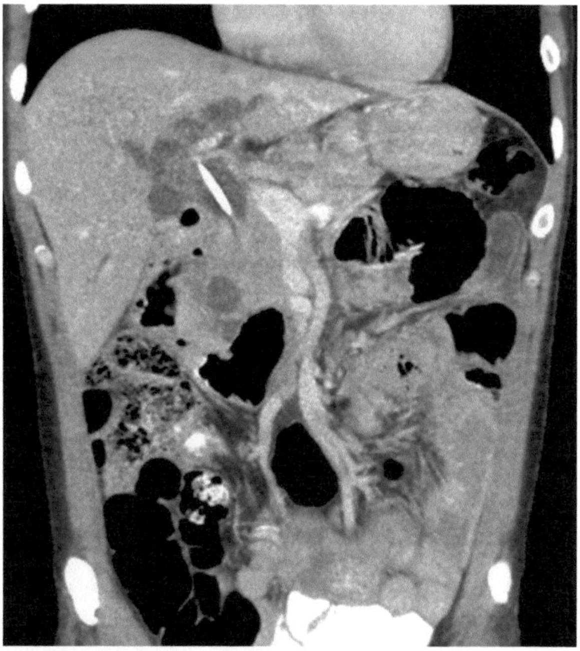

Fig. 40.3 CT scan, mass in duodenum with stent in the CBD

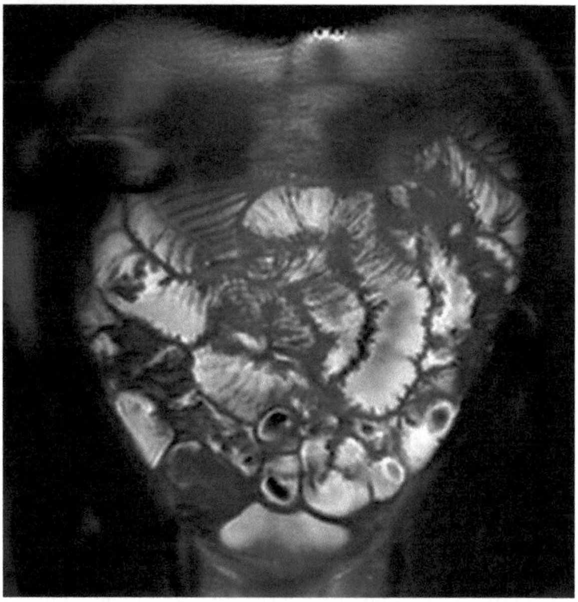

Fig. 40.4 MRI enteroclysis, polyps in jejunum and ileum

unfeasible. Despite a benign histological examination, the possibility of malignancy was considered and a transduodenal polypectomy or a Whipple procedure by laparotomy was decided on. Through subcostal laparotomy, locally resecting the huge

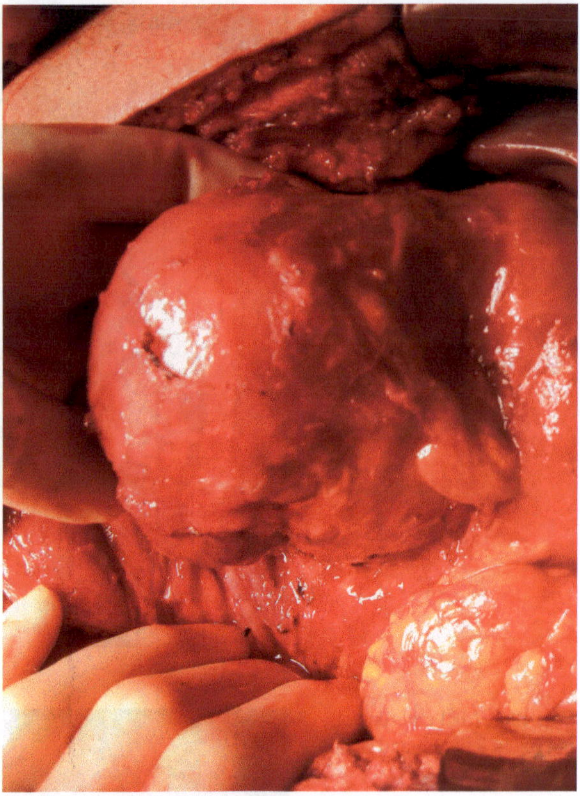

Fig. 40.5 Duodenum aspect during Whipple operation

tumor was considered unachievable without Whipple operation (Fig. 40.5). A duodenopancreatectomy was performed without technical problems and after operation patient was admitted to the general ward.

Postoperative Course: Identification and Treatment of the Complication

Two hours later, the patient started with hematemesis and become hemodynamically unstable. The on duty surgeon decided to reoperate directly due to abundant bleeding and hemodynamic instability. At laparotomy, a dilated gastric remnant was found with dilatation of the loop to the pancreas as produced by clots. The anastomosis to the pancreas was performed end to side and we opened the end loop of the anastomosis in order to inspect first the pancreaticojejunostomy. There was bleeding at the capsule of the pancreas, and we could fix it by means of stitches. The opening was closed in transversal direction in two layers and the stomach emptied of clots.

Pathology

Pathology examination of the specimen showed benign polyps typical for Peutz Jegher syndrome. Patient recovered well after this reoperation and 6 months later he was again operated to remove the small bowel polyps, endoscopically assisted by the gastroenterologist. All polyps were proven to be benign and patient is doing well. The rest of the colon polyps will be resected by colonoscopy program. The patient has no progeny but a genetic study has been performed regarding himself and family members.

Second Patient

Postoperative Intraabdominal Bleeding After Whipple Procedure

Diagnosis and Indication for Surgery

A 69-year-old female patient was evaluated because of silent obstruction jaundice. She had a pancreatic head tumor with double duct lesion suspect for carcinoma and because of a bilirubin less than 150 U/ml, a direct surgical exploration was carried out without previous drainage of the biliary duct.

Operation

A Whipple operation was performed without technical problems and the blood loss was 300 cc.

Postoperative Course: Identification and Treatment of the Complication

She went to the Medium Care Department and after a couple of hours, her blood pressure decreased to 70/40 mm Hg and her hemoglobin and hematocrit decreased 2 points to 5 and 23 % respectively. Coagulation tests were normal.

Her abdomen was painful and lightly distended and clots occluded the left drain.

After diagnosis of postoperative bleeding, a relaparotomy through the subcostal incision was again performed.

Especially in the subhepatic space, 1.5 L blood with clots were found. Inspection showed two venous bleeding points along the portal vein. These were sutured with care in order to maintain the pancreatic and biliary anastomosis without any changes.

A new drain was left in the subhepatic space and patient recovered without complications.

Comments

The lesson in these two patients with immediate postoperative bleeding after a Whipple procedure and hemodynamically instability is that an emergency relaparotomy can fix the problem. Important is that the same surgeon who did the operation will perform the reoperation.

Discussion

Postoperative hemorrhage is another serious complication after pancreatic resection with incidence rates varying from 2 to 20 % and mortality rates exceeding 50 % [1–3]. The variability in incidence and mortality is partly caused by the many different definitions that are being used. The International Study Group of Pancreatic Surgery (ISGPS) developed a definition and proposed the term postpancreatectomy hemorrhage (PPH) [2]. They classified postoperative bleeding based on three criteria: time of onset: early PPH occurring within 24 h postoperatively and late PPH >24 h; location: intraluminal or extraluminal; and severity and impact: mild PPH with a similar clinical impairment and severe PPH with sequential blood transfusions and radiological and/or surgical interventions.

Since the introduction of the ISGPS hemorrhage classification, a number of studies validated the scoring system which is currently generally accepted [3, 4].

Diagnosis and grading. Patients who develop PPH may present with hypotension, tachycardia, decreasing haemoglobin concentration, clinical deterioration, or blood loss through gastrointestinal tract or abdominal drains depending on the site of the bleeding: intraluminal or extraluminal.

Intraluminal bleeding is seen near the anastomotic site, vessels in that area, the surface of the pancreas, or near a gastric ulcus. It generally presents with blood loss through the gastrointestinal tract being hematemesis and melena and blood loss through the nasogastric tube. Intraluminal bleeding will usually manifest as an early hemorrhage. Consensus has been reached considering the cause of early hemorrhage which is likely due to technical failures during the index operation. In the case of intraluminal hemorrhage, endoscopy can be very useful since diagnosing and managing an anastomotic bleeding can be performed simultaneously. Angiography can be used to embolize bleeding from vessels. A recent analysis showed that angiography was performed in over 50 % of patients with PPH after pancreatic surgery and 18 % was subjected to an endoscopy. Both procedures were initially performed to detect the bleeding site [5]. All diagnostic interventions were performed provided that the patient was in a stable hemodynamic condition.

Extraluminal bleeding is seen in the abdominal cavity and may be evident by blood loss through the abdominal drain. The bleeding is caused by vascular erosion, anastomotic ulceration, arterial pseudoaneurysm, or disrupted suture-line caused by POPF, biliary leakage, or intra-abdominal infections and generally present as late PPH. When PPH is suspected, ultrasonography and CT can detect intra-abdominal collections (hematoma as well as abscesses) seen in 70–80 % in late PPH. Furthermore, both procedures can detect pseudoaneurysms. The diagnosis is confirmed by angiography [6].

Management and Outcome

Severe PPH asks for immediate treatment through either radiological intervention, e.g. angiography with embolisation or endoscopy with clips or sclerotherapy, or surgical intervention when the patients' condition is deteriorating rapidly or radiological interventions are unsuccessful or infeasible.

In a recent study on PPH 38 % of patients underwent primary surgery, 57 % underwent primary radiological intervention and 5 % was treated conservatively. More than half of the radiological interventions (54 %) were unsuccessful and a rescue laparotomy still had to be performed. The success rate of radiological coiling in terms of hemostasis was 80 % [5]. In this study endoscopic intervention was used in patients with early intraluminal bleeding realizing that a PJ bleeding generally is outside the reach of endoscopy but can also be managed by interventional angiography. Intraluminal bleeding can disrupt the anastomosis causing a "false" extraluminal bleed since blood is than seen in the abdominal cavity. Early extraluminal PPH (within 24 h after surgery) is generally managed immediately with relaparotomy.

Management of late PPH is different since it is often caused by pseudoaneurysms due to POPF or intra-abdominal infections. An earlier study conducted at the AMC showed that 69 % of patients with late PPH underwent primary surgery and only 9 % was managed by radiological embolisation. In half of all the surgical procedures a vessel ligation was performed. Completion pancreatectomy was performed because of persistent anastomotic leakage [6].

More recently embolisation is performed in the majority of patients.

A meta-analysis regarding the management of late PPH after PD showed 20 small case series with 163 patients in which 47.2 % of patients underwent primary surgery, 44.8 % underwent primary radiological intervention and 8 % was treated conservatively. No significant differences were found regarding to morbidity or mortality between relaparotomy and radiological intervention. Though late haemorrhage is often already associated with other complications, in particular leakage and sepsis, as mentioned earlier this combination is associated with a poor prognosis [7].

The pathophysiology of early PPH makes its management less complicated with better outcomes compared to late PPH. Identifying the importance of a sentinel bleed and an adequate aggressive approach towards the patients' clinical status will dictate the appropriate treatment. More research is needed to offer any standardized rules in the management of PPH.

References

1. Tol JAMG, van Gulik TM, Busch ORC, Gouma DJ. Prevention and treatment of major complications after duodeno-pancreatic head surgery. In: Cuesta MA, Bonjer HJ, editors. Treatment of complications after digestive surgery, chapter 14. London: Springer; 2013.
2. Wente MN, Veit JA, Bassi C, Dervenis C, et al. Postpancreatectomy hemorrhage (PPH): an International Study Group of Pancreatic Surgery (ISGPS) definition. Surgery. 2007;142:20–5.
3. Jagad RB, Koshariya M, Kawamoto J, et al. Postoperative hemorrhage after major pancreatobiliary surgery: an update. Hepatogastroenterology. 2008;55:729–37.
4. Puppala S, Patel J, McPherson S, et al. Hemorrhagic complications after Whipple surgery: imaging and radiologic intervention. AJR Am J Roentgenol. 2011;196:192–7.
5. Yekebas EF, Wolfram L, Cataldegirmen G, et al. Postpancreatectomy hemorrhage: diagnosis and treatment: an analysis in 1669 consecutive pancreatic resections. Ann Surg. 2007;246:269–80.
6. de Castro SM, Kuhlmann KF, Busch OR, et al. Delayed massive hemorrhage after pancreatic and biliary surgery: embolization or surgery? Ann Surg. 2005;241:85–91.
7. Limongelli P, Khorsandi SE, Pai M, et al. Management of delayed postoperative hemorrhage after pancreaticoduodenectomy: a meta-analysis. Arch Surg. 2008;143:1001–7.

Chapter 41
Case on Leakage of the Pancreato-Jejunostomy After a Whipple Procedure

Suzanne S. Gisbertz

Keywords Leakage • Pancreato-jejunostomy • Whipple • Duodenopancreatectomy • Leakage pancreatojejunostomy

Diagnosis and Indication for Surgery

A 72-year-old female patient was analyzed for silent jaundice and itchiness since 3 weeks. Her medical history revealed surgery for kidney stones and spinal disc hernia, hypertension, and dyslipidaemia, for which she used medication. Physical examination showed jaundice, scratch effects on the skin, and a palpable, non-tender gallbladder (Courvoisier's sign). Laboratory testing showed elevated levels of bilirubin, AF, and g-GT. Ultrasound, CT scan, and endoscopic ultrasound showed a double duct sign, with both dilated bile and pancreatic ducts. No masses or enlarged lymph nodes were identified. ERCP showed a normal papilla Vateri, and a distal obstruction was observed in the common bile duct. Because of high bilirubin rate >150 U/ml, a sphincterotomy was performed, followed by introduction of an endoprosthesis in order to drain the biliary duct before operation. Since no metastases were identified, this patient was scheduled for a Whipple procedure.

Operation

A duodenopancreatectomy according to Whi pple was performed, with and an end-side pancreaticojejunostomy, an end-side hepaticojejunostomy, and an end-side gastrojejunostomy. A low vacuum drain was placed at the anastomotic sides.

S.S. Gisbertz, M.D.
Department of Surgery, Academic Medical centre, Amsterdam, The Netherlands
e-mail: s.gisbertz@antoniusziekenhuis.nl

M.A. Cuesta, H.J. Bonjer (eds.), *Case Studies of Postoperative Complications after Digestive Surgery*, DOI 10.1007/978-3-319-01613-9_41,

Pathology

The surgical resection specimen showed a radical resected well-differentiated ductal adenocarcinoma with a maximum diameter of 2.8 cm. No lymph node metastases were identified. Therefore, the TNM classification was pT3N0M0.

Postoperative Course: Identification and Treatment of the Complication

The first 5 postoperative days were uneventful. On the 6th postoperative day, the patient clinically deteriorated. She developed abdominal pain, fever, and a tachycardia. Laboratory research showed a leukocytosis and elevated levels of C-reactive protein. An abdominal CT scan showed free fluid around the anastomoses and both left and right paracolic (Fig. 41.1a–c). A percutaneous drain was placed in the right paracolic space. The aspect was serous, and the amylase level was low (135 U/L). Additionally, broad-spectrum antibiotics were given intravenously and adjusted after positive cultures. Despite this treatment, the patient did not recover, and on the 10th, 13th, and 18th day, additional percutaneous drainages were performed subhepatic (amylase 9,503 U/L), left subfrenic and in the right lower quadrant (amylase 290 U/L), and left paracolic (amylase level not determined), respectively. Furthermore, a percutaneous transhepatic cholangiography (PTC) was performed on the 18th postoperative day, with the tip of the catheter through the hepaticojejunostomy (Figs. 41.2, 41.3 and Illustration 41.1). On the 24th day, the amylase drain fluid level reached its peak of 21,998 U/L. The first cultures of the drain fluids notably showed the same bacteria as on the peroperative bile culture: enterococcus species and *Candida albicans*. On the 27th day, blood was suddenly observed at the subhepatic drain. A CT-angiography and angiography did not show the source of bleeding and the problem spontaneously resolved. The patient remained hemodynamically stable throughout this episode. Slowly she could recover and regain strength with the aid of physical therapy and nutritional support. Eventually, she was discharged without any drains on the 49th postoperative day. Subsequently, she was readmitted twice with abdominal pain and fever based on an intra-abdominal abscess, treated with percutaneous drainage. On her last outpatient visit, 10 months after the initial operation, she displayed no symptoms of disease and no signs of recurrence. She regained her old weight, did not develop diabetes, but she does use pancreatic enzyme supplements.

Discussion

This patient with leakage from the pancreaticojejunostomy was treated with multiple percutaneous drainages, PTC, and antibiotics, without the need for surgical reintervention.

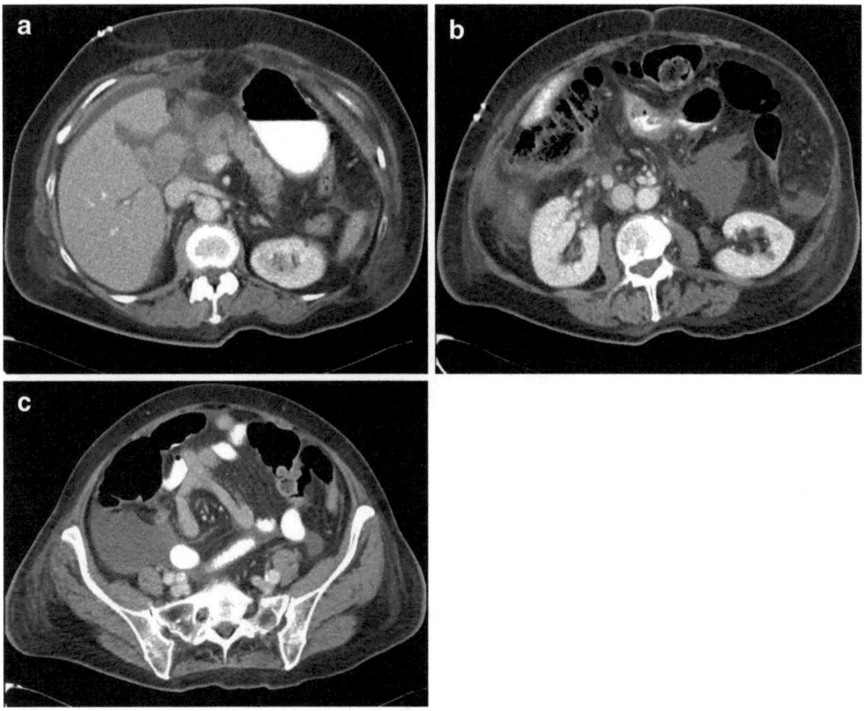

Fig. 41.1 (**a**) CT scan, Leakage of the pancreaticojejunostomy. (**b**) CT scan, Intra-abdominal free fluid. (**c**) CT scan, free fluid in the right paracolic space

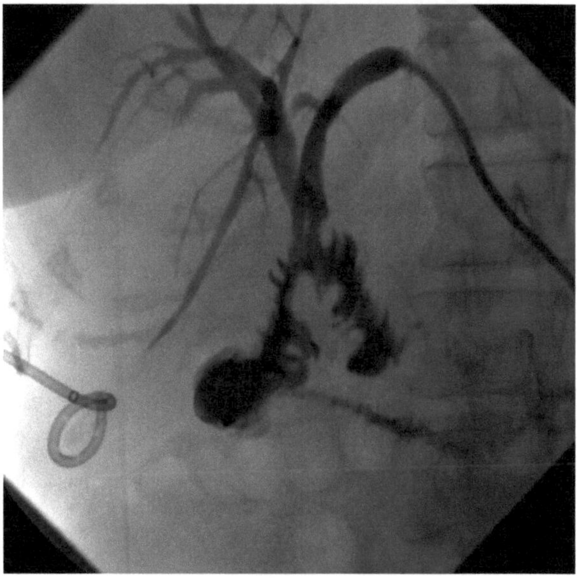

Fig. 41.2 Two percutaneous drains: a PTC drain and a subhepatic drain

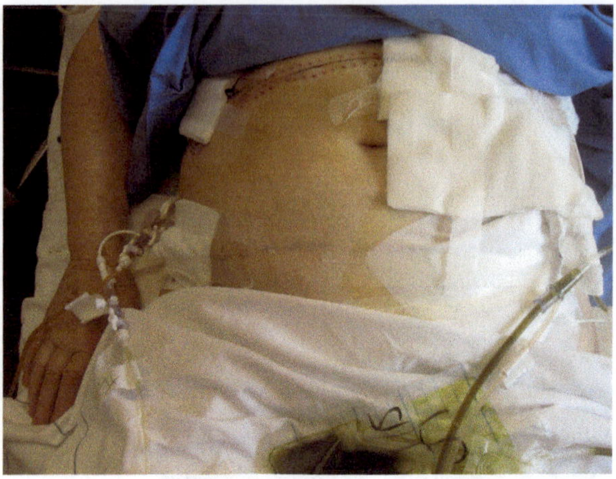

Fig. 41.3 Percutaneous transhepatic cholangiography (PTC) on the 18th postoperative day

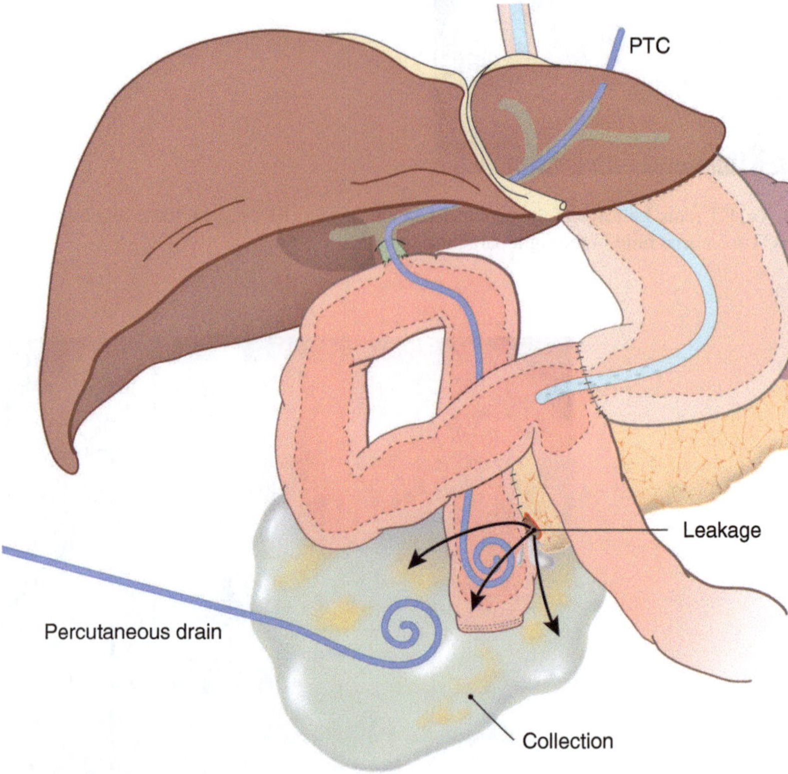

Illustration 41.1 Once diagnosed the leakage of the pancreaticojejunostomy, collection should be drained percutaneously, along a PTC drain placed in front of the anastomosis for drainage

Chapter 42
Case on Bile Leakage (and Portal Vein Thrombosis) After Whipple Procedure

Miguel A. Cuesta

Keywords Bile leakage • Portal vein thrombosis • Whipple procedure • Pancreatic head cancer

Diagnosis and Indication for Surgery

A 67-year-old female patient was referred because of a pancreatic head-uncinate process tumor with obstructive jaundice and pain in her back. She had already lost 6 kg. Concerning her back pain, she could not explain clearly if this pain was different from the chronic pain she had felt for years. US and CT scan and ERCP revealed a tumor locally invasive with no clear encasement of the superior mesenteric vein. Preoperatively, biliary tract was drained by means of sphincterotomy and stent. Biopsy showed adenocarcinoma and patient was scheduled for explorative laparotomy.

Operation

During subcostal laparotomy, a Whipple resection was performed with a wedge resection of the junction between the superior mesenteric and portal vein, because of small ingrowth of the tumor. The vein was closed in horizontal direction without necessity of a patch or mobilization.

M.A. Cuesta, M.D.
Department of Surgery, VU University Medical Center, Amsterdam, The Netherlands
e-mail: ma.cuesta@vumc.nl

M.A. Cuesta, H.J. Bonjer (eds.), *Case Studies of Postoperative Complications after Digestive Surgery*, DOI 10.1007/978-3-319-01613-9_42,

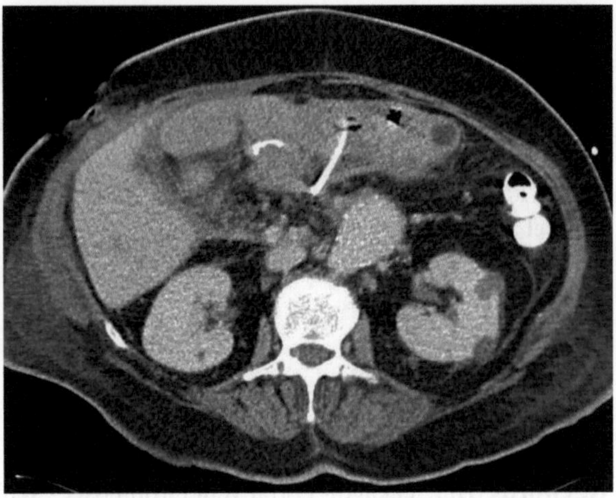

Fig. 42.1 CT scan, PTC drainage and open wound

Postoperative Course: Identification and Treatment of the Complication

Postoperatively, she experienced several complications. First, deep wound infection with biliary leakage through the wound, along the subhepatic drain, necessating exploration and debridement under general anesthesia. Here, drains were left in the subhepatic region and the wound was left open for adequate drainage. A PTC drainage was performed to drain conveniently the leakage of the hepaticojejunostomy (Fig. 42.1 and Illustration 42.1). Patient remained low grade septic; after blood cultures she was given broad spectrum antibiotics. Bleeding of the upper digestive tract was suspected because of melena, being diagnosed by gastroscopy as having an important hemorrhagic gastritis, and was treated by a stop of prophylactic heparin, correction of coagulation tests, and by proton inhibitors medication. Patient was initially treated by TPN and afterwards by jejunal tube feeding. A new control CT showed a portal vein thrombosis with hypoperfusion of the whole liver (Fig. 42.2). Radiological thrombectomy was considered but due to the general condition of patient, we decided to start carefully with anticoagulation by means of subcutan heparin. Situation of the patient incrementally improved and after a period of 2 months, she could be dismissed with a still open abdominal wound while having no more bile leakage.

Two years later patient appeared doing reasonably well with continuing back pain yet stable weight. CT scans requested by the gastroenterologist showed different kinds of enlarged lymph nodes in the subhepatic area, but no signs of local recurrence. The early diagnosed aneurysm in the infrarenal abdominal aorta has grown up to 6 cm and vascular surgeon has recently treated this aneurysm successfully by means of endovascular aneurysm repair (EVAR).

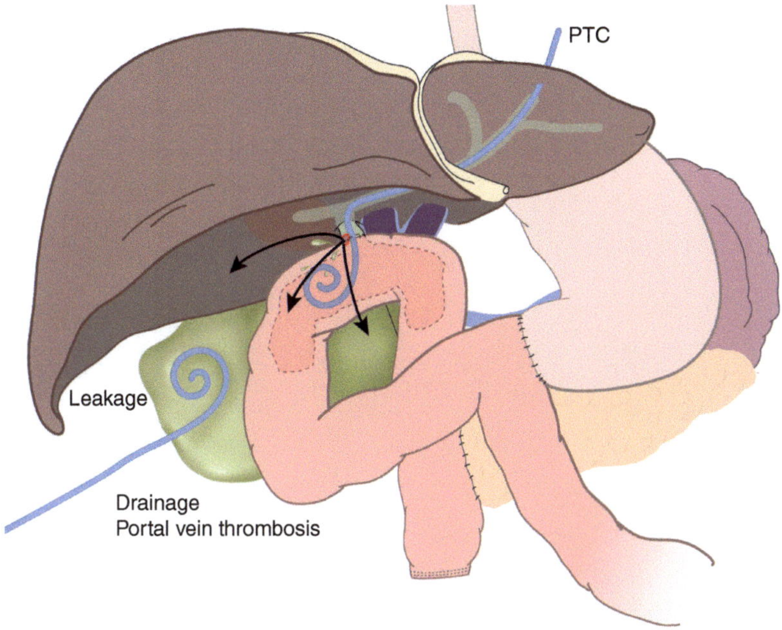

Illustration 42.1 Leakage of the hepaticojejunostomy has been shown treated by PTC and percutaneous drainage of the subhepatic collection. Moreover, the portal vein thrombosis with impaired irrigation of liver was treated conservatively with success

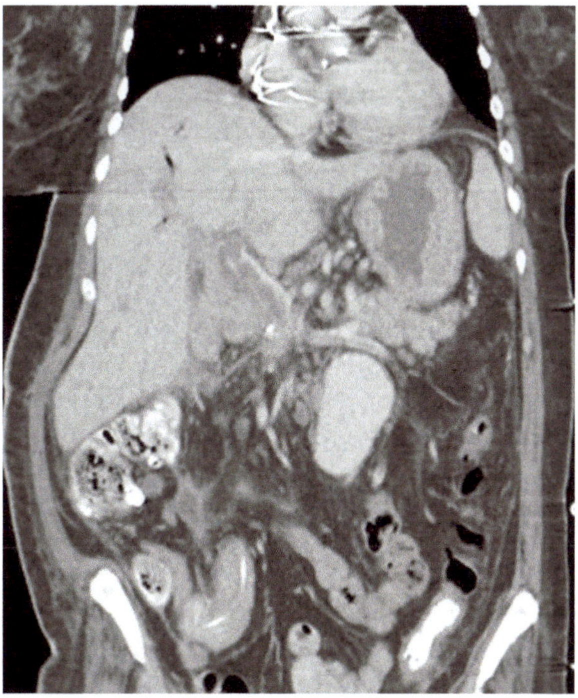

Fig. 42.2 CT scan, portal vein thrombosis and subhepatic collection

Chapter 43
Case on Bleeding in the Small Remnant of the Head of the Pancreas After Duodenum Preserving Resection for Middle Pancreatic Tumor

Suzanne S. Gisbertz and Rutger J. Lely

Keywords Pancreatic Cystadenoma • Laparoscopic TME • Rectum cancer • Pancreatic resection • Whipple operation

Diagnosis and Indication for Surgery

A 68-year-old man presented with blood in feces and tenesmus and was diagnosed with a mid-rectal cancer 8 cm from the anal verge. During screening for metastases, a cystadenoma of the junction between pancreatic head and body of pancreas was found on the CT scan (Fig. 43.1).

Operation

After radiotherapy, 5×5 Grays, he underwent 6 weeks later a laparoscopic TME with LAR. The specimen was radical, T2N0M0 with a response Mandard type 2. Protective ileostomy was closed 6 weeks after operation without complications.

Deliberation began when to operate the cystadenomatous pancreatic lesion.

Three months later, it was decided to operate the lesion by means of a median upper laparotomy. After dissection of the pancreas, a central pancreatectomy was performed, leaving a small strip of the head of the pancreas with the duodenum

S.S. Gisbertz, M.D. (✉)
Department of Surgery, Academic Medical Centre, Amsterdam, The Netherlands
e-mail: s.gisbertz@antoniusziekenhuis.nl

R.J. Lely, M.D.
Department of Radiology, VU Medical Center, Amsterdam, The Netherlands
e-mail: r.lelij@vumc.nl

M.A. Cuesta, H.J. Bonjer (eds.), *Case Studies of Postoperative Complications after Digestive Surgery*, DOI 10.1007/978-3-319-01613-9_43,

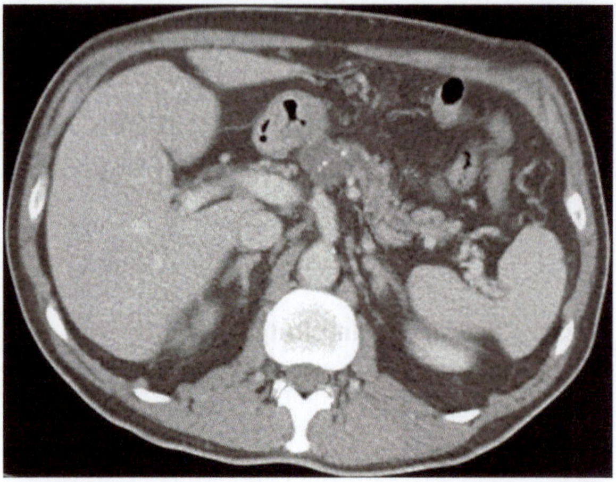

Fig. 43.1 Preoperative CT scan with tumor in the pancreas

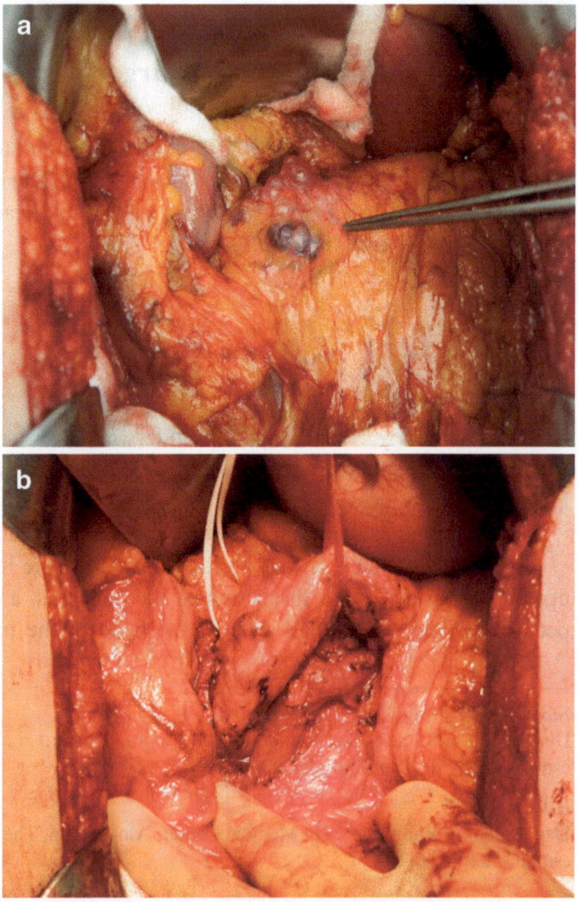

Fig. 43.2 (**a**) Aspect of the tumor during laparotomy. (**b**) Dissection of pancreas

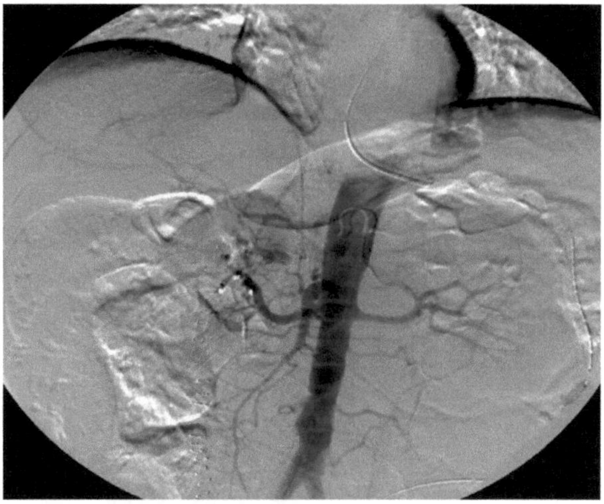

Fig. 43.3 Angiography and blush at the duodenum

being sutured. The start of the pancreas was anastomosed, end to side by means of a Roux-en-Y anastomosis (Fig. 43.2a, b). Pathology showed a serous cystadenoma of 5 cm, radical resected.

Postoperative Course: Identification and Treatment of the Complication

Patient recovered well and went home. The day after the first control at the outpatient clinic, he was admitted to the emergency department because of hematemesis and melena.

Evaluation by emergency gastroscopy and by CT angiography showed that the bleeding was caused (blush) in the small rest of the head of the pancreas (Figs. 43.3 and 43.4)

An attempt to coil the bleeding site—the bleeding probably coming from pancreaticoduodenal arteries—was considered impossible because the celiac trunk was seriously stenosed/obstructed (Illustration 43.1). A second attempt to coil the bleeding through the superior mesenteric artery was also considered impossible because of the difficult angle to localize the bleeding point.

Due to hemodynamic instability, it was decided to perform a relaparotomy and devascularize the head of the pancreas. Some arteries were found around the duodenum and were subsequently fixed with stitches. Next day, bleeding recurred again with hemodynamic instability in spite of coagulation correction and transfusions and a relaparotomy was decided on. A clot of 7 cm was found near the second and third part of duodenum and rest of pancreas with active bleeding present, and so we decided to perform an acute Whipple resection. Anatomy was difficult to recognize, especially the relation with the superior mesenteric vessels. Anastomosis with the common hepatic duct and the stomach was completed.

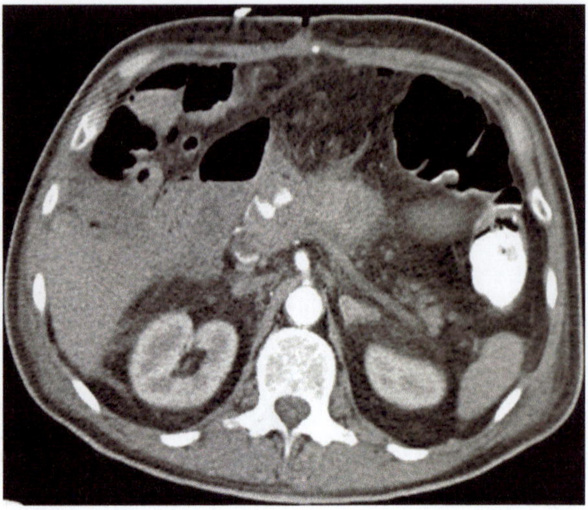

Fig. 43.4 Clots and bleeding at the duodenum–pancreas rest

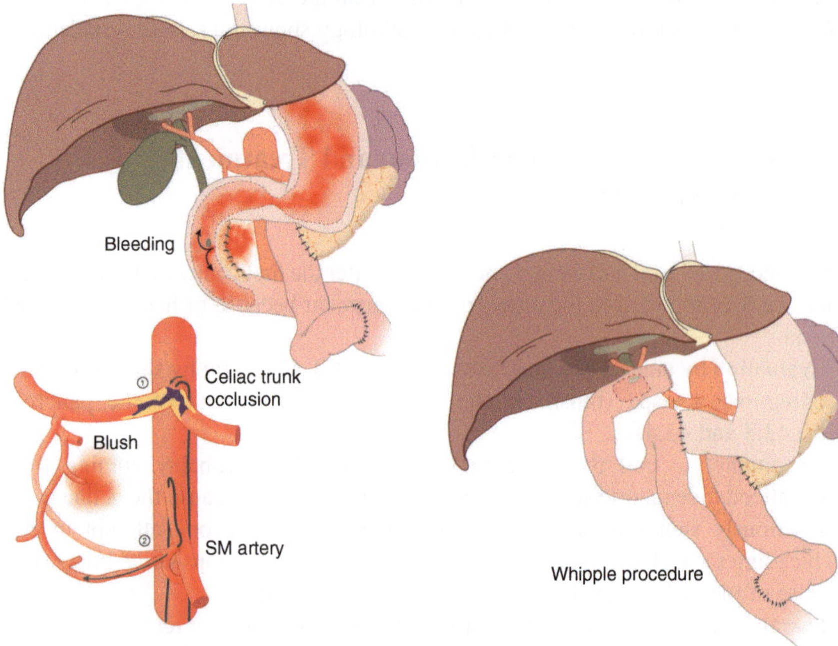

Illustration 43.1 Bleeding of the remnant of the pancreas head. Angiography and coiling were not possible because of occlusion of the celiac trunk

Patient was ventilated on the IC, yet was hemodynamically stable. After 2 days he could be disconnected from mechanical ventilation. Pathology showed rest of necrotizing pancreatitis with fat necrosis. He recovered and after 2 years is doing very well.

Chapter 44
Case on Impaction of Enteral (Bezoars) During Enteral Feeding After Whipple Procedure

Miguel A. Cuesta

Keywords Whipple • Bezoar • Impacted • Jejunostomy • Pancreatic head cancer • Enteral nutrition

Diagnosis and Indication for Surgery

An 80-year-old man, in good general condition, was referred to us for a Whipple operation because of pancreatic head cancer. He had lost seven kg weight. On CT scan and ERCP a double duct sign became visible. Due to very high bilirubin values and itching, a stent was placed after sphincterotomy.

Operation

The Whipple resection occurred without problems, and the patient was fed postoperatively by means of a jejunostomy tube placed during the operation.

Postoperative Course: Identification and Treatment of the Complication

In the first postoperative days, 1.5 l high fiber feeding was administered by jejunostomy along with some oral feeding. On the seventh postoperative day, the patient suddenly became septic, experiencing general abdominal pain and vomiting.

M.A. Cuesta, M.D.
Department of Surgery, VU University Medical Center, Amsterdam, The Netherlands
e-mail: ma.cuesta@vumc.nl

M.A. Cuesta, H.J. Bonjer (eds.), *Case Studies of Postoperative Complications after Digestive Surgery*, DOI 10.1007/978-3-319-01613-9_44,

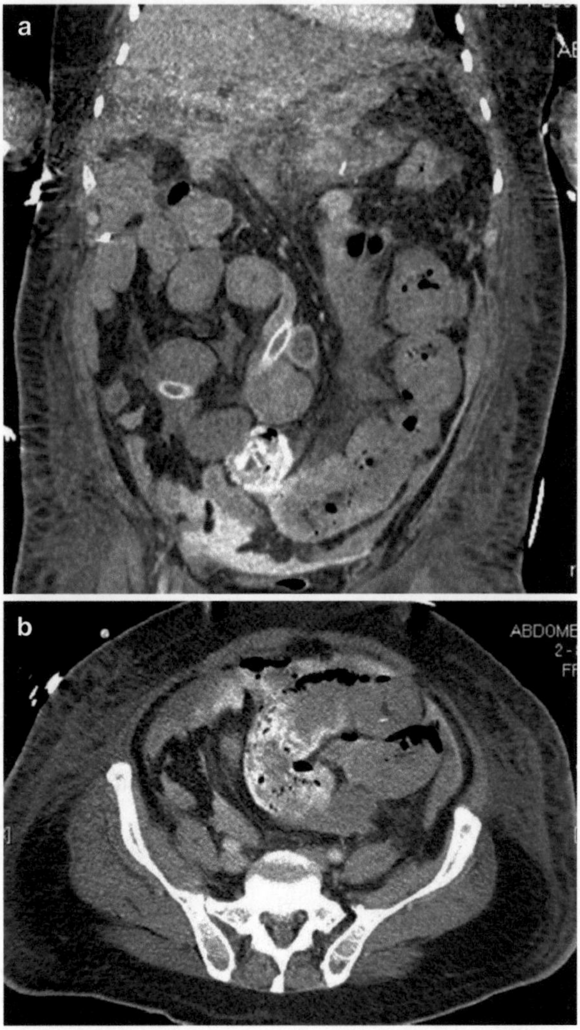

Fig. 44.1 (**a**, **b**) CT scan showing impaction of intestinal contents, ischemia of the wall, and leakage of contrast in peritoneal cavity

A CT scan showed impaction of intestinal contents, ischemia in the intestinal wall, and leakage of contrast in peritoneal cavity (Fig. 44.1a, b). Decision was taken to operate the patient immediately.

During relaparotomy, an impaction of the high fiber feeding (bezoars) was found in the small bowel in a length of 50 cm, middle jejunum with dilatation, and necrosis (Figs. 44.2 and 44.3). Proximal and distal jejunum and ileum were dilated but considered well vascularized. The impacted necrotic bowel segment was resected and primary anastomosis followed. Despite risk of leakages, the patient could be weaned from the mechanical ventilation. After a slow recovery and rehabilitation, he went home.

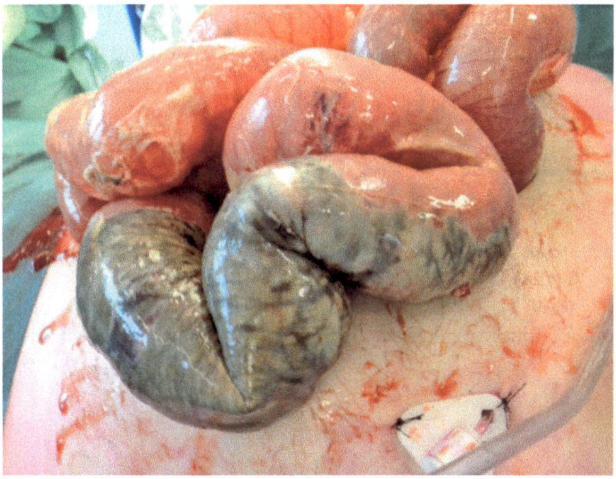

Fig. 44.2 During laparotomy, ischemia/necrosis small bowel

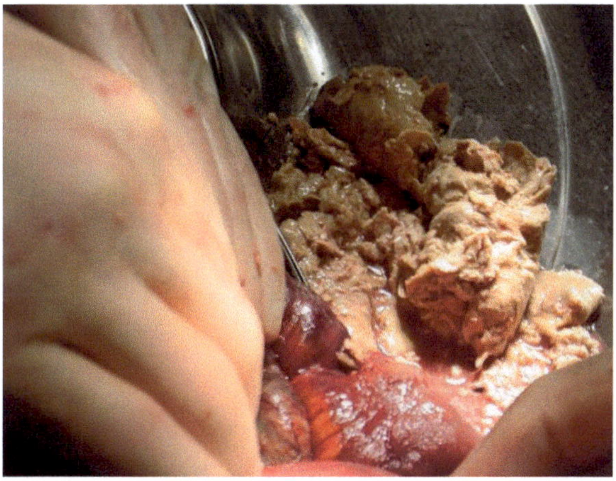

Fig. 44.3 Extraction of bezoar from the bowel

Discussion

Several reports have described different complications in the early postoperative period in relation to enteral synthetic feeding through jejunostomy. Not only intestinal obstruction but also bowel necrosis has been reported. In our patient, in the period between fifth and seventh postoperative days, an intestinal obstruction and a septic situation led to a relaparotomy. At relaparotomy an impacted bezoar of enteral feeding was found as cause for the obstruction and ischemia. This bezoar may have been caused by denatured nutrition formula distal to the catheter tip [1]. Possible relation with high fiber enteral feeding has been also discussed. Explaining the cause of mesenteric ischemia with bowel necrosis proved more difficult. Mesenteric ischemia may present in up to 3.5 % of all enteral-fed surgical patients [2] and associated mortality approaches almost

100 %. A high index of suspicion for diagnosis is necessary. As in our case, prompt relaparotomy and bowel resection provided the only chance for survival.

References

1. Dedes KJ, Schiesser M, Schafer M, Clavien PA. Postoperative bezoar ileus after early enteral feeding. J Gastrointest Surg. 2006;10:123–7.
2. Melis M, Fichera A, Ferguson MK. Bowel necrosis associated with early jejunal tube feeding: A complication of postoperative enteral nutrition. Arch Surg. 2006;141:701–4.

Chapter 45
Case on Gastric Bleeding Caused by a Necrotizing Pancreatitis with Extensive Pseudocyst Formation

Rutger J. Lely and Miguel A. Cuesta

Keywords Pancreatitis • Pseudocyst • Pancreatitis • Pseudoaneurysm • Splenic artery • Gastroduodenal artery

Diagnosis and Indication for Surgery

A 32-year-old law student known with a severe systemic lupus erythematosus (SLE- like) disease had been treated with high doses of prednisone and supportive care. Now she was admitted in the hospital, at first on the gastroenterology Department and after on the Medium Care because of progressive abdominal pain, hypotension, elevated amylase, and lipase in serum. After fluid reposition, a CT scan with double contrast was performed showing an extensive acute necrotizing pancreatitis.

Course and Identification of the Complication

After conservative treatment, there initially was clinical improvement. Because no signs were seen of infection, she was conservatively treated by means of nasogastric tube, initially total parenteral nutrition, and broad-spectrum antibiotics. Situation of patient evolved unchanged for 4 weeks, with the usual ups and downs. Pneumonia

R.J. Lely, M.D. (✉)
Department of Radiology, VU Medical Center, Amsterdam, The Netherlands
e-mail: r.lelij@vumc.nl

M.A. Cuesta, M.D.
Department of Surgery, VU University Medical Center, Amsterdam, The Netherlands
e-mail: ma.cuesta@vumc.nl

M.A. Cuesta, H.J. Bonjer (eds.), *Case Studies of Postoperative Complications after Digestive Surgery*, DOI 10.1007/978-3-319-01613-9_45,

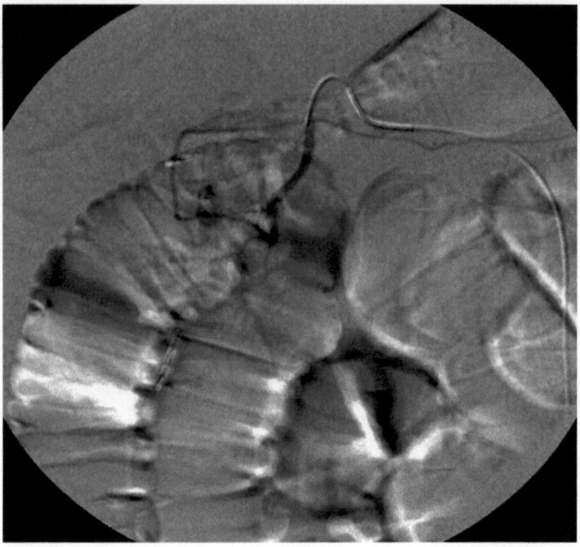

Fig. 45.1 Identification bleeding splenic artery during angiography

was diagnosed and consequently treated. Moreover, CT scans showed the necrosis with pseudocysts in lesser sac, along the pancreas in the direction of the spleen and descending colon. Abdomen of the patient was distended and many doctors involved with her treatment pushed surgeon and radiologist to drain the cysts because of mechanical complaints such as abdominal distention and threatening respiratory insufficiency. Pseudocysts were not drained, but 5 weeks after admission she developed an important hematemesis and melena with hypovolemic shock. Taking into regard gastric bleeding from a rupture of a pseudoaneurysm of the splenic artery, a CT angiography was performed, where a blush was seen at splenic artery and subsequently angiography was performed. A bleeding was observed at the middle level of the splenic artery with leakage of blood at the level of the greater curvature, thereafter being successfully coiled (Figs. 45.1, 45.2, 45.3, and 45.4; Illustration 45.1). Bleeding was under control, but patient stayed for 8 weeks, at first admitted on medium care, thereafter on intensive care because mechanical ventilation proved needed, and finally back to the ward. She went on for revalidation because of an important neuropathy. After 4 months, she was again admitted with recurrent acute pancreatitis. Currently, she can walk with crutches and she has partially reinitiated her activities, still following physiotherapy.

Discussion

The lesson in this case is the need to think immediately about this complication. Many times a warning bleeding will get ahead of the important bleeding. Whatever, in any upper gastrointestinal bleeding experienced by a patient having

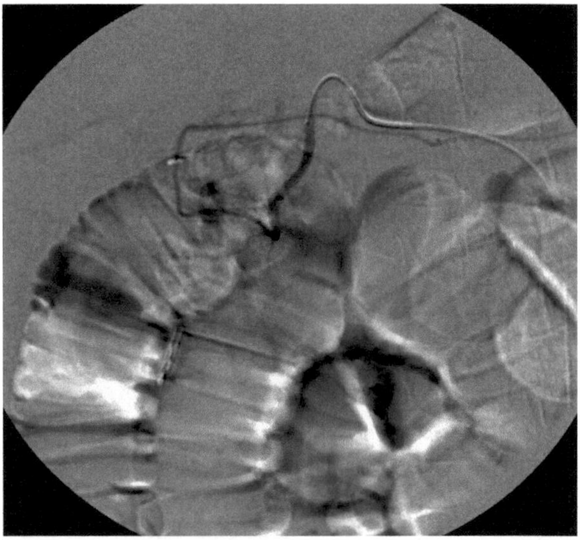

Fig. 45.2 Blush splenic artery

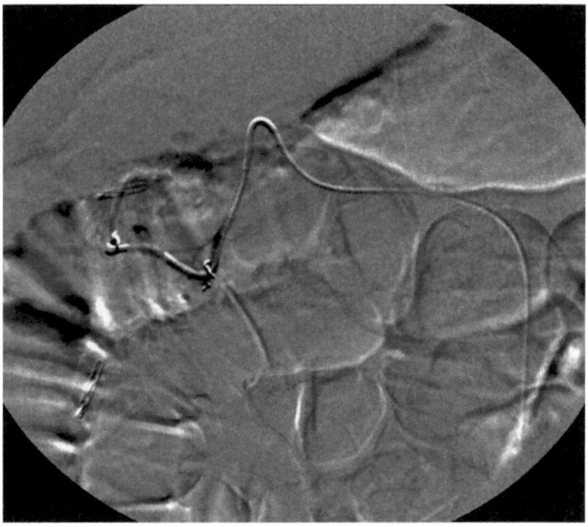

Fig. 45.3 Starting coiling

an acute necrotizing pancreatitis, interventionist radiologists and surgeons have to consider the likelihood of a rupture of a pseudoaneurysm at the level of splenic artery or gastroduodenal artery. The role of the intervention radiologist is quite crucial here. Identifying the blush and using coils to occlude the corresponding artery will control the bleeding. If coiling is not possible, surgical intervention will be necessary. Using packing and to identify bleeding point after suturing should—if possible—come to form the treatment. Postoperative follow-up will be very complicated.

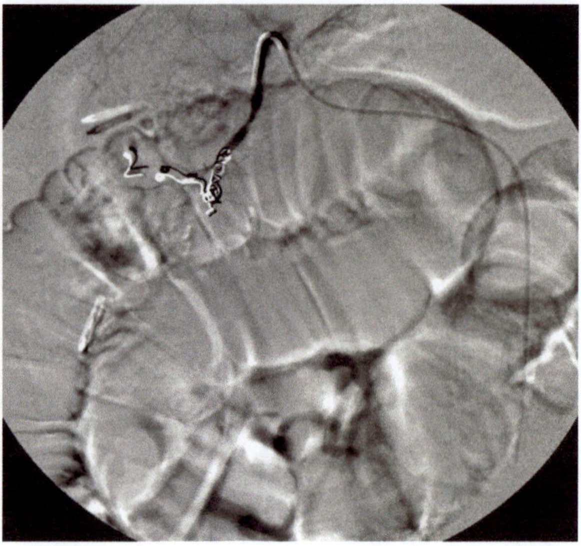

Fig. 45.4 Artery coiled

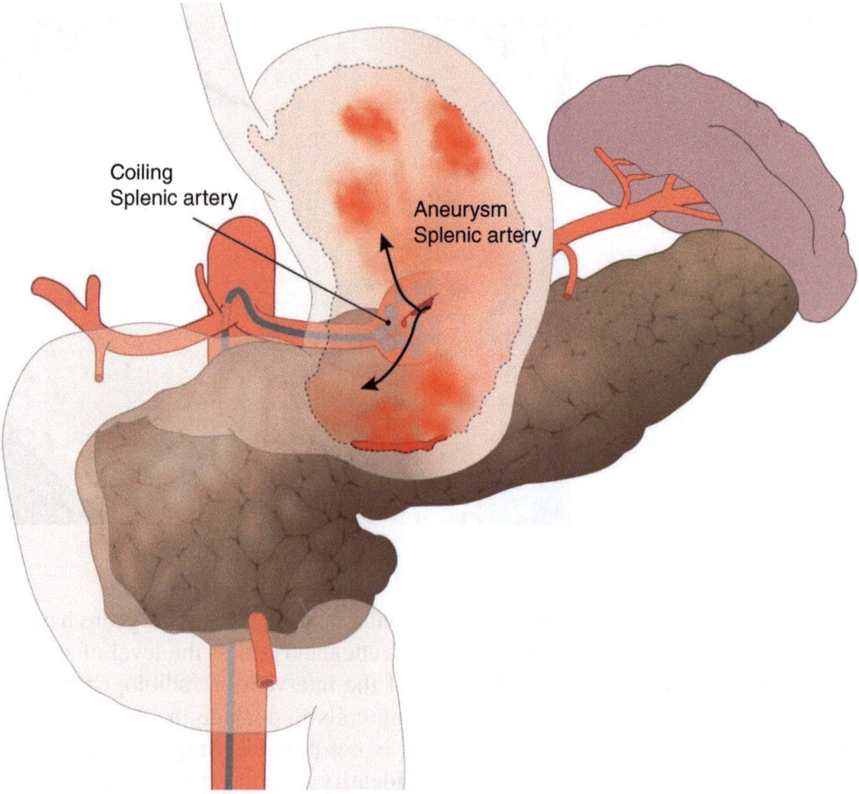

Illustration 45.1 Splenic artery pseudoaneurysm will cause bleeding thorough gastric erosion. Angiography after identification of the blush will fix the complication by successful coiling of the artery

Chapter 46
Case on Necrotizing Acute Pancreatitis: "Infection Is Not Found But Patient Is Becoming Worse"

Marc Besselink

Keywords Acute Pancreatitis • Stones • Necrosectomy • Infected necrotizing pabncreatitis • Fine needle aspiration

Infected necrotizing pancreatitis is a severe complication of acute pancreatitis and occurs in 5–10 % of cases. Whereas the median mortality of sterile necrotizing pancreatitis in the literature is 12 %, the mortality of infected necrotizing pancreatitis is 30 % [1]. Since intervention is only indicated in case of infection, it is of utmost importance to distinguish between sterile and infected necrotizing pancreatitis.

Patient

A 65-year-old male with a history of mild chronic obstructive pulmonary disease and hypertension presented at the emergency room with severe upper abdominal pain since 4 h. During physical examination the patient was in mild respiratory distress, had tachycardia (110/min), experienced upper abdominal pain without signs of peritonitis, and had a subfebrile temperature.

Laboratory analysis demonstrated that serum amylase and lipase levels were both more than three times the upper limit of normal elevated, bilirubin was slightly elevated but less than 40 μmol/L (2.3 mg/dL), and C-reactive protein was higher than 150 mg/L. Imrie score was 5 and APACHEII score was 11. Abdominal ultrasound demonstrated multiple small stones in the gallbladder but no dilatation of the common bile duct.

M. Besselink, M.D., Ph.D.
Department of Surgery, Academic Medical Center, Amsterdam, The Netherlands
e-mail: m.besselink@amc.uva.nl

M.A. Cuesta, H.J. Bonjer (eds.), *Case Studies of Postoperative Complications after Digestive Surgery*, DOI 10.1007/978-3-319-01613-9_46,

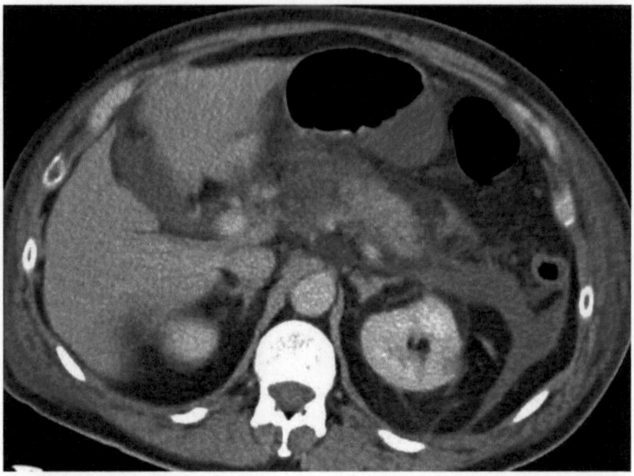

Fig. 46.1 CT 1 week after onset of disease demonstrating pancreatic parenchymal necrosis as well as signs of peripancreatic necrosis. No walled-off collection or impacted gas bubbles are visible

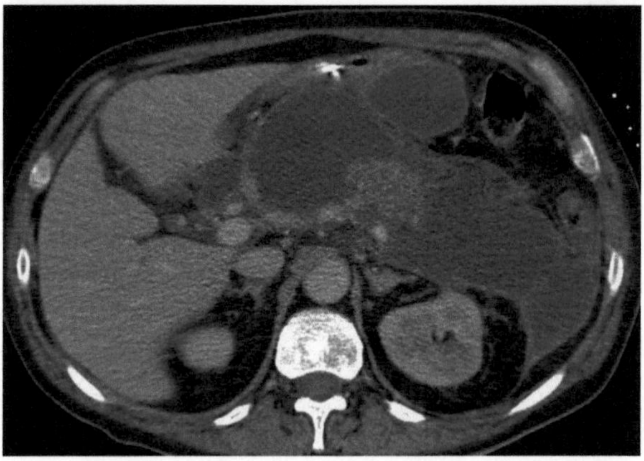

Fig. 46.2 CECT 4 weeks after onset of disease demonstrating a walled-off peri-pancreatic collection with central viable pancreatic parenchyma and surrounding necrosis and fluid

Based on the above-mentioned findings the patient was diagnosed with "predicted severe biliary pancreatitis without cholestasis or cholangitis."

Since there was no apparent cholestasis, there was no urgent indication to perform endoscopic retrograde cholangiography/sphincterotomy [2], and the patient was transferred to the medium care unit. There, despite optimal fluid therapy with a goal diuresis of more1 mL/kg/h, within 12 h he quickly deteriorated and was transferred to the intensive care unit for intubation and respiratory support. New physical examination revealed no signs of peritonitis or abdominal compartment syndrome and it was decided to continue nonsurgical supportive management. After 1 week, the condition had not improved and a contrast-enhanced computed tomography (CECT) was performed (Fig. 46.1).

The condition of the patient remained stable for 3 more weeks and the pulmonary condition improved somewhat, but patient remained intubated and ventilated. Four weeks after initial presentation, the patient's condition deteriorated with signs of infection and vasopressors had to be started. A new CECT was performed under the suspicion of infected necrosis (Fig. 46.2). This CECT did not demonstrate impacted gas bubbles, a pathognomic sign of infection.

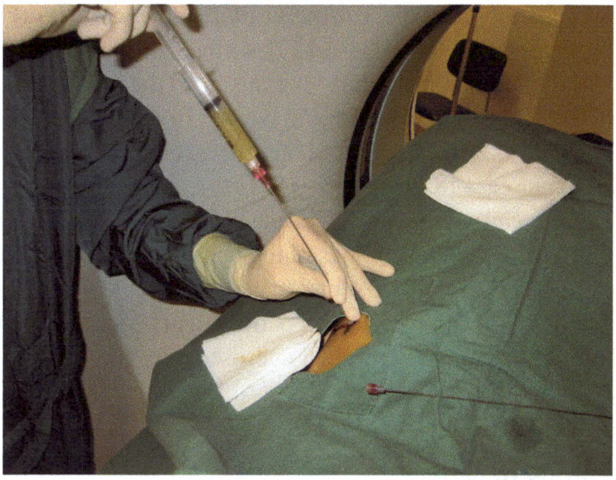

Fig. 46.3 CT-guided fine needle aspiration of a peripancreatic collection. The patient is in prone position, and the needle is placed through the left retroperitoneal, suprarenal space

CECT underestimates necrosis in peripancreatic collections.

Fine needle aspiration of the collection was performed (Fig. 46.3), but no bacteria could be demonstrated. There were no apparent other sources of infection (e.g., pneumonia, line sepsis) or intra-abdominal catastrophes (e.g., abdominal compartment syndrome, peritonitis). There was an extensive discussion as to whether intervention was indicated in this patient as the necrosis appeared to be sterile. Eventually, it was decided that the culture results might have been false negative and the collection was drained percutaneously. The cultures of the drainage procedure did demonstrate infection with *Escherichia coli*. The patient's condition improved without further necrosectomy and, 2 months after admission, he was discharged in good clinical condition.

Discussion

Diagnosing infected necrotizing pancreatitis requires insight not only in the disease but also in the value of fine needle aspiration and CT imaging. Although infection may occur as early as in the first week of the disease, it is typically diagnosed after 3–4 weeks [3]. Fine needle aspiration may produce false-negative results as is described in the current case. Although impacted gas bubbles are pathognomic for infection in necrotizing pancreatitis, this is only seen in approximately 50 % of cases. Consequently, absence of gas bubbles does not exclude infection.

In the first randomized trial on intervention in infected necrotizing pancreatitis (PANTER, a Dutch multicenter trial), no routine fine needle aspiration was used. The decision to intervene was rather based on a clinical suspicion of infection (i.e., clinical deterioration despite maximal conservative support); the results of this strategy proved excellent with a 95 % infection rate, the highest ever reported [4].

Typically, the most difficult clinical scenario to diagnose infected necrotizing pancreatitis is in the case as described in this chapter: a patient is admitted with severe pancreatitis and needs transfer to the ICU where the condition of the patient does not improve over several weeks. In these cases a fine needle aspiration may be helpful. As described one should be aware that the test results may be false negative as in our case [5].

Once infection is diagnosed, it is probably beneficial to postpone intervention with the help of antibiotics until such a time that the infected collection has become "walled off," typically seen after some 4 weeks [5]. After the infected collection has "walled off," up to half of all patients can be treated with only percutaneous catheter drainage, without additional necrosectomy [6].

References

1. Banks PA, Freeman ML. Practice guidelines in acute pancreatitis. Am J Gastroenterol. 2006;101:2379–400.
2. Van Santvoort HC, Besselink MG, De Vries AC, et al. Early endoscopic retrograde cholangio-pancreatography in predicted severe acute biliary pancreatitis: a prospective multicenter study. Ann Surg. 2009;250:68–75.
3. Besselink MG, Van Santvoort HC, Boermeester MA, et al. Timing and impact of infections in acute pancreatitis. Br J Surg. 2009;96:267–73.
4. Van Santvoort HC, Besselink MG, Bakker OJ, et al. A step-up approach or open necrosectomy for necrotizing pancreatitis. N Engl J Med. 2010;362:1491–502.
5. Besselink MG, Verwer TJ, Schoenmaeckers EJ, et al. Timing of surgical intervention in necrotizing pancreatitis. Arch Surg. 2007;142:1194–201.
6. Van Baal MC, Van Santvoort HC, Bollen TL, et al. Systematic review of percutaneous catheter drainage as primary treatment for necrotizing pancreatitis. Br J Surg. 2011;98:18–27.

Chapter 47
Case on Pseudocyst of the Pancreas, Endoscopically or Surgical Treatment?

Suzanne S. Gisbertz and Maarten A.J.M. Jacobs

Keywords Pseudocyst • Pancreas • Endoscopy • Surgery • Laparotomy • Gastroscopy • Stent

First Patient

Noninfected giant pancreatic pseudocyst, drained transgastrically.

Diagnosis and Indication for Operation

A 32-year-old obese male patient (BMI 35), known with hyperlipidemia, was admitted to the hospital because of abdominal pain and fever. Patient was in shock and was admitted to the Medium Care department. He was feeling sick and had a heart frequency of 140 PM, blood pressure of 90/45 mmHg, and temperature of 38.7 °C. Abdominal exploration was painful with tenderness in the upper abdomen. After reposition of fluids with good response, a CT scan was performed. There an acute pancreatitis was seen, and no gallstones. No necrotizing component was observed, but the patient was continually observed at the Medium Care department. His reaction to fluids remained satisfactory, but his abdominal pain and fever persisted. One week later, a new CT scan showed a pseudocyst of the pancreas at a retrogastric position (Fig. 47.1). Enteral feeding was given through a duodenal tube.

S.S. Gisbertz, M.D.
Department of Surgery, Academic Medical Centre, Amsterdam, The Netherlands
e-mail: s.gisbertz@antoniusziekenhuis.nl

M.A.J.M. Jacobs
Department of Gastroenterology, VU University Medical Center, Amsterdam, The Netherlands

M.A. Cuesta, H.J. Bonjer (eds.), *Case Studies of Postoperative Complications after Digestive Surgery*, DOI 10.1007/978-3-319-01613-9_47,

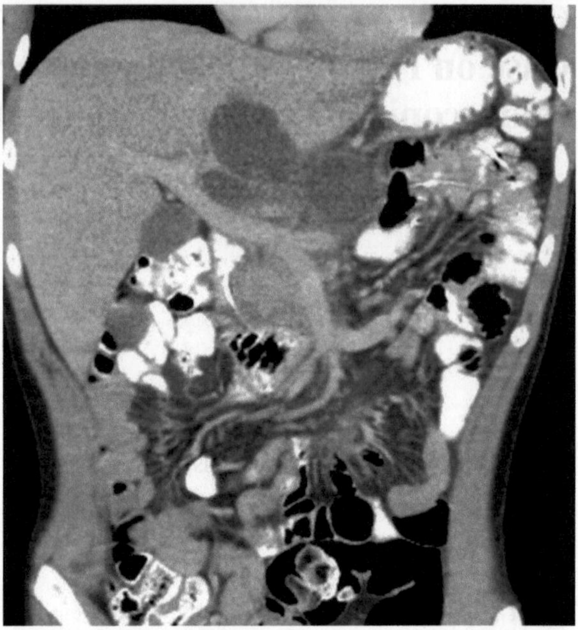

Fig. 47.1 CT scan, the pseudocyst in retrogastric position to subhepatic area

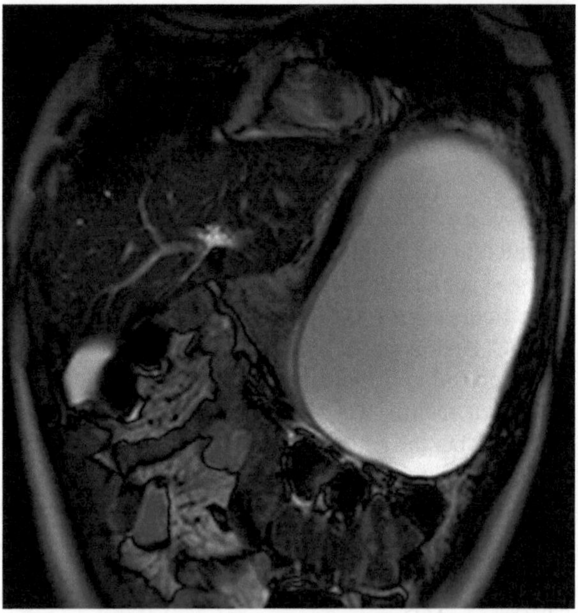

Fig. 47.2 MRCP: pancreatic pseudocyst becoming larger

Weekly controls showed an increasing growth of the cyst with important elevation of the diaphragm and respiratory worsening (Fig. 47.2). Given that there were no signs of infection, our approach was initially conservative. However, due to the increasing abdominal distension and respiratory problems, it was decided to drain the pseudocyst transgastrically by endoscopy.

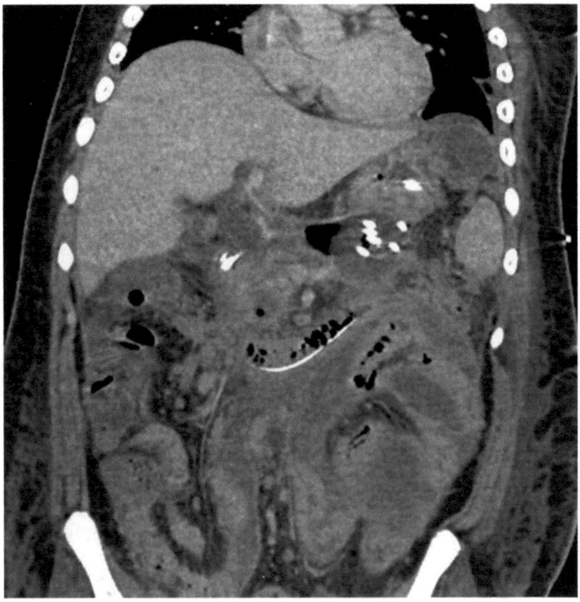

Fig. 47.3 CT scan after transgastric drainage

Operation

This was performed without problems, draining almost three liters of pancreatic fluid. Various stents were left to communicate the stomach and cyst. Important clinical and imaging improvements were seen immediately after drainage (Fig. 47.3 and Illustration 47.1).

Second Patient

Noninfected giant pancreatic pseudocyst, drained by laparotomy following failed drainage by gastroscopy.

Diagnosis and Indication for Operation

A young obese architecture student, 29-year-old, known with diabetes mellitus type I and insulin treatment, presented acutely with abdominal pain, high amylase, and lipase in the serum. Patient felt sick, had tachycardia, and an upper abdominal tenderness could be palpated. Differential diagnosis was made amongst either acute cholecystitis, duodenal perforation, or acute pancreatitis.

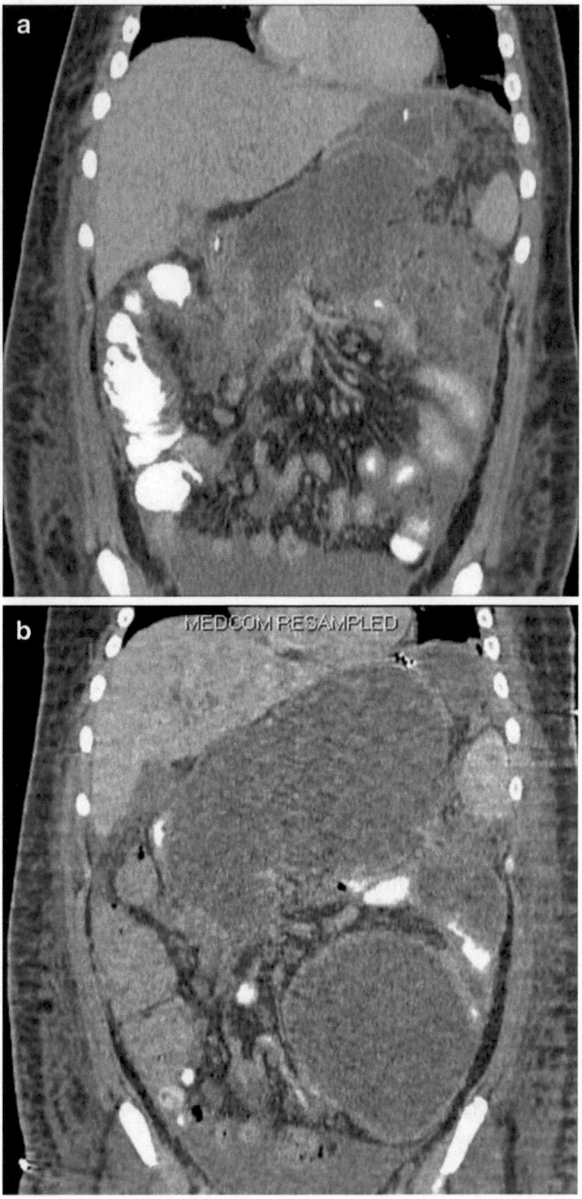

Fig. 47.4 (**a**) CT scan, necrotizing acute pancreatitis with pseudocyst forming. (**b**) CT scan, pancreatic pseudocyst behind stomach

On the CT scan, a necrotizing acute pancreatitis-type Balthazar stage E (score 4), with extensive necrosis score 6, was seen. He was admitted to the Medium Care department and treated initially with oxygen, broad spectrum iv antibiotics, TPN, and physiotherapy. Yet, the situation of the patient worsened, involving fever and more abdominal distension, without respiratory insufficiency. Each ensuing week a control CT scan showed different images. Eventually a growing pseudocyst with retrogastric position was observed (Fig. 47.4a, b). No signs of infection could be

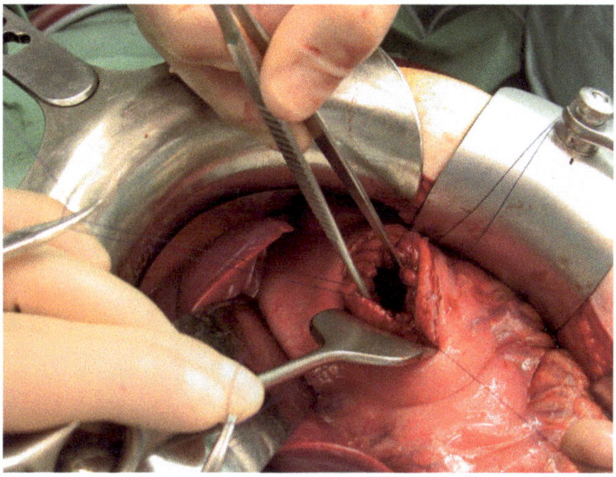

Fig. 47.5 Open transgastric drainage of a pancreatic pseudocyst

seen, but respiratory problems with fever arose. At the multidisciplinary sessions this patient was repeatedly discussed, with a conservative attitude displayed by our side and a more aggressive stance held by the gastroenterologist. The issue was whether to engage transgastric drainage because of the size of the cyst (20 cm), abdominal distension, and progressive respiratory difficulties. Finally 5 weeks after admission, a decision was taken to drain the cyst.

Operation

During gastroscopy and after localizing the cyst, it was possible to pass a guide into the cyst. Yet while putting in the first stent, the patient developed hypotension with gastric bleeding. The gastroenterologist considered the possibility of arterial damage or gastric damage with bleeding and so a decision was made to operate the patient immediately. At upper abdomen laparotomy, bleeding was found present along the small gastric curvature, with damage along the curvature (Fig. 47.5). After repair of this by stitches transgastrically, the huge cyst was drained by opening the posterior gastric wall (Illustration 47.1). Patient recovered on the Intensive Care unit, and his cyst decreased significantly, but did not disappear entirely, being reduced to 5 cm. He is now stable, at home, and resuming his studies.

Discussion

In comparison with the past, surgical attitude to pancreatic pseudocyst has changed to conservative treatment. Pseudocysts do vary by shape and size during the whole acute process and should be controlled by ultrasonography or CT scan. Those that have become infected should be percutaneously drained. The two patients here presented each had a huge growing noninfected pseudocyst while increasingly

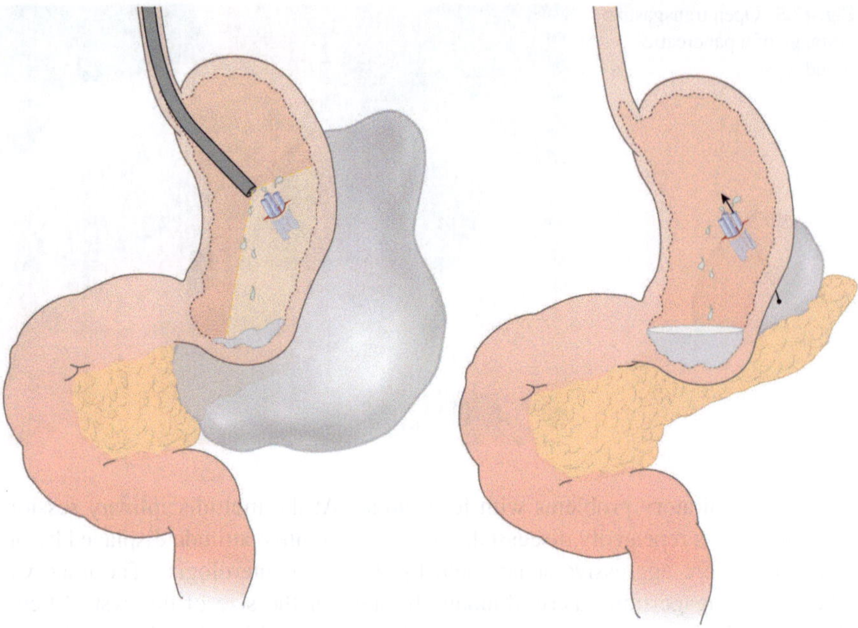

Illustration 47.1 In the case that a huge pseudocyst should be drained the first option will be endoscopically. If failed or because of complications, surgical transgastric drainage should be done

experiencing respiratory problems. In spite of an initial conservative attitude in both cases, drainage was decided. Endoscopic transgastric drainage appears to be the right choice, but in the case of complications the surgeon should always stand by.

Chapter 48
Case on Pancreatic Pseudocyst Far from the Stomach

Mariëlle L.A.W. Vehmeijer-Heeman

Keywords Pancreatic pseudocyst • Acute necrotizing pancreatitis • Cystojejunostomy

Diagnosis and Indication for Surgery

A female patient of 32 years of age (previously presented above in case 47), and who now had been diagnosed with SLE-like autoimmune necrotizing acute pancreatitis that was complicated by several pseudocysts, finally went home after a stay of 6 months at the hospital, largely in the Intensive Care department. During her revalidation period, the patient had developed a mechanical bowel obstruction with important abdominal distension. CT scan demonstrated an increase in diameter of the known pseudocyst in the left abdominal cavity. Three months before, she experienced a short period of blood loss in the feces with significant diarrhea. At that time, we did not dare to perform a colonoscopy because the descending colon was located at the wall of the pseudocyst and the bleeding had no hemodynamic consequences. The patient was then transfused with two erythrocyte concentrated units. At readmission, an MRI showed the pseudocyst with a maximum diameter of 20 by 15 cm in the left abdominal cavity. Because of the mechanical problems caused by the pseudocyst, a decision was taken to drain the cyst by laparotomy.

M.L.A.W.Vehmeijer-Heeman, M.D.
Department of Surgery, VU University Medical Center,
Amsterdam, The Netherlands
e-mail: m.heeman@vumc.nl

M.A. Cuesta, H.J. Bonjer (eds.), *Case Studies of Postoperative Complications after Digestive Surgery*, DOI 10.1007/978-3-319-01613-9_48,

Operation

The problem was considered how to drain the pseudocyst far from the stomach. Percutaneous drainage was not considered an option, because of the high chance of recurrence. Through an infraumbilical laparotomy, the pseudocyst was drained (2,300 ml debris was evacuated and cultured), followed by a Roux-en-Y reconstruction at the lowest aspect of the cyst with proximal jejunal loop, and leaving a drain along the anastomosis. An *Enterococcus faecalis* was cultured and the antibiotic therapy was iv administered.

Postoperative Course: Identification and Treatment of Complication

On the first postoperative day, she had an acute onset of abdominal pain with tenderness, local peritonitis, fever, and drain of cyst content through the drain. Relaparotomy showed a normal anastomosis but leakage of the cystic wall as caused by perforation of the drain. After repair, she recovered and was discharged 1 month after surgery without symptoms. After 6 months, follow-up control showed no recurrence of symptoms.

Discussion

Approximately 75–80 % of the cystic lesions of the pancreas are pancreatic pseudocysts. There is a difference in pathogenesis of the several pseudocysts [1, 2]. The most common etiologies for pancreatic pseudocysts include chronic pancreatitis (40 %), acute pancreatitis, pancreatic trauma, pancreatic duct obstruction, and pancreatic malignancies. Complications of pancreatic pseudocyst include infection, hemorrhage (caused by a leaking pseudoaneurysm of the splenic artery), rupture, gastric outlet obstruction, and biliary obstruction.

A pseudocyst is a localized fluid collection that contains pancreatic enzymes and necrotic tissue. Pseudocysts have a non-epithelialized wall consisting of fibrous and granulation tissue and therefore are distinguished from true cysts with epithelial lining.

Pseudocysts are usually in continuity with the pancreas. Most frequently, the pseudocysts are located in the lesser peritoneal sac behind the stomach. Large pseudocysts may extend beyond the lesser sac and become remote from the pancreas in the area of the paracolic gutters, the pelvis, and the mediastinum. The traditional guidelines for management of larger pseudocysts call for drainage after a 6-week observation period. As a vast majority of the pseudocysts resolve spontaneously, asymptomatic pseudocysts should therefore not be drained. In case of complications or persistent symptoms, pseudocysts should be treated. Pseudocysts can be

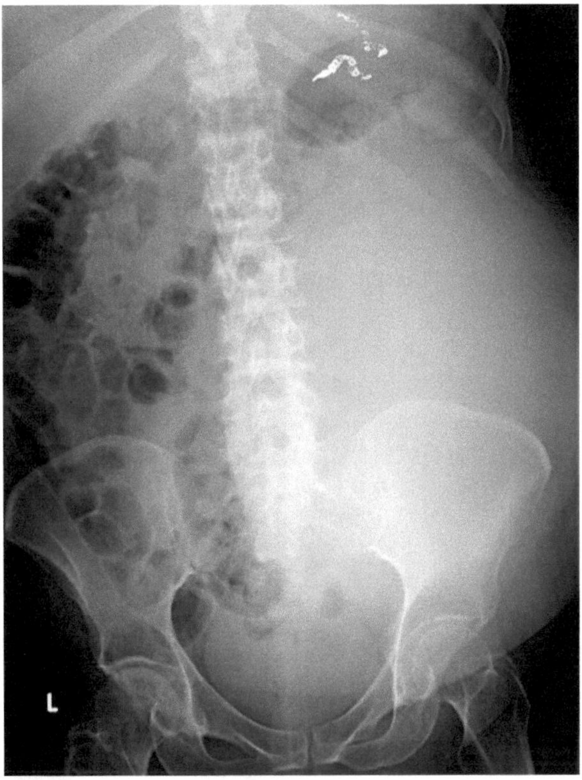

Fig. 48.1 Abdomen X-ray showing the pseudocyst in the left lower abdomen with compression of descending colon

managed by several types of interventions. Three different types of interventions are available: endoscopic drainage, imaging guided percutaneous drainage, and laparoscopic or open cystogastrostomy or cystojejunostomy (Figs. 48.1, 48.2, and 48.3). When possible, an endoscopic drainage through the stomach is preferred as it provides high success and low complication rates. Feasibility of endoscopic drainage is highly dependent on the anatomy and topography of the pseudocyst, considering the relation with the posterior wall of the stomach and local vessels (see cases 47). In this current case, involving a pseudocyst far from the stomach in the left abdominal cavity, applying an endoscopic procedure, was not an option. Imaging-guided percutaneous drainage may give rise to a significant number of complications such as a high risk of infection, persistent leakage from the drain, and repositioning of the drain. However, percutaneous drainage is useful if the pseudocyst has become infected. The type of surgical procedure to follow depends on the location of the cyst. When a retrogastric cyst is not attached to the stomach, high suspicion for malignant process should be in order. And finally, if the pseudocyst is not in contact with the stomach, a Roux-Y-reconstruction needs to be performed. Generally speaking, an operation of pseudocysts might be complicated by anastomosis leakage, postoperative bleeding, and in some cases a mistaken diagnosis as in cystadenocarcinoma.

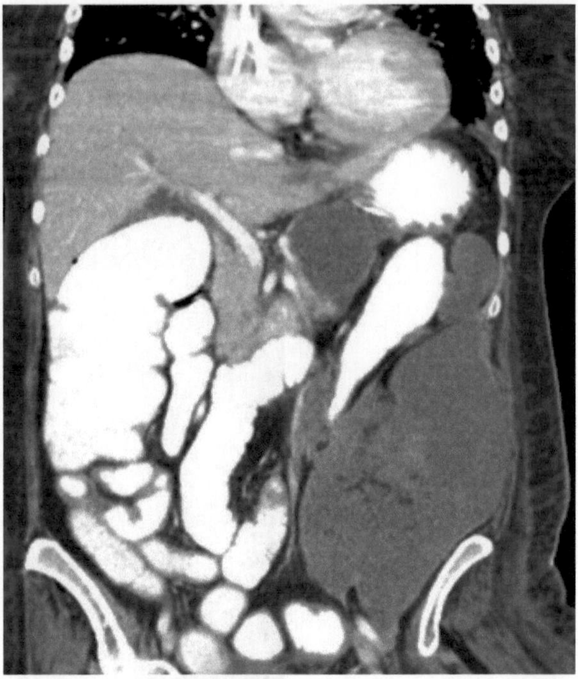

Fig. 48.2 MRI showing preoperative imaging of the cyst and relation with descending colon

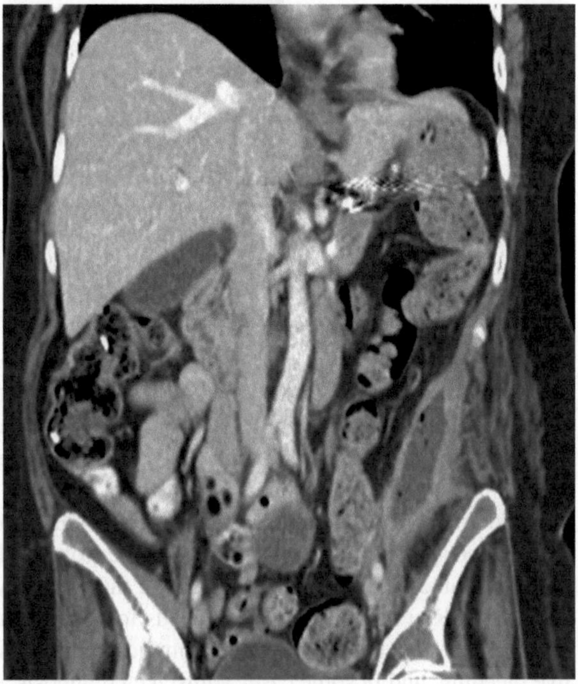

Fig. 48.3 MRI after surgical drainage of the pseudocyst

So far, no prospective controlled studies have been reported contrasting the different drainage approaches. Several retrospective studies compared these approaches and showed slightly higher morbidity and mortality in the surgical group as compared with endoscopic intervention. Because of the heterogeneity in the groups, these results are not comparable. In addition, there is also an enormous difference in morbidity between emergency operations versus elective procedures. Most important is that the preferred intervention varies particularly on the localization and the surrounding anatomy of the pseudocyst and may also depend on personal expertise. In this case, based on the location and the large size of the pseudocyst, an open cystojejunostomy was the preferred option. Aljarabah et al. published a review study about successful laparoscopic approaches [3]. Again, as there have been no prospective randomized trials, it is very difficult to compare the short- and long-term outcome of laparoscopic versus open procedures.

References

1. Behrns K. Surgical therapy of pancreatic pseudocysts. J Gastrointest Surg. 2008;12:2231–9.
2. Aghdassi A, Mayerle J, Kraft M, et al. Diagnosis and treatment of pancreatic pseudocysts in chronic pancreatitis. Pancreas. 2008;36:105–12.
3. Aljarabah M, Ammori BJ. Laparoscopic and endoscopic approaches for drainage of pancreatic pseudocysts: a systematic review of published series. Surg Endosc. 2007;21:1936–44.

Chapter 49
Case on Intra-abdominal Bleeding with Shock as Consequence of Necrotizing Pancreatitis

Miguel A. Cuesta

Keywords Acute Necrotizing pancreatitis • Intra-abdominal bleeding • Hypovolemic Shock • Gallstones

Diagnosis and Indication for Surgery

A 55-year-old man was presented to the First Aid department because of abdominal pain and shock.

Patient was resuscitated by intubation and ventilation, and abundant fluid reposition. His amylase in serum was high (2,500 U/ml), and the possibility of his having an acute pancreatitis rose. A CT scan confirmed acute pancreatitis, Balthazar type C with gallstones, and no aneurysm of the abdominal aorta (Fig. 49.1a). He was admitted to the Intensive Care department and the following day he developed a hypovolemic shock with low hemoglobin rate. An angiography showed no blush and no aneurysms in the visceral arteries (Fig. 49.1b). Because of hemodynamic instability, the surgeon decided to operate him.

Operation

At laparotomy, an acute necrotizing pancreatitis was found with abundant blood and clots in the lesser sac. A central bleeding was observed possibly coming from the left of the celiac trunk, possibly a pseudoaneurysm of the splenic artery, and different stitches were done to fix the bleeding.

M.A. Cuesta, M.D.
Department of Surgery, VU University Medical Center, Amsterdam, The Netherlands
e-mail: ma.cuesta@vumc.nl

M.A. Cuesta, H.J. Bonjer (eds.), *Case Studies of Postoperative Complications after Digestive Surgery*, DOI 10.1007/978-3-319-01613-9_49,

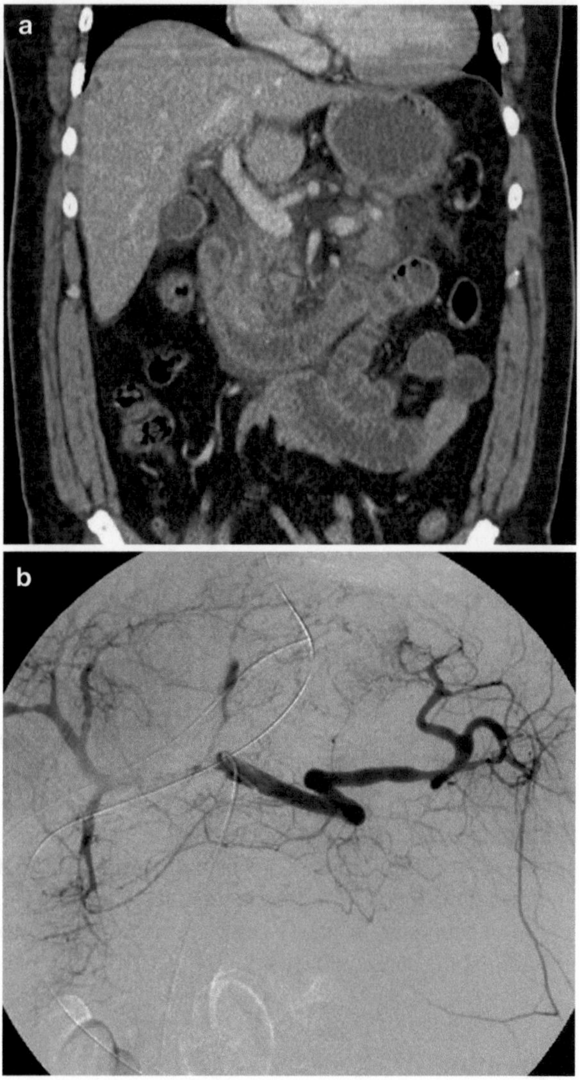

Fig. 49.1 (**a**) CT scan on admission acute pancreatitis and cholelithiasis. No aorta aneurysm. (**b**) Angiography of celiac trunk and SMA, no blush

Postoperative Course and Identification of the Complication

The patient was mechanically ventilated and the sepsis treated by iv broad spectrum antibiotics, iv noradrenaline and total parenteral nutrition. His wound became infected and dehiscent and abundant pus drained spontaneously. Vacuum system therapy was considered but because of the presence of bowels on the surface of the wound was not performed. Wound cleansing was performed. During the course of 6 weeks, because of the low-grade septic situation, various CT scans were performed in which different intra-abdominal abscesses were percutaneously drained

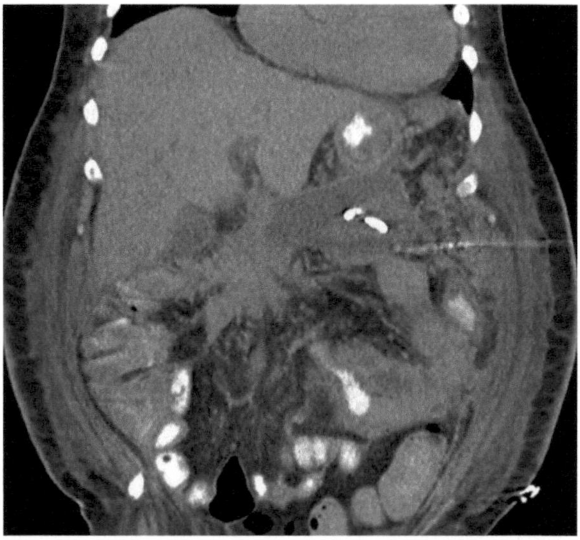

Fig. 49.2 Central abscess in pancreas, percutaneously drained

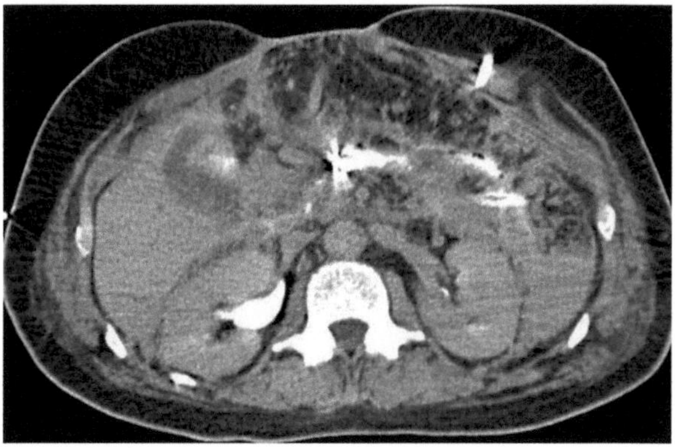

Fig. 49.3 Abscesses are becoming quite. Open abdomen approach

(Fig. 49.2). After a long period of 4 months during which he developed psychosis with deliriums, he was admitted to the psychiatric unit at the hospital. He recovered completely (Fig. 49.3) and 3 months later a cholecystectomy and repair of the cicatricial hernia by means of polypropylene mesh were performed.

Discussion

The lesson of this case is that at presentation, a differential diagnosis was made between rupture of aorta aneurysm or necrotizing acute pancreatitis. After resuscitation, a CT scan established the proper diagnosis. Because of intra-abdominal bleeding, an angiography was done without visualization of a blush. Intervention was considered necessary because of no blush and hemodynamic instability. At emergency laparotomy, it was a difficult procedure to fix the bleeding. Consequently infection of the necrosis, multiple abscesses, open wound approach, and psychosis were adequately treated during a very long hospital stay. Mortality may be very high with this approach.

Chapter 50
Case on Recurrence of Infection After Video-Assisted Retroperitoneal Debridement

Marc Besselink

Keywords Retroperitoneal debridement • Infection • Dutch PANTER trial • Step-up approach • Drainage • Necrosectomy

After the publication of the Dutch PANTER trial [1], the "step-up approach" is now considered the reference standard for treating infected necrotizing pancreatitis. When infection is diagnosed or suspected, antibiotic treatment is started with the aim to postpone intervention up to 4 weeks, as most collections have become "walled-off" by that time. The first step is percutaneous catheter drainage, preferably retroperitoneal. In the PANTER trial, 35 % of patients could be treated with only percutaneous drainage. Additionally, a recent systematic review suggested that half of all patients with infected necrotizing pancreatitis can be treated with percutaneous drainage only [2]. In patients in whom percutaneous drainage fails, either because they do not improve or because their condition deteriorates after initial improvement, the next step is drain-guided video-assisted retroperitoneal debridement (VARD). In this technique, a 5 cm retroperitoneal incision is made and the drain is followed into the collection with infected necrosis and pus [3]. The debridement is performed under videoscopic assistance. It is not the goal to remove all necrosis; some necrosis may be left for the patient to deal with. In this way the risk of bleeding is minimized. We describe a case in which the step-up approach was used.

M. Besselink, M.D., Ph.D.
Department of Surgery, Academic Medical Center, Amsterdam, The Netherlands
e-mail: m.besselink@amc.uva.nl

M.A. Cuesta, H.J. Bonjer (eds.), *Case Studies of Postoperative Complications after Digestive Surgery*, DOI 10.1007/978-3-319-01613-9_50,

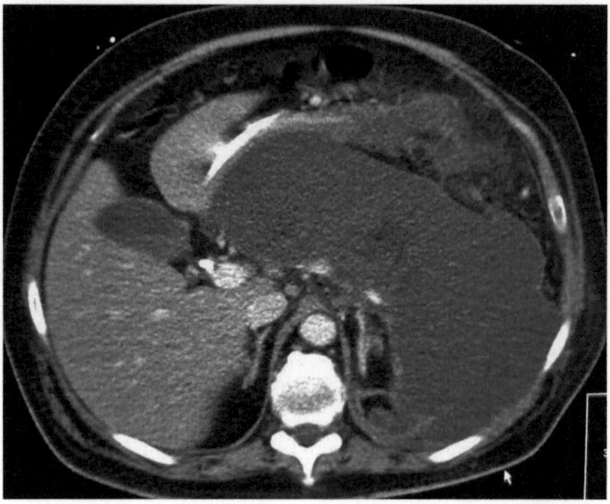

Fig. 50.1 CECT 4 weeks after onset of disease, demonstrating a large peri-pancreatic collection with necrosis and fluid

Patient

Diagnosis and Indication for Surgery

A 50-year-old male with alcoholic pancreatitis was treated conservatively on the surgical ward with enteral nutrition. After 4 weeks, his clinical condition deteriorated with clinical and laboratory signs of infection. A contrast-enhanced computed tomography (CECT) revealed a large peri-pancreatic collection with necrosis and fluid (Fig. 50.1).

Because of the clinical suspicion of infected necrotizing pancreatitis and the fact that the majority of the collection had become "walled off," percutaneous retroperitoneal catheter drainage was performed. Immediately after drainage, some 500 ml of pus and small necrotic particles drained and in a few days the clinical condition of the patient clearly improved. One week after drainage a repeat CECT was performed according to protocol of a CECT (Fig. 50.2).

One week after the drainage procedure, the clinical condition of the patient deteriorated again with new clinical and laboratory signs of acute infection. A repeat CECT was performed and is shown in Fig. 50.3.

It was decided to perform a VARD procedure as initial percutaneous drainage had clinically failed and the remaining collection seemed to contain almost no drainable fluid. Figure 50.4 shows the removal of the first necrosis encountered during the VARD procedure.

Again, the patient's condition improved. One week after the VARD procedure, the patient again demonstrated clinical signs of infection. A new CECT was performed (Fig. 50.5).

As there was necrosis remaining in the collection and the patient experienced symptoms of infection it was decided to perform a second VARD procedure. During this procedure, several large pieces of infected necrosis were removed under videoscopic assistance. Figure 50.6 shows the necrosis that was removed.

After this second VARD procedure, the patient's condition improved rapidly and 3 weeks later he left the hospital in a good clinical condition.

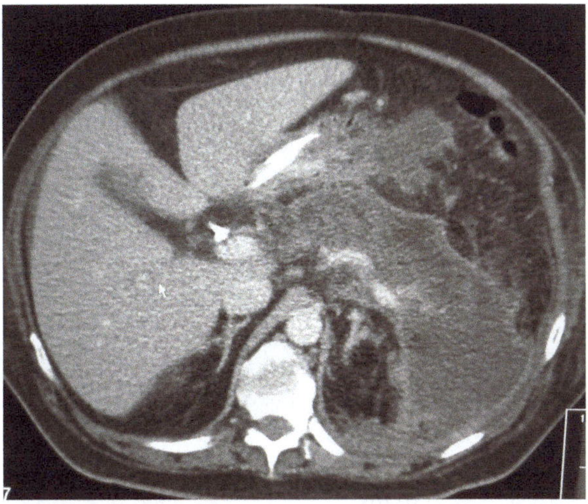

Fig. 50.2 CECT 5 weeks after onset of disease and 1 week after percutaneous retroperitoneal catheter drainage of infected necrotizing pancreatitis, the collection has clearly diminished in size

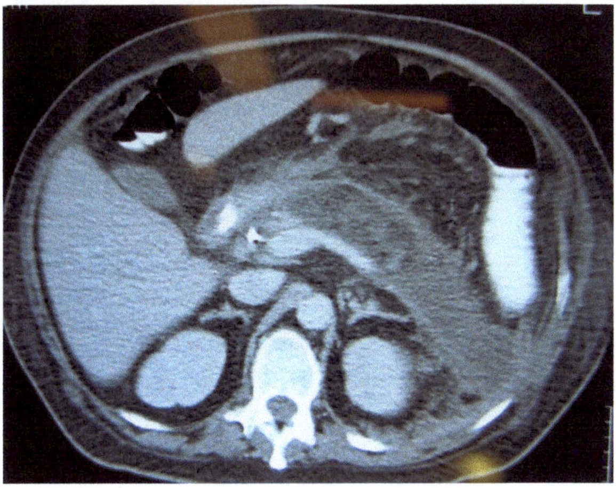

Fig. 50.3 CECT 6 weeks after onset of disease and 2 weeks after percutaneous retroperitoneal catheter drainage of infected necrotizing pancreatitis

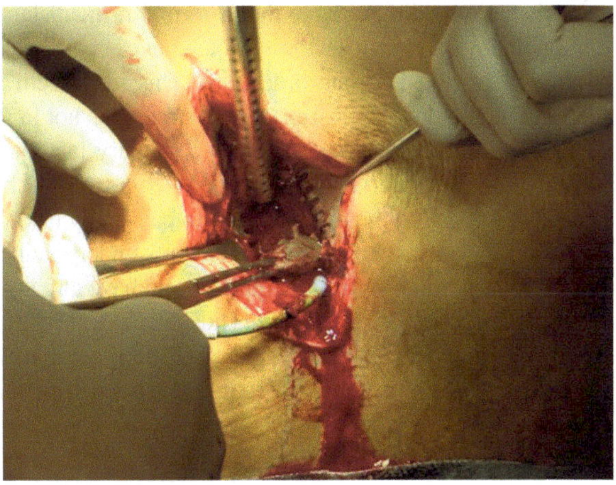

Fig. 50.4 VARD procedure: a small incision is made in the left flank next to the retroperitoneal drain. The drain is followed into the infected collection and the first necrosis encountered is removed. Later, video-assistance is used to clear the collection of necrosis and two surgical drains are placed for continuous postoperative lavage

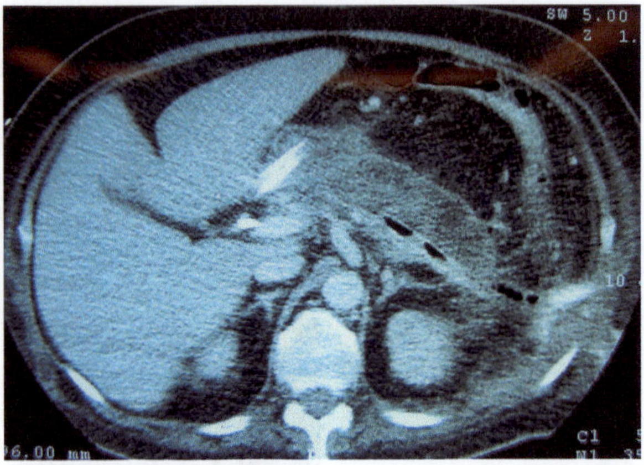

Fig. 50.5 CECT 7 weeks after onset of disease, demonstrating the surgical drain in the collection and residual necrosis

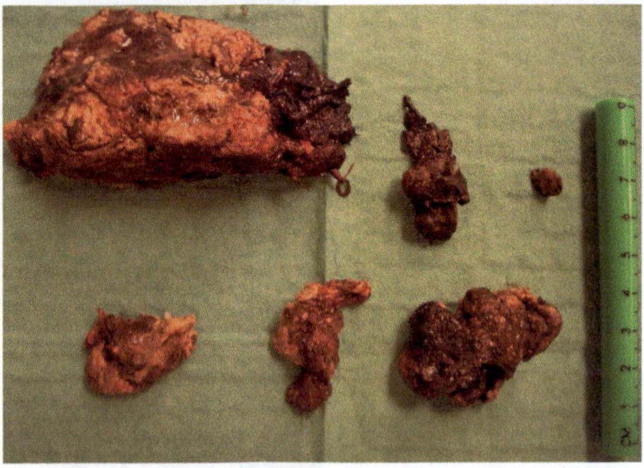

Fig. 50.6 Necrosis removed during the second VARD procedure, 7 weeks after onset of disease

Discussion

Several drainage and necrosectomy procedures may be required to remove all infected necrosis and pus. Some argue that a formal primary laparotomy, without drainage or minimally invasive necrosectomy, would have been a better option as all necrosis would have been removed in one procedure. This may seem as a valuable argument, but, according to the PANTER trial, such a strategy is not in the best interest of the patient. The PANTER trial demonstrated that a primary laparotomy leads to more new onset organ failure after intervention than the "step-up approach" [1]. The reason for this may be the larger "hit" to the immune system caused by laparotomy as compared to (multiple) minimally invasive procedures. Patients undergoing interventions for infected necrotizing pancreatitis are usually quite ill and have already been hospitalized for several weeks, weakening their condition. Thus, the least invasive approach is likely to be beneficial, or rather less harmful. Apparently, the fact that with these minimally invasive approaches more procedures are required is not detrimental to the patient's condition.

This case also clearly describes the use of repeat CECT for optimal planning of the optimal treatment strategy. When performing CECT in necrotizing pancreatitis, one should be very aware of the fact that CECT is not capable of detecting necrosis in fluid-predominant collections. Imaging modalities that are capable of doing so are magnetic resonance imaging and ultrasound.

References

1. Van Santvoort HC, Besselink MG, Bakker OJ, et al. A step-up approach or open necrosectomy for necrotizing pancreatitis. N Engl J Med. 2010;362:1491–502.
2. Van Baal MC, Van Santvoort HC, Bollen TL, et al. Systematic review of percutaneous catheter drainage as primary treatment for necrotizing pancreatitis. Br J Surg. 2011;98:18–27.
3. Van Santvoort HC, Besselink MG, Horvath KD, et al. Videoscopic assisted retroperitoneal debridement in infected necrotizing pancreatitis. HPB (Oxford). 2007;9:156–9.

Chapter 51
Case on Splenic and Portal Vein Thrombosis After Splenectomy

Miguel A. Cuesta and H. Jaap Bonjer

Keywords Splenectomy • Giant spleen • Myelofibrosis • Portal vein thrombosis • Portal hypertension

First Patient

Diagnosis and Indication for Surgery

A 65-year-old man was diagnosed 10 years before with myelofibrosis involving a significantly enlarged spleen. Patient was treated by the internist and hematologist conservatively. The only treatment options had been largely supportive without an alteration of the disease, including *folic acid*, *allopurinol*, *blood transfusions*, and *dexamethasone*. He underwent a progressive growth of the spleen, occupying his entire abdomen, having produced important scoliosis with deformity that impeded him in walking properly. Moreover, there was an important depression of the bone marrow function and changes in fibrosis. Indication for splenectomy was considered because of the mechanical complaints with rest dyspnea. On the US and CT scan, a splenomegaly of 30 by 25 cm was seen with enlarged veins around the spleen (Fig. 51.1). No portal hypertension was observed and neither were esophageal varices seen on the gastroscopy.

M.A. Cuesta, M.D. (✉) • H.J. Bonjer, M.D., Ph.D., F.R.C.S.C.
Department of Surgery, VU University Medical Center,
Amsterdam, The Netherlands
e-mail: ma.cuesta@vumc.nl; j.bonjer@vumc.nl

M.A. Cuesta, H.J. Bonjer (eds.), *Case Studies of Postoperative Complications after Digestive Surgery*, DOI 10.1007/978-3-319-01613-9_51,

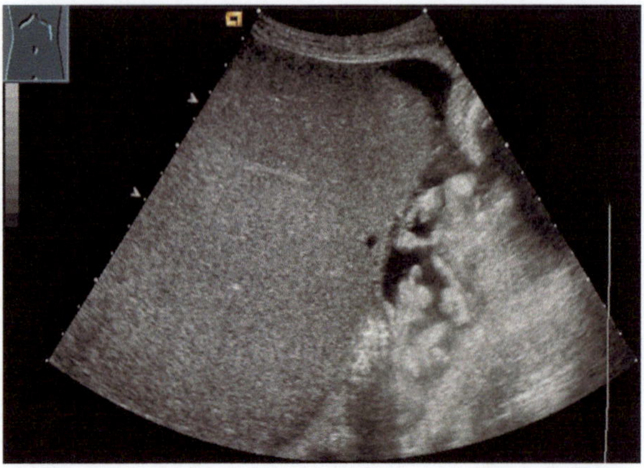

Fig. 51.1 Splenomegaly on the US

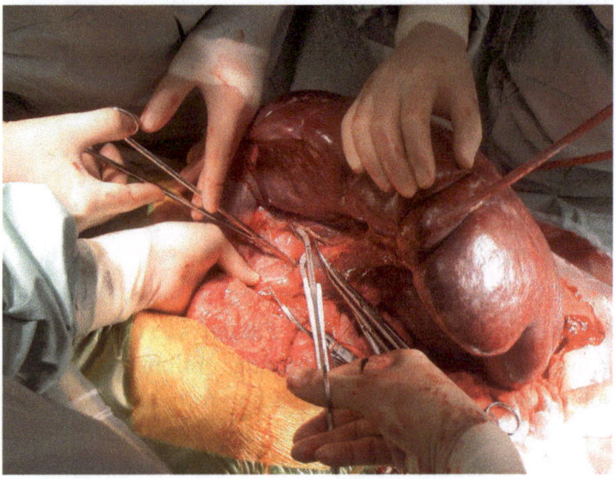

Fig. 51.2 View of operative field during open splenectomy for a giant spleen

Operation

At laparotomy, 1 l of ascites was found, and the liver was hard on palpation and enlarged; moreover the spleen was giant, larger than 30 cm. After careful mobilization and division of short vessels, the hilar vessels, first the artery and then the vein, 30 mm in size, were taken down by ligatures (Fig. 51.2). Platelet suspension was transfused once the enlarged splenic vein was divided. The spleen weighed 8.2 kg. The splenorenal and phrenosplenic ligaments were already calcified and this disturbed the course of the operation.

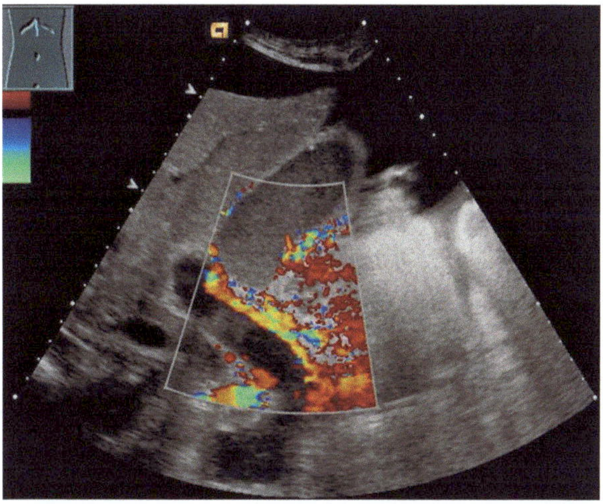

Fig. 51.3 Two days postoperative US-Doppler, portal vein open

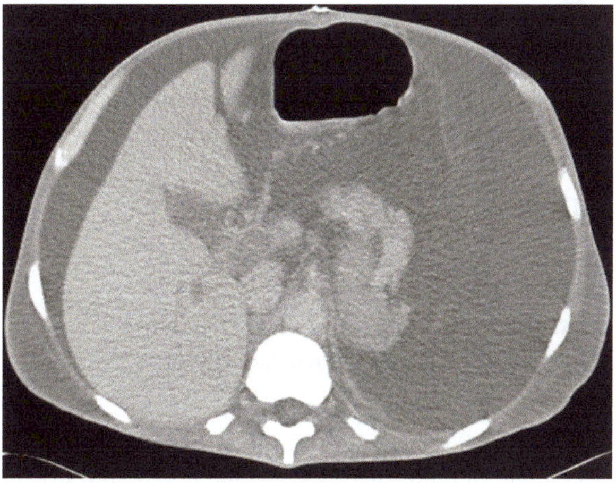

Fig. 51.4 Portal vein thrombosis and ascites

Postoperative Course: Identification and Treatment of Complication

Postoperative course of the patient was initially undisturbed, yet thrombocytosis came about and he was then treated with double doses of sc Fraxiparin®. Because of abdominal distention an Echo-Doppler was performed showing an open portal vein (Fig. 51.3). Seven days after operation the patient developed important ascites and abdominal distension. On a CT scan, thrombosis of the splenic and portal vein was seen (Fig. 51.4). Treatment was started with iv heparin in therapeutic doses and adequate feeding. Apparently the situation stabilized, and partial reopening of the portal vein was seen on the CT scan. After 2 weeks, the situation of the patient worsened; he became septic, refused surgical treatment, and died. At autopsy, mesenteric ischemia/necrosis was found.

Second Patient

Diagnosis and Indication for Surgery

A 33-year-old patient with morbid obesity and a BMI of 50 had been operated in other hospital by means of a laparoscopic gastric bypass.

Operation

According to surgeon, the operation went from the technical point of view without incidences, but patient had to be reoperated immediately after the initial operation because of hypovolemic shock and low hemoglobin rate. By laparotomy, postoperative bleeding appeared that was caused by a splenic bleeding and splenectomy was performed.

Postoperative Course: Identification and Treatment of Complication

Patient developed important ascites after operation. On the CT scan at postoperative day three, thrombosis of the splenic portal vein was observed with some thickness of small bowel loops (Fig. 51.5). Leukocyte rate was normal and the lactate increased to 2.6 mmol/l. The day of the transfer to our department and suspecting some grade of mesenteric ischemia, a relaparotomy was performed. Bowels were found to be normal and the surgeon decided not to perform thrombectomy of the thrombosed superior mesenteric and portal vein and hence treated the patient conservatively by anticoagulation in the form of iv heparin (Fig. 51.6). Patient recovered completely and went home.

Discussion

Van 't Riet et al. reviewed 563 splenectomies and found nine (2 %) that were complicated by symptomatic portal vein thrombosis (Illustration 51.1a, b) [1]. All the patients of these cases had either fever or abdominal pain. Two of 16 patients

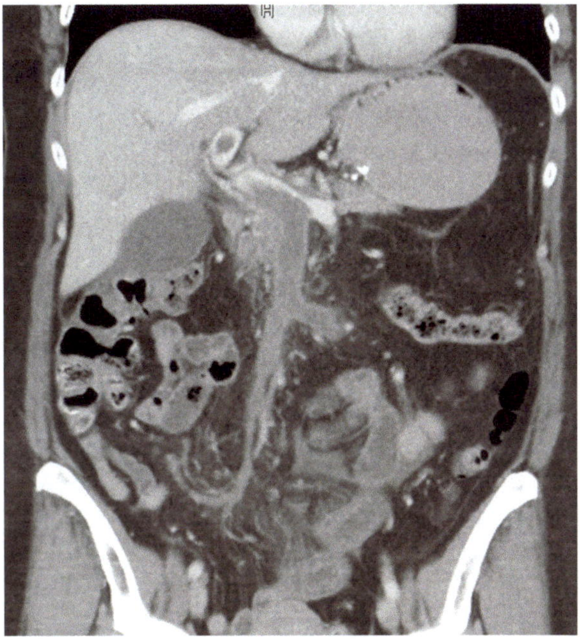

Fig. 51.5 Thrombosis vena porta, superior mesenteric vein and splenic vein

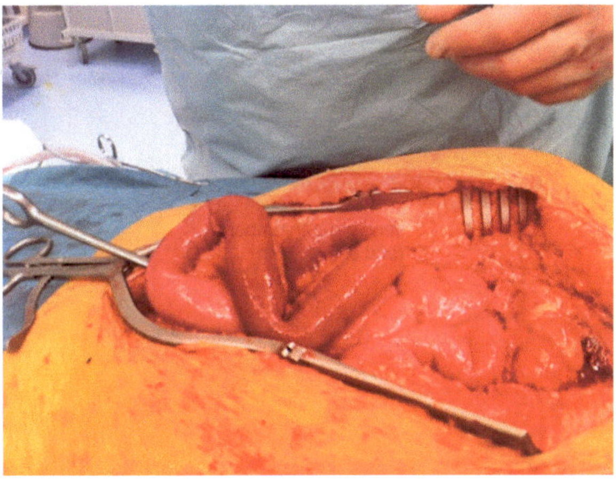

Fig. 51.6 Aspect of the bowels during explorative laparotomy

with a myeloproliferative disorder developed portal vein thrombosis after splenectomy ($P=0.03$) and 4 of 49 patients with hemolytic anemia ($P=0.005$). Portal vein thrombosis should be suspected in a patient with fever or abdominal pain after splenectomy. Prophylactic anticoagulants should be given. Patients with a myeloproliferative disorder or hemolytic anemia are at higher risk; they might benefit from early detection by a routine Doppler ultrasonography after splenectomy.

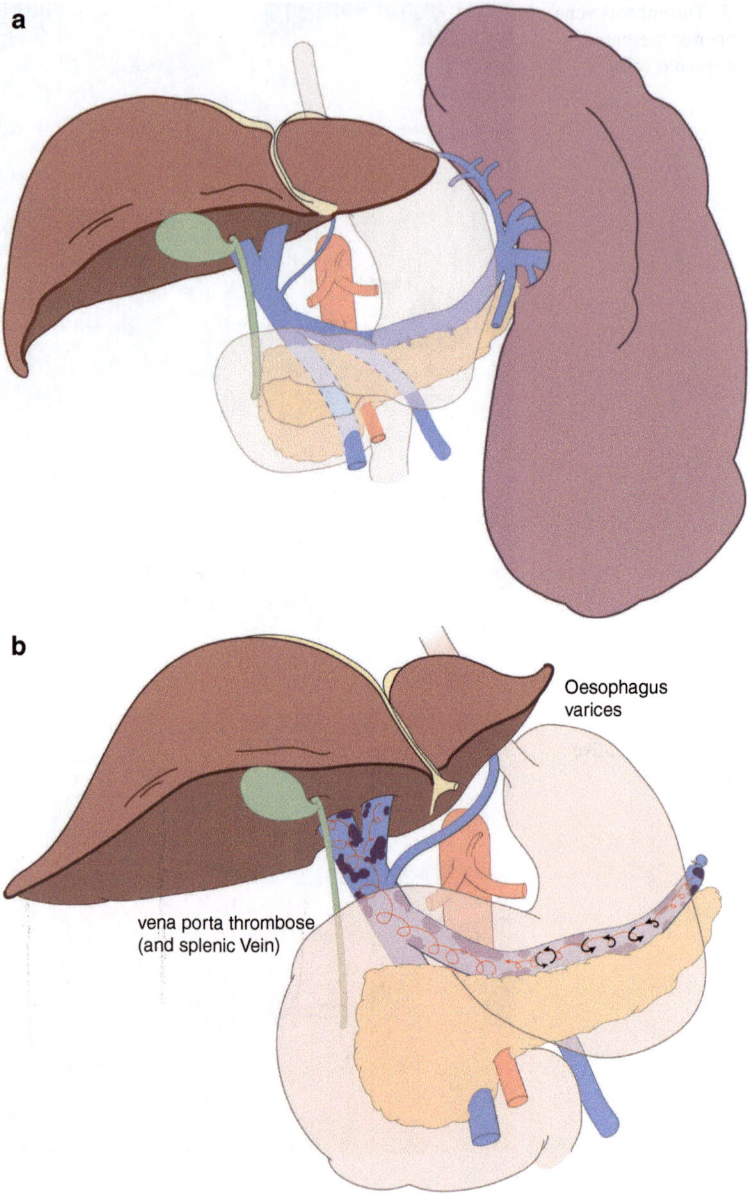

Illustration 51.1 (**a**, **b**) Postoperative thrombosis of the splenic and portal vein is a frequent complication after splenectomy for giant spleens. It should always be considered and prevented by prophylactic anticoagulation. Turbulence in the flow and postoperative thrombocytosis may be the cause. Portal thrombosis can lead to portal hypertension

Reference

1. Van 't Riet M, Burger JW, van Muiswinkel JM, et al. Diagnosis and treatment of portal vein thrombosis following splenectomy. Br J Surg. 2000;87:1229–33.

Chapter 52
Case on Rebleeding After Initial Coiling of Spleen Trauma

Rutger J. Lely and Miguel A. Cuesta

Keywords Spleen • Splenic trauma • Angiography and coiling • Rebleeding

Diagnosis and Indication for Angiography

A 48-year-old male patient was admitted to the hospital after a scooter-to-car accident. Patient had abdominal pain, the physical and radiological examinations revealed his two lowest ribs broken, the CT scan showed the spleen ruptured (Fig. 52.1), hemoglobin was low 6.5, and the patient became hemodynamically stable after fluid reposition. A decision was taken to perform angiographic examination and coiling. On CT-angiography, a blush was seen in the splenic artery, it being coiled successfully on angiography (Fig. 52.2a, b). Patient recovered and went home 3 days later, being stable and having adequate pain treatment.

Follow-Up: Identification and Treatment of Complication

Two months later, he was acutely readmitted on to the ward, because of a large mass in the left upper abdomen and abdominal pain. On the CT scan, some sort of splenic fluid collection or cyst of 15 cm was observed that was attached to the inferior aspect of the spleen (Fig. 52.3). Patient was hemodynamically stable, but his hemoglobin

R.J. Lely, M.D.
Radiology, VU University Medical Centre, Amsterdam, The Netherlands
e-mail: r.lelij@vumc.nl

M.A. Cuesta, M.D. (✉)
Department of Surgery, VU University Medical Center, Amsterdam, The Netherlands
e-mail: ma.cuesta@vumc.nl

M.A. Cuesta, H.J. Bonjer (eds.), *Case Studies of Postoperative Complications after Digestive Surgery*, DOI 10.1007/978-3-319-01613-9_52,

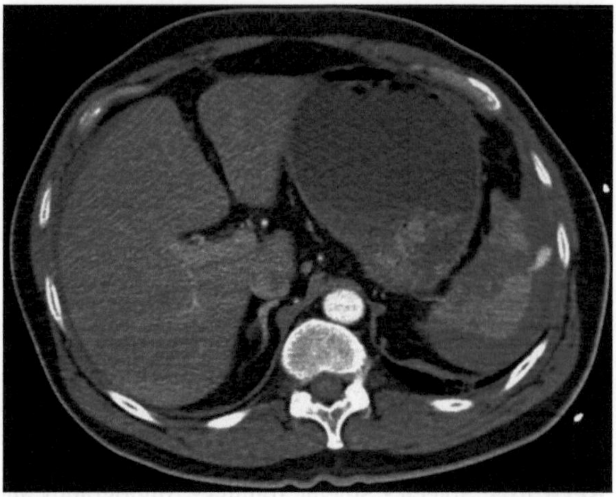

Fig. 52.1 CT-angiography scan on admission, bleeding splenic rupture

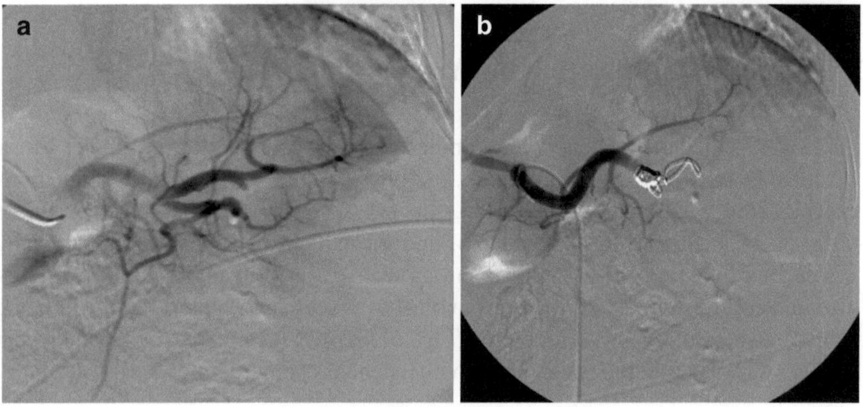

Fig. 52.2 Angiography pre- (**a**) and post-coiling (**b**) splenic artery

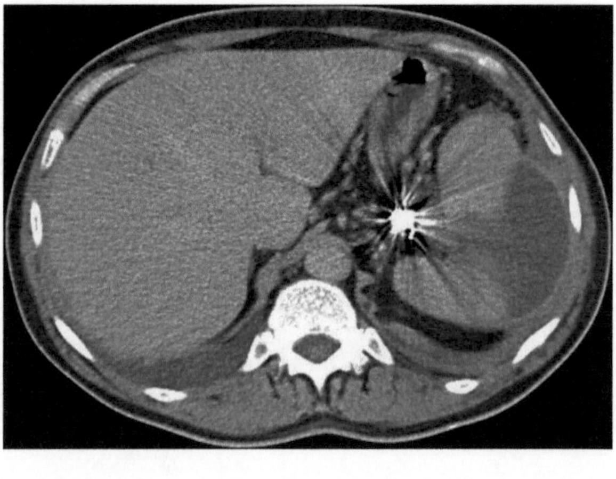

Fig. 52.3 CT scan on readmission, showing the hemorrhagic cyst

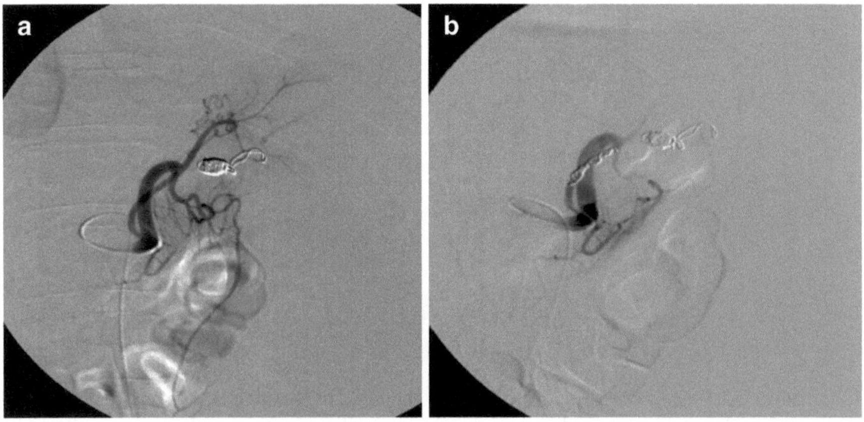

Fig. 52.4 Pre- (**a**) and post-coiling (**b**) short vessel with blush

Fig. 52.5 Percutaneous drainage of the splenic cyst

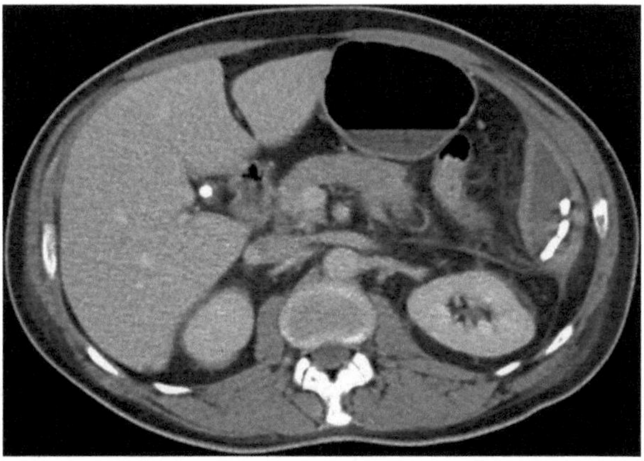

was 7.3. A new angiography was performed, and it revealed a large branch of the short vessels going to the splenic old ruptured surface. This was considered the cause for the bleeding and it was subsequently coiled (Fig. 52.4a, b). In retrospect, at the first angiography this short vessel had been seen producing a blush. The next day, the cyst was drained by means of a percutaneous drain, evacuating 1.5 l old blood (Fig. 52.5). After 2 days, the drain was retired and patient could go home.

Discussion

Angiographic coiling is becoming the standard approach for this blunt abdominal trauma. Only those hemodynamic unstable patients who are not reacting to fluid reposition or having associated traumatic lesions should be considered for explorative laparotomy. During angiography, all blush should be coiled. In the present

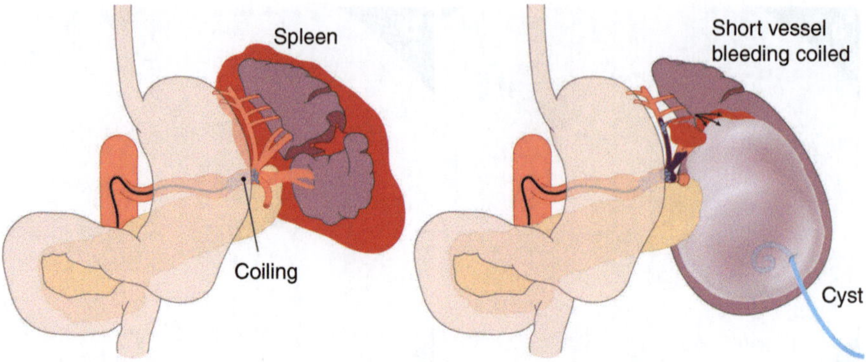

Illustration 52.1 Spleen trauma is frequently conservatively treated. CT-angiography scan showing a blush should be treated by angiography and coiling. In the case that patient is hemodynamically unstable and does not react to fluids, surgical approach is indicated. Moreover if multitrauma patient, surgical treatment of the splenic trauma should be done

case, only the splenic artery bleeding had been initially coiled, whereas in retrospection also a blush was present at one short vessel. Patient developed a slow bleeding with a hemorrhagic cyst. During the second admission a new angiography showed the bleeding. This was coiled and the cyst percutaneously drained (Illustration 52.1) [1].

Reference

1. Bhullar IS, Frykberg ER, Siraqusa D, et al. Selective angiographic embolization of blunt splenic traumatic injuries in adults decreases failure rate of nonoperative management. J Trauma Acute Care Surg. 2012;72:1127–34.

Chapter 53
Case on Adrenal Insufficiency (Addison Syndrome), After Removal of an Adenocarcinoma of the Adrenal Gland

Miguel A. Cuesta and H. Jaap Bonjer

Keywords Adrenal carcinoma • Thrombus caval vein • Addison crisis

Diagnosis and Indication for Surgery

A 30-year-old female patient was referred to our department because of a tumor of the right adrenal with ingrowth in the inferior vena cava. Since 4 months, she had complaints of tiredness and loss of weight. Recently she had been admitted to the referral hospital because of thoracic pain, edematous legs, and dyspnoea; her complaints were possibly caused by pulmonary emboli. Pulmonary emboli were not found, though, but a tumor of $8 \times 5 \times 7$ cm in the right adrenal with ingrowth into the inferior vena cava (IVC) (Fig. 53.1). There were no distance metastases, but on the CT scan of her abdomen an extensive thrombus was seen in the IVC up to the right atrium and into the right hepatic vein (Figs. 53.2a, b and 53.3a, b). During high fever, a blood culture showed a not-yet specified Streptococcus, but on the endo-ultrasound there were no signs of endocarditis. Moreover, on the PTC a positive tumor and thrombus were found with central necrosis (Fig. 53.4a, b). Hormonal assessment showed normal aldosterone and epinephrines, but high cortisol 0.5 μmol/L, normal 0.03 and 0.28. Diagnosis was established as cortisol-releasing adrenal carcinoma on the right side with thrombus in the ICV. At admission, she was heparinized and an operation plan was made with the cardio surgeon to resect the tumor and thrombus as radical operation.

M.A. Cuesta, M.D. (✉) • H.J. Bonjer, M.D., Ph.D., F.R.C.S.C.
Department of Surgery, VU University Medical Center, Amsterdam, The Netherlands
e-mail: ma.cuesta@vumc.nl; j.bonjer@vumc.nl

M.A. Cuesta, H.J. Bonjer (eds.), *Case Studies of Postoperative Complications after Digestive Surgery*, DOI 10.1007/978-3-319-01613-9_53,

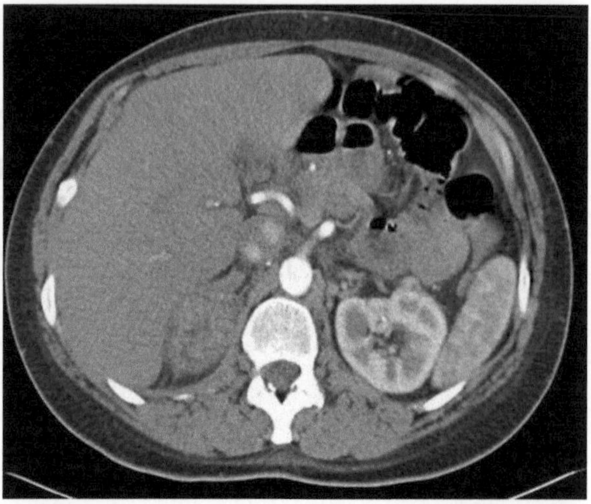

Fig. 53.1 CT scan showing the tumor in the right adrenal and vena cava

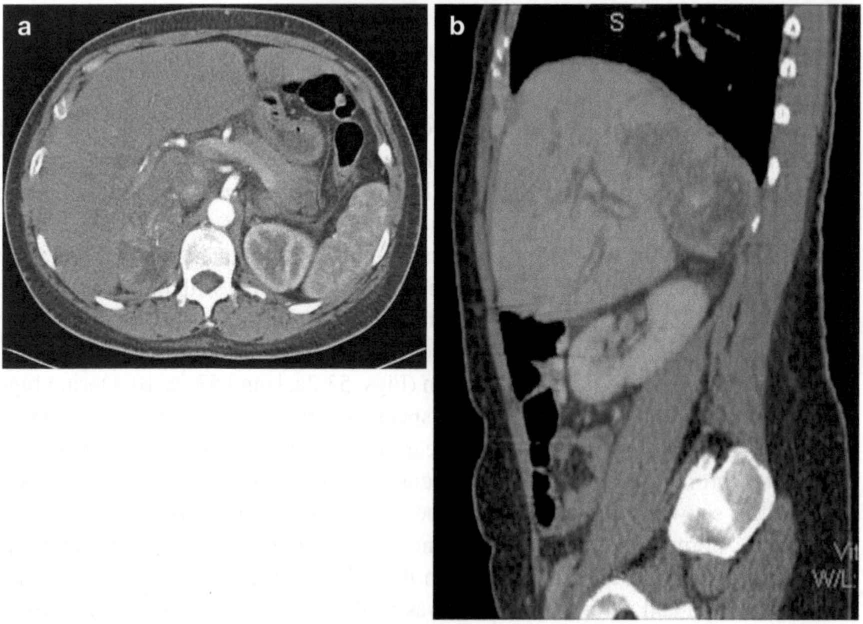

Fig. 53.2 (**a**, **b**) CT scan showing the tumor in contact with the right hepatic vein

Operation

At operation, by subcostal right phrenolaparotomy and sternotomy, a resection was performed on the right adrenal and the thrombus in the vena cava after control of the suprahepatic vena cava at the level of the right auricle and proximal of the hepatic veins. Also a Pringle maneuver was done. The tumor and the thrombus were resected en bloc. The thrombus was taken out by a cavotomy. Because of

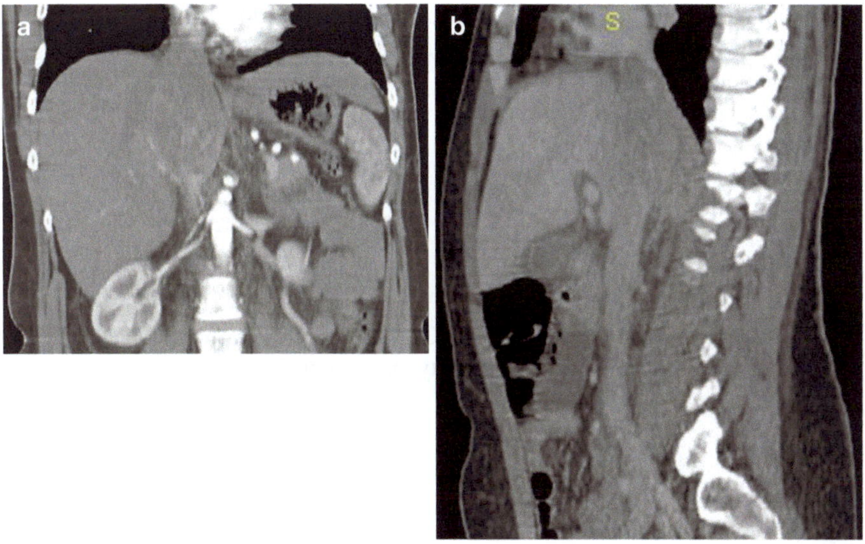

Fig. 53.3 (**a**, **b**) CT scan showing the tumor with thrombus in the vena cava in direction to right auricle

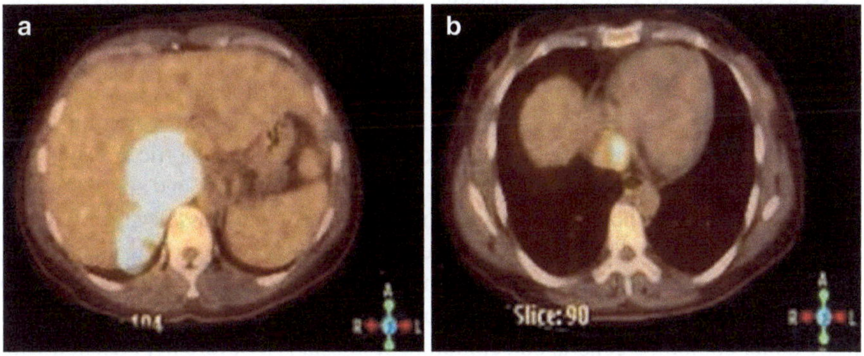

Fig. 53.4 (**a**, **b**) PET-CT showing avid spot in the tumor and vena cava

ingrowth in the right hepatic vein, a small part was resected and consequently occluded. Pathology showed a radical resected adrenocortical carcinoma with high mitosis index and areas of necrosis and hemorrhage.

Postoperative Course: Identification and Treatment of Complication

Patient was admitted postoperatively on the IC, where a period of shock occurred and oliguria was observed. Differential diagnosis was made between (a) sepsis (started with iv broad spectrum antibiotics), (b) postoperative bleeding,

(c) thrombosis of the hepatic veins, and (d) presence of Addison crisis (started with hydrocortisone iv). Blood cultures were negative, US showed permeable hepatic veins, and hemoglobin was constant. The Addison crisis was treated by an iv hydrocortisone scheme. Patient went home 11 days after operation with hydrocortisone treatment.

Pathology

A 7-cm adrenocortical carcinoma (ACC) was found. The tumor was radically resected but showed a high mitotic activity and venous invasion.

Discussion

Currently, Addison crises are not frequently found in surgical practice. The cause of Addison crisis in this patient is that no corticosteroid scheme was given preoperatively. In spite of a precise diagnosis and preparation of the operation, nobody had taken account of this important point during preparation of patient for surgery. This was especially important in this case because of corticosteroid production of the tumor, the other being adrenal and probably atrophic. Functional variants of ACC have been reported to be more common than the nonfunctional types, and patients mainly present with Cushing syndrome. Recently data suggest that nonfunctional ACCs are more common than the functional types. Adrenocortical carcinoma accounts for approximately 5–10 % of cases of Cushing syndrome and approximately 40 % of patients with both Cushing syndrome and an adrenal mass have an ACC.

Cassinello Ogea et al. described a 70-year-old obese, hypertensive woman taking angiotensin-converting enzyme (ACE) inhibitors and chlorthalidone but with no history of corticosteroid treatment. She underwent a nephrectomy and adrenalectomy under combined general and epidural anesthesia [1]. Severe hypotension with oliguria developed during surgery and persisted during postoperative recovery, with anuria, metabolic acidosis, hyponatremia, and hyperpotassemia. The anuria, metabolic acidosis, hyponatremia, and hyperpotassemia led the authors to consider a diagnosis of an Addison crisis. The patient responded to corticosteroids treatment and low cortisol levels confirmed the diagnosis of adrenal insufficiency.

Reference

1. Cassinello Ogea C, Giron Nombiela JR, Ruiz Tramazaygues J, et al. Severe perioperative hypotension after nephrectomy with adrenalectomy. Rev Esp Anestesiol Reanim. 2002;49:213–7.

Chapter 54
Case on Leakage After Left Pancreatic Resection

Joris J.G. Scheepers

Keywords Mucinous cystadenoma • Left pancreatectomy • Enucleation • Pancreatic leakage • Pancreatic stump

First Patient

Diagnosis and Indication for Surgery

A 63-year-old lady was admitted to the hospital and studied by US and CT scan because of pain in the epigastric region. A tumor was found in the body of the pancreas with aspect of a cyst, possibly mucinous (Fig. 54.1). It was proposed to resect the cyst by laparoscopic approach.

Operation

During laparoscopy, the tumor was considered superficial and probably serous. After laparoscopic US it was enucleated. The tumor was found at distance of 5 mm from the pancreatic duct (PD). A drain was left along the pancreas.

J.J.G. Scheepers, M.D.
Department of Surgery, Ranier de Graaf Hospital, Delft, The Netherlands
e-mail: j.scheepers@rdgg.nl

M.A. Cuesta, H.J. Bonjer (eds.), *Case Studies of Postoperative Complications after Digestive Surgery*, DOI 10.1007/978-3-319-01613-9_54,

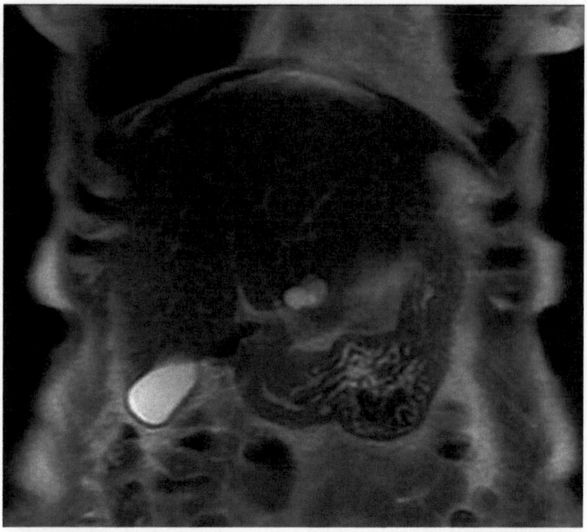

Fig. 54.1 MRI, showing preoperative tumor in the pancreas

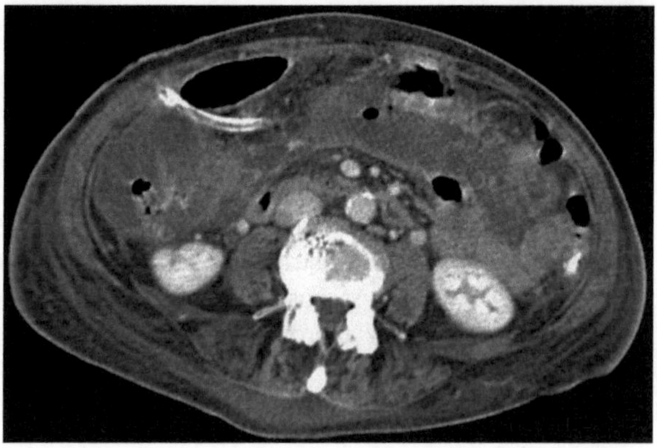

Fig. 54.2 Postoperative CT scan. Fluid in lesser sac drained

Postoperative Course

Postoperatively from the first day a progressive high production of the drain was observed ranging from 500 cc to 1 L, with amylase rate of 10,000 U/mL. Because of increasing pain and fever, a CT scan again was performed and a fluid collection in the lesser sac percutaneously drained (Fig. 54.2). Because of the high production, it was clear that the leakage could be caused by a leak of the PD or a direct branch; hence it was decided to stent the duct by means of an ERCP (Fig. 54.3). This was

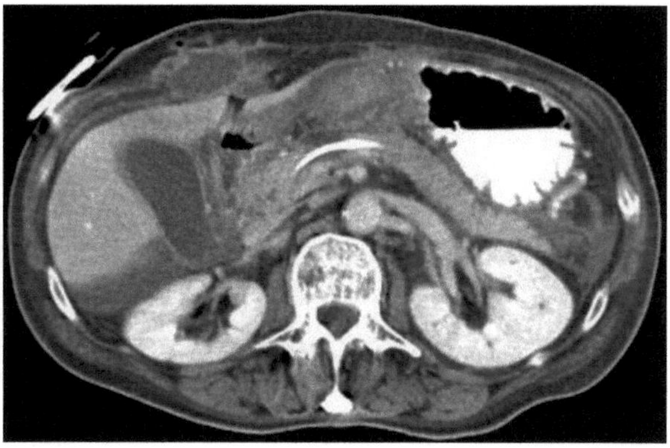

Fig. 54.3 Drain in pancreatic duct

done the ninth postoperative day with success. Production decreased and finally the two drains could be taken out.

Pathology of the cyst showed a pancreatic serous cystadenoma radically resected.

Second Patient

Diagnosis and Indication for Surgery

A 58-year-old male butcher was admitted to the hospital because of acute pancreatitis localized in the tail of the pancreas by the CT scan. Complaints disappeared after 3 days and no cause was found for the pancreatitis, neither gallstones nor alcohol abuse.

After a period of 3 months, pain in the left upper abdomen returned without other symptoms. Amylase and lipase were normal and on the CT scan a suspected image for tumor was found in the area between body and tail of pancreas. Imaging was not typical for chronic pancreatitis or pseudocyst but more for a nonclassified tumor of 3 cm and it was proposed for it to be resected.

Operation

By laparotomy, the tumor was resected along with the spleen without problems and the stump of the pancreas closed by stitches. A drain was left in the area. After 2 days the drain was taken out. Patient was discharged at the fifth postoperative day.

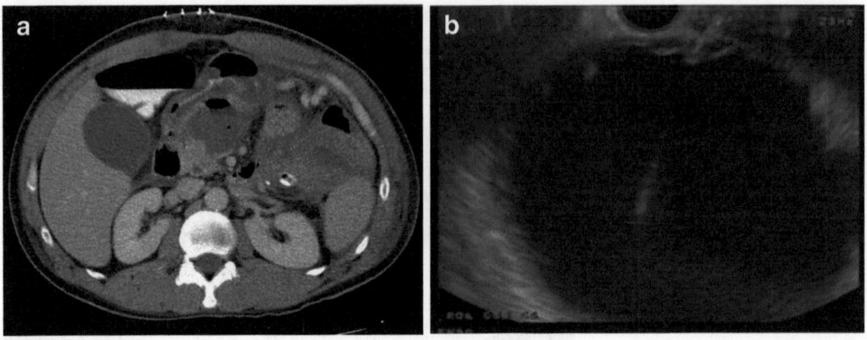

Fig. 54.4 (**a**, **b**) CT scan showing the leak collection. Transgastric US. First stent along the guide wire

Postoperative Course: Identification and Treatment of Complication

At the outpatient clinic at the14th postoperative day, the patient had abdominal pain and discomfort. The laboratory study showed the amylase to be normal, but CRP was increased up to 310 mg/L. A CT scan showed a fluid collection of 8 cm at the resection area and it was proposed to be drained transgastrically (Fig. 54.4a).

Through gastroscopy and endoscopic US, fluid collection was localized retrogastrically (Fig. 54.4b), being drained transgastrically, leaving three stents between stomach and fluid collection (Fig. 54.5a–c). Complaints did not disappear completely and because of fever a new CT scan was performed showing a collection at the pancreatic area (Fig. 54.5d). A pancreatic duct stent was placed by ERCP and the collection was percutaneously drained (Fig. 54.5e). Four days later the patient could be discharged. Pathology of the tumor showed a mucinous cystadenoma, radically resected.

Discussion

These two cases illustrate the uncertainty the surgeon can experience following such operations whether or not postoperative leakage is taking place. There are different ways to close the surface of pancreas and—protocols are ongoing to establish the best way. In the first case, enucleation was done and probably a direct branch of the PD was damaged. In the case of stump leakage with complaints, there are two possibilities for drainage, the transgastric and the percutaneous route. If leakage persists, then the pancreatic duct should be drained (Illustration 54.1) [1].

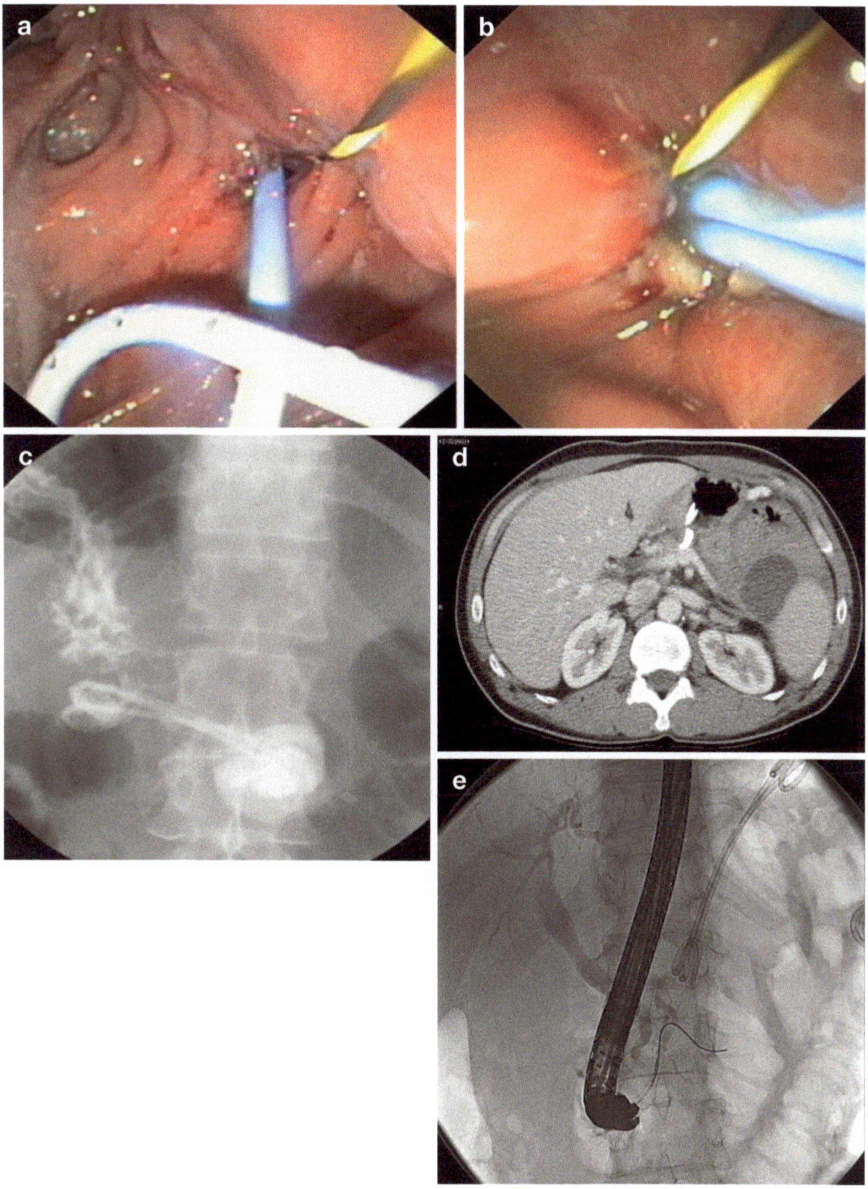

Fig. 54.5 (**a–c**) First stent along the guide wire and stents between collection and stomach; control gastric X-ray showing the stents. (**d**, **e**) Control CT scan showing persisting collection, being drained by pancreatic duct drainage and percutaneous drainage

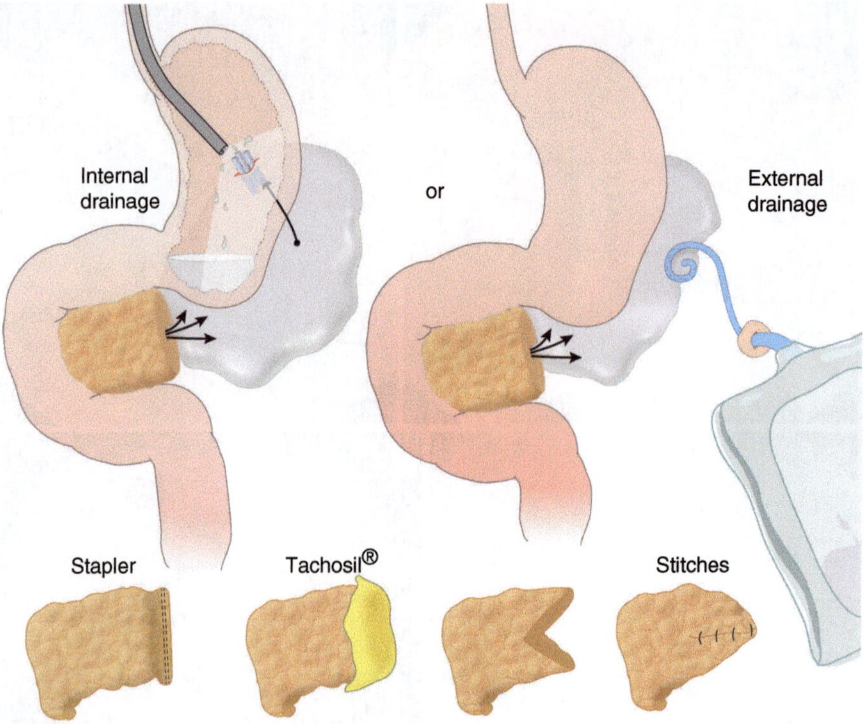

Illustration 54.1 Pancreatic leakage after resection with symptoms can be drained percutaneously or transgastrically depending on the localization. Both approaches are complementary. Different methods to close the pancreatic stump

Reference

1. Goh BKP, Tan YM, Chung YFA, et al. Critical appraisal of 232 consecutive distal pancreatectomies with emphasis on risk factors, outcome and management of the postoperative pancreatic fistula. Arch Surg. 2008;143:956–65.

Chapter 55
Case on Postoperative Shock After Laparoscopic Appendicectomy

Joris J.G. Scheepers

Keywords Bleeding • Abdominal wall • Acute appendicitis • Laparoscopic appendectomy • Epigastric arteries

Diagnosis and Indication for Surgery

A 36-year-old lady was admitted to the hospital because of acute appendicitis. Clinically but also on the CT scan the diagnosis was clear (Fig. 55.1).

Operation

Patient underwent a laparoscopic exploration by means of a three-trocar approach, one of 10 mm under the umbilicus, a second of 5 mm suprapubic, and the third of 10 mm localized between the umbilicus and the anterior superior left iliac spine. The operation was converted to a MacBurney incision because of bleeding from the appendicular artery, and that was difficult to fix. The appendix was taken out and bleeding fixed with stitches. After closure, the patient went into shock and she did not react on saline and colloids. The surgeon thought of the possibility of a re-bleeding from the appendicular artery and decided to reoperate the patient immediately. During the exploration through the MacBurney incision, the patient went deeply into shock and surgeon called upon a senior surgeon to assist him. It was clear that the appendicular artery was not the cause for the bleeding, but the abdomen was filled with blood and clots. The surgeons decided to perform a median

J.J.G. Scheepers, M.D.
Department of Surgery, Ranier de Graaf Hospital, Delft, The Netherlands
e-mail: j.scheepers@rdgg.nl

M.A. Cuesta, H.J. Bonjer (eds.), *Case Studies of Postoperative Complications after Digestive Surgery*, DOI 10.1007/978-3-319-01613-9_55,

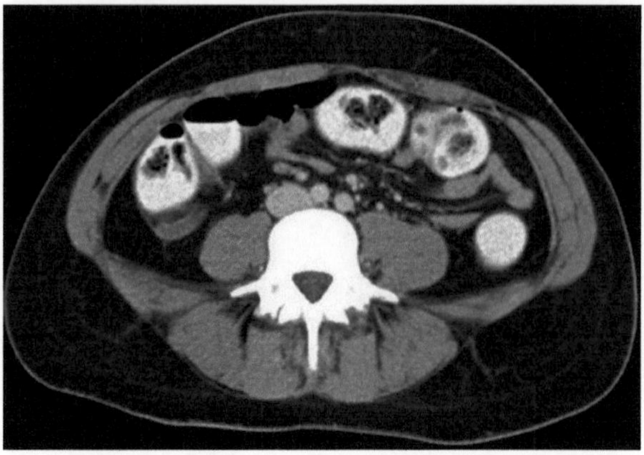

Fig. 55.1 CT scan with diagnosis of acute appendicitis

laparotomy and it became clear that the bleeding was not coming from the liver or the spleen but from a lesion of the left inferior epigastric artery and vein right on the place of the last trocar between the umbilicus and the spine. Bleeding was fixed by means of transfixion stitches and clots removed. Patient recovered after transfusion of 4 packed cell units.

Discussion

The lesson of this case is that every step during laparoscopy, including insertion of trocars, is very important and will be safe. Especially, lateral of the midline introduced trocars are at risk for lesions of the vessels of the abdominal wall. Saber et al. studied by CT scan the at-risk zones for bleeding in the abdominal wall and determined that the inferior epigastric vessels are usually located in the area between 4 and 8 cm from the midline [1]. Avoiding this area will determine the safe zone of entry of the anterior abdominal wall. But it is not always possible to obviate this zone and it is possible by visualization to see the epigastric vessels during insertion of trocars and the corresponding bleeding [2]. Moreover, this is a complication not frequently described in the literature, probably occurring more frequent than published [3]. The patient here presented summarizes all problems in relation with lesion of the epigastric vessels during laparoscopy: bleeding during operation, patient in shock, and difficult differential diagnosis. Take care during creation of insufflation and insertion of trocars !

References

1. Saber AA, Meslemani AM, Davis R, Pimentel R. Safety zones for anterior abdominal wall entry during laparoscopy: a CT scan mapping of epigastric vessels. Ann Surg. 2004;239: 182–5.
2. Hurd WW, Amesse LS, Gruber JS, et al. Visualization of the epigastric vessels and bladder before laparoscopic trocar placement. Fertil Steril. 2003;80:209–12.
3. Valera Sánchez Z, Morales Conde S, López Bernal F, Cadet Dussort H. A large hematoma in the abdominal wall after trocar insertion. Rev Esp Enferm Dig. 2008;100:64–6.

Chapter 56
Case on Postoperative Abscess After Appendicectomy

Suzanne S. Gisbertz

Keywords Acute appendicitis • Laparoscopic appendicectomy • Percuatneous drainage • Abscess

Diagnosis and Operation Description

Six weeks before, this 58-year-old female manager had undergone a laparoscopic appendectomy because of a phlegmonous-inflamed appendix (Fig. 56.1). Through three trocars her appendix had been removed by using an endostapler white. The appendix was deposited in an endobag and consequently exteriorized. Hemostasia was good, and after closure of the trocar sites, the operation was completed.

Postoperative Course: Identification and Treatment of Complication

During the same hospital stay, her postoperative course was complicated by a small bowel ileus and fever. On the CT scan, an abscess was seen in the right paracolic area, being subsequently percutaneously drained (Fig. 56.2a, b). Patient improved, and once the drain was removed, she went home.

Presenting now some weeks later at the outpatient policlinic, she claimed not feeling well, having a poor intake, and diarrhea. She was readmitted to the hospital, now sick, with temperature 38.1 °C, heart rate 94 bpm, and on physical examination having localized pain in the right lower abdomen. The CRP was 250, and

S.S. Gisbertz, M.D.
Department of Surgery, Academic Medical Centre, Amsterdam, The Netherlands
e-mail: s.gisbertz@antoniusziekenhuis.nl

M.A. Cuesta, H.J. Bonjer (eds.), *Case Studies of Postoperative Complications after Digestive Surgery*, DOI 10.1007/978-3-319-01613-9_56,

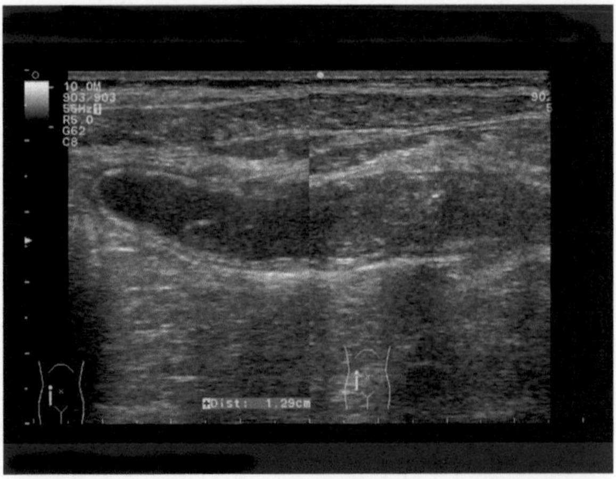

Fig. 56.1 US diagnosis acute appendicitis

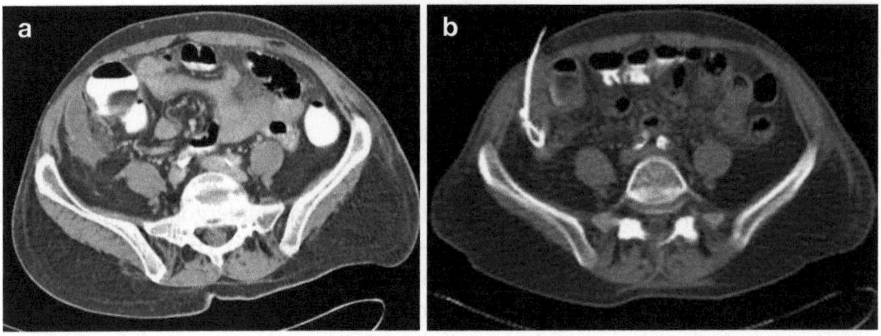

Fig. 56.2 (**a**) CT scan showing an abscess around cecum. (**b**) CT scan, percutaneous drainage abscess

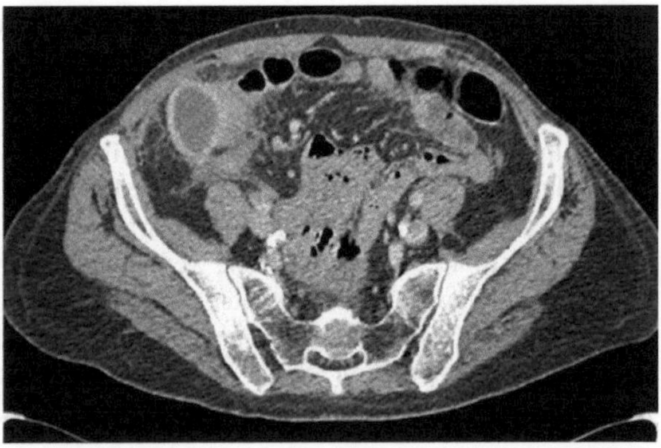

Fig. 56.3 CT scan, new abscess, 3 weeks after 1st operation

leukocytosis of 12.5×10^9/l. On the CT scan an abscess was found paracolic space right, again being drained (Fig. 56.3) and treated by iv broad spectrum antibiotics (AB). Nutrition and general condition improved, and after retiring the drain, she could return home at the 10th day following readmission.

Discussion

The Cochrane reviews and meta-analysis comparing rates of open and laparoscopic appendectomies of postoperative abscesses show rates slightly higher for the laparoscopic group [1].

Pertaining lesson of this case is perhaps that before the first discharge following the requirement for checking clinically and by imaging whether the abscess has completely disappeared. Instead—after pressure by the patient to return home for reinitiating her work—this control had been omitted.

Reference

1. Sauerland S, Jaschinski T, Neugebauer EA. Laparoscopic versus open surgery for suspected appendicitis. Cochrane Database Syst Rev. 2010;6(10).

Chapter 57
Case on Carcinoid Discovered in the Appendix

Miguel A. Cuesta and Maria Conde Rodriguez

Keywords Appendix tumor • Appendix • Carcinoid tumor

First Patient

Diagnosis and Indication for Surgery

A 47-year-old male schoolteacher was admitted to the department because of abdominal pain in the lower abdomen and vomiting. He had fever of 39.2 °C and leukocytosis of 13,000 and a CRP of 61 mg/l. On physical examination the patient was sick and had a clear peritonitis sign on the right lower abdomen. On the US, an imaging was suspected for acute appendicitis and the patient was proposed for a laparoscopic appendectomy (Fig. 57.1).

Operation

A perforated appendicitis was found with local pus in Douglas space—thereafter being drained. Patient received a 5-day administration of iv antibiotics and recovered slowly. On pathological examination, a perforated acute appendicitis was seen with a carcinoid tumor of 8 mm, radically resected.

M.A. Cuesta, M.D. (✉)
Department of Surgery, VU University Medical Center, Amsterdam, The Netherlands
e-mail: ma.cuesta@vumc.nl

M.C. Rodriguez
Department of Surgery, Hospital Clinico, Universidad de Madrid, Spain

M.A. Cuesta, H.J. Bonjer (eds.), *Case Studies of Postoperative Complications after Digestive Surgery*, DOI 10.1007/978-3-319-01613-9_57,

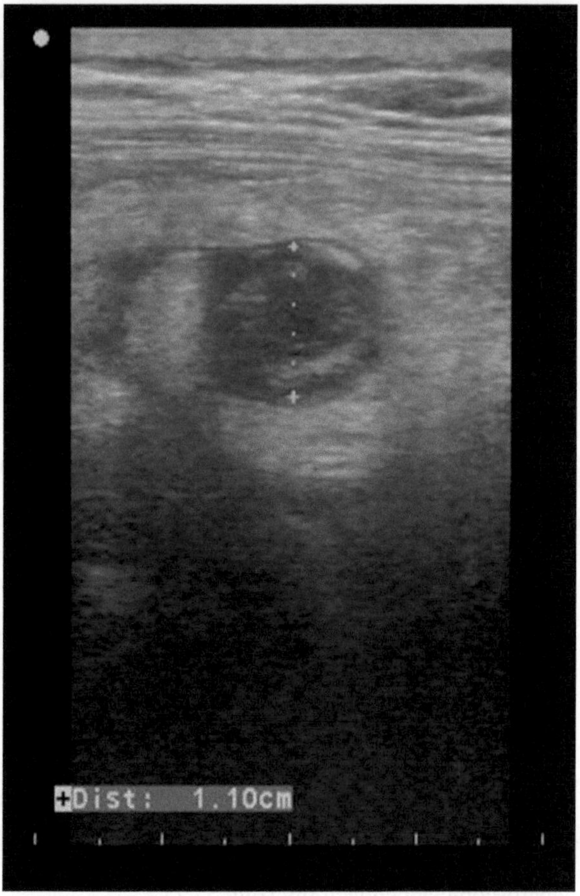

Fig. 57.1 US diagnosis of acute appendicitis with possible tumor

The patient was told that no interventions were necessary, and he recovered. Outpatient clinic control was ended after 1 year.

Second Patient

Diagnosis and Indication for Surgery

A 66-year-old retired man, known with Bechterew's disease and diabetes mellitus type II, was admitted to the hospital with a worsening of abdominal pain, and vomiting. Since a year he had complained of progressive abdominal distension, colic pain, and change of defecation pattern. On the day of admission, physical examination showed a moderately sick patient with 37.8 °C temperature, abdominal distension, and intestinal obstruction type peristalsis. Laboratory tests included a leukocytosis

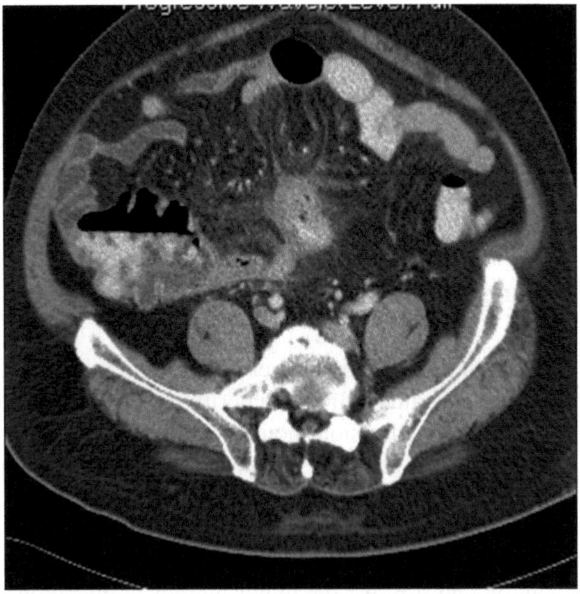

Fig. 57.2 CT scan, intestinal obstruction with an abscess located on the right lower abdomen possibly of appendicular origin

of 15,000 with CRP of 75. On the plain X-ray of the abdomen, small bowel dilatation was observed. On the CT scan, a small bowel intestinal obstruction was found with an abscess located on the right lower abdomen possibly of appendicular origin (Fig. 57.2).

Operation

Because of the intestinal obstruction, the surgeon decided to operate on the patient through a midline incision, and so a perforated appendicitis was found with an abscess of 7 by 7 cm. This was the cause of the intestinal obstruction. After appendectomy and abscess drainage, intestinal loops were freed and abdomen closed leaving a drain.

Postoperative Course

Antibiotics were given iv for 7 days, and TPN (parenteral nutrition) until recovery of the intestinal transit. Patient recuperated. Histological examination showed a goblet cell carcinoid, growing diffuse over a trajectory of 4 cm with ingrowth through the muscularis propria. Serosa and mesoappendix were free of tumor. Moreover, an acute appendicitis with perforation was found.

On the postoperative CT scan, there were no distance metastases and after recovery patient was proposed for colonoscopy and right hemicolectomy based on the histological outcome. Six weeks later, a right hemicolectomy was performed with no special postoperative events. No metastases and no lymph node involvement of the central mesentery were observed. On histological examination no rest of the carcinoid tumor was seen and all the lymph nodes (17) were negative.

After 6 years of follow-ups, with regularly held CT scans of abdomen and controls of serotonin in platelets, the patient could be discharged.

Discussion

A lesson drawn from both cases is that a carcinoid in the appendix can present itself as acute appendicitis. In the majority of cases, the pathologist will reveal the diagnosis and then a decision should be done what to do.

Questions do arise. First, what to do during operation if suspicion arises of the presence of a (malignant) tumor of the appendix? Second, what to do once the pathology report confirms the type of tumor and staging?

Concerning the first question, my answer would be: If the tumor is larger than 2 cm, one must resect the tumor by radical operation—in most of the cases by an ileocecal or right hemicolectomy resection. If in doubt or in the case of a small tumor, being less than 2 cm, one must wait for the pathological report of the appendix. If the location of the tumor is in the base of the appendix at the cecum, then one must do an ileocecal resection (Figs. 57.3 and 57.4, Illustration 57.1).

Concerning the second matter, the different histological types and subsequent treatment and behavior of malignant tumors of the appendix, Turaga et al. studied all patients ($n = 5{,}655$) with appendiceal malignancies and found in the Surveillance, Epidemiology, and End Results (SEER) database from 1973 to 2007 [1]. The tumors were classified as malignant carcinoid, goblet cell carcinoid, colonic type adenocarcinoma, mucinous adenocarcinoma, and signet ring cell type. The 5-year disease-specific survival rates were 93 % for malignant carcinoid, 81 % for goblet cell carcinoid, 55 % for colonic type adenocarcinoma, 58 % for mucinous

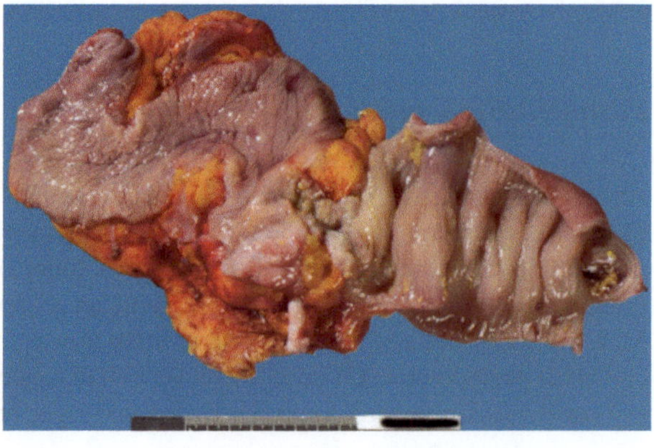

Fig. 57.3 Globet cell carcinoid of the appendix. Open specimen of ileocecal resection

adenocarcinoma, and 27 % for signet ring cell type. Histologic subtype is an important predictor of disease-specific survival and overall survival in patients with appendiceal tumors. Moreover, prognosis depends on the radicality of the appendectomy but also of the size of the tumor. Especially carcinoids smaller than 2 cm and radically operated do not require other complementary treatment, whereas tumors > 2 cm or not radical will need a right hemicolectomy to assure the completeness.

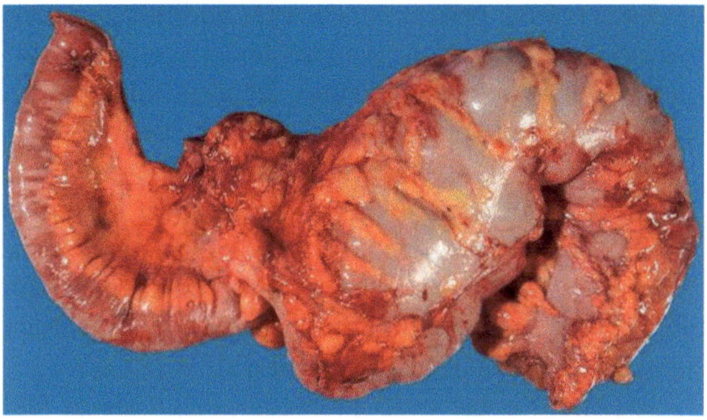

Fig. 57.4 Goblet cell carcinoid located at the origin of the appendix in the cecum, 1 cm. Radically resected, but 5 positive lymph nodes

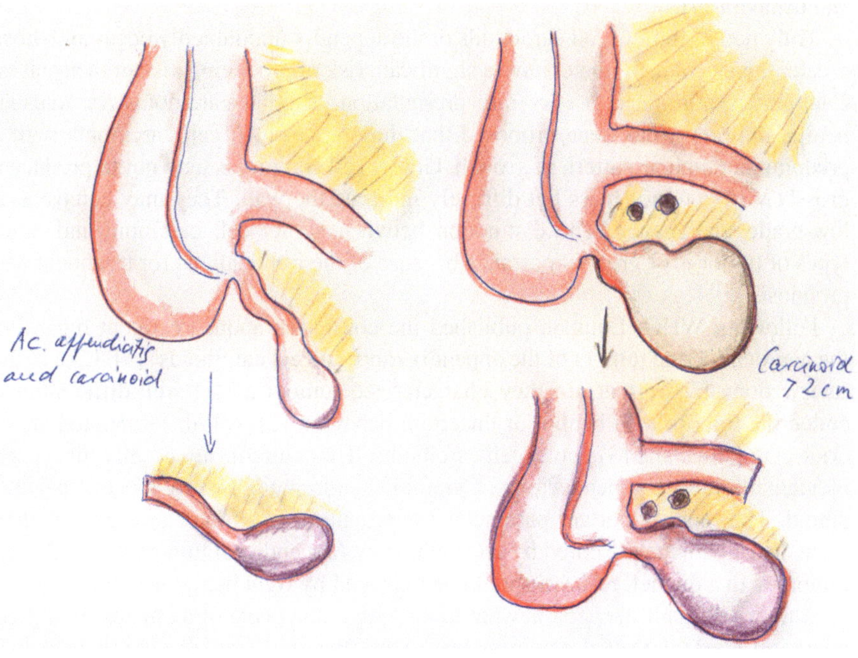

Illustration 57.1 In case that a carcinoid is found in the appendicectomy specimen, and the tumor is less than 2 cm and radically resected, no more surgical resection should be added. If the tumor is >2 cm or not radically resected, a right hemicolectomy should be proposed

Concerning frequency of carcinoid tumors found in appendectomy specimens and posterior policy, In't Hof et al. performed a retrospective review of 1,485 appendectomies operated on in two centers in the Rotterdam area, during a period of 6 years [2]. Demographic data, clinical presentation, histopathology, operative reports, and survival rates were scored and compared with the literature. Carcinoid tumors were identified in three women and four men (0.47 %); their mean age was 32.7 years (range of 20–59). In all cases the clinical presentation resembled the symptoms of acute appendicitis. Laparoscopic appendectomy was the treatment of choice in five patients; in one of these patients, a conversion to laparotomy became necessary. Five patients underwent additional surgery after the pathology report became available. Four patients underwent ileocecal resection; one other patient underwent right hemicolectomy. In none of the reoperation specimens was a residual carcinoid tumor detected. After a mean follow-up of 65 months (age range of 25–92), all patients were alive and disease and symptom free. The authors concluded that carcinoid tumors of the appendix most often present as acute appendicitis. They also emphasized the value of histopathological analysis of each appendix removed. The long-term prognosis of incidentally found carcinoid tumors of the appendix is good. Butte et al. by analyzing 8,903 appendectomy specimens confirmed the results of In't Hof et al. [3].

Important is the exact pathology diagnosis of the different types of carcinoid tumors. Carr et al. reviewed these neuroendocrine tumors and their different types and behavior [4].

Truly neoplastic EC cell carcinoids of the appendix undoubtedly occur and those greater than 2 cm in diameter have a significant risk of producing distant metastases. Carcinoid syndrome is a very rare presentation. Tubular carcinoids are unusual benign tumors; it has been proposed that they represent L cell carcinoids with a predominant tubular pattern of growth. Goblet cell carcinoids tend not to produce a grossly visible tumor mass but diffusely infiltrate the wall. They may behave as a low-grade malignancy. The distinction between goblet cell carcinoid and other types of tumor is of great importance because of the implications for treatment and prognosis.

Following WHO, Louthan published the consensus about treatment regarding the neuroendocrine tumors of the appendix (appendiceal carcinoids) [5]. Like in the review done by Carr et al., they characterized tumors as (1) well-differentiated endocrine tumors with benign or uncertain behavior, (2) well-differentiated endocrine carcinoma, and (3) goblet cell carcinoma. These tumors are usually diagnosed incidentally during appendectomy. Carcinoid syndrome is rare in appendiceal carcinoid. The most important parameter for prognosis is a tumor size greater than 2 cm. Most patients are cured by appendectomy (appendiceal tumors < or = 2 cm); tumors with a diameter > 2 cm should be managed by right hemicolectomy [5].

Another difficult decision is what to do with a mucocele of an appendix during operation. Caracappa et al. found in their review that it is a rare disease (0.3 % of all appendectomies) and is characterized by the accumulation of mucoid material in the appendiceal lumen [6]. Four entities can be distinguished on the basis of histopathological epithelial characteristics: (1) simple appendiceal mucocele (AM),

(2) mucocele with epithelial hyperplasia, (3) cystadenoma, and (4) cystadenocarcinoma; the last two subgroups representing neoplastic forms. Dissemination of neoplastic cells and mucoid material in abdominal cavity, caused by appendiceal perforation, will clinically result in pseudomyxoma peritonei, which is the dramatic evolution in 10–15 % of cases. Clinically it can remain either asymptomatic for long time or it can manifest with abdominal pain that can be associated with the presence of a palpable mass, pain, and abdominal distension. Preoperative diagnosis is rare, while it is more frequently intraoperative. Therapy is fundamentally surgical: appendectomy is curative for simple AM, for AM with epithelial hyperplasia, and for cystadenoma with intact appendiceal base; ileocecal resection is indicated and with larger implantation a right hemicolectomy should be performed. Notable though is that Gonzalez-Moreno and Sugarbaker recently demonstrated the validity of right hemicolectomy as definitive treatment only if it is performed for obtaining complete cytoreduction, if there is lymph node involvement, or if histopathological examination indicates non-mucinous type. This is based on clinical data of 501 patients with epithelial malignancy of the appendix, which had been collected prospectively [7]. All patients examined had peritoneal seeding at the time of referral and were treated by cytoreductive surgery and perioperative intraperitoneal chemotherapy (HIPEC). The main independent variable for statistical analysis was the surgical procedure used to resect the primary cancer (appendicectomy alone versus right hemicolectomy). Median follow-up after the initial diagnosis was 4 years. The authors concluded that right hemicolectomy does not confer a survival advantage in patients with mucinous appendiceal tumors with peritoneal seeding. Their study suggests that right hemicolectomy should be avoided unless the metastatic involvement of the appendiceal or distal ileocolic lymph nodes is documented by biopsy, or when the resection margin is inadequate.

References

1. Turaga KK, Pappas SG, Gambling TC. Importance of histologic subtype in the staging of appendiceal tumors. Ann Surg Oncol. 2012;19:1379–85.
2. In't Hof KH, van der Wal HC, Kazemier G, Lange JF. Carcinoid tumors of the appendix: an analysis of 1485 consecutive emergency appendectomies. J Gastroinest Surg. 2008;12: 1436–8.
3. Butte JM, Garcia Huidobro MA, Torres J, et al. Long term survival in carcinoid tumor of the appendix. An analysis of 8903 appendectomies. Gastroenterol Hepatol. 2009;32:537–41.
4. Carr NJ, Sobin LH. Neuroendocrine tumors of the appendix. Semin Diagn Pathol. 2004;21: 108–19.
5. Louthan O. Neuroendocrine tumors of the appendix. Vnitr Lek. 2009;55:1051–5.
6. Caracappa D, Gulla N, Gentile D, et al. Appendiceal mucocele. A case report and literature review. Ann Ital Chir. 2011;82:239–45.
7. Gonzalez Moreno S, Sugarbaker PH. Right hemicolectomy does not confer a survival advantage in patients with mucinous carcinoma of the appendix and peritoneal seeding. Br J Surg. 2004;91:304–11.

Chapter 58
Case on Complications After Conservatively Treated Appendicular Phlegmon

Miguel A. Cuesta

Keywords Cecal cancer • Intestinal obstruction • Recurrent acuta appendicitis • Appendicular plastron

First Patient: Intestinal Obstruction

Diagnosis and Indication for Surgery

A dentist of 66 years asked for a second opinion regarding his conservatively treated appendicular phlegmon (Fig. 58.1). The patient had been admitted 1 week earlier at another hospital because of pain in right lower abdomen and fever of 39.5 °C. On physical examination and CT scan, an appendicular phlegmon had been seen with a small abscess of two cm. He then was treated conservatively with iv antibiotics. Patient did well, recovered the intestinal transit, and his temperature normalized. Yet, he asked for a second opinion and went home.

On physical examination, an appendicular plastron was palpated, not painful, and we proposed him to continue with current policy and after a period of 4 weeks to perform a colonoscopy to exclude a cecal cancer.

Meantime, the patient developed again an intestinal obstruction and was readmitted to our hospital. On physical examination, he was not sick, and had no fever but a distended abdomen with high peristalsis. On the abdominal X-ray and CT scan, a small bowel intestinal obstruction was observed with retraction at the ileocecal area (Fig. 58.2).

M.A. Cuesta, M.D.
Department of Surgery,
VU University Medical Center, Amsterdam, The Netherlands
e-mail: ma.cuesta@vumc.nl

M.A. Cuesta, H.J. Bonjer (eds.), *Case Studies of Postoperative Complications after Digestive Surgery*, DOI 10.1007/978-3-319-01613-9_58,

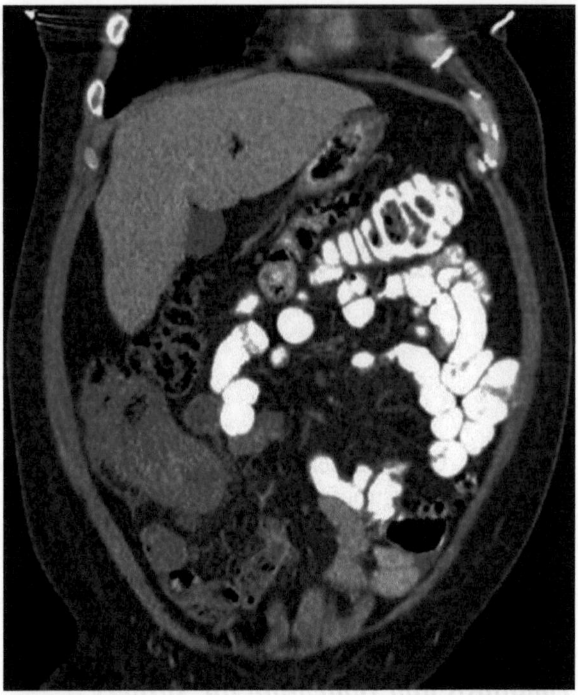

Fig. 58.1 CT scan, acute appendicitis and phlegmon

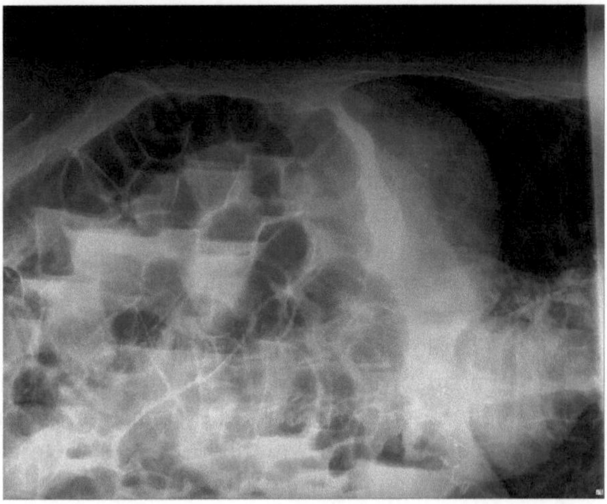

Fig. 58.2 X-ray abdomen, intestinal obstruction after appendicular phlegmon

Operation

Through a midline laparotomy, an inflamed fibrotic tumor was palpated at the ileocecal area as cause of the intestinal obstruction. An ileocecal resection was performed with a side-to-side anastomosis. Resection was not at all easy because of the fibrosis. Pathological examination showed an intense fibrotic area with no appendix in the specimen and old rests of inflammation and some mucus areas. Because of mucus after histological examination, a discussion arose about the possibility of appendiceal mucocele. This diagnosis was not made and patient remained under control on the outpatient polyclinic.

Postoperative Course

Nine months later, he was again admitted because of an intestinal obstruction; after a couple of days he recovered with conservative treatment. A new CT scan showed no mucus or recurrence of any tumor. Patient is doing well.

Second Patient: Recurrent Acute Appendicitis

Diagnosis and Indication for Surgery

A 37-year-old garage technician was admitted to the emergency department because of acute appendicitis.

He had been admitted 1½ years earlier with an appendicular phlegmon and consequently had been treated conservatively. Because he then had no complaints, he had been advised not to operate. However, now at the new admission it was clear that he had local peritoneal signs in the right lower abdomen and on the CT scan an acute appendicitis with a fecalith free in abdominal cavity was visible. Laparoscopic was started and an ileocecal resection was performed after conversion to a McBurney incision because of fibrosis and inflammation. Pathological examination revealed fibrosis and acute inflammation. Patient recovered.

Third Patient: Having a Cecal Cancer

Diagnosis and Indication for Surgery

A 71-year-old man went to outpatient polyclinic because of abdominal pain and diarrhea. He had no fever, leukocytes were normal, and no peritoneal signs on abdominal exploration. Patient was discharged. Four weeks later he was readmitted because of melena, fever, and vomiting. On physical examination, a temperature of 38.5 °C, leukocytosis of 12,000, and a painful palpable mass on the right lower abdomen were found. On US and CT scan an abscess in an appendicular mass was seen and percutaneously drained (Fig. 58.3a). Two weeks later, because of melena

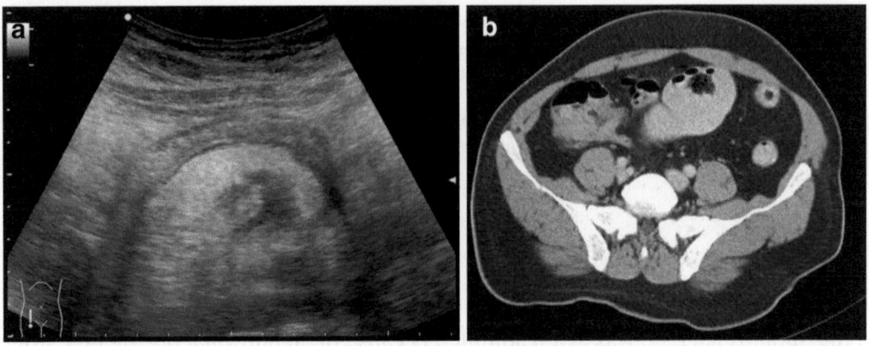

Fig. 58.3 (**a**) US acute appendicitis with an abscess? (**b**) CT scan, cecal cancer considered appendicular phlegmon in the previous CT scan

with slight decrease of hemoglobin from 7.5 to 6.5, a colonoscopy was performed. There a cecum tumor was seen and biopsied. By biopsy the diagnosis of adenocarcinoma was established. On CT scan no distance metastases were found (Fig. 58.3b). Through a transverse laparotomy a right hemicolectomy was performed with excision of all inflammatory mass and peritoneum, because of suspicion for tumor perforation. A pT3N2Mo was diagnosed and patient proposed for postoperative chemotherapy. Two years later all controls appeared normal and patient is doing well.

Discussion

The lesson of these three cases is that an appendicular phlegmon may initially be treated conservatively and in the most of cases will not bring about further complaints and hence no elective appendectomy is necessary. Moreover, it is important to treat patients according to their complaints. Chronic pain on the right lower abdomen will be indication for elective appendectomy, but also intestinal obstruction, or recurrence of acute appendicitis is an indication for surgical exploration. And not to forget, in patients older than 40 years, a control colonoscopy has to be done 4–6 weeks after discharge to exclude a cecal cancer.

Chapter 59
Case on Anastomotic Leakage Following Small Bowel Resection

Cornelius G. Niels Vos

Keywords Small bowel • Anastomosis leakage • Peritonitis • Ileostomy

Anastomotic leakage can be a disastrous complication of small bowel resection. In this section, two cases of anastomotic leakage following small bowel resection will be described and therapeutic management options will be discussed.

First Patient

Diagnosis and Indication for Surgery

A 57-year-old male with a medical history of refractory celiac disease type II was admitted to the intensive care unit with respiratory insufficiency because of bilateral pneumonia. On abdominal CT, performed because of abdominal pain, a thickening of the small intestinal bowel wall and multiple enlarged intra-abdominal lymph nodes were visible. He underwent a gastro-duodenoscopy to rule out gastrointestinal lymphoma (associated with his celiac disease). Following the procedure, the patient developed acute abdominal pain and on physical examination signs for peritonitis. A plain abdominal X-ray demonstrated massive free intra-abdominal air, suggestive of a perforation.

C.G.N. Vos, M.D.
Department of Surgery, VU University Medical Center, Amsterdam, The Netherlands
e-mail: n.vos@vumc.nl

M.A. Cuesta, H.J. Bonjer (eds.), *Case Studies of Postoperative Complications after Digestive Surgery*, DOI 10.1007/978-3-319-01613-9_59,

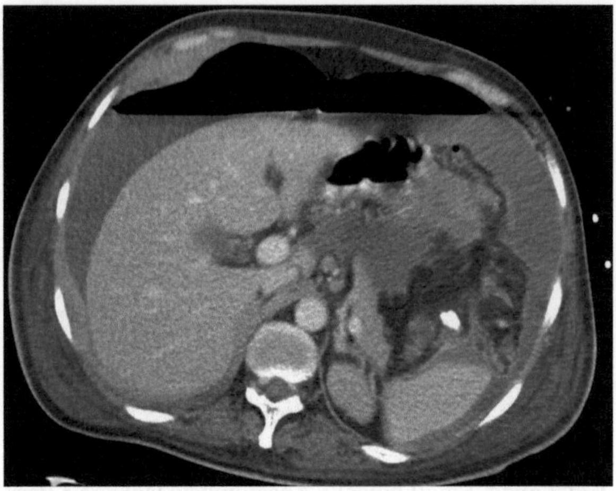

Fig. 59.1 Abdominal CT scan before the second laparotomy of first patient demonstrating large amounts of ascites and free intra-abdominal air

Operation

At laparotomy, a large perforation of the proximal jejunum was found in a bowel affected with intestinal lymphoma. The perforation did not have the appearance of a recent iatrogenic perforation but was considered to be an older covered perforation, which had opened again by introduction of air during gastro-duodenoscopy. The affected segment of jejunum was *resected* and a side-to-side anastomosis performed.

Postoperative Course: Identification and Treatment of Complication

On the 9th postoperative day, patient developed acute abdominal pain and hemodynamic instability. An abdominal CT scan was performed which demonstrated free intra-abdominal air and free fluid (Fig. 59.1). A relaparotomy was performed and an anastomotic leakage of the side-to-side anastomosis was found. The anastomotic leak was primarily closed and a deviating loop jejunostomy was created. Despite this intervention, the patient deteriorated. Because of his general condition, his T-cell lymphoma with poor prognosis, and the lack of therapeutic options, further treatment was ceased and the patient died on the 4th postoperative day.

Second Patient

Diagnosis and Indication for Surgery

A 77-year-old male with a medical history of Kahler's disease and a right hemicolectomy, 1 year ago, because of a T3N0M0 colon carcinoma, presented with weight loss and abdominal pain. Abdominal CT scan demonstrated a mass in the jejunum. Double-balloon enteroscopy showed apparently no abnormalities.

Operation

An explorative laparotomy was performed and a large mass was found in the right half of the abdominal cavity with ingrowth in the ileum. In addition, multiple peritoneal deposits were found. Frozen sections demonstrated adenocarcinoma. Therefore, the right abdominal mass was not resected and the involved ileum was bypassed by a side-to-side jejunum-ileum entero-enterostomy, leaving a blind loop of ileum in place.

Postoperative Course: Identification and Treatment of Complication

On the third postoperative day, the patient developed acute abdominal pain and on physical examination with signs for peritonitis. Abdominal CT scan demonstrated free intra-abdominal air and fluid. A relaparotomy was performed and leakage from a defect in the blind loop was found. The side-to-side entero-enterostomy anastomosis was intact. The blind loop was resected, en bloc with the tumor. Postoperative course was complicated by a pneumonia that was successfully treated with antibiotics after which the patient could be discharged.

Discussion

In case of anastomotic leakage after small bowel resection, there are several management options. The easiest option is primary closure of the defect in the anastomosis. This can be performed if there is no doubt about the vitality of the anastomosis and the patient is hemodynamically stable. If the anastomosis is of poor quality, another option is to make a new anastomosis after resection of the old anastomosis (Illustration 59.1). If the patient is septic, hemodynamically instable, or in a bad general condition, a better option includes disconnecting the anastomosis and creating a double proximal and distal loop stoma. Closure will be ideally performed after 8 weeks, but if the proximal stoma is very proximal in the jejunum and production very high, then the concept of control damage can here be applied. After some days, a relaparotomy can be performed and continuity of the tract restored. Another infrequent option performed is to create a deviating or protective stoma after closure of the defect in a difficult located anastomosis. This protective stoma will reduce the risk of leakage—although conflicting results are reported in the literature. Nonetheless, clinical consequences of leakage are less severe when a protective stoma is used and the risk of needing a reoperation is reduced.

Important to keep in mind is that a conservative approach may be the proper decision in case the abdominal wall is closed and the leakage drained completely through the abdominal wound, with the so-called controlled fistula, in a complicated inaccessible abdomen. Treatment will include a correct protection of the skin

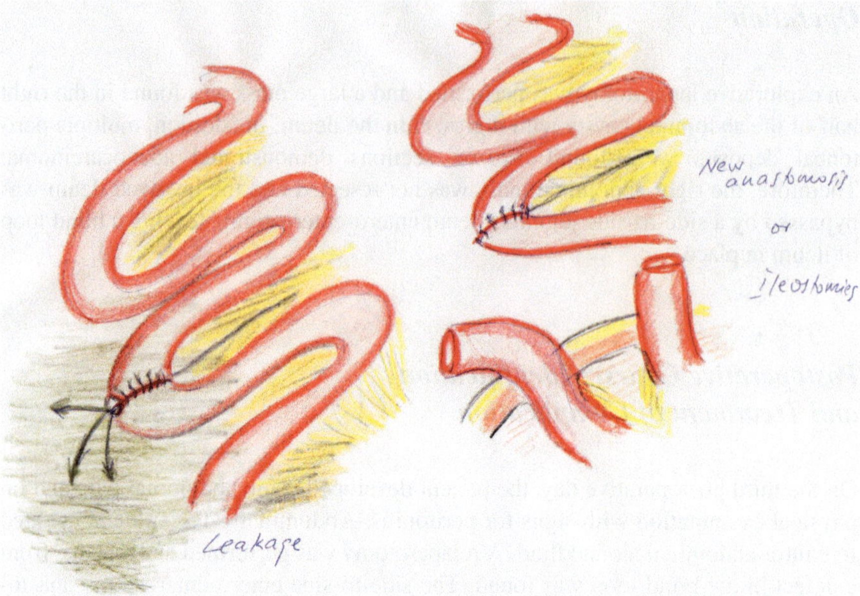

Illustration 59.1 If after a small bowel resection with primary anastomosis, patient has a leakage of the anastomosis with peritonitis, patient should be operated on. If hemodynamically stable and purulent peritonitis, a new anastomosis may be considered. If unstable or with fecal peritonitis, stoma deviation should be done

by means of a VAC system or adequately stoma devices, total parenteral nutrition, somatostatine to decrease production, and eventually percutaneous drainage of intra-abdominal fluid collections/abscesses. If fistulas are drained optimally, and the continuity of the bowel is good without further mechanical obstruction, the fistula will close naturally.

Chapter 60
Case on Recurrence of Crohn's Disease

Adriaan A. van Bodegraven

Keywords Crohn's disease • Recurrent Crohn disease • Intestinal obstruction • Intestinal resection

First Patient

Diagnosis and Indication for Surgery

During military service in the midst of the 1980s, a 23-year-old male patient known with Crohn's disease presented with symptoms of stenosis of small bowel. Crohn's disease had been localized in the small bowel (Montreal classification L1+L4). Patient was operated on; the disease was surgically removed "completely"—according to medical opinion holding for that era of time—at two instances, the first in 1984 involving extended ileocecal resection and the second in 1987 involving partial jejunum resection. Documentation was scarce, but according to histology reports, at least 1.5 m of small bowel was removed. From 1990 on, the patient had experienced relapse of obstructive symptoms, due to recurrence of disease, notwithstanding maintenance therapy with varying dosages of corticosteroids (between 5 and 20 mg prednisolone o.d.) (Fig. 60.1). He presented at our third-line referral hospital and was refereed by another gastroenterologist because of a recurrence of multiple stenosis in remaining jejunum and ileum.

He was advised to adapt his diet to frequent, preferably liquid, small meals. This was carefully monitored for recurrent follow-up of symptoms and laboratory studies to assess inflammatory parameters and drug-related toxicity. Intercurrent occlusion

A.A. van Bodegraven
Department of Gastroenterology, VU University Medical Center, Amsterdam, The Netherlands
e-mail: v.bodegraven@vumc.nl

M.A. Cuesta, H.J. Bonjer (eds.), *Case Studies of Postoperative Complications after Digestive Surgery*, DOI 10.1007/978-3-319-01613-9_60,

of central retinae vein of the right eye occurred (Fig. 60.2), an uncommon but well-known extra-intestinal manifestation of IBD, decreasing the sight in that eye to less than a 30 %. Later, in addition, cornea dysplasia of both eyes was diagnosed.

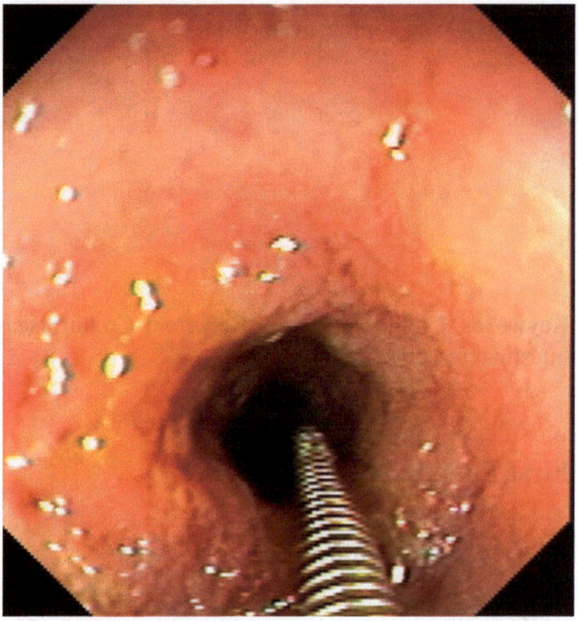

Fig. 60.1 Colonoscopy showing Crohn's disease, being biopsied

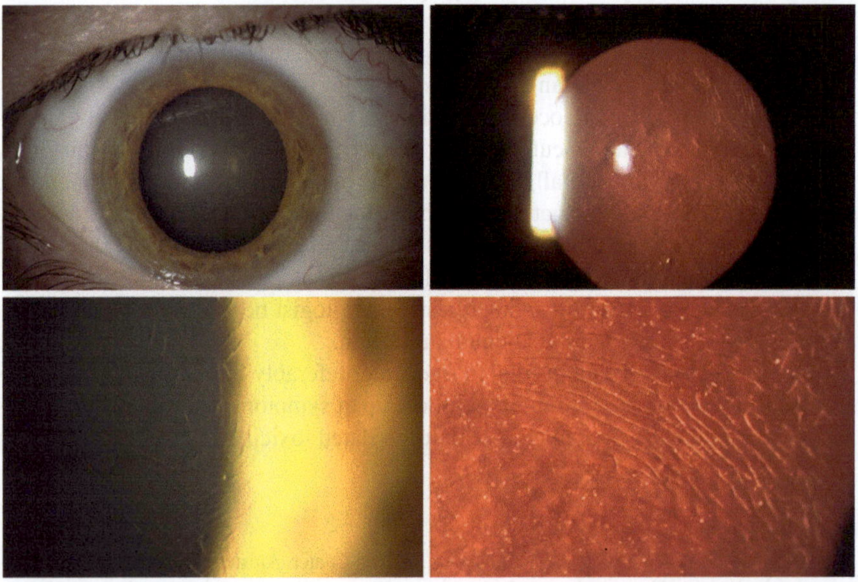

Fig. 60.2 Cornea dysplasia of both eyes

Nevertheless, symptoms increased, and in the absence of inflammation, surgical therapy was again advised.

Operation

Laparotomy followed in 1996 to address the symptomatic and quiescent (cold) stenosis in order to perform bowel-sparing procedures, and five stricturoplasties were performed; whereas the most proximal stenosis over 10 cm length was treated by a side-to-side anastomosis. After this operation, he maintained quite well his general condition and was able to work adequately.

Postoperative Course

Nevertheless, recurrence of complaints and disease activity returned in 2002 (Fig. 60.3), prompting another laparotomy during which two other stricturoplasties and resection of the neo-terminal ileum, 15 cm, were performed. Approximately 180 cm of small bowel remained. This procedure was complicated by a leakage, and so relaparotomy was performed, and an ileostomy and colonic fistula were created.

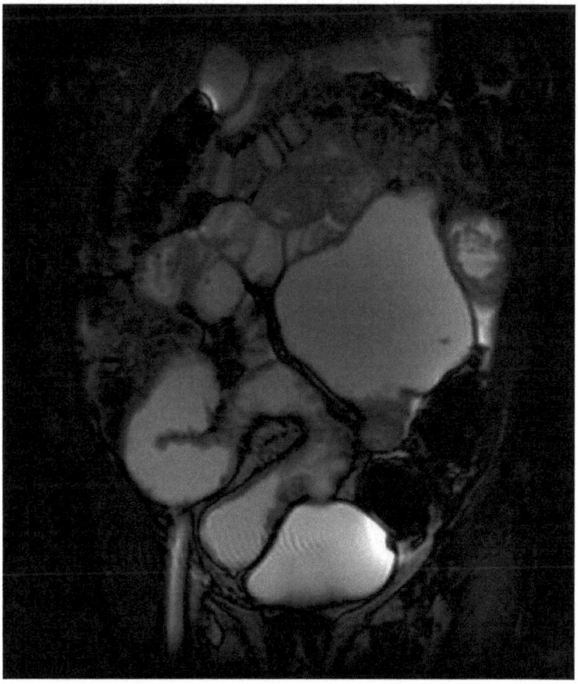

Fig. 60.3 MRI enteroclysis: dilatation jejunum and thickness intestinal wall

Two relaparotomies were performed shortly after drain and rinse of the peritoneal cavity. Late in 2003, intestinal continuity was performed without further complications.

After the latest operations, patient persistently produced voluminous stools and had a slow but progressive loss of weight. Treatment consisted nonetheless in hyperphagia based on a calculated and measured energy need and corrected for fecal energy losses (indirect calorimetry and fecal bomb calorimetry). Finally, a percutaneous endoscopic gastrostomy was placed to warrant continuous dripping of predigested enteral feeding allowing for 24-h nutrition via a pump device.

Currently, his weight is stable. However, again stenotic symptoms do occur, and again in the neo-terminal ileum, active Crohn's disease has been diagnosed (Fig. 60.4a), notwithstanding treatment with at first subcutaneous methotrexate, later in combination with infliximab, and now monotherapy with adalimumab 40 mg o.w. Patient has recently been operated, finding a fibrotic mass around the distal anastomosis (Fig. 60.4b). Twenty-centimeter resection has been performed with side-to-side anastomosis. Seventy centimeters of small bowel and from the transverse colon are remaining.

Discussion

"Complete" resection of Crohn's disease has been abandoned since long, as it does not preclude recurrence of disease in the remaining bowel. Therefore, current surgical approach in Crohn's disease comprises minimal resection and preferably so minimally invasive, the latter referring to laparoscopic techniques being preferable over open approach [1]. In general, a patient with Crohn's disease has a chance of 70–80 % to be operated once, whereas 50 % may encounter a second procedure. Extensive resection of the (small) bowel must be avoided whenever possible. Therefore, prior to surgery the disease should preferably be in a quiescent stage, and infiltration, abscesses, and other complicating factors should be treated by means of antibiotics and enteral feeding or percutaneously by drains, whenever possible. There is debate whether the total length of the small bowel is generally less in patients with Crohn's disease, even before surgery. This factor in itself might contribute to a higher chance of getting clinically significant short bowel syndrome, which is leading to nutritional and energetic deficiencies. Anyhow, following each surgical procedure for Crohn's disease, remaining small bowel length has to be carefully documented (with or without duodenum, Bauhin's valve, and length of remaining colon) to have an indication of the functional bowel and estimation for

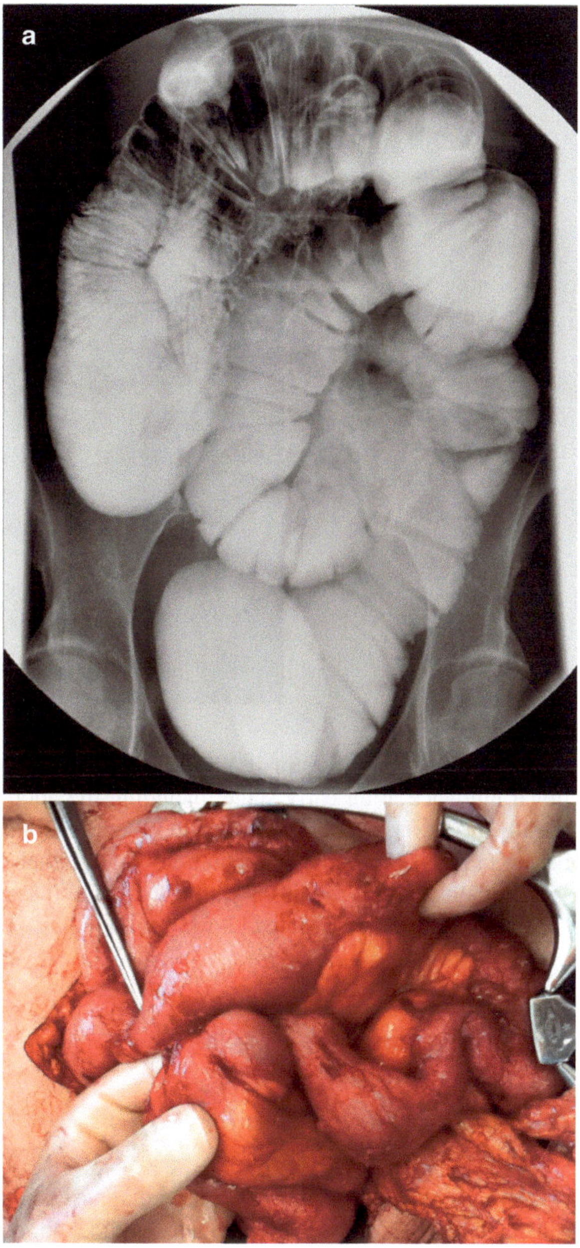

Fig. 60.4 MRI enteroclysis: small bowel dilatation, recurrence Crohn's disease

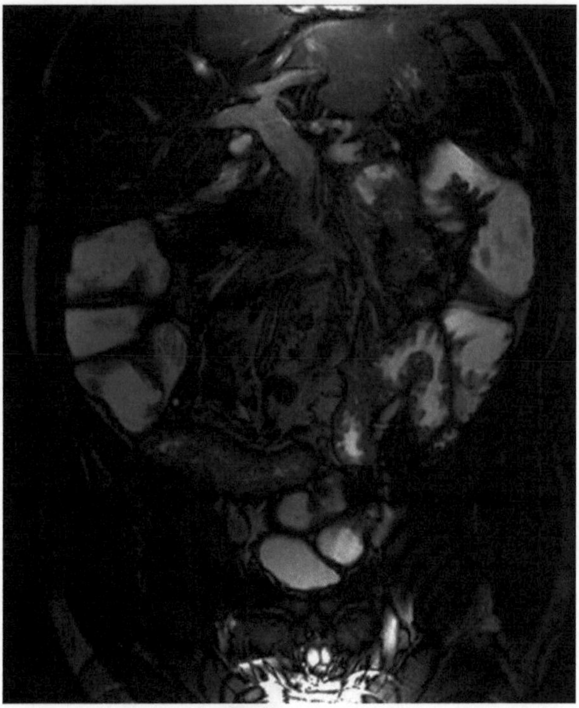

Fig. 60.5 MRI enteroclysis showing stenosis neo-terminal ileum

clinically significant intestinal failure. This might prompt commencing with nutritional guidance at an early stage, including the adoption of medical therapy that usually has lower bioavailability due to suboptimal intestinal absorption, sometimes necessitating different administration routes (subcutaneously, intravenously). Additionally, careful monitoring of postsurgical intestinal function by a dedicated (nutritional) team is warranted [2–6].

Second Patient

Diagnosis and Indication for Surgery

A 19-year-old patient had in 1990 been diagnosed with Crohn's disease of the terminal ileum. Stenosis of this segment, without inflammatory signs in laboratory studies or at radiography, was treated by open ileocecal resection in 1992. Recurrence of stenotic disease necessitated reresection of the neo-terminal ileum in 1999, and again in 2006 (Figs. 60.5 and 60.6). The latest operation included a right-sided

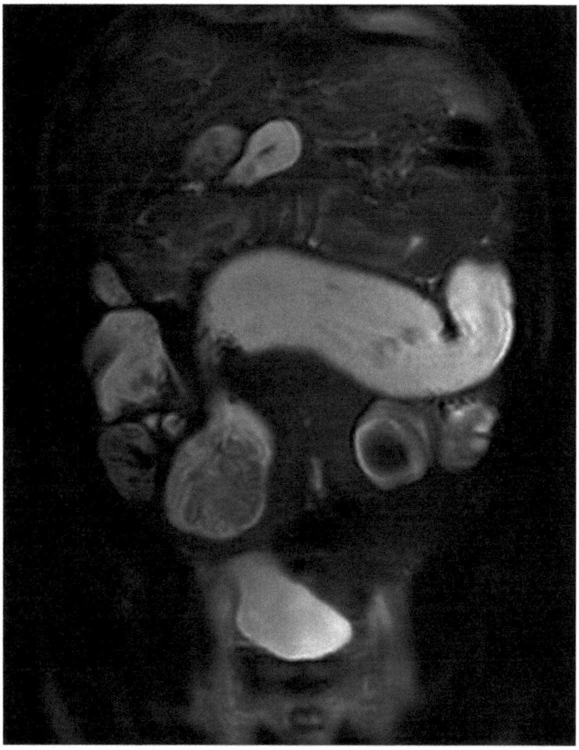

Fig. 60.6 MRI enteroclysis showing restenosis of the neo-terminal ileum

hemicolectomy due to a spontaneous enterocutaneous fistula formation. Furthermore, a perianal abscess had to be drained in 1998.

Besides Crohn's disease, this patient was diagnosed with HLA-B27-negative sacroiliitis, fitting with an IBD-associated spondyloarthropathy, and osteopenia. Supplementation of vitamin B12 was initiated after the first surgical procedure.

All surgical procedures were uneventful. Following operation, symptoms disappeared for long period of time. At the time of recurrence with symptoms including usually a combination of inflammatory signs, right under quadrant pain especially following meals and general depression, medical treatment was reinitiated, whereas in the asymptomatic periods, adherence to medical treatment was suboptimal. Although induction to remission of disease activity was repetitively successful, remaining complaints obliged to reoperations, the last one in an extended form to remove the described fistula. Currently, the patient suffers from active Crohn's disease of the neo-terminal ileum with abdominal cramps following large meals, notwithstanding potent anti-TNF alpha therapy (adalimumab 40 mg o.w.).

Discussion

Crohn's disease is phenotypically characterized by age of diagnosis, localization of disease, and disease behavior in the so-called Montreal classification [7]. Initially, this classification intended to be helpful in prediction of disease course, but its accuracy is limited in this respect. Lifetime chance for operation, when diagnosed with Crohn's disease, is approximately 70–80 % with a 50 % chance of reoperation within the next 10 years. Clinically, specifically stenotic type of disease behavior is associated with recurrent surgery. Up till now, no medical therapy has clearly been demonstrated to decrease relapse leading to surgical reintervention, in particular when taking adverse response, as with metronidazol or imidazol derivatives, or costs, as with anti-TNF alpha therapy, are taken into consideration. Anyhow, only a relative small number of studies addressed this issue. Additionally, there is a high diversity in phenotype of Crohn's disease patients with a different "a priori" chance of surgical relapse. In order to predict recurrence of disease, Rutgeerts et al. suggested to assess an endoscopic score of mucosal lesions of the neo-terminal ileum, following ileocecal resection, being a biomarker of mucosal inflammation, clinical recurrence, and eventually surgical relapse, respectively [8]. This procedure might be performed in the 6–12 months following first operation. Currently fecal calprotectin bears potential as a biomarker of recurrence of mucosal damage after resection and, thus, might be considered as simple biomarker [9]. Nevertheless, up till now, no clear-cut medical treatment strategy is known to avoid second or more surgical interventions.

References

1. Maartense S, Dunker MS, Slors JF, et al. Laparoscopic assisted versus open ileocolic resection for Crohn's disease: a randomised trial. Ann Surg. 2006;243:143–9.
2. Ambe R, Campbell L, Cagir A. Comprehensive review of strictureplasty techniques in Crohn's disease: types, indications, comparisons, and safety. J Gastrointest Surg. 2012;16:209–17.
3. Lewis RT, Maron DJ. Efficacy and complications of surgery for Crohn's disease. Gastroenterol Hepatol (NY). 2010;6:587–96.
4. Spinelli A, Sacchi M, Fiorino G, et al. Risk of postoperative recurrence and postoperative management of Crohn's disease. World J Gastroenterol. 2011;17:3213–9.
5. Thompson JS, Iyer KR, DiBaise JK, et al. Short bowel syndrome and Crohn's disease. J Gastrointest Surg. 2003;7:1069–72.
6. Donohoe CL, Reynolds JV. Short bowel syndrome. Surgeon. 2010;8:270–9.
7. Satsangi J, Silverberg MS, Vermeire S, Colombel JF. The Montreal classification of Inflammatory bowel disease: controversies, consensus and implications. Gut. 2006;55:749–53.
8. Daperno M, D'Haens G, Van Assche G, et al. Development and validation of a new, simplified endoscopic activity score for Crohn's disease: the SES-CD. Gastrointest Endosc. 2004;60:505–12.
9. D'Haens G, Ferrante M, Vermeire S, et al. Fecal calprotectin is a surrogate marker for endoscopic lesions in inflammatory bowel disease. Inflamm Bowel Dis. 2012;18:2218–24.

Chapter 61
Case on Short Bowel Syndrome

Adriaan A. van Bodegraven

Keywords Crohn's disease • Short Bowel Syndrome

Diagnosis and Indication for Surgery

Another patient presenting with a highly complicated, but generally considered, benign course of Crohn's disease is currently 52-year-old man with a length of 1.85 m and with an initial bodyweight of approximately 90 kg. The patient's initial symptoms and diagnosis had already been encountered in 1988—he then was 29 years of age. His steroid-refractory ileocolonic disease led to partial colectomy of the descending colon. Once he presented at our hospital, the active colonic disease had recurred, even though postoperatively azathioprine had been prescribed to prevent postsurgical relapses. Moreover, Crohn's disease was at that time complicated by an enterovesical fistula.

Operation Description

A low anterior resection, fistulectomy, closure of the bladder, and creation of colostomy had then been performed.

A.A. van Bodegraven
Department of Gastroenterology, VU University Medical Center,
Amsterdam, The Netherlands
e-mail: v.bodegraven@vumc.nl

M.A. Cuesta, H.J. Bonjer (eds.), *Case Studies of Postoperative Complications after Digestive Surgery*, DOI 10.1007/978-3-319-01613-9_61,

Postoperative Course

Two years later, the terminal ileum had become so stenosed that he was admitted because of an ileus; consequently, an ileocecal resection was performed with a side-to-side anastomosis. During the following years, the course of the disease proved uneventful, with use of azathioprine and short courses of corticosteroids, leading to a gradual increase of bodyweight up to 101 kg. In 2000, his complaints returned, involving colics as caused by a stenosis of the neo-terminal ileum. Compassionate use of infliximab—introduced at that time in the Netherlands—failed to relieve his symptoms, necessitating another resection of the stenosed neo-terminal ileum with end-to-end anastomosis, and approximately 20 cm of colon remaining. Due to adhesions, recovery was delayed by postoperative ileus, which 3 weeks later necessitated a relaparotomy involving adhesiolysis and resection of the distal part of the jejunum. The patient's clinical recovery during the next 2 years remained incomplete, due to his recurrent abdominal pains and decreased appetite, as evidenced by a slow decrease of his weight to 84 kg.

Two years afterward, once again small bowel disease recurred, primarily of the stenotizing type, which induced symptomatology such as cramps and abdominal pain, loss of weight, and ileus-like episodes. It was then decided to perform stricturoplasty; however, this was complicated by postoperative leakage through the laparotomy wound. This complication was treated by an open abdominal approach with enteral nutrition, the frequent use of antibiotics, and by opiates. The combination of the preoperative and relatively short bowel length, together with the presence of at least three enterocutaneous fistulas, induced a full-blown intestinal failure. Enteral feeding was insufficient to maintain the patient's bodyweight and additional parenteral feeding became required. Yet, due to chronic inflammation induced catabolism and feeding problems his weight continued to decrease to 64.5 kg. After approximately 1 year of supportive nutritional therapy, in combination with methotrexate monotherapy, and allergic reaction to infliximab, we decided to close the enterocutaneous fistulas, one of them localized above the left anterior spine. Although most inflammation and scar tissue could be removed and intestinal continuity was completed, once again a postoperative fistula formed. Three months later, it was closed by a new laparotomy. The remaining small bowel was considered to be 70–80 cm, with 30 cm colon and rectum. Then, finally, the intestinal disease and Crohn's manifestations went into remission, leaving the patient with a short bowel syndrome. A period of hyperphagia with supplemental vitamin and trace elements was introduced to adapt the remainder of the intestine. Over time, TPN and supplements could be discontinued, and his bodyweight slowly increased. Following this strategy, in 2006 his bodyweight had risen to 86 kg, and adalimumab therapy was given to treat recurrence of inflammatory luminal disease. Since then, no further manifestations of Crohn's disease have required other surgical procedures. Remarkably, the patient's current weight is 108 kg, apparently brought about by solely hyperphagia and combined with several vitamin and mineral (in particular Mg) supplements.

Discussion

This patient is an excellent example of the relatively few medical options we have to treat Crohn's disease postoperatively, thereby preventing new surgical procedures. On top of that, an abdominal operation for alleviating Crohn's itself carries risks for complications requiring additional surgical interventions. Surely, this may lead to intestinal failure and to short bowel syndrome [1–3]. The latter condition is generally considered to be directly related to the length of the remaining intestine. Interestingly, patients with Crohn's disease appear to start with a shorter total small bowel length even before any surgery has been performed [1, 3]. Total length of the intestines, it must be noted, is one of the characteristics of successful digestion. Once the ileum has been removed, its function cannot be restored, whereas the ileum can adapt to jejunal functions if the latter has been resected. Furthermore, the presence or absence of the valve of Bahuin is pivotal for increasing the capacity of the small intestines to digest. Also, the length and function of the colon contribute primarily via the absorption of bacteria-generated and short-chain fatty acids to the nutritional balance of energy (and water and salts).

When short bowel syndrome develops following surgical resections, the therapeutic and clinical approach comprises three phases, specified below (Tables 61.1 and 61.2).

Table 61.1 Intestinal remnants and nutritional risks

Intestinal parts remaining	Characteristic risks regarding nutrition
Duodenum, >2 m jejunum, and colon	Oral intake will suffice
Duodenum, jejunum, ileum, of which 60–100 cm resected	Malabsorption vitamin B12, bile salts pool intact by increased production in liver
Duodenum, jejunum, ileum > 1 m resected	Decreased bile salt pool, thus fat maldigestion and decrease in fat-soluble vitamins
<1 m jejunum	Excessive fluids and mineral losses, oral intake will be lost concomitantly
>1.5 m small bowel + ileostomy or 60–90 cm small bowel + most of colon	Initial TPN dependent, but high probability of (partial) weaning into enteral nutrition
<60 cm small bowel + intact colon	Probably ongoing dependence on TPN
<100–140 cm small bowel, no colon	Probably ongoing dependence on TPN
<115 cm small bowel + jejunostomy	Probably ongoing dependence on TPN
<60 cm + jejunocolonic or ileocolonic anastomosis	Probably ongoing dependence on TPN
<35 cm small bowel + duodenostomy or jejunostomy	Probably ongoing dependence on TPN

Table 61.2 Three-phase therapeutic–nutritional strategy in short bowel syndrome

	Parenteral	Enteral	Complications
Phase 1 (acute)	TPN, preferably following indirect calorimetry Fluids and minerals to compensate for excessive loss	No enteral challenges as long as fluid homoeostasis is compromised Commonly introduction small amount of complex food (fat) at day 4–5 postoperatively	Hemodynamic instability Mineral disturbances
Phase 2 (adaptation)	TPN initially to cover all nutritional needs, up till assessment of intestinal absorption capacity Calculated decrease in TPN may follow Follow-up by regular anthropometric measurements (fat-free mass, muscle strength, indirect calorimetry)	Increase of enteral feeding, as clinically accepted Proton pump inhibition High-dose vitamin D and calcium Social reintegration	Malnutrition Vitamin deficiencies Osteoporosis Calcium oxalate kidney stones Bacterial overgrowth TPN complications
Phase 3 (maintenance)	Ideally, total weaning of TPN If not, balanced TPN and enteral feeding scheme If possible, oral scheme with nutritional supplements	Personalized dietary advices regarding enteral feeding needs and supplemental oral feedings Follow-up by long-term nutritional assessments, usually at yearly basis Social reintegration	Malnutrition Osteoporosis Vitamin deficiencies, usually fat soluble Zinc and magnesium deficiency

1. Acute phase

   - This is the period directly following surgery and it is characterized by an imbalanced water and mineral homeostasis
   - In this phase of an approximate duration of 1 month, the total parenteral nutrition and supplementation of excessive losses of water and minerals are warranted to stabilize the patient

2. Adaptation phase

   - A phase to stimulate intestinal adaptation by a gradual increase of intestinal nutrient exposure, preferably of complex foods (fat)
   - This phase may take at least 1 year, but probably up to as much as 2–3 years for gaining a maximal result in terms of digestive capacity

- Predicting the necessity of either parenteral or enteral supplemental feeding is difficult and the outcome depends, among other matters, on quality and anatomy of the remaining intestine

3. Maintenance phase

- This phase gradually comes about in the wake of the adaptation phase
- It concerns the permanent dietetic treatment done on an individual basis and comprises all macronutrients and micronutrients
- The careful monitoring of postsurgical intestinal functions as carried out by a dedicated (nutritional) team is warranted [4, 5]

References

1. Keller J, Panter H, Layer P. Management of the short bowel syndrome after extensive small bowel resection. Best Pract Res Clin Gastroenterol. 2004;18:977–92.
2. Wierdsma NJ, van Bodegraven AA. Energetische verliezen uit een korte darm; meer dan alleen vet (Short bowel energy-loss-more than just fats). Ned Tijdschr Geneeskd. 2005;19:149–54.
3. Borowiec AM, Fedorak RN. Predicting, treating and preventing postoperative recurrence of Crohn's disease: The state of the field. Can J Gastroenterol. 2011;25:140–6.
4. Estívariz CF, Luo M, Umeakunne K, et al. Nutrient intake from habitual oral diet in patients with severe short bowel syndrome living in the south-eastern United States. Nutrition. 2008;24:330–9.
5. Elriz K, Palascak-Juif V, Joly F, et al. Crohn's disease patients with chronic intestinal failure receiving long-term parenteral nutrition: a cross-national adult study. Aliment Pharmacol Ther. 2011;34:931–40.

Chapter 62
Case on Recurrence of Intestinal Obstruction Because of Adhesions

Miguel A. Cuesta and Rebecca P.M. Brosens

Keywords Sigmoid resection • Diverticulitis • Intestinal obstruction • Recurrence obstruction

First Patient

Diagnosis and Indication for Surgery

A 70-year-old man was readmitted, now for the third time to hospital. Two years before he had undergone without problems a sigmoid resection due to recurrent diverticulitis with stenosis. But 6 months after that, he underwent a relaparotomy because of small bowel intestinal obstruction caused by adhesions. One year later, again he was admitted to hospital because of intestinal obstruction (Fig. 62.1). He was treated conservatively for 4 days without success, and because of increasing abdominal pain, he was again operated.

Operation

During the relaparotomy, an important multiadherential process was found without a real intestinal caliber difference. Extensive adhesiolysis was performed with some perforation of small bowel loops, all being closed.

M.A. Cuesta, M.D. (✉) • R.P.M. Brosens
Department of Surgery, VU University Medical Center,
Amsterdam, The Netherlands
e-mail: ma.cuesta@vumc.nl

M.A. Cuesta, H.J. Bonjer (eds.), *Case Studies of Postoperative Complications after Digestive Surgery*, DOI 10.1007/978-3-319-01613-9_62,

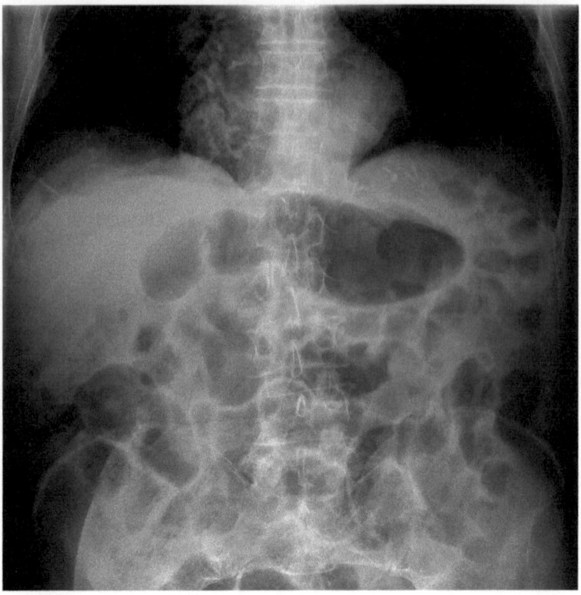

Fig. 62.1 AP view of intestinal obstruction on the plain X-ray of abdomen

Postoperative Course

Patient had a difficult postoperative recovery, involving use of a nasogastric tube for 1 week and total parenteral nutrition (TPN). Two months later, he was admitted again with small bowel intestinal obstruction and then it was decided to await recovery of the transit. Conservative treatment consisted of applying a nasogastric tube for emptying the upper gastrointestinal tract, TPN, and enemas. Patient was mobilized in order to stimulate the peristalsis that seemed to be absent. Problem was that he had progressive pain, the nasogastric tube was not productive, and patient did not pass any gas or stools.

A plain abdomen X-ray and a new CT scan showed important distension of the small bowel with some degree of intestinal pneumatosis (Fig. 62.2a, b). This sign, together with rising leukocytes, prompted us to explore the abdomen again by laparotomy in order to exclude any ischemia of the intestines. During this relaparotomy, the bowels seemed a block, showing adhesion between loops. A long procedure was engaged to inspect the entire bowel. Several perforations and serosa lesions were closed. No ischemia was found, even though an important distension. Bowels were decompressed and a conservative treatment was started. Patient experienced difficult periods, having ups and downs with much pain, but finally after a period of 2 weeks, he could start with oral feeding and go home.

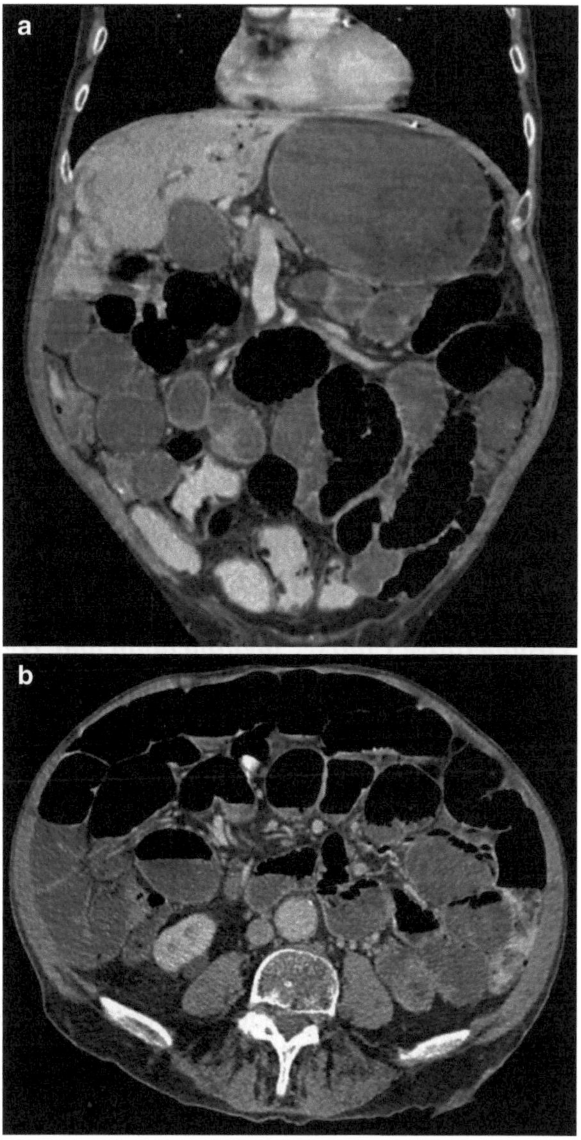

Fig. 62.2 (**a**, **b**) CT scan showing intestinal obstruction with pneumatosis

Second Patient

Diagnosis and Indication for Surgery

A 70-year-old man was referred to us after different abdominal operations because of recurrent intestinal obstruction. He was known with chronic ischemia in the lower extremities taking as medication Ascal®. Using plain abdomen X-ray and CT scan, a small bowel intestinal obstruction was diagnosed. He had been operated on 6 months before because of cecal cancer by means of right hemicolectomy. Because of leakage he underwent a relaparotomy involving dismantling of the anastomosis and ileostomy. Reversal of the stomas led to a torsion of the anastomosis with intestinal obstruction and a new reoperation. Three months later—because of intestinal obstruction and lack of improvement after 2 days of conservative treatment—the surgeon decided to operate him again. Through a median laparotomy, multiple adhesions were taken down, but a clear obstruction was not observed. Quality of the bowels was considered normal, but multiple serosa defects were repaired.

Postoperative Course: Identification and Treatment of Complication

During the postoperative period, the abdomen remained distended for a period of 2 weeks without any activity or peristalsis. Patient was treated by nasogastric tube and total parenteral nutrition. He had abdominal pain, and since the operation he had been receiving opiates. Suspicion about mesenteric ischemia led to performing a CT angiography that revealed an important stenosis of the celiac trunk and the superior mesenteric artery (SMA) (Fig. 62.3a, b).

Under a diagnosis of chronic mesenteric ischemia, the patient was referred to us. We decided to perform an angiography and to stent the stenosis in order to increase the arterial flow in an attempt to normalize the intestinal peristalsis (Fig. 62.4a, b). Conservative treatment was continued, all opiates were stopped, and finally after a period of 2 weeks, passage recovered. Following treatment by coumarin as anticoagulant, the patient could be discharged.

Discussion

Lessons of these cases are twofold. Many centers hold as principle to operate a small bowel obstruction after applying 24 h of conservative treatment. Immediate operation holds only for those patients having strangulation complaints at admission,

Fig. 62.3 (**a**, **b**) CT angiography showing stenosis of the superior mesenteric artery (SMA)

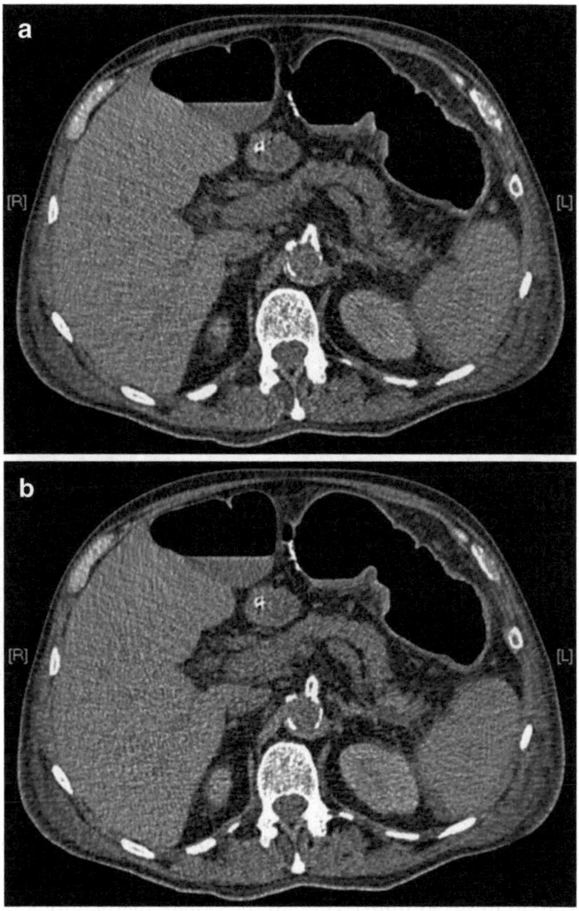

pain, unrest, leukocytosis, and eventually high lactate levels; such patients should be operated on immediately because of the danger for ischemia of bowels included in adhesions, internal hernia, or volvulated loops. Other patients with quiet abdomen can be treated conservatively.

The pertaining question now is: How many days involved doing such? My rule will be that if there is a progression to normality, less distension, and less production by the nasogastric tube, I would prefer to continue with conservative therapy. In the case of no changes, diagnosis should be done. However, the "24-h rule" no longer holds. In the case of a recurrent operation because of already known adhesions, we prefer to wait longer, using conservative treatment with nasogastric tube and TPN. Too easily decided-on reoperations will harm the patient, establish more adhesions, and generate difficult operations in the future. Before considering a reoperation,

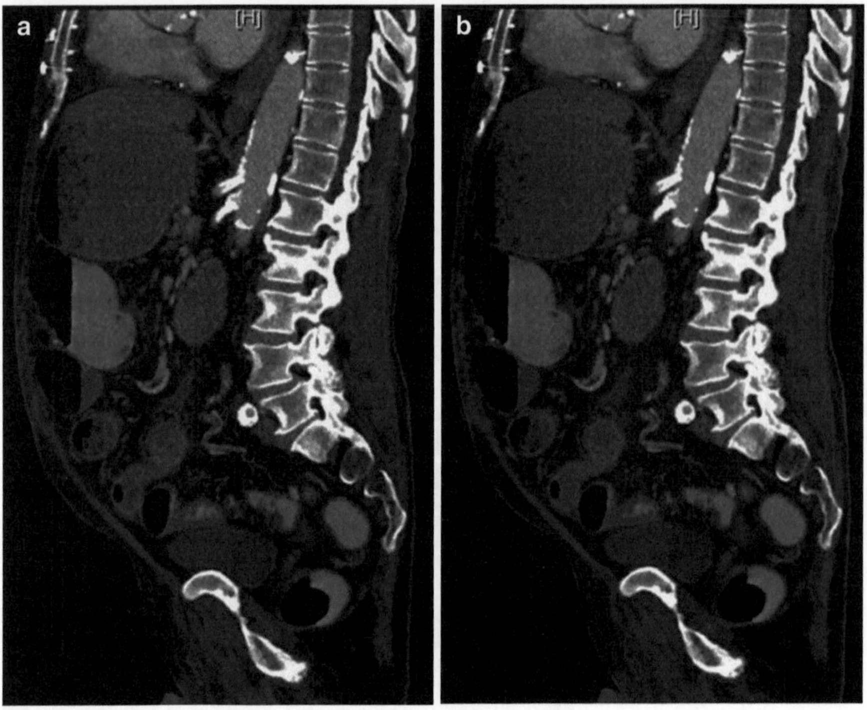

Fig. 62.4 (**a**, **b**) Celiac trunk and SMA have been stented

a CT scan should be done to look for complications of the last operations or a cause for the ileus (as portrayed in the second patient with mesenteric ischemia). Importantly, administering all the opiate medications should be stopped.

Chapter 63
Case on Inadvertent Small Bowel Lesion During Laparoscopic Operation

Laura Gonzalez Sanchez

Keywords Laparoscopic hysterectomy • Uterus fibroid • Intestinal lesion • Laparoscopy

Diagnosis and Indication for Surgery

A 44-year-old homemaker with a history of four prior deliveries was operated by the gynecologist using laparoscopic hysterectomy to alleviate recurrent bleeding produced by a uterus fibroid of 12 cm in length. The operation was successful and blood loss amounted to 200 cc.

Postoperative Course: Identification and Treatment of Complication

A drain was left in Douglas cavity and on the first postoperative day it produced a suspicious fluid. It was not typical of small bowel contents and its analysis revealed 19,800 mg/dl amylase! Gynecologist and internist considered a pancreatic fistula, probably constituting an operation trauma to the pancreas, so she was initially treated with conservative management. The next day, the patient was presented to the surgeon on duty because of progressive abdominal pain, high fever, and leukocytosis of 23,000 cell/field. Under suspicion of high small bowel perforation, the surgeon decided to perform a CT scan (Figs. 63.1 and 63.2). On the CT scan an

L. Gonzalez Sanchez, M.D.
Department of Surgery, Hospital J. Negrin, Tenerife, Spain
e-mail: lgsanchez08@gmail.com

M.A. Cuesta, H.J. Bonjer (eds.), *Case Studies of Postoperative Complications after Digestive Surgery*, DOI 10.1007/978-3-319-01613-9_63,

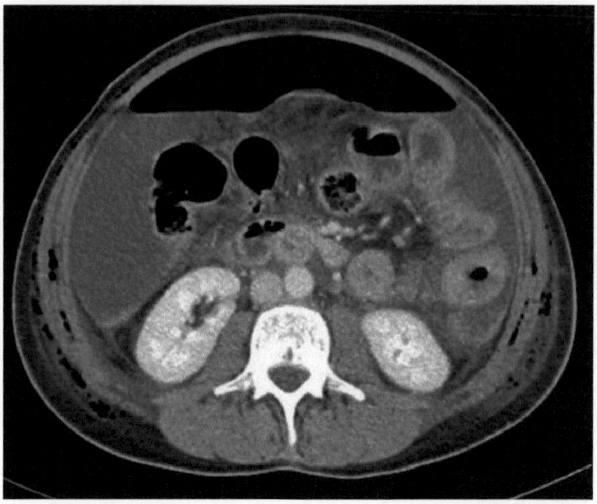

Fig. 63.1 CT scan showing fluid collection in whole abdomen and pneumoperitoneum

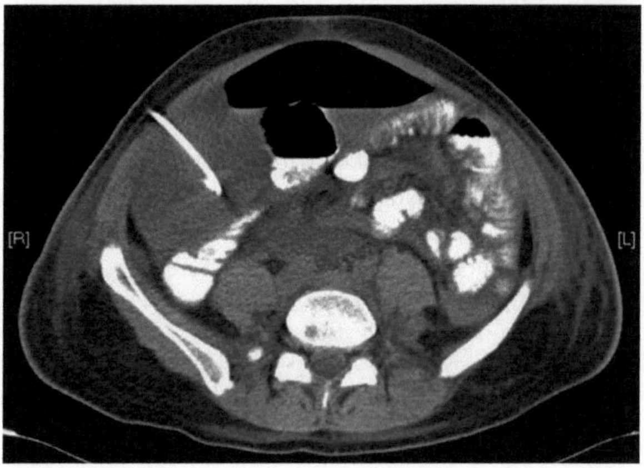

Fig. 63.2 CT scan showing fluid collection and pneumoperitoneum. Drain was left during operation

important pneumoperitoneum and moderate quantity of free fluids in abdomen were observed and it was decided to operate immediately. At laparotomy, peritonitis produced by perforation on anterior and posterior wall was found at 15 cm from ligament of Treitz. Perforations were one cm in size and the bowel was vital and nor destroyed, and surgeon decided to close both lesions with interrupted suture. Bowel was patent and vital and the pancreas was normal; abdomen was rinsed and closed and a drain was left behind. The course of the first two postoperative days was complicated by fever, but peristalsis recovered quickly. The patient only was frustrated by the complications. After drainage of a small wound abscess, she recovered and went home. Pathology of the uterus was uterus myoma.

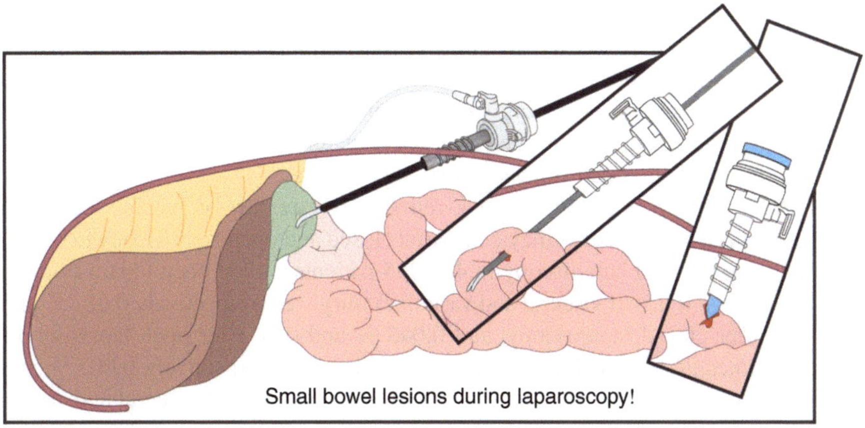

Illustration 63.1 To sum up, if we have a patient who has been operated by laparoscopic surgery, who develops postoperatively fever, tachycardia, abdominal pain, or any other sepsis or peritonitis signs, then bowel damage must be excluded by a CT scan, followed by emergency reintervention

Discussion

Currently, the laparoscopic approach is used more frequently; its advantages are clear, but its use is not completely free of risks. Especially when gaining access to the abdominal cavity by means of Veress needle, trocars, and such instruments, certain accidents are likely, such as inadvertent vascular lesions and hollow organ perforations, thereby putting patients at an important risk for their lives (Illustration 63.1).

Schafer et al.—reporting on behalf of The Swiss Association for Laparoscopic and Thoracoscopic Surgery (SALTS)—prospectively collected data on 14,243 patients undergoing various standard laparoscopic procedures between 1995 and 1997 [1]. The database contained 22 trocar and four needle injuries (incidence, 0.18 %). Nineteen lesions involved visceral organs; the remaining seven were vessel injuries. The small bowel was the single most affected organ (six cases) followed by the large bowel and the liver. Nineteen trocar injuries were recognized intraoperatively; diagnoses of two small bowel injuries and one bladder injury were made postoperatively. Needle injuries were all diagnosed intraoperatively. Only five injuries could be repaired laparoscopically; the remaining lesions were repaired openly. Four patients underwent an open reoperation, and another patient needed five reoperations. There was one death (4.0 %).

Schafer et al. concluded that trocar and needle injuries constitute rare complications of laparoscopy. However, if unrecognized intraoperatively and not repaired immediately, these induce increased morbidity and mortality. Both the open- and closed establishment of the pneumoperitoneum are related to a potential danger of perforating lesions. By inserting the first trocar under direct vision, an early recognition and immediate repair of lesions may be possible.

In 1997, Bonjer et al. published a retrospective review of the literature and authors' experience, whereby they compared closed and open laparoscopy [2]. Data were culled on closed laparoscopy in 489,335 patients and on open laparoscopy in 12,444 patients. Rates of visceral and vascular injury were respectively 0.083 % and 0.075 % after closed laparoscopy, and 0.048 % and 0 % after open laparoscopy. Mortality rates after closed and open laparoscopy were respectively 0.003 % and 0 %. They found a statistically significant difference in terms of visceral and vascular injury between closed and open laparoscopy, there being no such difference for mortality rates. Their conclusion was that open establishment of pneumoperitoneum should be advocated in laparoscopic surgery, because it is safer than the closed method.

Establishing the pneumoperitoneum and inserting the working ports remain the most crucial steps in the laparoscopic approach. Fifty percent of laparoscopic complications are entry related. In order to mitigate laparoscopic entry mishaps and improve patient safety, several international surgical corporations, including European Association of Surgeons (EAES), have published clinical practice guidelines for laparoscopic entry practice [3].

Which of the two methods—the open or the closed using the Veress needle—used for gaining access to the abdomen is safer remains a subject of controversy.

Moreover, the outcome of injuries is strongly related to the type of anatomical structure damaged (bladder, bowel, vessels, etc.), its immediate recognition, and meticulous repair, which usually necessitates a conversion to a laparotomy [4].

Inadvertent small bowel perforation in laparoscopic surgery seems underreported [4–6]. There is no evidence of the influence of the type, size, or shape of trocars [4]. However, there are several conditions that can increase the risk of bowel lesions, such as:

- Obesity (for needing to exert more pressure when inserting working ports)
- Extreme thinness (caused by the short distance between the skin and anatomical structures)
- Dilated bowel loops (e.g., in case of intestinal obstruction)
- Previous history of abdominal or pelvic surgery

That last issue is the most important factor. In fact, the probability of bowel injury is ten times greater if patient has had three previous laparotomies or more [6].

Inadvertent small bowel perforation is potentially a lethal complication of laparoscopic surgery; the mortality rate for bowel injuries being between 3 and 4 % [4–6].

To sum up, if we have a patient who has been operated by laparoscopic surgery, who postoperatively develops fever, tachycardia, abdominal pain, or any other sepsis or peritonitis signs, then bowel damage must be excluded by a CT scan, followed by emergency reintervention [4]. Nevertheless, we should not forget that sometimes—as in the case of our patient above—clinical symptoms are poorly visible and that patients should maintain an acceptable general situation. Because of that, diagnosis can be very complicated and should certainly involve recognizing that this complication may be diagnosed several days after the first procedure.

References

1. Schafer M, Lauper M, Krahenbuhl L. Trocar and Veress needle injuries during laparoscopy. Surg Endosc. 2001;15:275–80.
2. Bonjer HJ, Hazenbroek EJ, Kazemier G, et al. Open versus closed establishment of pneumoperitoneum in laparoscopic surgery. Br J Surg. 1997;84:599–602.
3. Neudecker J, Sauerland S, et al. The European Association for Surgery. Clinical practice guideline on the pneumoperitoneum for laparoscopic Surgery. Surg Endosc. 2002;16:1121–43.
4. Steven J, Binenbaum MD, Michael A, Goldfarb MD. Inadvertent enterotomy in minimally invasive abdominal surgery. JSLS. 2006;10:336–40.
5. Tinelli A, et al. Laparoscopy entry in patients with previous abdominal and pelvic surgery. Surg Innov. 2011;18:201–5.
6. Orlando R, Lirussi F. Delayed recognition of inadvertent gut injury during laparoscopy. Surg Endosc. 2000;14:1188–9.

Chapter 64
Case on Small Bowel Ischemia During Neoadjuvant Chemotherapy for Gastroesophageal Junction Cancer

Miguel A. Cuesta and Donald L. van der Peet

Keywords Hernia • Duodenum • Colon • Necrosis • Complication • Paraesophageal hernia • Esophageal cancer • Neoadjuvant chemotherapy • Intestinal ischemia

Diagnosis and Identification of Complication

A 60-year-old man was referred to us because of progressive dysphagia complaints. Three years before he had been operated on twice because of paraoesophageal hernia and postoperative dysphagia. Finally, a Nissen fundoplication was created with no further swallowing complaints until now. By endoscopy, a gastroesophageal junction adenocarcinoma was found with no signs of metastases on the CT scan of thorax and abdomen (Fig. 64.1). An endoscopic ultrasonography had staged the tumor as T3N1. Patient was proposed for neoadjuvant chemotherapy, the MAGIC study. After the third cycle, patient was admitted to the Department of Oncology because of progressive sickness with bone marrow depression and abdominal pain. On the CT scan, an image of distended small bowel was observed with pneumatosis intestinalis (Fig. 64.2a, b).

Treatment of Complication

Patient was proposed for an exploratory laparotomy, but oncologists accentuated the risks for laparotomy because of bone marrow depression and the possibility of spontaneous recovery with antibiotics and a wait-and-see policy.

M.A. Cuesta, M.D. (✉) • D.L. van der Peet
Department of Surgery, VU University Medical Center, Amsterdam, The Netherlands
e-mail: ma.cuesta@vumc.nl

M.A. Cuesta, H.J. Bonjer (eds.), *Case Studies of Postoperative Complications after Digestive Surgery*, DOI 10.1007/978-3-319-01613-9_64,

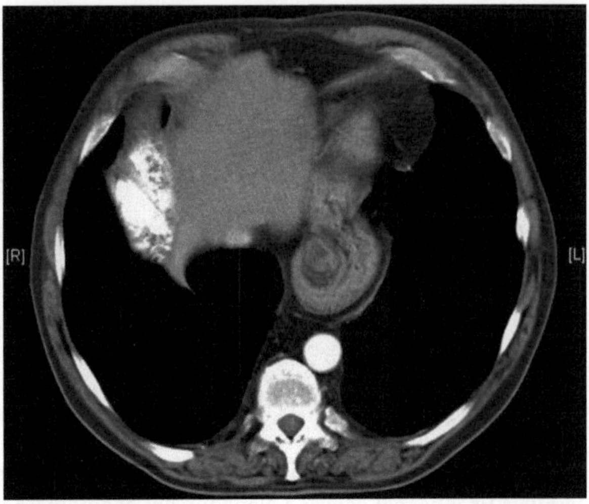

Fig. 64.1 CT scan showing the tumor at the gastroesophageal junction with the Nissen fundoplication

At laparotomy, an extensive ischemia/necrosis of the entire small bowel was found (Fig. 64.3). The superior mesenteric artery was patent with pulsations up to the bowel. No resection was considered but to await some demarcation of the necrosis. Decision was taken to perform a second look after 24 h.

Patient seemed stabilized and the next day at laparotomy, the necrosis was found patchy, including the duodenum and ascending colon. Considering the situation, no further aggressive treatment was provided.

Discussion

Lesson of this case is that currently the neoadjuvant therapy has an important role in the treatment of many gastrointestinal cancers such as esophageal and gastric. The expected response to neoadjuvant therapy and reasonably good prognosis after surgery never should exclude the possibility that these may cause as such high toxicity resulting in morbidity and even mortality, as took place in the present case. Toxicity and morbidity are clearly reported, but mortality rate exclusively due to the neoadjuvant therapy is not clearly reported.

In the MAGIC trial, they randomly assigned patients with resectable adenocarcinoma of the stomach, esophagogastric junction, or lower esophagus to either perioperative chemotherapy and surgery (250 patients) or surgery alone (253 patients) [1]. Chemotherapy consisted of three preoperative and three postoperative cycles of intravenous epirubicin and cisplatin, and a continuous intravenous infusion of fluorouracil. The primary end point was overall survival.

ECF-related adverse effects were similar to those previously reported among patients with advanced gastric cancer. Rates of postoperative complications were similar in the perioperative-chemotherapy group and the surgery group (46 % and 45 %, respectively), as were the numbers of deaths within 30 days after surgery. They reported that with a median follow-up of 4 years, 149 patients in the

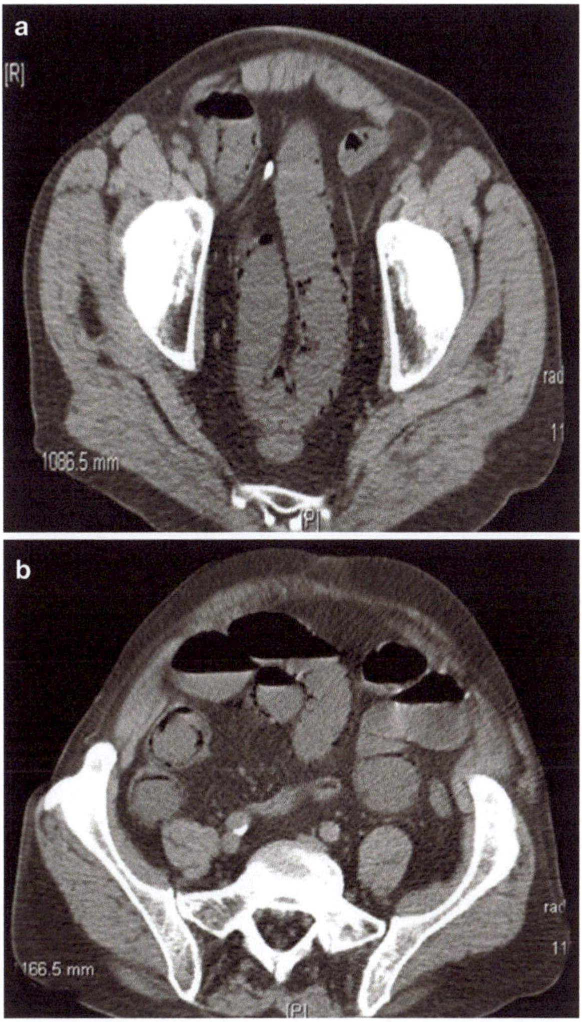

Fig. 64.2 (**a**, **b**) Intestinal dilatation with pneumatosis intestinalis

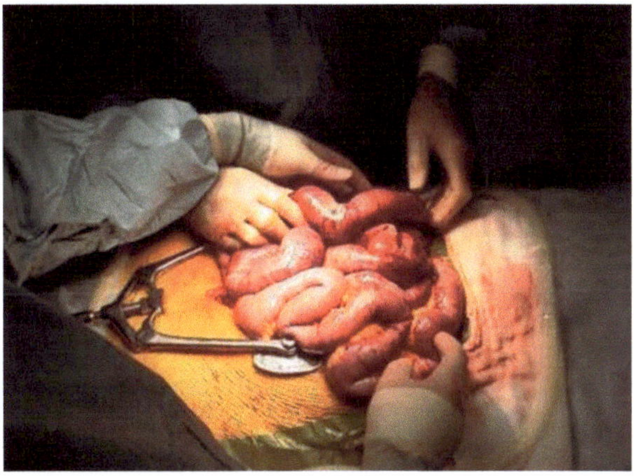

Fig. 64.3 Operative picture. Extensive patchy ischemia of the small bowel

perioperative-chemotherapy group and 170 in the surgery group had died. As compared with the surgery group, the perioperative-chemotherapy group had a higher likelihood of overall 5-year survival rate and of progression-free survival. In conclusion there are enough arguments to use the neoadjuvant therapy without forgetting that it will be the cause of such a complication.

Reference

1. Cunningham D, Allum WH, Stenning SP, et al. Perioperative chemotherapy versus surgery alone for resectable gastroesophageal cancer. N Engl J Med. 2006;355:11–20.

Chapter 65
Case on Complications of Intestinal Malrotation

Miguel A. Cuesta

Keywords Intestinal obstruction • Colopexy • Midgut malrotation • Adult malrotation

Diagnosis and Indication for Surgery

A 29-year-old nurse was referred to us from a regional hospital because of intestinal obstruction. She had never been operated on before and the physical examination revealed no inguinal or femoral hernias. Three years before this patient did have an episode of some hours of intense pain in her abdomen, explained then by the GP as a colic condition.

On the X-ray of her abdomen and on the CT scan, a gastric dilatation was seen and also that the distended small bowel was displaced to the right side of the abdomen and the right colon to the left hemiabdomen, suggesting the existence of a midgut malrotation in an adult patient (Figs. 65.1 and 65.2a–c).

Operation

After initial conservative treatment by nasogastric tube and parenteral feeding, she was operated on laparoscopically in order to take down the Ladd's bands. The bands were not clearly found by laparoscopy and operation was converted to upper

M.A. Cuesta, M.D.
Department of Surgery, VU University Medical Center, Amsterdam, The Netherlands
e-mail: ma.cuesta@vumc.nl

M.A. Cuesta, H.J. Bonjer (eds.), *Case Studies of Postoperative Complications after Digestive Surgery*, DOI 10.1007/978-3-319-01613-9_65,

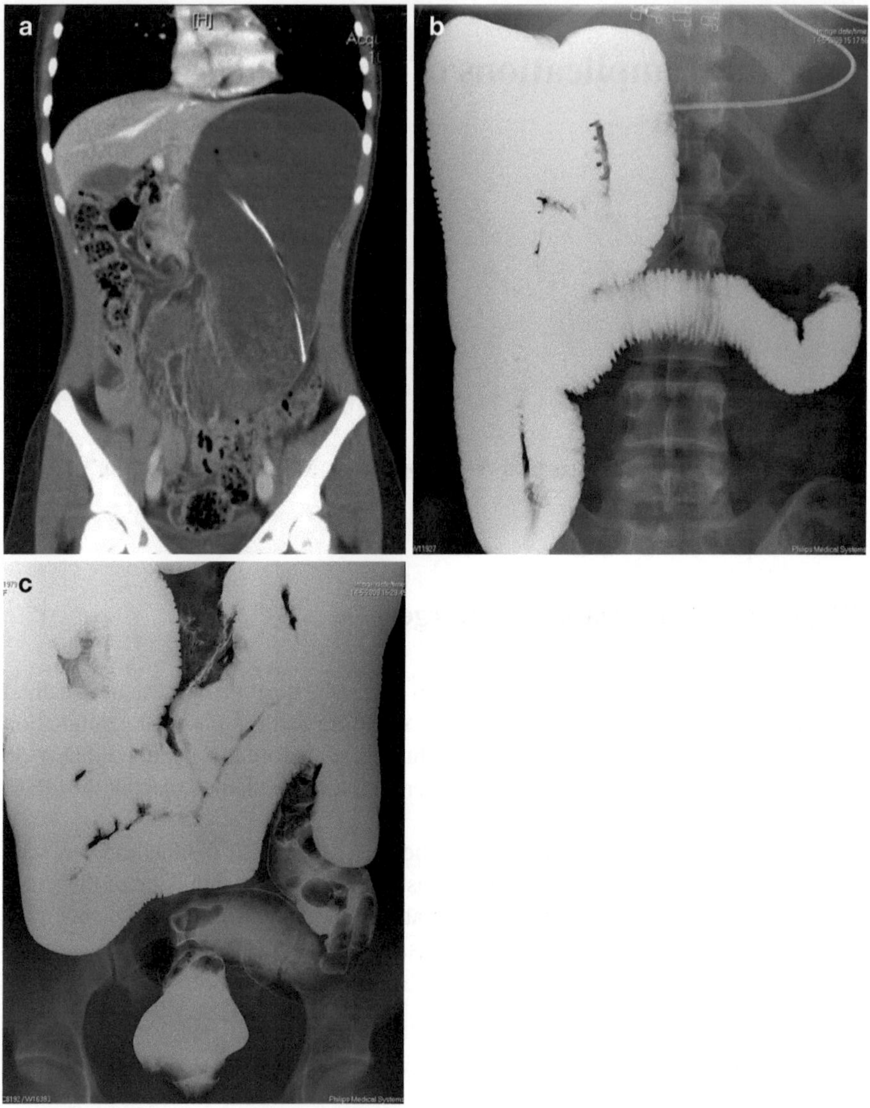

Fig. 65.1 (**a**) CT scan, midgut malrotation showing small bowel to the *right*, colon *left*, and gastric dilatation probably due to Ladd's bands. (**b**) Contrast through tube introduced in small bowel showing the bowels on the *right side*. (**c**) Small bowel *right*, duodenojejunal junction on the *right*, and colon *left*

laparotomy because of a difficult anatomy. After exploring the abdomen, the Ladd's bands were found and divided, small bowel volvulus derotated, and an appendectomy performed.

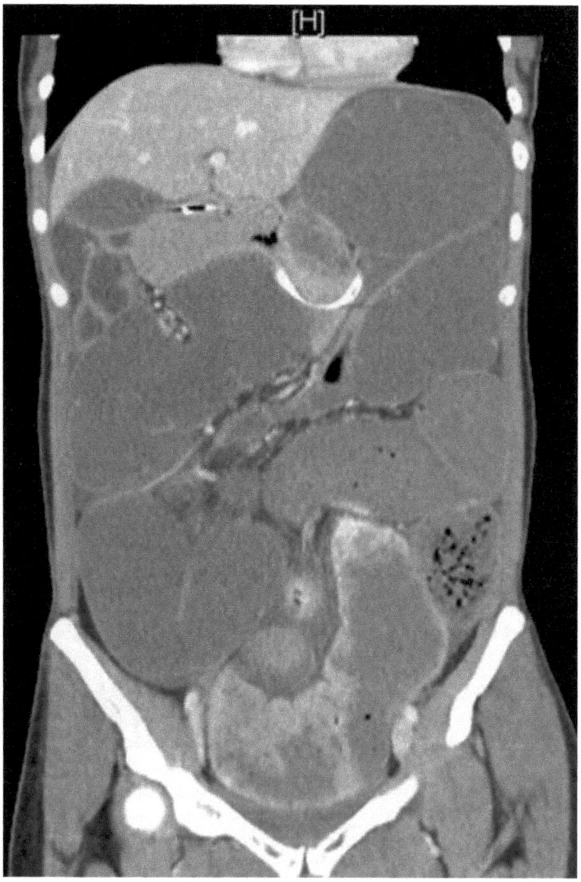

Fig. 65.2 Plain abdominal X-ray. 2011. Distended colon

Postoperative Course: Identification and Treatment of Complication

Patient was readmitted 6 months later due to the same clinical picture of intestinal obstruction and abdominal pain. On a CT scan, the image of a volvulus of the colon was observed and patient was reoperated. During the operation, the colon was attached to the left abdominal wall by stitches, permitting the small bowel to remain free at the right side of the abdomen.

A long period of 2 years followed with intermittent abdominal pain, the patient in the meantime having delivered a child.

One year later, a period followed of intense abdominal pain and obstruction; on the CT scan an important colon distension of 13 cm was seen (Fig. 65.2). At relaparotomy a bride crossed over the colon at the place where the colopexy was performed 2 years previously. The bride was taken down and the colon recovered after decompression. The patient recovered and is nowadays stable (Fig. 65.3).

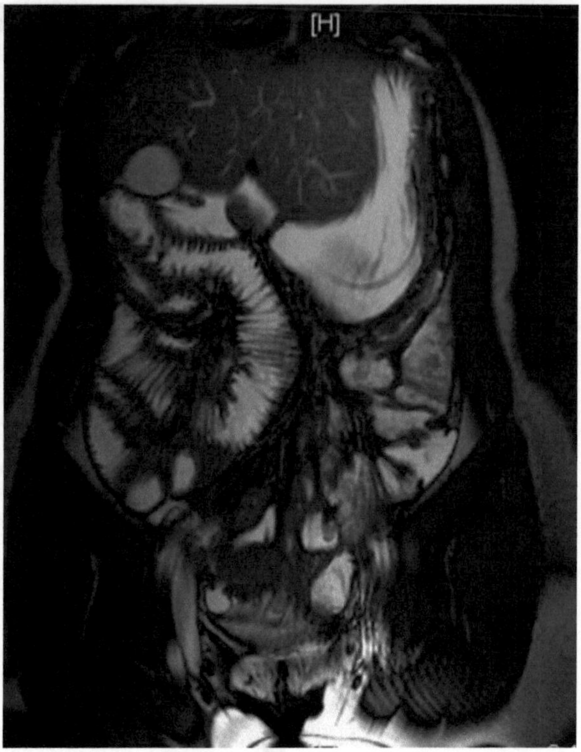

Fig. 65.3 MRI showing stable situation. Midgut malrotation

Discussion

Lesson of this case is how difficult is to manage and operate an adult patient with malrotation.

First described by Ladd in 1932 involving children [1], Pickhardt et al. have described extensively the radiology diagnosis of the midgut malrotation in adults. Midgut malrotation has been estimated to occur in approximately one in 500 live births [2–4]. Reportedly, 64–80 % of patients present the symptoms within the first month of life. In older children and adults, malrotation is rarely suspected on clinical grounds and is generally first visible on imaging studies or at laparotomy. Conventional radiography is neither sensitive nor specific for malrotation. The upper gastrointestinal barium series remains accurate for detection; the duodeno-jejunal junction fails to cross the midline and lies below the level of the duodenal bulb. The enema findings are also nonspecific because cecal location can be variable without malrotation. Enhanced CT scan with oral contrast serves best to diagnose this condition. Obstruction at duodenojejunal junction produced by the

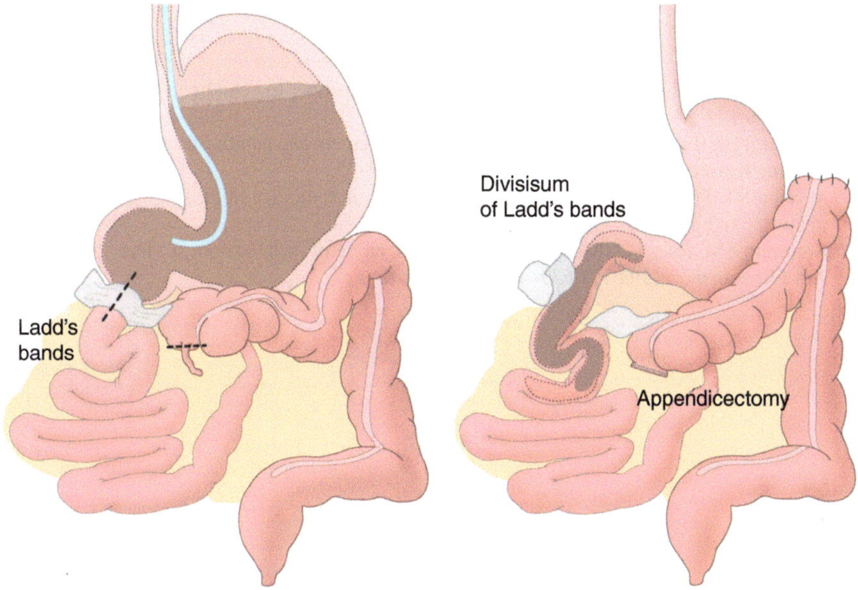

Illustration 65.1 Malrotation in adults is a rare condition, but if an acute abdomen occurred it is important to know the embryological principles of its cause and what to do ?. Gastric dilatation caused by Ladd's bands, midgut malrotation, and internal hernias are the three most important clinical situations

Ladd's bands, small bowel displaced to the right abdomen, the colon to the left and inverted relationship between superior mesenteric artery, and superior mesenteric vein are important findings to establish the diagnosis of midgut malrotation (Illustration 65.1).

Midgut volvulus is a complication of malrotation in which clockwise twisting of the bowel around the SMA axis occurs because of the narrowed mesenteric attachment This life-threatening condition is a clear indication for emergency surgery. The clinical diagnosis of midgut volvulus in adolescents and adults is difficult because the presentation is usually nonspecific and malrotation is rarely considered. Recurrent episodes of colicky abdominal pain with vomiting over a period of months or years are typical and may eventually lead to imaging [2–4].

Fortunately, the CT findings of malrotation with midgut volvulus are characteristic. The CT whirl or whirlpool sign describes the swirling appearance of bowel and mesentery twisted around the SMA axis. Additional CT findings include duodenal obstruction, congestion of the mesenteric vasculature, and evidence of underlying malrotation The presence of intestinal ischemia or necrosis is an ominous sign.

Surgical treatment should be performed if volvulus, duodenal obstruction (division of Ladd's bands), and internal hernia (Illustration 65.1) are factors.

References

1. Ladd WE. Congenital obstruction of the duodenum in children. N Eng J Med. 1932;206:277–83.
2. Pickhardt PJ, Bhalla S. Intestinal malrotation in adolescent and adults. Spectrum of clinical and imaging features. Am J Roentgenol. 2002;179:1429–35.
3. Maxson RT, Franklin PA, Wagner CW. Malrotation in the older child: surgical management, treatment and outcome. Am Surg. 1995;61:135–8.
4. Bernstein SM, Russ PD. Midgut volvulus: a rare cause of acute abdomen in an adult patient. Am J Roentgenol. 1998;171:639–41.

Chapter 66
Case on Leakage After Right Hemicolectomy

Nike M. Hanneman

Keywords Colon cancer • Laparoscopic hemicolectomy • Leakage anastomosis • Peritonitis

First Patient

Diagnosis and Indication for Surgery

A 61-year-old man with anemia was sent to a gastroenterologist, who diagnosed a disc-shaped anomaly at the Bauhin's valve. Biopsy showed a tubulovillous adenoma with severe dysplasia—most likely an intestinal adenocarcinoma. The additional CT scan showed no evidence for metastatic disease.

Operation

A laparoscopic right hemicolectomy was performed with a side-to-side stapled anastomosis.

N.M. Hanneman, M.D.
Department of Surgery,
Medisch Centrum, Alkmaar, The Netherlands
e-mail: n.hanneman@mca.nl

M.A. Cuesta, H.J. Bonjer (eds.), *Case Studies of Postoperative Complications after Digestive Surgery*, DOI 10.1007/978-3-319-01613-9_66,

Postoperative Course: Identification of Complication

Two days postoperative, the patient developed fever with tachycardia and abdominal tenderness. The CT scan showed a leakage of the blind ileum loop. A laparotomy showed a local purulent peritonitis, so it was decided to resect the anastomosis and perform a new side-to-side anastomosis. The pathology showed a T2N0M0. The patient left the hospital 12 days after his last operation.

Second Patient

Diagnosis and Description of Operation

A 76-year-old lady, known with auricular fibrillation and taking coumarin, underwent a laparoscopic extended right hemicolectomy because of an adenocarcinoma located proximal of the hepatic flexure. Course of operation was uncomplicated, dissection was adequate, blood loss 100 cc, and after retrieval of the specimen through a transumbilical incision, anastomosis was performed extra-corporeally manually in side-to-side fashion. Stage of tumor was T3N0.

Postoperative Course: Identification of Complication

Initially, she was treated postoperatively according to fast track principles, but the third day postoperative a paralytic ileus developed and treatment was changed in nasogastric tube and Total Parenteral Nutrition. Vicissitudes followed in this situation up to the eighth day postoperative when she developed fever and abdominal pain. CRP values were 270 and she had a leukocytosis of 18,000. Patient was sick, and the whole abdomen showed signs of peritonitis. Blood pressure was normal, auricular fibrillation of 124 bpm and oliguria of 25 cc/h. Patient was admitted to the Medium Care ward and a CT scan performed. The CT scan showed free air and fluid collections on the right more than left abdomen and a leakage of contrast through the anastomosis (Fig. 66.1). Emergency laparotomy followed; important purulent peritonitis was found with leakage of 2 cm at the ileum side of anastomosis. Patient was unstable during operation, and we decided to disconnect the anastomosis and create an ileostomy in the right lower abdomen, the transverse colon being closed by staplers. Patient was admitted to the Intensive Care Unit, was mechanically

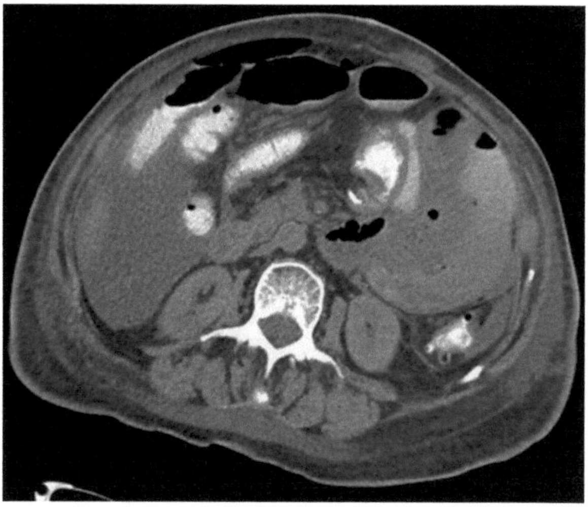

Fig. 66.1 CT scan showing intraabdominal fluids, leakage of contrast, and pneumoperitoneum

ventilated, and was noradrenaline dependent. Digoxin was given to control the fibrillation and on the 1st postoperative day, cardioversion became necessary to control the atrial fibrillation. After 3 days, her situation improved and gradually she could be weaned off the mechanical ventilator. Initially, ileostomy production was high, 2,300 cc necessitating fluids reposition and NaCl. Patient was dismissed after 30 days. Six months later through a laparotomy ileostomy was reversed by a new ileotrasversostomy. Patient is doing well and cancer control is good.

Discussion

Right-sided or proximal colon cancers are increasing; as of today, 34–44 % of all colon cancers are proximal to the splenic flexure. The incidence in the Netherlands is about 50 cases per 100,000 inhabitants per year. The most dreaded complication of operation is anastomotic leakage. The percentage of occurrence of anastomotic leakage for the colon holding for the Netherlands in the year 2010 has been 7 %. There are many risk factors categorized as patient specific and intraoperative. Surgical treatment includes resection of the anastomosis or fecal diversion via ileostomy (Illustration 66.1). With a small degree of contamination the right-sided colonic leaks can often be reanastomosed and drained. With more extensive contamination, resection with ileostomy should be performed. There is no place for simple local repair [1].

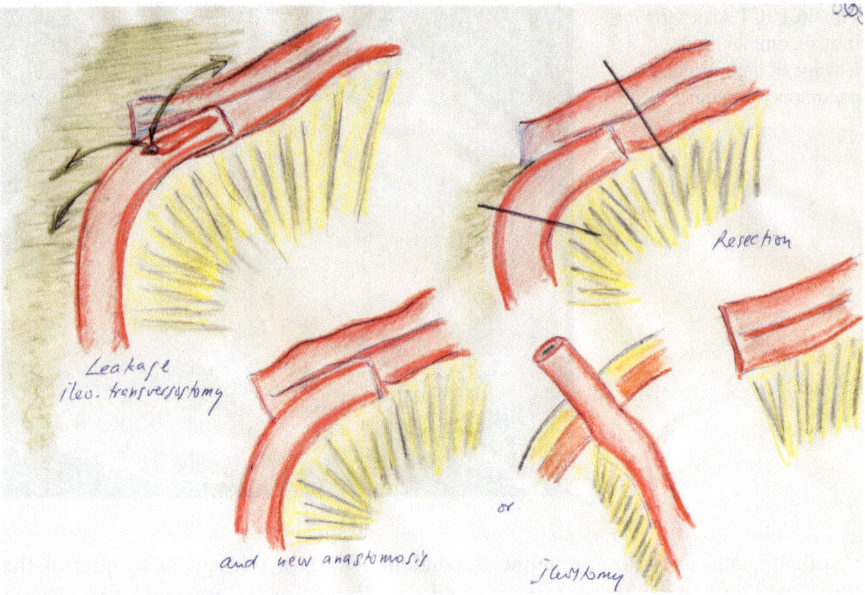

Illustration 66.1 In the case of anastomosis leakage after right hemicolectomy, surgical treatment includes resection of the anastomosis or fecal diversion via ileostomy. With a small degree of contamination, the right-sided colonic leaks can often be reanastomosed and drained. With more extensive contamination, resection with ileostomy should be performed. There is no place for simple local repair

Reference

1. Snijders HS, Wouters MW, van Leersum NJ et al. Meta-analysis of the risk for anastomotic leakage, the postoperative mortality caused by leakage in relation to the overall postoperative mortality. Eur J Surg Oncol. 2012;38:1013–9.

Chapter 67
Case on Anastomotic Rotation After Laparoscopic Right Hemicolectomy for Colonic Cancer

Bastiaan R. Klarenbeek

Keywords Cecal cancer • Intestinal obstruction • Laparoscopic right hemicolectomy • Torsion anastomosis

Diagnosis and Indication for Surgery

An otherwise healthy 69-year-old male patient without a medical history was referred to the outpatient clinic of Internal Medicine because of fatigue and energy-loss based on a microcytic anemia. A colonoscopy during the study revealed an ulcerative cecal carcinoma. A thoracic X-ray and a four-phase intravenous contrast abdominal CT scan showed no distant metastases. Patient was scheduled for a laparoscopic right hemicolectomy.

Operation

Operation coursed without incidents; blood loss was less than 50 cc and through a well-protected trans umbilical incision, specimen was retrieved without division of ileum and transverse colon, division followed outside. After division by means of staplers, anastomosis was performed in a side-to-side fashion using a hand-sewn one-layer running suture technique. The defect in the mesentery was closed by an absorbable suture and the bowel was repositioned in the abdomen.

B.R. Klarenbeek
Department of Surgery, MC Leeuwarden, Leeuwarden, The Netherlands
e-mail: bas.klarenbeek@znb.nl

M.A. Cuesta, H.J. Bonjer (eds.), *Case Studies of Postoperative Complications after Digestive Surgery*, DOI 10.1007/978-3-319-01613-9_67,

Postoperative Course: Identification and Treatment of Complication

Postoperatively, the patient developed at once an ileus, which did not resolve with conservative measures during the first 10 days (Fig. 67.1). Clinically, he was not sick, no fever, abdomen distended yet not painful, light leukocytosis, and a stable CRP of 120. An abdominal CT scan showed no signs of anastomotic leakage, but an obstructive ileus with a transition zone at the anastomotic site (Fig. 67.2). Pathology study showed a T3N0M0 cecal carcinoma.

Because of the clinical and CT scan findings, a laparotomy was performed at day 11.

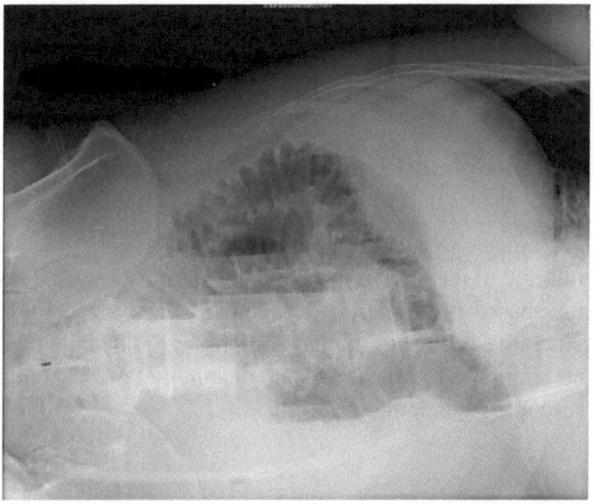

Fig. 67.1 X ray of abdomen showing postoperative small bowel obstruction

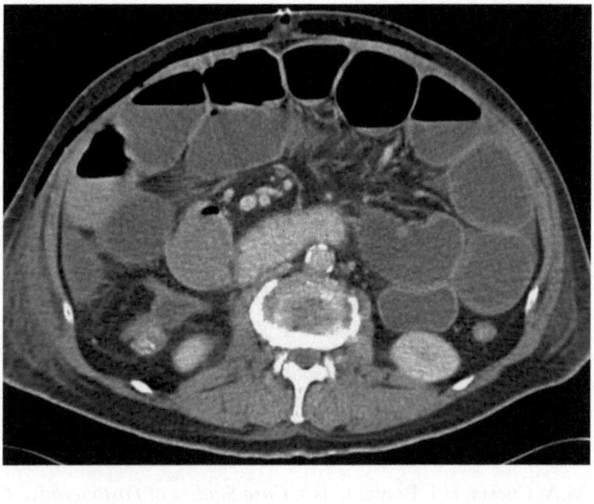

Fig. 67.2 CT scan with small bowel obstruction at the level of the anastomosis

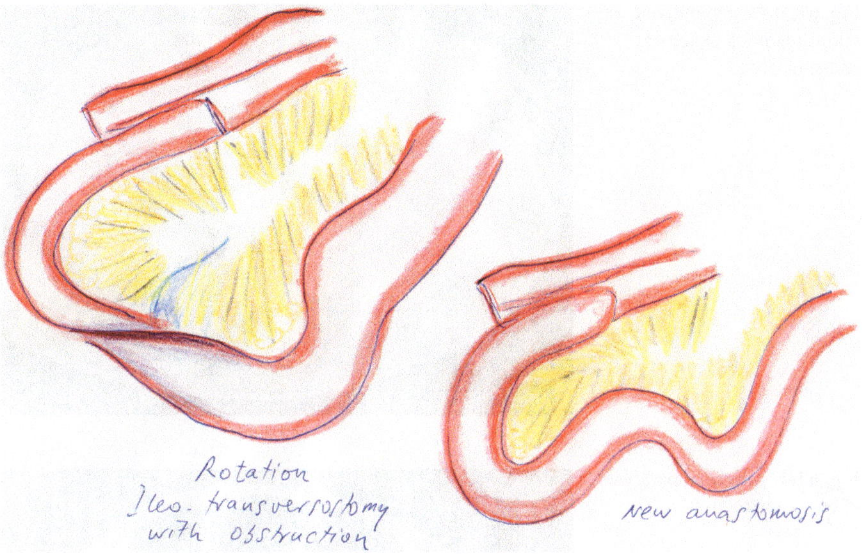

Illustration 67.1 Twist of the anastomosis after right hemicolectomy is an infrequent complication. During laparoscopy perhaps it is more frequent. It is very important during extracorporeal resection not to twist the small bowel! Before anastomosis check that the small bowel is in good position and not twisted

During operation, a complete rotation of the anastomosis was found without vascular compromise or ischemia, but with an important proximal distension. Resection of the anastomosis was performed, followed by the creation of a new hand-sewn end-to-side anastomosis (Illustration 67.1). Care was being taken that no rotation or vascular compromise was present.

Outcome

Unfortunately, the patient developed progressive signs of abdominal sepsis with multiple organ failure. Another abdominal CT scan with oral contrast showed evidence of air and contrast leakage, supporting the suspicion of an anastomotic leakage (Fig. 67.3). A relaparotomy was performed to take down the anastomosis and create an ileostomy and mucous fistula at the transverse colon. The same day, another laparotomy was performed because of postoperative hypovolemic shock due to a laceration of the spleen, and a splenectomy was performed. After long recovery at the intensive care unit, the patient could be discharged from the hospital 6 weeks postoperative. After 6 months, continuity of the bowel was restored together with reconstruction of the abdominal wall, by means of sub-lay mesh. A long period of postoperative intestinal paralysis followed (Fig. 67.4). At the most recent visit of the outpatient clinic, the patient had an acceptable bowel function, and routine follow-up for colon cancer will be carried out.

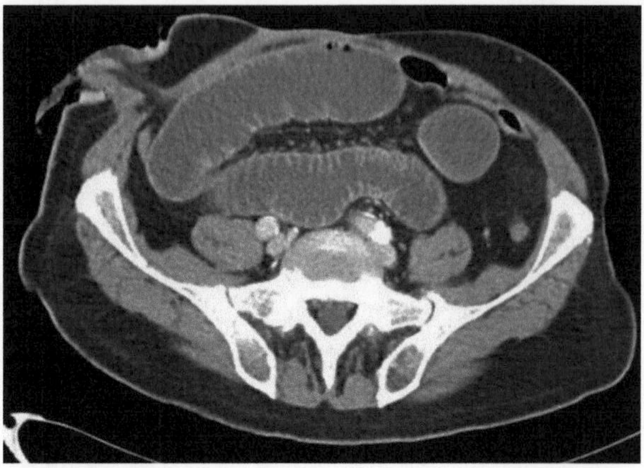

Fig. 67.3 Postoperative CT scan showing leakage of anastomosis

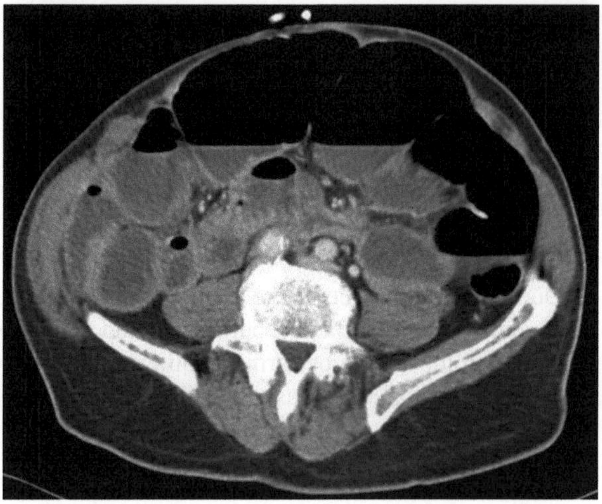

Fig. 67.4 Intestinal paralysis after reconstruction

Discussion

Anastomotic misalignment is a very rare complication in colorectal surgery. Laparoscopic surgery might have increased this risk of rotation, because the bowel is exteriorized through a small incision. The creation of an extracorporeal anastomosis through the same small incision might facilitate misalignment. However, current literature shows only four reports of this complication after laparoscopic colectomy. Two retrospective cohort studies report one case each (0.5–0.8 %) [1, 2]. Also, two case reports describe cases of anastomotic rotation: one after right hemicolectomy [3] and another after anterior resection [4]. Presumably, these figures are an underestimation of anastomotic misalignment, because probably if rotation is less than 180° that is clinically not significant. It seems that only a more than 180° rotation or more will most certainly give obstructive complaints and vascular compromise to some extent. In our case, there was no recovery of bowel function after initial surgery and reoperation took place during the same hospital admission. Two other cases in literature report initial intestinal passage and posterior discharge, with readmission after several weeks up to 2 years because of bowel obstruction. This partial recovery might reflect a subtotal obstruction, with peristaltic compromise causing recurrent symptoms. Identification of anastomotic misalignment seems difficult; CT scans and colonoscopy will not always reveal the origin of the bowel obstruction. Surgical re-intervention appears to be the only way to correct this complication. Whether a new anastomosis or an ileostomy should be created depends on individual factors, such as the extent of vascular compromise and the general condition of the patient.

References

1. Lacy AM, Garcia-Valdecasas JC, Delgado S, et al. Postoperative complications of laparoscopic-assisted colectomy. Surg Endosc. 1997;11:119–22.
2. Croce E, Olmi S, Azzola M, et al. Laparoscopic colectomy: indications, standardized technique and results after 6 years experience. Hepatogastroenterology. 2000;47:683–91.
3. Bonjer HJ, Lange JF. Rotation of the terminal ileum in laparoscopic right hemicolectomy. Surg Endosc. 1993;7:534–9.
4. Lynes K, Takacs K, Paice AG, Trotter G. Delayed presentation of a 360-degree rotational anastomotic misalignment following laparoscopic anterior resection. Colorectal Dis. 2010;12: 1268–71.

Chapter 68
Case on Leakage After Ileocecal Resection for Crohn's Disease

Hugo W. Nijhof

Keywords Crohn's disease • Laparoscopic ileocecal resection • Anastomosis leakage • Abdominal abscess

Diagnosis and Indication for Surgery

A 20-year-old healthy female patient presented to the surgical outpatient clinic elsewhere. For the last 3 years, she had been conservatively treated for ileocecal Crohn's disease. However, since her disease with developing of symptomatic stenosis did not successfully respond to medical treatment, a laparoscopic ileocecal resection was proposed.

Operation

The procedure was performed in a standard fashion with antibiotic prophylaxis. By laparoscopy, a disease was localized in the ileocecal area. By using four trocars, ascending colon and ileum were mobilized, exteriorized through a transumbilical incision, resected, and anastomosed in side-to-side isoperistaltic stapled anastomosis, which was overseen with PDS 3-0.

Postoperative Course: Identification and Treatment of Complication

The initial postoperative period was without complications. However, the patient suffered from a continuing paralytic ileus, which was at first

H.W. Nijhof, M.D.
Department of Surgery, Kennemer Gasthuis, Haarlem, The Netherlands
e-mail: hw.nijhof@kg.nl

M.A. Cuesta, H.J. Bonjer (eds.), *Case Studies of Postoperative Complications after Digestive Surgery*, DOI 10.1007/978-3-319-01613-9_68,

conservatively managed with fluid resuscitation and gastric tube drainage. Nonetheless, at the 17th postoperative day, she developed fever with increased infection parameters. A contrast-enhanced CT scan of the abdomen was performed that showed a fluid collection at the anastomotic site without signs of contrast extravasation (Fig. 68.1). A CT-scan-guided drainage was performed, after which the drain remained in place for 10 days (Fig. 68.2). The drain had become accidentally dislocated, after which the patient's condition deteriorated with continuous episodes of spiked fever. On her request, she was finally transferred to our hospital.

Presentation in our department, at the 12th postoperative day, revealed a patient in poor nutritional condition, septic with a fever of 38.5 °C, respiratory rate of 30, pulse of 124, and abdominal tenderness in the right abdomen. A CT scan of the abdomen was performed, which showed a large pelvic and right paracolic abscess. Because of her septic condition, we did not opt for a CT scan-guided drainage, but for an explorative laparotomy, which revealed the large

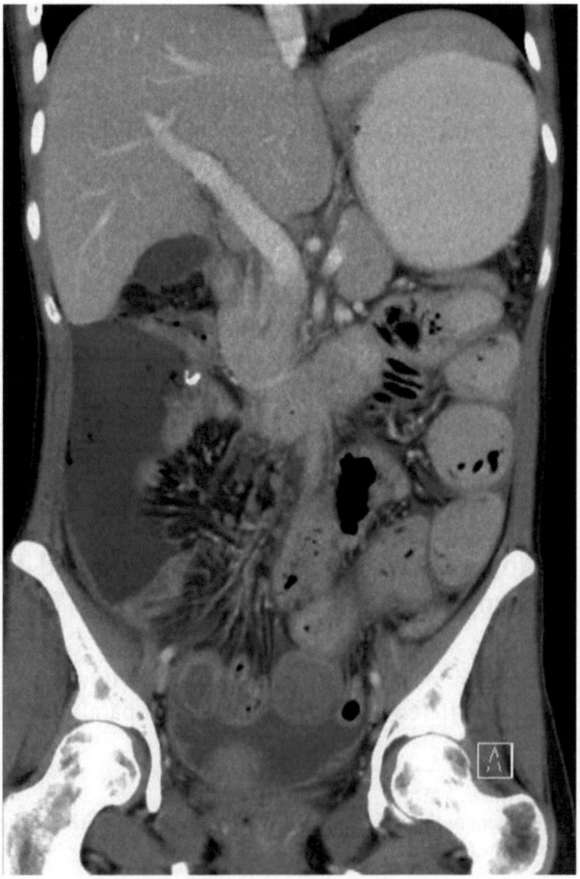

Fig. 68.1 CT scan showing a large pelvic and right paracolic fluid collection

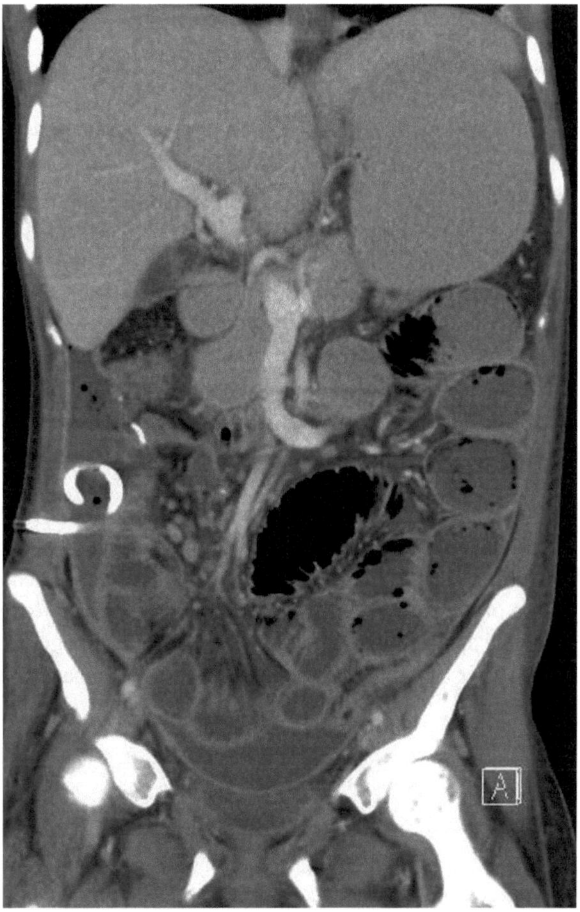

Fig. 68.2 CT abdomen showing the percutaneous placed drain in the right paracolic fluid collection

abscesses. Already depicted with CT scan, these were an almost complete anastomotic dehiscence, the rest being converted in an inflammatory plastron. Dissection was difficult, yet an ileostomy without eversion and colostomy could be performed. After extensive rinsing of the abdominal cavity two large drains were left, after which the abdominal wall was closed. Antibiotic treatment was continued for 7 days.

Postoperatively the patient's condition improved steadily. Oral intake improved and the drains were removed. Two weeks after the last laparotomy she was discharged. Nasogastric tube feeding was continued at home because of her poor nutritional condition.

Five months later, her ileostomy could be closed as well as the resection of a small enterocutaneous fistula that she had developed. Further recovery was without complications. Progressively, she has gained weight and recently she has married.

Discussion

Although much care is always given to an bowel anastomosis, leakage still may occur. The lowest rates are found after ileocolic anastomosis; however, these nonetheless occur in 1–3 %. Although patients with Crohn's disease may be at risk for leakage because of the immunosuppressive medication used, yet leakage while performing a side-to-side stapled or manual anastomosis remains low [1]. Usually leakage presents itself between postoperative days 5–7; however, later manifestation can occur [2, 3]. There is no clear definition of radiological or clinical anastomotic leakage. As in the present case, the CT scan of abdomen initially revealed no clear anastomotic leakage of contrast, but fluid (or gas) collections were presented early as signs of anastomotic leakage. Together with clinical signs as pain, fever, tachycardia, and peritonitis, we regard anastomotic leakage as more likely [4]. Management of the leakage, however, is diverse and is dependant on many factors.

With non-septic patients, their small abscesses (<3 cm) can merely be treated by antibiotics. With larger intra-abdominal abscesses, an attempt is usually made to perform a radiologically guided drainage of the collection [5]. However, if the condition of the patient fails to improve, deteriorates—or as in this case—develops into general sepsis, time must not be wasted for drainage to be completed. In such a case, explorative surgery for drainage and a new anastomosis or deviation stomas are necessary.

References

1. Resegotti A, Astegiano M, Farina EC, et al. Side-to-side stapled anastomosis strongly reduces anastomotic leak rates in Crohn's disease surgery. Dis Colon Rectum. 2005;48:464–8.
2. Dietz DW, Bailey HR. Postoperative complications. In: Church JM, Beck DE, Wolff BG, Fleshman JW, Pemberton JH, editors. The ASCRS textbook of colon and rectal surgery. New York: Springer; 2007. p. 143.
3. Hyman N, Manchester TL, Osler T, et al. Anastomotic leaks after intestinal anastomosis: it's later than you think. Ann Surg. 2007;245:254–63.
4. Law WI, Chu KW, Ho JW, Chan CW. Risk factors for anastomotic leakage after low anterior resection with total mesorectal excision. Am J Surg. 2000;179:92–8.
5. Phitayakorn R, Delaney CP, Reynolds HL, International Anastomotic Leak Study Group, et al. Standardized algorithms for management of anastomotic leaks and related abdominal and pelvic abscesses after colorectal surgery. World J Surg. 2008;32:1147–52.

Chapter 69
Case on Leakage After Ileoanal Pouch Anastomosis

Miguel A. Cuesta

Keywords Ulcerative colitis • Proctocolectomy • Ileoanal pouch • Leakage IAPA pouch

First Patient

Diagnosis and Indication for Surgery

A 25-year-old male student underwent a total proctocolectomy and ileoanal pouch anastomosis (IAPA) because of an intractable ulcerative colitis by conservative means.

Operation

The operation was performed totally laparoscopically, that means that the Panproctocolectomy was followed by the extracorporeal formation of a J-pouch through a well-protected incision in the right lower abdomen. The pouch was anastomosed to the anal canal by a circular stapler, without protective ileostomy.

Postoperative Course: Identification of Complication

Patient had a long postoperative ileus period without fever or increased inflammatory parameters (Fig. 69.1a, b). In this period he received TPN. After 2 weeks a CT scan

M.A. Cuesta, M.D.
Department of Surgery, VU University Medical Center, Amsterdam, The Netherlands
e-mail: ma.cuesta@vumc.nl

M.A. Cuesta, H.J. Bonjer (eds.), *Case Studies of Postoperative Complications after Digestive Surgery*, DOI 10.1007/978-3-319-01613-9_69,

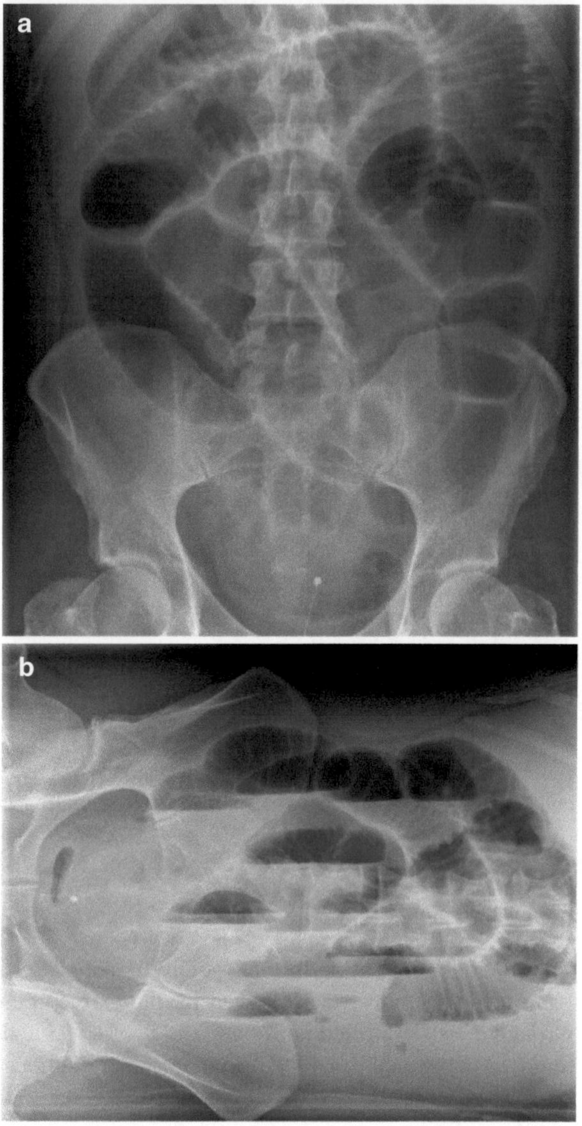

Fig. 69.1 (**a**) Abdominal X-ray showing a postoperative intestinal obstruction. (**b**) Lateral X ray showing intestinal obstruction

was performed showing a progressive imaging of a leakage of the ileoanal anastomosis with an ischiorectal abscess around the pouch and the anastomosis (Fig. 69.2). Patient developed fever, lower abdominal pain, and a high CRP of 325. We decided to drain the abscess transanally under anesthesia. Inspection revealed a defect on the posterior side of the anastomosis, and through it the abscess could be drained whereby a Penrose-like drain was left in the collection (Illustration 69.1). Thereafter, a laparoscopic loop ileostomy was created. Postoperatively, the abscess had to be drained two more times and rinsed under anesthesia. During this period, the patient was fed by

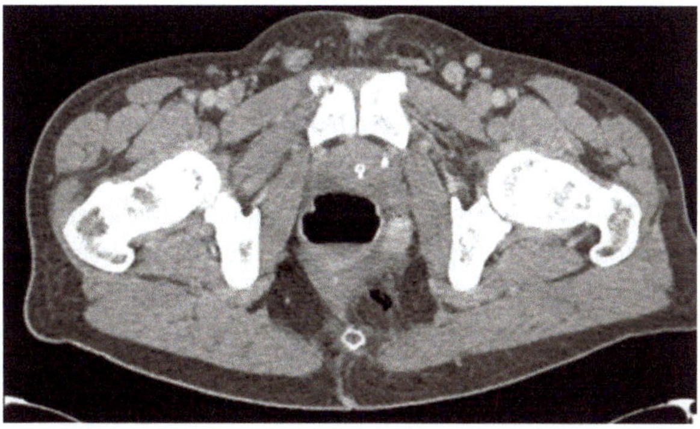

Fig. 69.2 CT scan, leakage, and ischiorectal abscess left side

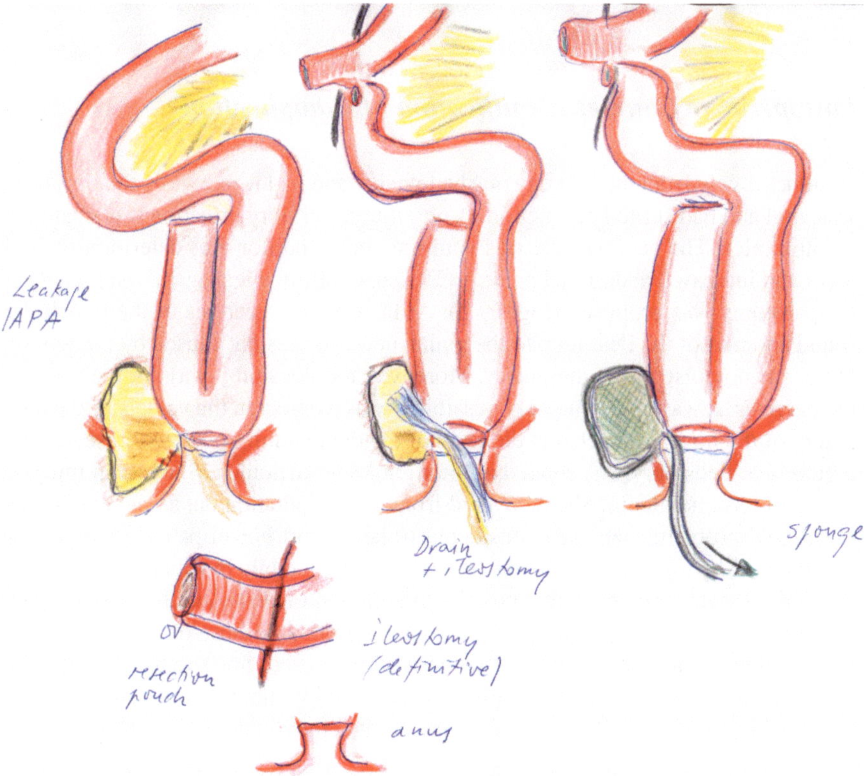

Illustration 69.1 Septic complications after IPAA should be treated by local drainage and diverting ileostomy. It is not clear what will be the ideal operation with or without diverting ileostomy. The ileostomy can protect the pouch and anastomosis during the immediate postoperative course, but it is also cause of high morbidity

enteral feeding by duodenal tube, and finally after a period of 6 weeks he recovered. Once the CT scan had demonstrated that there was no more abscess or leakage, the anastomosis was dilated before taking down of the ileostomy 3 months later.

Second Patient

Diagnosis and Indication for Surgery

A 17-year-old high school girl underwent a panproctocoletomy and ileoanal pouch anastomosis with protective loop ileostomy because of ulcerative colitis and not reacting on conservative therapy. She was known with UC since her 13th year. Operation was performed laparoscopically and hand assisted, that means that the colon was resected by hand assistance followed by the resection of the rectum through a Pfannenstiel incision. Through it the J-pouch was created followed by a stapled ileoanal pouch anastomosis with a protective ileostomy.

Postoperative Course: Identification of Complication

Postoperatively from the first day on she felt sick and had fever, while the ileostomy was vital and had started production. A possible respiratory infection was treated by iv antibiotics. The next day she was vomiting and condition was deteriorating with fever and increased abdominal pain. A CT scan confirmed leakage of the pouch and a laparotomy was proposed (Fig. 69.3). At laparotomy, necrosis of the pouch was found and part of the ileal loop to the pouch necrosis was not caused by torsion, but there was no pulse in the mesentery. Moreover, the ileostomy was not the cause of the necrosis; it was vital. The only possibility was a defect in the vessels of the mesentery of the pouch dissected at the level of the duodenum. Pouch was resected and a definitive ileostomy was created at the right lower abdomen. She lost in this way 75 cm of terminal ileum. She recovered from this reoperation but as she maintained nutritional problems, she was considered to be a short bowel patient. Nutrition is enteral, but she was followed by the special outpatient clinic in which not only feeding and elements are controlled but also production of ileostomy by imodium and cholestyramine. One year later she was again admitted because of abdominal pain. On the plain X-ray, intestinal obstruction was diagnosed. She reacted very quickly to conservative therapy and has until now recovered without pain. During this time she finished high school and began her university study in the faculty of Law.

Discussion

Diverting ileostomy has been considered mandatory for minimizing the effects of septic complications in pelvic pouch surgery. Nowadays, it is a trend to do the operation without diverting ileostomy, apparently with no increase of sepsis or pouch complications on the short and long term. Two questions arise in a discussion of these two patients. First, what is the frequency of septic complications after the

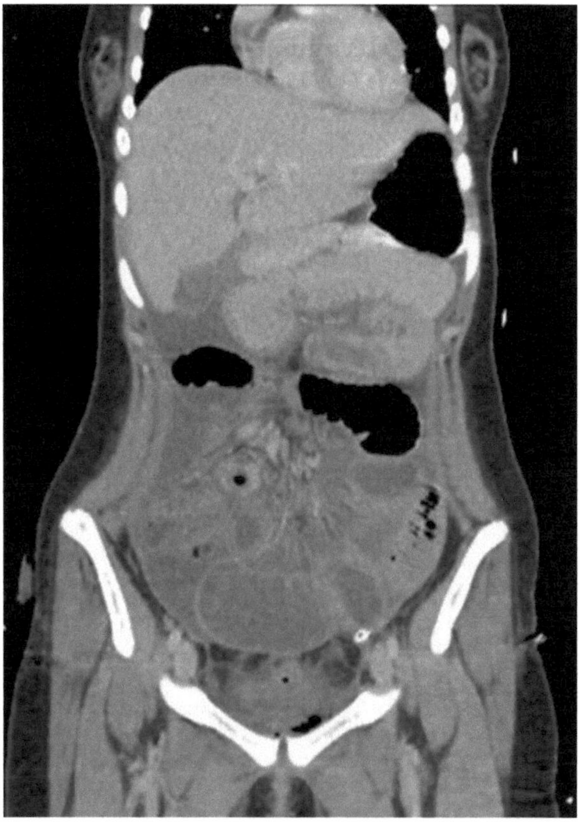

Fig. 69.3 CT scan showing leakage of the IAPA

IAPP procedure? Second, what is the need for a diverting ileostomy? Kiely et al. studied the frequency and consequences of pelvic sepsis after IPAA [1]. Two hundred (6.2 %) of 3,234 patients developed pelvic septic complications within 3 months of IPAA. They compared the complications in two groups of patients with and without septic complications after IPAA. Patients with pelvic sepsis had higher rates of postoperative hemorrhage (13.5 % versus 3.7 %), anastomotic leakage (35 % versus 3.7 %), and fistula formation (37 % versus 7.1 %). The overall median follow-up was 7 years. Moreover, pelvic sepsis was associated with greater pouch failure (19.5 % versus 4 %), incontinence, and worse quality-of-life score.

Gunnarsson et al. studied the complications of a diverting loop ileostomy in the context of an IAPP intervention [2]. They studied complications following diverting loop ileostomies in 143 patients subjected to restorative pelvic pouch surgery. In the period between discharge after pelvic pouch surgery and closure of the loop ileostomy, 20 (14 %) patients were hospitalized because of excessive stoma flow and 19 (13 %) patients were treated for other surgical complications, of whom 10 (7 %) required surgical intervention. In the early postoperative period (within 30 days) after closure of the loop ileostomy, 18 (13 %) patients suffered complications necessitating surgery. Another 12 (8 %) patients were hospitalized because of intestinal obstruction that could be treated conservatively. They concluded that the proportion of complications associated with diverting loop ileostomies in pelvic pouch surgery was considerable. A randomized controlled multicentre study was considered ethically defensible and recommended. Yet, this randomized study never appeared.

References

1. Kiely JM, Fazio VW, Remzi FH, et al. Pelvic sepsis after IPAA adversely affects function of the pouch and quality of life. Dis Colon Rectum. 2012;55:387–92.
2. Gunnarsson U, Karlbom U, Docker M, et al. Proctocolectomy and pelvic pouch-is a diverting stoma dangerous for the patient? Colorectal Dis. 2004;6:23–9.

Chapter 70
Case on Leakage After Sigmoid Resection

Hugo W. Nijhof

Keywords Laparoscopic sigmoid resection • Leakage anastomosis • Colostomy • Diverticulitis

First Patient

Diagnosis and Indication for Surgery

At issue is a 46-year-old window cleaner, who after a persistent period of acute diverticulitis including recovery and recurrence, now underwent an elective laparoscopic sigmoid resection.

Operation

This operation went well; no technical problems appeared, although the splenic flexure was not mobilized. Anastomosis was performed end to end on the level of the promontory.

H.W. Nijhof, M.D.
Department of Surgery, Kennemer Gasthuis, Haarlem, The Netherlands
e-mail: hw.nijhof@kg.nl

M.A. Cuesta, H.J. Bonjer (eds.), *Case Studies of Postoperative Complications after Digestive Surgery*, DOI 10.1007/978-3-319-01613-9_70,

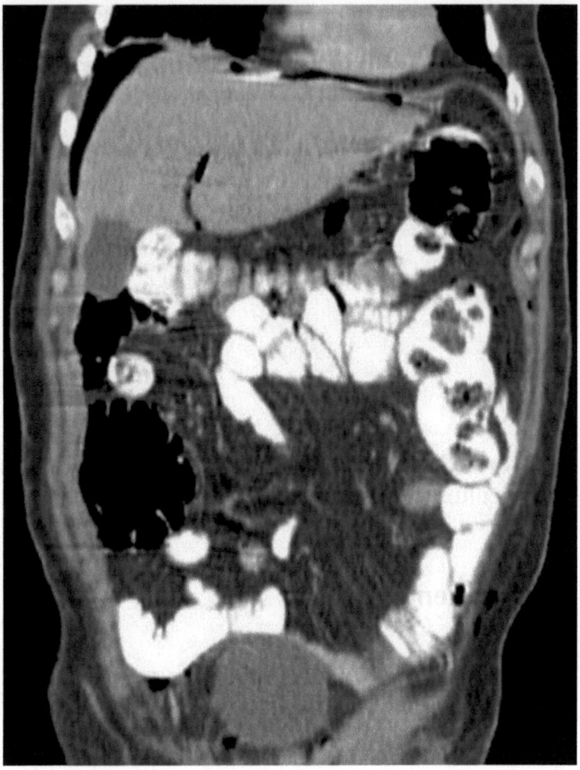

Fig. 70.1 CT scan, leakage of anastomosis with pneumoperitoneum

Postoperative Course: Identification and Treatment of Complication

On the 4th postoperative day, the condition of the patient worsened, with abdominal pain, fever, and abdominal distension.

A CT scan with contrast was performed and a leakage of the anastomosis was found with an abscess in the lower abdomen and with free air under the diaphragm (Fig. 70.1).

Patient underwent a median laparotomy; the leakage was located and the anastomosis was dismantled with creation of a colostomy and closure of the rectal stump. Basis of the decision was that the leakage included fecal peritonitis and because the patient showed signs of hemodynamic instability.

After operation, patient developed a deep wound infection and after its drainage, he recovered. As a consequence of this, he developed an important incisional hernia. He could not work because of the combination of hernia and colostomy. Six months later, a new operation was proposed; an anastomosis was performed after mobilization of the splenic flexure and the incisional hernia repaired by means of an onlay Marlex® mesh. The patient recovered and returned to work after a period of 3 months after operation.

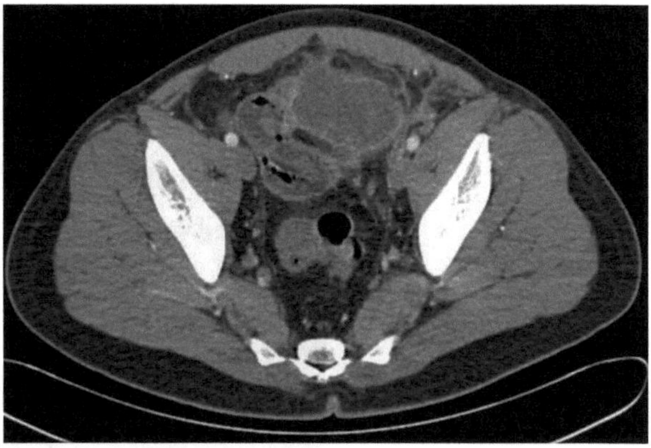

Fig. 70.2 CT scan, leakage with intraabdominal abscesses

Second Patient

A 41-year-old male patient with two recurrences of acute diverticulitis was operated on elsewhere by means of laparoscopic sigmoid resection. Patient was sent to home the 4th postoperative day in good general condition, yet having a temperature of 38 °C. Two days after discharge, he was readmitted because of abdominal pain, fever, and sepsis. On the CT scan, free air was observed with fluid collections in the four abdominal quadrants (Fig. 70.2) Under a diagnosis of general peritonitis, he was reoperated by median upper and lower laparotomy. One-third of anastomosis was found leaking with fecal peritonitis, and the anastomosis was dismantled with creation of a colostomy in the left lower abdomen. Patient was treated by mechanical ventilation for 2 days in the intensive care ward. There he developed a dehiscence of the abdominal wound that led to an open abdomen approach. He developed two intraabdominal abscesses, being drained percutaneously (Fig. 70.3a, b). These abscesses became two intestinal fistulas at the edge of the huge incisional hernia (Fig. 70.4). Referred to our unit, the rectal stump and the rest of colon were assessed by colonoscopy, showing a stump of 15 cm with good patency. The two fistulas were found connected to the terminal ileum and rectal stump (Fig. 70.5). Six months after the discharge from the other hospital patient was again operated. After excision of the split skin used to close the granulation wound and adhesiolysis, the two fistulas were found and treated by a small terminal ileum resection and partial resection of recto-sigmoid stump. After mobilization of splenic flexure an end-to-side anastomosis was performed without tension and good donuts. Thereafter, we used a double Vycril® mesh to repair the huge defect of abdominal wall, in an onlay position.

Surprisingly, the patient recovered very quickly and could go home 10 days after the operation with a supporting corset. Because of the very weak abdominal wall, he requested its repair. He is currently on the waiting list to undergo an components separation technique of the abdominal wall.

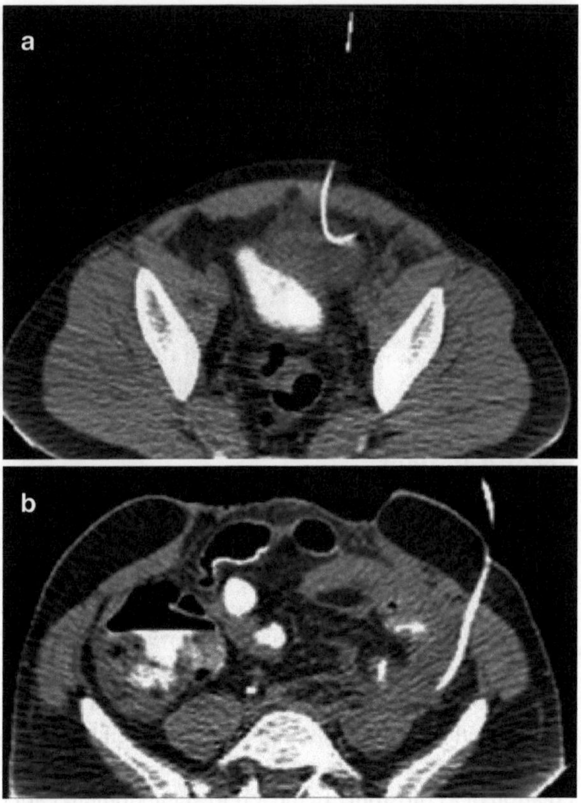

Fig. 70.3 (**a**) CT scan-guided drainage abscess median lower abdomen. (**b**) CT scan-guided drainage abscess left paracolic gutter

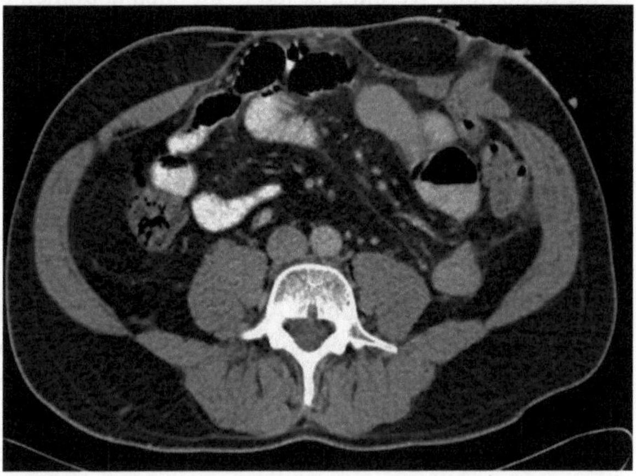

Fig. 70.4 CT scan showing open abdomen and colostomy (Hartmann procedure)

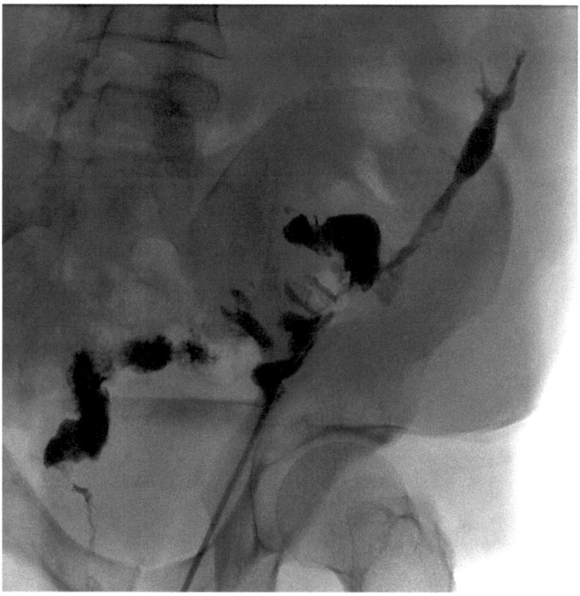

Fig. 70.5 Fistulogram, two tracks terminal ileum and rectal stump

Discussion

The main lesson of these two cases is to be careful using the indication for sigmoid resection in case of diverticulitis. A clear policy warns being more conservative using this indication and also not selecting patients for operation on the basis of the number of episodes of acute diverticulitis. The second lesson is that a proper operative technique should be used, meaning that sigmoid should be divided at the level of promontory distally and at the level of a healthy descending colon-sigmoid proximally. Anastomosis should be performed without any tension; otherwise, splenic flexure should be mobilized. And third, a leakage developing in 5 % of the anastomosis at this level should be treated by dismantling the anastomosis with the temporary creation of a colostomy [1, 2].

References

1. Snijders HS, Wouters MW, van Leersum NJ, et al. Meta-analysis of the risk for anastomotic leakage, the postoperative mortality caused by leakage in relation to the overall postoperative mortality. Eur J Surg Oncol. 2012;38:1013–9.
2. van Leersum NJ, Snijders HS, henneman D, et al. The Dutch Surgical Colorectal Audit. Eur J Surg Oncol. 2013;18. Available online.

Chapter 71
Case on Leakage After LAR and Coloanal Anastomosis

Hugo W. Nijhof and Miguel A. Cuesta

Keywords Rectal cancer • Low anterior resection • Laparoscopy • Leakage anastomosis • Ileostomy

First Patient

Diagnosis and Indication for Surgery

A 68-year-old male with no previous medical history was referred to our outpatient surgical clinic by the gastroenterologist. He had suffered from abdominal pain and change in stools since a few months. Physical examination showed no abnormalities; however, rectal examination revealed a tumor that was palpable at the tip of the finger. A colonoscopy was performed, which revealed a tumor located at the posterior wall of the rectum approximately 8 cm from the anus. The biopsy report showed adenocarcinoma. Further radiological investigation, by means of CT thorax and abdomen, showed no distant metastases and the MRI showed a 5-cm-long tumor, at 9 cm from the anus, being classified as a T2-3N0M0 rectum carcinoma. According with the location of the tumor, he was treated by short radiotherapy scheme of 5×5 Gys with a long interval to operation of 6 weeks. Preoperative colon preparation was done using two enemas and prophylactic antibiotics.

H.W. Nijhof, M.D. (✉)
Department of Surgery, Kennemer Gasthuis, Haarlem, The Netherlands
e-mail: hw.nijhof@kg.nl

M.A. Cuesta, M.D.
Department of Surgery, VU University Medical Center, Amsterdam, The Netherlands
e-mail: ma.cuesta@vumc.nl

M.A. Cuesta, H.J. Bonjer (eds.), *Case Studies of Postoperative Complications after Digestive Surgery*, DOI 10.1007/978-3-319-01613-9_71,

Operation

A laparoscopic low-anterior resection was performed, according to the TME principles after a low tie of the IMA. After mobilization of the sigmoid and descending colon, it was evident that not enough length was available for an adequate distal anastomosis. Therefore, splenic flexure was mobilized before completion of a side-to-end double-stapled anastomosis. There were no tensions at the anastomosis; the donuts were intact and methylene blue test showed no leakage at all. No deviating ileostomy was performed.

Postoperative Course: Identification and Treatment of Complication

The initial postoperative period was uncomplicated. However, 3 days after surgery, the patient complained of abdominal pain. At physical examination there was tenderness in the lower abdominal region. Diuresis was minimal and he had developed a fever of 40 °C. Laboratory tests showed elevated CRP of 280 and Leukocytosis of 18,000 and an additional performed chest X-ray revealed a large amount of abdominal free air (Fig. 71.1). A CT abdomen was performed that showed anastomosis leakage with fluid collections in the whole abdomen and free air (Fig. 71.2).The patient was reoperated, thereby enlarging the earlier performed small Pfannenstiel incision. Free air was present, with initial signs of purulent peritonitis. The anastomosis was identified, which revealed a ventral perforation of 1.5 cm. Policy became to secure the perforation with additional sutures. The abdominal cavity was rinsed and drained using two large-caliber silicon drains. Moreover, a protective loop ileostomy was performed. The further postoperative course was uncomplicated.

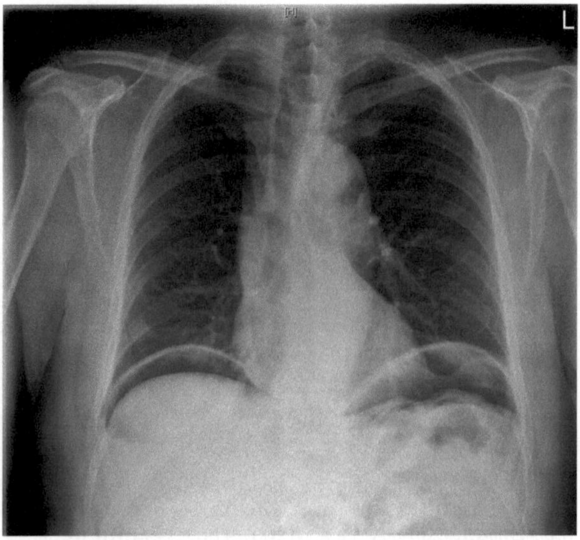

Fig. 71.1 Pneumoperitoneum

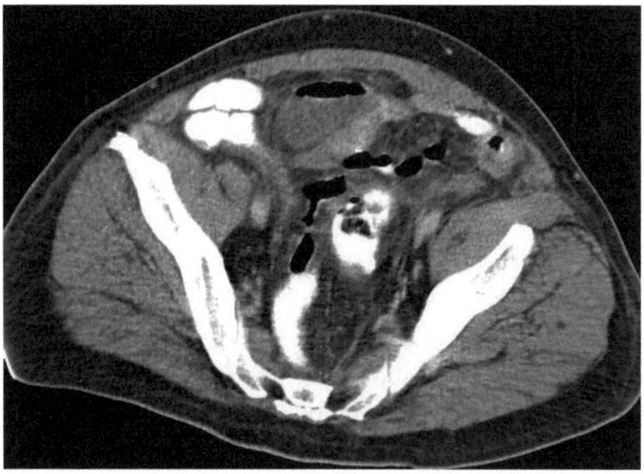

Fig. 71.2 CT scan showing leakage of the end-to-side anastomosis

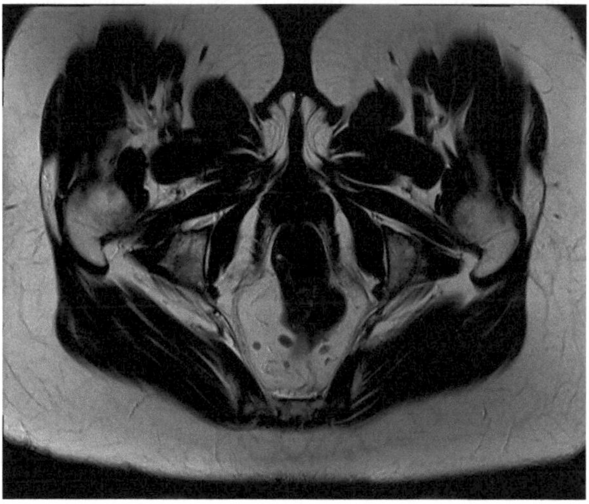

Fig. 71.3 MRI showing a mid rectal T3 rectal tumor

Five months later the loop ileostomy was closed, which happened uneventfully.

Second Patient

Diagnosis and Indication for Surgery

A 60-year-old female patient was diagnosed having distal rectal cancer. She had symptoms of tenesmus and rectal blood loss since 2 months, and the tumor was palpated by rectal examination on the posterior aspect of the rectum, being found as not fixed. Colonoscopy showed no pathology in the rest of colon, and biopsies showed a well-differentiated carcinoma. The tumor was staged as T3N0M0 by CT scan and MRI (Fig. 71.3). Importantly, there was no ingrowth of tumor in the external sphincter or pelvic floor muscles. Vagina wall was also free. As a consequence, the patient was told the chance of performing a sphincter-sparing operation was considered higher than 50 %. She was treated by neoadjuvant radiotherapy and 5 days of 5 Grays; the operation was scheduled 6 weeks later. In meantime, a new MRI and rectal examination showed an important response of the tumor to radiotherapy.

Operation

Mechanical preparation was not given, but prior to operation, two enemas were given: the first the evening before operation and the second early the next morning.

At anesthesia, rectal examination confirmed the possibility of a coloanal anastomosis. A laparoscopic TME dissection was performed with mobilization of the splenic flexure. Distal dissection was performed distal of the pelvic floor, followed by a transanal division of the rectum at 2 cm proximal of the dentate line. Specimen was retrieved transanally, followed by side-to-end anastomosis, manually performed. The presacral space was drained.

Postoperative Course: Identification and Treatment of the Complication

Five days after operation, the patient developed lower abdominal pain and fever. CRP was high and on the CT scan fluid was seen in the peritoneal cavity with huge amounts of free air (Fig. 71.4). With the diagnosis of leakage of anastomosis, her reoperation was performed through an enlarged Pfannenstiel incision. Small leakage was seen by injection of methylene blue through rectum at the left aspect of the anastomosis. Abdomen was rinsed and drained, then followed by creation of a loop ileostomy.

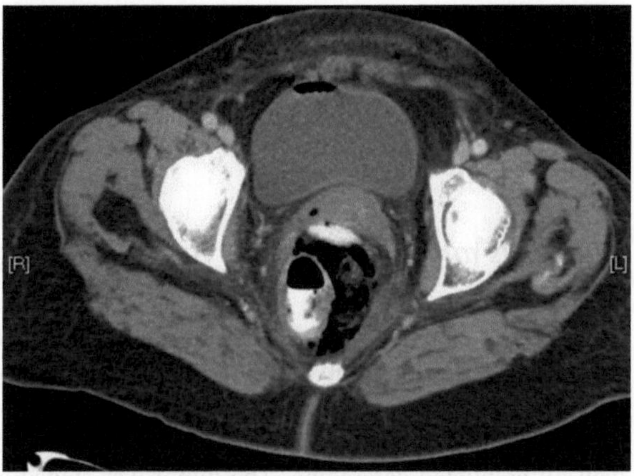

Fig. 71.4 CT scan showing leakage anastomosis after LAR

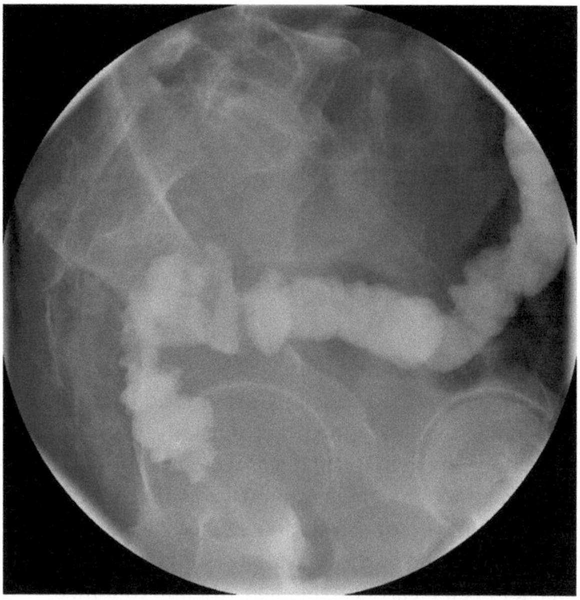

Fig. 71.5 Colon enema, good patent, and no leakage or sinus

Patient recovered and could go home after 10 days. After 3 months, anastomosis was patent with no leakage (Fig. 71.5) and the ileostomy was closed. Patient retained a good continence and cancer controls still show good results.

Third Patient

Diagnosis and Indication for Surgery

A 57-year-old entrepreneur was operated on after a short-scheme radiotherapy, 5×5 Grays by an open TME, followed by a coloanal anastomosis, manually transanally performed and a deviating loop ileostomy. Tumor was staged as pT2N0 by pathological study.

Postoperative Course and Identification of Complication

At the sixth postoperative day, patient was diagnosed as having a dehiscence of anastomosis with signs of general peritonitis confirmed by CT scan.

At relaparotomy purulent peritonitis was found, as caused by leakage of one-third of the anastomosis. Patient was hemodynamically stable and wished to preserve the sphincter-saving anastomosis. At laparotomy, after mobilization of splenic flexure, a transanally pull-through was performed after rinsing of the abdomen and drainage. Patient recovered after 2 days on the Intensive Care department. At the eighth postoperative day while under anesthesia, the prolapsed colon was resected leaving a small stump of 2 cm at the dentate line. This has healed without stenosis and acceptable defecation was possible after closure of ileostomy. At 4 years after operation, patient is still happy with this solution.

Discussion

Unfortunately, anastomotic leakages are inevitable in colorectal surgery, even though they are performed by experienced surgeons. The incidence rises when the anastomosis is performed more distally, with the highest rates of 10–20 % after operations in the mid and distal rectum, followed by distal anastomosis [1].

An extraperitoneal anastomosis, as performed in the above-mentioned cases, is therefore at risk for anastomotic dehiscence and leakage. Risk factors are the perfusion and tension of the anastomosis, male gender, and neoadjuvant radiotherapy. It has not been clearly established when to mobilize "a priory" the splenic flexure. It is our experience to commence with this in the case of planned anterior resection with small sigmoid loop and always in the case of LAR and coloanal anastomosis. Subject of debate concerns the creation of protective ileostomy after these operations, but an indication to do so is quite liberal and it is left up to the surgeon. The majority of surgeons are creating a protective ileostomy in those cases. Moreover, the definition and grade of anastomotic leakage following anterior resection of the rectum has been defined by the International Study Group of Rectal Cancer [2, 4]. Anastomosis leakage has been defined as a defect of the intestinal wall at the level of anastomosis leading to a communication between the intra- and extraluminal compartments. A pelvic abscess close to anastomosis is also considered anastomotic leakage. There are three categories (a to c) including the treatment adopted: (a) requiring no active therapeutic intervention; (b) requiring intervention, but manageable without relaparotomy; and (c) requiring relaparotomy. Clinically, if patient is getting worse, a CT scan with transanal and iv contrast will show fluid (or gas) collections as signs of leakage, even with or without contrast extravasation, as was the case in the first patient [3, 4]. Management strategies of leakage are diverse [3, 4]. If the leakage is subclinical, or if small abscesses are present (type a), conservative management with antibiotics and bowel rest can be performed. Contained leakage with large abscess mostly located in the presacral area must be drained transanally through anastomosis or percutaneously. The best is through anastomosis with creation of an ileostomy, if not done during the first operation. If drainage is done percutaneously, this can lead to a fistula to the perineum, with difficult treatment. Drainage through laparotomy is the last option. In case of general peritonitis, relaparotomy should be done. Management of a dehiscent anastomosis depends on the size of the defect and the contamination of the abdominal cavity. Small defects usually can be salvaged by an additional suture and/or protective loop ileostomy and adequate local drainage. Larger defects, or extensive fecal contamination, in a hemodynamically unstable patient mostly require dismantling of the anastomosis and creation of a permanent colostomy. The solution for the third case remains exciting [5, 6].

References

1. Komen N, Slieker J, de Kort P, et al. High tie versus low tie in rectal surgery: comparison of anastomotic perfusion. Int J Colorectal Dis. 2011;26:1075–8.
2. Rahbari NN, Weitz J, Hohenberger W, et al. Definition and grading of anastomotic leakage following anterior resection of the rectum: A proposal by the International Study Group of Rectal Cancer. Surgery. 2010;147:339–51.
3. Breukink SO, Pierie JPEN, Grond AJK, et al. Laparoscopic versus open total mesorectal excision: a case control study. Int J Colorectal Dis. 2005;20:428–33.
4. Phitayakorn R, Delaney CP, Reynolds HL, International Anastomotic Leak Study Group, et al. Standardized algorithms for management of anastomotic leaks and related abdominal and pelvic abscesses after colorectal surgery. World J Surg. 2008;32:1147–52.
5. Veenhof AAFA, van der Peet DL, Sietses C, Cuesta MA. Pull-through procedure as treatment for coloanal anastomotic dehiscence following TME. Dis Colon Rectum. 2007;50:1271–4.
6. Snijders HS, Wouters MW, van Leersum NJ, et al. Meta-analysis of the risk for anastomotic leakage, the postoperative mortality caused by leakage in relation to the overall postoperative mortality. Eur J Surg Oncol. 2012;38:1013–9.

Chapter 72
Case on Presacral Abscess and Sinuses After LAR

Alexander A.F.A. Veenhof

Keywords Sarcoma pelvis • Rectal cancer • Leakage anastomosis • Low anterior resection • Presacral abscess

First Patient

Diagnosis and Indication for Surgery

Presacral abscess following LAR because of sarcoma in the lower pelvis.

A 60-year-old female patient presented with anemia and lower abdominal pain. Colonoscopy and gastroscopy were normal. Double balloon endoscopy (DBE) showed an ulcerating tumor 120 cm past the ligament of Treitz. Biopsies could not prove malignancy or infection. An additional CT scan of the abdomen showed a large tumor in the lower pelvis (Fig. 72.1). Differential diagnosis was established between GIST tumor, gynecological tumor, and sarcoma.

Operation

In January 2011, an en bloc resection of the tumor, both ovaries, a loop of 20 cm jejunum, and low anterior resection (LAR) were performed. Continuity was restored by a jejunojejunostomy and an end-to-side colorectal stapled anastomosis. This last anastomosis was protected by a loop ileostomy.

A.A.F.A. Veenhof, M.D.
Department of Surgery, VU University Medical Centre, Amsterdam, The Netherlands
e-mail: a.veenhof@vumc.nl

M.A. Cuesta, H.J. Bonjer (eds.), *Case Studies of Postoperative Complications after Digestive Surgery*, DOI 10.1007/978-3-319-01613-9_72,

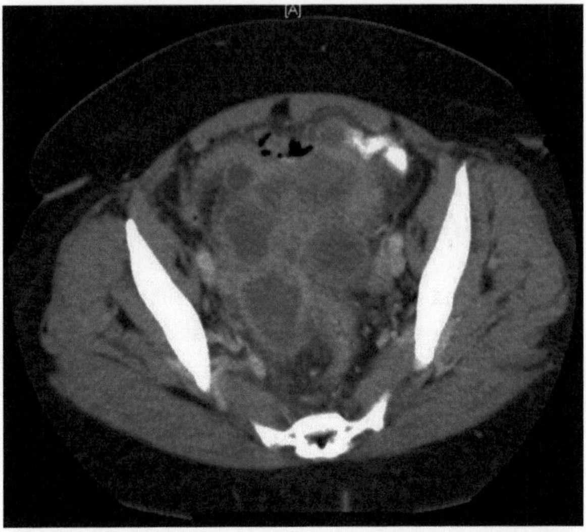

Fig. 72.1 CT scan showing a rectosigmoid sarcoma in the pelvis

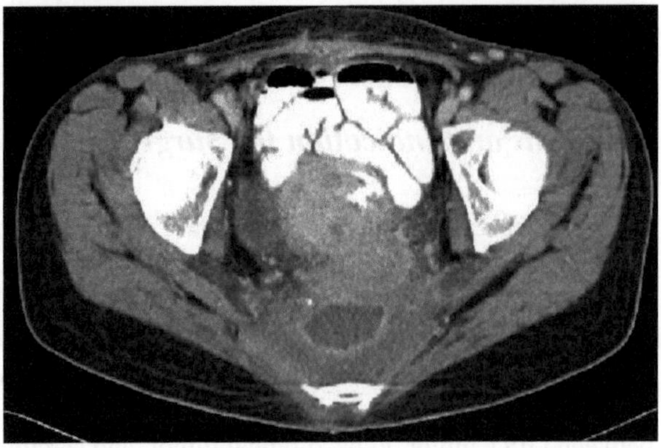

Fig. 72.2 CT scan, presacral abscess

Postoperative Course: Identification and Treatment of Complication

One week postoperatively, the patient developed fever and abdominal pain. A CT scan of the abdomen showed a presacral abscess of 6 cm without clear signs of anastomotic leakage (Fig. 72.2). Under anesthesia the abscess was transrectal drained through the anastomosis. Following the latter intervention, no complications were observed.

The pathology result showed a radically removed sarcoma and 17 lymph nodes without metastases. After control of anastomosis by enema, ileostomy was reversed 6 months later. Patient is doing well.

Second Patient

Diagnosis and Indication for Surgery

A 48-year-old male patient was diagnosed having a T2 N0 M0 adenocarcinoma at 12 cm of anal verge. He had blood loss in the stools since 3 months.

Operation

Patient was proposed to have a LAR after a mechanical colon preparation. The operation was conventionally performed without protecting ileostomy. Anastomosis was created in an end-to-side fashion at the level of the pelvic floor.

Postoperative Course: Identification and Treatment of Complication

On the seventh postoperative day the patient's health became worse, and he was reoperated on because of a suspicion of leakage. At the relaparotomy, a leakage of anastomosis was found with a huge abscess around the anastomosis (Fig. 72.3). The abdomen was rinsed, drained, and a double colostomy was done in sigmoid colon. After stabilization patient was referred to us with the question if a restoration of continuity was possible. At proctoscopy (Fig. 72.4a, b) it became clear that a presacral abscess was still present with pus discharge and consequently treated by an VAC Endo-sponge. Pus discharge disappeared and

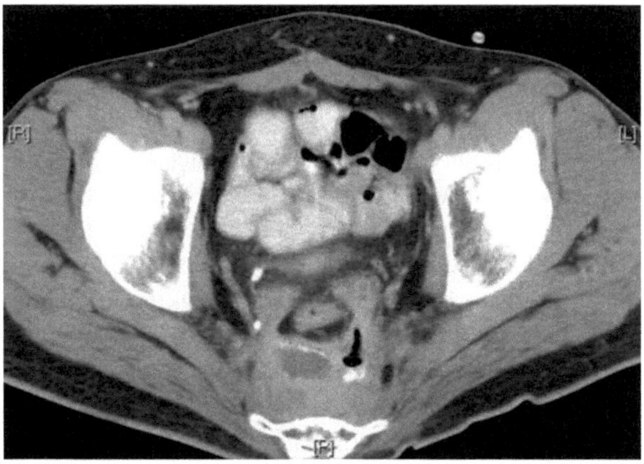

Fig. 72.3 MRI, T2 N0 rectal cancer

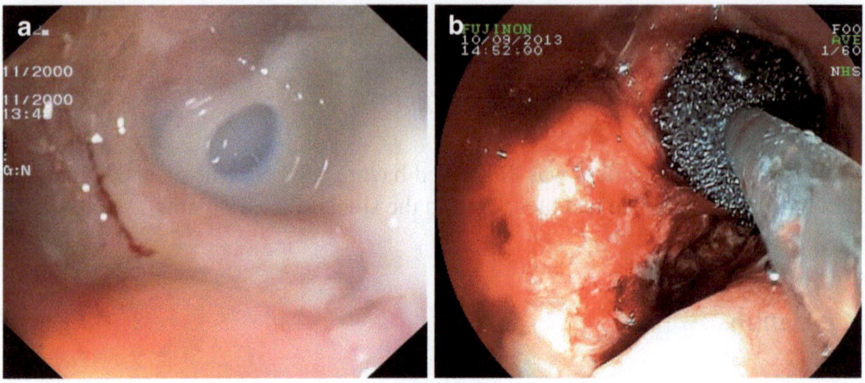

Fig. 72.4 (**a, b**) Proctoscopy showing leakage of the anastomosis with abscess and treatment with Endo-sponge

we proposed a waiting period of 6 months, after which the sinus still persisted but now without pus discharge. Under diagnosis of chronic presacral sinus, we decided to restore the continuity by taking down the colostomy. Initially, the patient had complaints of tenesmus and some fever, but finally he recovered. His defecation remains irregular but continent.

Discussion

Few articles are available regarding the approach of the presacral abscesses following LAR. Total mesorectal excision after neoadjuvant radiotherapy or chemoradiotherapy remains the first choice of treatment with a low local recurrence rate (<5 %) and the high 5-year survival rate (80 %) in patients with mid- and low-rectal cancer [1, 2]. In 2006, van der Vaart reported higher incidences of presacral abscesses following the onset of neoadjuvant therapy [3]. The incidence following total mesorectal excision is believed to be approximately 10 % [4]. No real evidence exists on whether the presacral abscess develops following an infected presacral hematoma, or an anastomotic leakage, or following both. Higher incidences of presacral abscesses have been found in patients receiving neoadjuvant therapy, patients in poor condition, and patients with large tumors [4]. In our experience, the presacral abscess is best managed by drainage through the anastomosis following LAR or through the perineal suture line following abdominoperineal resection. The need for a concomitant diverting colo-/ileostomy is subject to debate. No evidence exists to support any decision making. If on pre-drainage CT scan with rectal and oral contrast no anastomotic leak can be objectified, then diversion stoma may be unnecessary. In this case, an abscess is most likely based on an infected presacral hematoma. However, if anastomotic leakage is observed, then diversion stoma should be done after drainage of the abscess. The VAC Endo-sponge has been

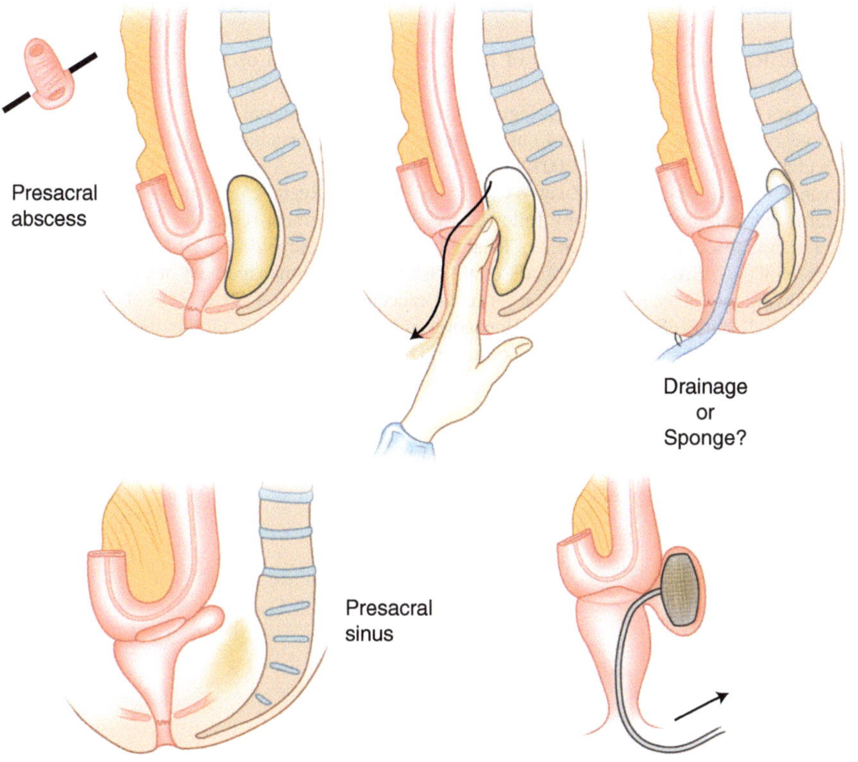

Illustration 72.1 No evidence exists to support any decision making concerning the treatment of presacral abscess. If on CT scan with rectal and oral contrast no anastomotic leak can be objectified, then diversion stoma may be unnecessary. In this case, an abscess is most likely based on an infected presacral hematoma. However, if anastomotic leakage is observed, then diversion stoma should be done after drainage of the abscess. The VAC Endo-sponge has been introduced in the last years in patients with a content distal rectal anastomosis leakage in order to create an optimal suction system leading to a quick closure without presacral sinus

introduced in the last years for patients having a content distal rectal anastomosis leakage in order to create an optimal suction system leading to a quick closure without presacral sinus (Illustration 72.1). In spite of favorable initial rapports, more evidence is necessary before further implementation [5].

The final question concerns, What to do with a chronic presacral sinus, like in case number 2? If we close the ileostomy/colostomy, will the abscess recur?

If the presacral sinus is huge and deep, probably the best policy will be to reconvert the LAR in a coloanal anastomosis or a pull-through procedure with omentum or muscle plasty in the presacral space. In the case of a small chronic sinus, probably reversal of ileostomy/colostomy will be enough.

References

1. Heald RJ, Karanjia ND. Results of radical surgery for rectal cancer. World J Surg. 1992; 16:848–57.
2. Peeters KCMJ, Marijnen CAM, Nagtegaal ID, et al. The TME trial after a median follow-up of 6 years. Increased local control but no survival benefit in irradiated patients with resectable rectal carcinoma. Ann Surg. 2007;246:693–701.
3. van der Vaart MG, van der Zwet WC, Arends JW, et al. Rectal carcinoma treated with short-term preoperative radiotherapy followed by abdominoperineal resection. Significantly more presacral abscesses with absence of local recurrence. Dig Surg. 2006;23:173–7.
4. Veenhof AA, Brosens R, Engel AF, et al. Risk factors and management of presacral abscess following total mesorectal excision for rectal cancer. Dig Surg. 2009;26:317–21.
5. Verlaan T, Bartels SAL, van Berge Henegouwen MI, et al. Early, minimally invasive closure of anastomotic leaks: a new concept. Colorectal Dis. 2011;13:18–22.

Chapter 73
Case on Stenosis After Low Anterior Resection

Miguel A. Cuesta and Hugo W. Nijhof

Keywords Low anterior resection • Stenosis anastomosis • Endoscopic dilatation

First Patient

Diagnosis and Indication for Surgery

A 74-year-old female patient presented to our surgical outpatient clinic. Her prior history stated an abdominal hysterectomy because of benign disease. Several times previously she had been admitted with abdominal pain, situated in the left lower quadrant. Earlier assessment had already revealed diverticular disease of the sigmoid for which conservative management had always been successful. Nonetheless, due to repeated complaints and repetitive hospital admittance, a definite therapy by means of sigmoid resection was agreed upon.

Operation

A laparoscopic sigmoid resection was initially intended; however, due to massive adhesions a conversion to a classic sigmoidectomy by laparotomy was performed.

M.A. Cuesta, M.D. (✉)
Department of Surgery, VU University Medical Center, Amsterdam, The Netherlands
e-mail: ma.cuesta@vumc.nl

H.W. Nijhof, M.D.
Department of Surgery, Kennemer Gasthuis, Haarlem, The Netherlands
e-mail: hw.nijhof@kg.nl

M.A. Cuesta, H.J. Bonjer (eds.), *Case Studies of Postoperative Complications after Digestive Surgery*, DOI 10.1007/978-3-319-01613-9_73,

The affected segment could be removed and enough length was obtained for creating a tension-free side-to-end anastomosis.

Postoperative Course: Identification and Treatment of Complication

The postoperative recovery was in the beginning uneventful. However, after 7 days the patient developed a fever and increased infection parameters, as revealed in her laboratory results. A CT scan of the abdomen was performed that showed fluid and gas collection, suggestive of anastomotic leakage. A relaparotomy was performed that revealed an anastomotic leakage. Because of the large anastomotic defect as well as abdominal fecal contamination, anastomosis was dismantled and definite colostomy was performed. Further clinical admission occurred without complications, and the patient could be discharged 2 weeks later. Six months after her last surgery, restoration of bowel continuity was decided on, especially so since she expressed complaints, which were caused by a large parastomal hernia. Surgery was performed in a standard fashion in which the bowel continuity was restored by means of a circular stapling device. Further hospital admittance was uneventful and during initial follow-ups the patient's condition steadily improved.

Four months later, she presented to our emergency ward with an acute onset of abdominal pain, preceded by cramps for some time. She was admitted and on CT scan of the abdomen with rectal contrast, a stenosis at the anastomotic site with fecal impaction was observed (Fig. 73.1). She was treated with laxatives

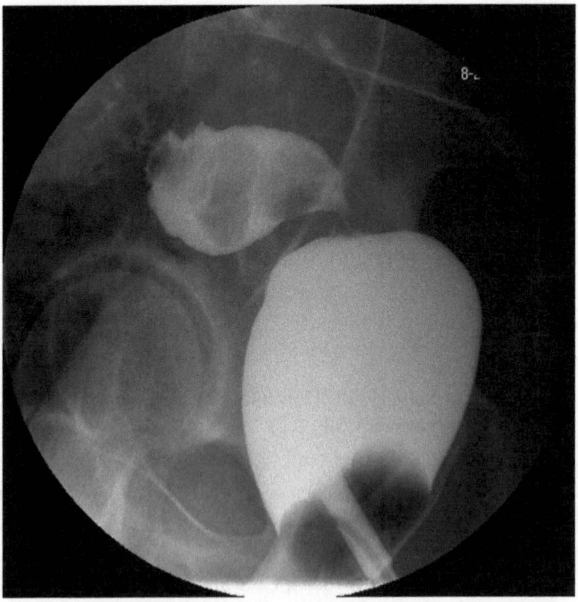

Fig. 73.1 Enema showing stenosis of anastomosis after anterior resection

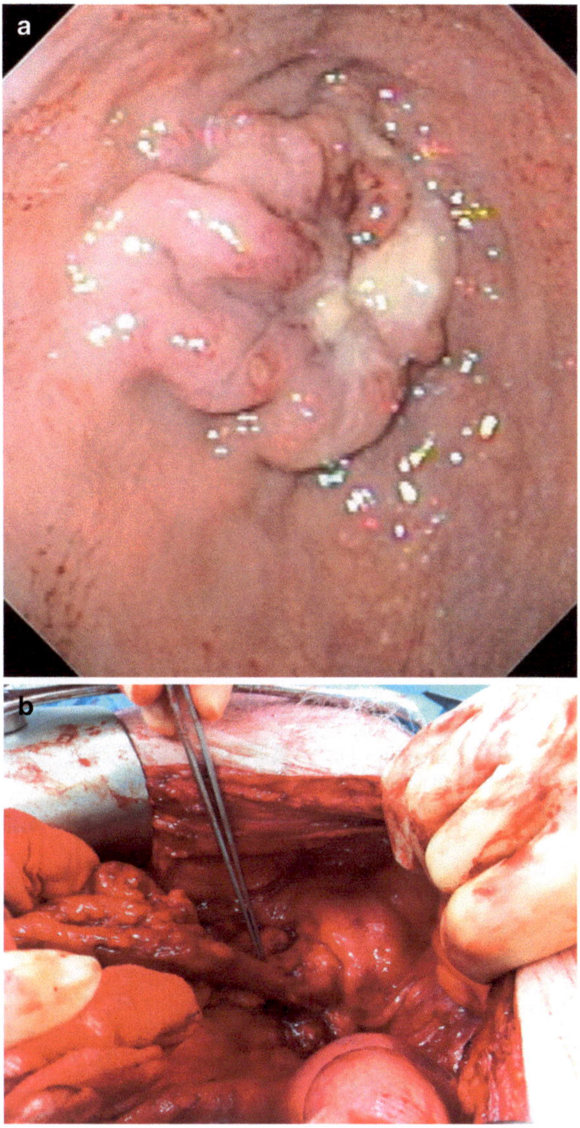

Fig. 73.2 (**a**) Stenosis of the anastomosis by colonoscopy. (**b**) At reoperation, stenotic segment will be resected

after which normal defecation was restored. At colonoscopy, the stenosis was treated by sequential endoscopic dilations (Fig. 73.2a). During follow-up the stenosis remained and complaints persisted. Finally, it was decided to perform a re-anastomosis.

Surgery took place in a standard fashion, and the earlier performed anastomosis was resected (Fig. 73.2b). A side-to-end circular stapled anastomosis was performed combined with a protective loop ileostomy. Her recovery was quick and further hospital stay uneventful. The pathology report showed no signs of

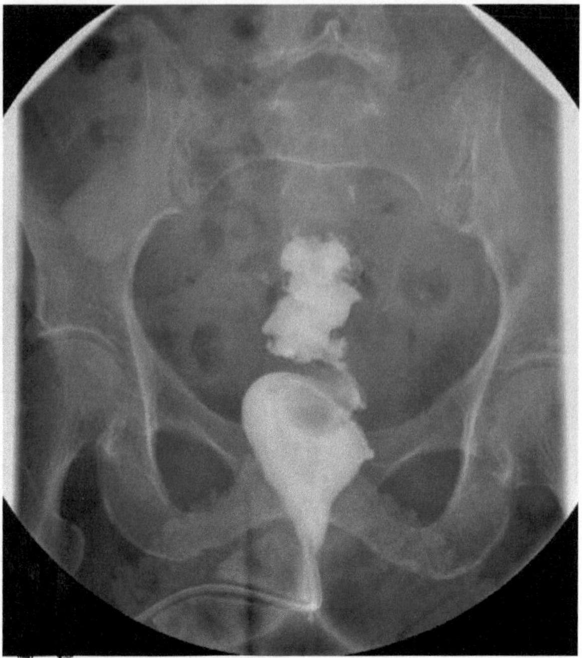

Fig. 73.3 Enema showing re-stenosis anastomosis

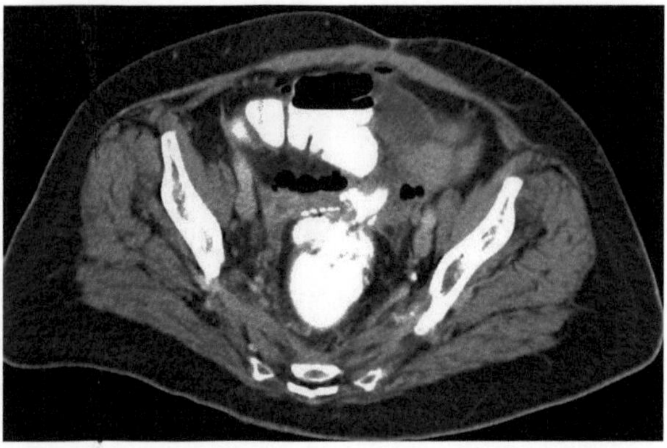

Fig. 73.4 CT scan showing leakage at the place of stenosed anastomosis

malignancy. Unfortunately, after a few months the original complaints returned. A colonic X-ray with rectal contrast was performed. This showed a stenotic anastomosis, necessitating repetitive endoscopic dilations again (Fig. 73.3). The last endoscopic dilation had caused a small perforation, for which she was readmitted. A CT abdomen revealed a covered perforation, which could be managed conservatively (Fig. 73.4).We then finally decided to perform a definite colostomy and closure of the loop ileostomy, after which the patient was without complaints.

Second Patient

Diagnosis and Indication for Surgery

A 32-year-old secretary could not work for long periods because of endometriosis complaints. Eventually, she was diagnosed having stenosis of the proximal rectum with the endometriosis at the level of the recto-vaginal septum (Fig. 73.5). Hormonal activity was blocked by Lukrin® but patient had defecation complaints and a desire to have children.

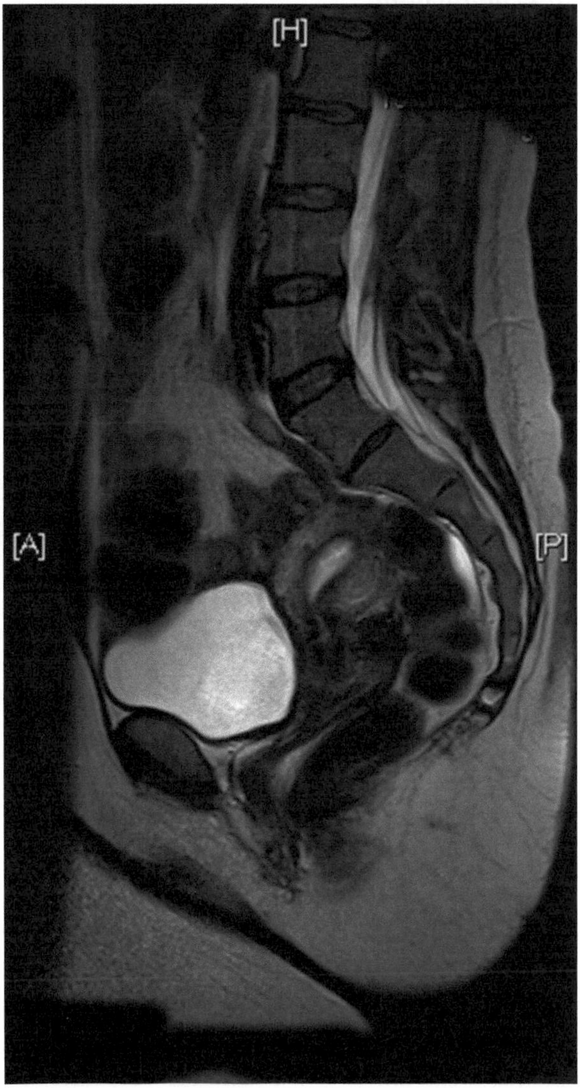

Fig. 73.5 MRI, recto-vaginal endometriosis

Operation

Therefore, a laparoscopic operation was performed elsewhere, in which a partial rectal resection had been performed along with a small resection of vaginal wall. The vaginal wall was closed and rectal continuity was done by circular stapled anastomosis.

Postoperative Course: Identification and Treatment of Complication

Patient developed a recto-vaginal fistula and had to be treated by a loop ileostomy. After referral, 6 months later a relaparotomy was performed, dissection of rectum distal of the fistula was done, the vaginal wall closed, and an end-to-side anastomosis with omentum interposition performed. After 3 months following a control by rectal and vaginal examination, the loop ileostomy was closed. During the postoperative period, the patient complained of thin defecation with constipation. Referred to gastroenterologist for proctoscopy, he scheduled a dilatation program after finding stenosis of anastomosis (Figs. 73.6 and 73.7). After three dilatations to 1.5 cm patient was again referred to us because

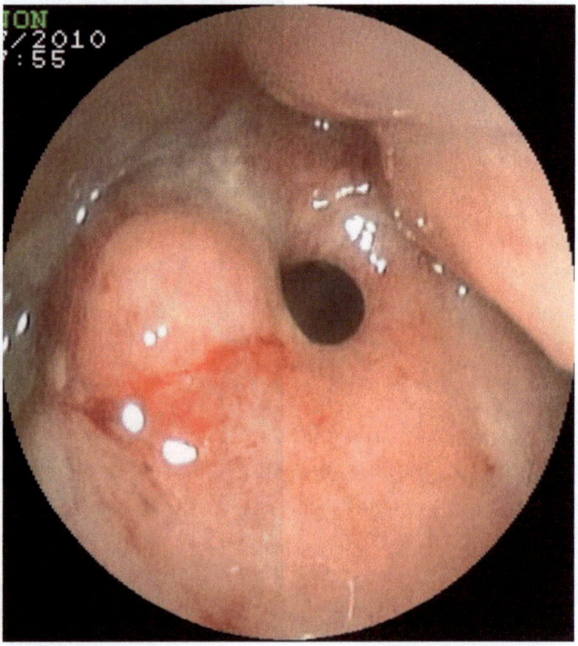

Fig. 73.6 Stenosis by colonoscopy of the anastomosis after LAR

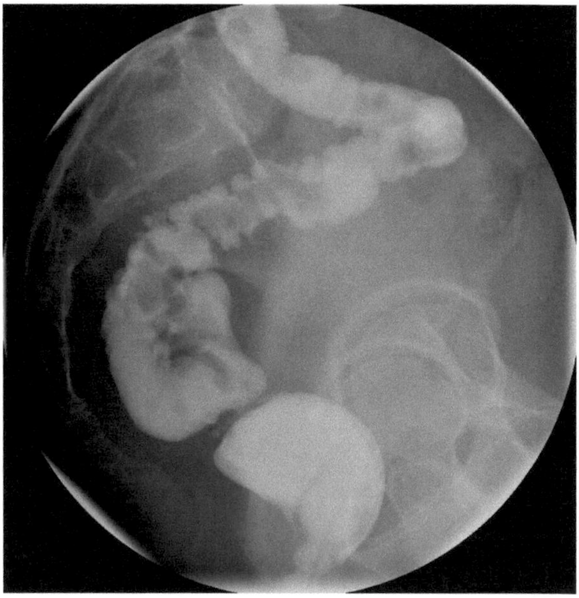

Fig. 73.7 Enema showing the distal stenosis

dilatation was not possible due to fibrotic ring. At rectal examination, stenosed anastomosis was palpated at 4 cm from the anus and we proposed to perform digital or by Hegar's dilatation under anesthesia. Under anesthesia, the stenosis could be dilated until an optimal size was gained without problems. Control of anastomosis at 3 months remains patent.

Discussion

Anastomotic stenosis after colorectal resection occurs in up to 30 % of patients; however, only 4–10 % of these are symptomatic [1,2]. Risk factors are male gender and the use of a stapling device, which is nowadays used for most patients [3]. However, the majority of them do not need any intervention, and for those who do, such can usually be managed by means of endoscopic dilatation. Success rates vary, but are usually in the range of 88–100 % for benign strictures [2,4,5]. Complications after endoscopic dilatation can be re-stenosis (11 %) and local perforation (5 %), which both occurred in the first case. If the patient is refractory to repeated endoscopic dilatation, resection of the affected anastomosis is usually the next step (Illustration 73.1). A permanent colostomy, as was the case of the first patient, is rarely necessary, though. Moreover, if stenosis is palpable by digital examination, doing digital dilatations under anesthesia qualifies as a good and effective treatment.

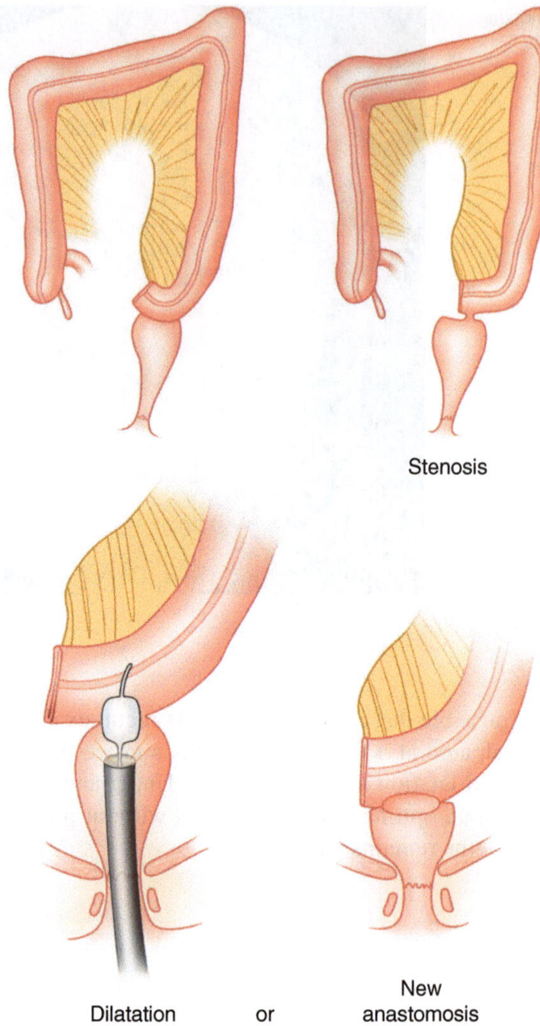

Illustration 73.1 Symptomatic stenosis of an anastomosis after LAR should be treated by endoscopic dilatations. If not successful, resection of the anastomosis should be done. If stenosis is palpable by digital examination, digital dilatation under anesthesia is a good and effective treatment

References

1. Schlegel RD, Dehni N, Parc R, et al. Results of reoperations in colorectal anastomotic strictures. Dis Colon Rectum. 2001;44:1464.
2. Bannura GC, Cumsille MA, Barrera AE, et al. Predictive factors of stenosis after stapled colorectal anastomosis: prospective analysis of 179 consecutive patients. World J Surg. 2004;28:921.
3. Matos D, Atallah ÁN, Castro AA, Silva Lustosa SA. Stapled versus handsewn methods for colorectal anastomosis surgery. Cochrane Database Syst Rev. 2008;2:CD003144.

4. Suchan KL, Muldner A, Manegold BC. Endoscopic treatment of postoperative colorectal anastomotic strictures. Surg Endosc. 2003;17:1110–7.
5. Ambrosetti P, Francis K, De Peyer R, Frossard JL. Colorectal anastomotic stenosis after elective laparoscopic sigmoidectomy for diverticular disease: a prospective evaluation of 68 patients. Dis Colon Rectum. 2008;51:1345–9.

Chapter 74
Case on Problems After Coloanal Anastomosis (Stenosis Coloanal Anastomosis and Frequent Stools and Soiling)

Miguel A. Cuesta

Keywords Rectal cancer • Coloanal anastomosis • Stenosis anastomosis • Difficult defecation • Incontinence

First Patient

Diagnosis and Indication for Surgery

A 62-year-old man was diagnosed of distal rectum cancer because of complaints of tenesmus and blood in feces. A tumor was located very low, at 4 cm of the anal canal and staged as T3-T4, N1 M0 by CT scan and MRI. The MRI revealed that the tumor was not growing into the pelvic floor or in the external sphincter (Fig. 74.1). Chemoradiation was proposed as neoadjuvant therapy followed by surgery 6 weeks later. After chemoradiation, clinically and on MRI, it became clear that the tumor showed a good regression grade.

Operation

An open TME resection was performed, the splenic flexure mobilized, and an end-to-side anastomosis transanally performed (Fig. 74.2). A deviation ileostomy was created during the same operation.

M.A. Cuesta, M.D.
Department of Surgery, VU University Medical Center, Amsterdam, The Netherlands
e-mail: ma.cuesta@vumc.nl

M.A. Cuesta, H.J. Bonjer (eds.), *Case Studies of Postoperative Complications after Digestive Surgery*, DOI 10.1007/978-3-319-01613-9_74,

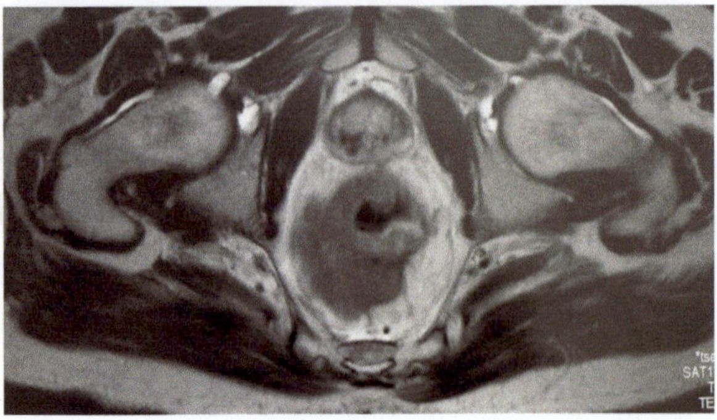

Fig. 74.1 MRI, distal rectal cancer T3

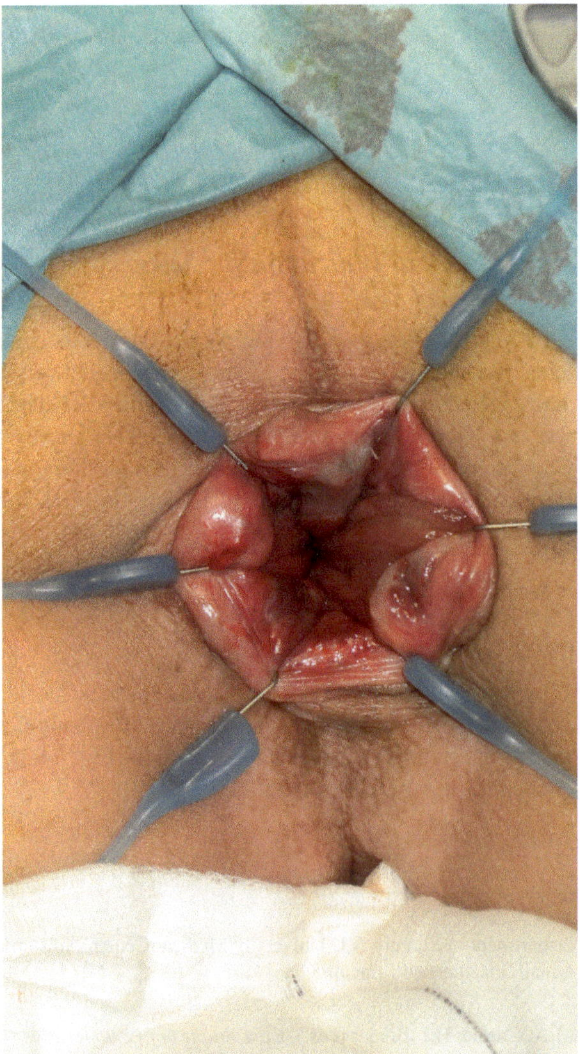

Fig. 74.2 At operation, coloanal anastomosis

Postoperative Course: Identification and Treatment of the Complication

Patient did well and went home after 10 days. At the outpatient policlinic, it became clear from the beginning that the anastomosis was importantly stenosed (Fig. 74.3); consequently, attempts were made to dilate it under anesthesia. Because of the difficulties to dilate it with Hegar's dilators, a decision was taken to introduce a guide wire and use the Savary's dilatators, followed by manual dilations by means of the finger (Illustration 74.1). The dilatation program took several weeks during which biopsies were taken to rule out a recurrence of cancer. Finally, anastomosis was considered open by rectal examination and proposed to close the ileostomy. After 5 months we could take down the ileostomy. Currently, the patient is doing fine, despite some soiling, but still very happy that a definitive colostomy was not necessary. He also is visiting the urologist regularly for treatment of a mild impotency.

Second Patient

Diagnosis and Indication for Surgery

A 63-year-old female patient was diagnosed with having a distal adenocarcinoma of the rectum. She suffered from claustrophobia and so it was very difficult to convince

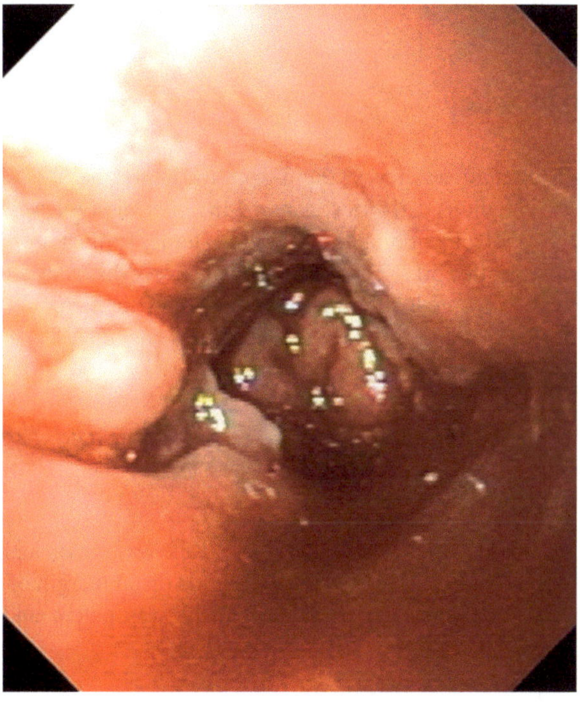

Fig. 74.3 Proctoscopy showing the stenosis of a coloanal anastomosis

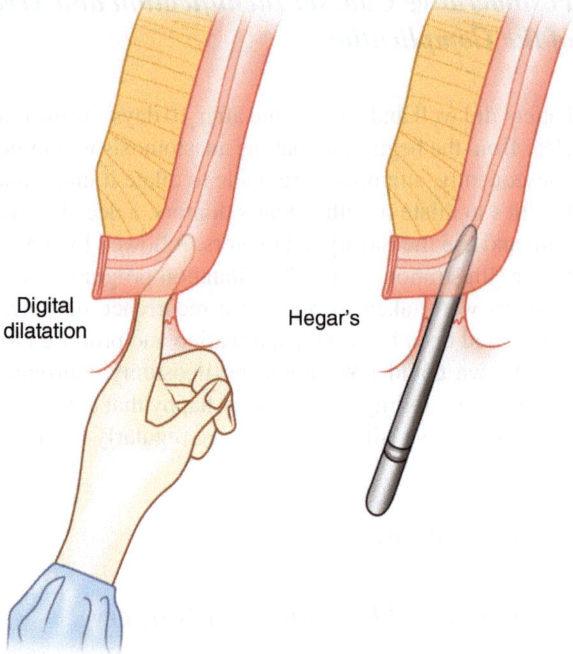

Illustration 74.1 Stenosis of a coloanal anastomosis should be dilated by means of digital dilatations or Hegar's dilators. If digital dilatations are not possible, Savary's should be used. In a patient with soiling and frequent defecation after coloanal anastomosis, lavage procedure should be advised

her to undergo all studies and posteriorly to administer the neoadjuvant therapy in the form of 5×5 Grays followed by intervention 6 weeks later. She had a younger partner and wished to undergo an operation without definitive stoma.

Operation

The tumor was low, 3.5 cm from the anal canal, but she had good sphincters after two previous deliveries. A new MRI after radiotherapy showed again that there was no involvement of a tumor in the external sphincter or pelvic floor. Patient was told that she had 50 % chance for getting a very distal anastomosis. A laparoscopic TME was performed, after mobilization of splenic flexure followed by a coloanal anastomosis. An ileostomy for deviation was created.

Postoperative Course: Identification and Treatment of the Complication

The patient did well, recovered, and she was put on a physiotherapy program for the pelvic floor. Pathology showed a good distal margin of 1.5 cm and a CRM of 4 mm. Three months later, the anastomosis was patent and the ileostomy was closed.

Thereafter, a difficult period for the patient took place, not due to incontinence but caused by difficult defecation in spite of laxatives. Defecation was either interrupted or diarrhea and we discussed with her the possibility of creating a colostomy. A lavage of the neorectum was proposed and contrary to what we expected, the patient is very happy with this therapy. All controls of cancer are good.

Discussion

These two cases illustrate certain difficulties surrounding a coloanal anastomosis. Important is to remark, that being this operation far from ideal,it is for many patients a better solution than a APR. But is an operation with technical problems and functional difficulties. Starting with the radiotherapy, radiotherapists will radiate not only the intra-abdominal rectum but also the perineum. It is a difficult issue, but my conjecture is that a radiated perineum will develop fibrosis and stenosis. Second, an optimally vascularized descending colon is the most optimal segment of colon for an anastomosis in an end-to-side fashion, protected by an ileostomy. The development of a presacral abscess can invalidate the advantages of a coloanal anastomosis; thus, a good drainage of the space is important. Third, it is important to avoid the development of stenosis, by carrying out rectal examination control. Moreover, pelvic floor physiotherapy and fiber intake are important for an optimal defecation.

In my opinion, the second case shows the functional difficulties female patients have with coloanal anastomosis. Incontinence and disturbed defecation are the most known problems. No definitive study about this point is available. Lavage of the neorectum may be a good therapy for a patient with these problems.

Chapter 75
Case on Ureter Lesion During Laparoscopic Low Anterior Resection

Miguel A. Cuesta

Keywords Rectal cancer • Ureter lesion • Ureter stent • Ureterography • Nephrectomy

First Patient

Diagnosis and Indication for Surgery

A 52-year-old healthy man was diagnosed having a high rectal cancer, staged as T3N0M0, and was proposed to undergo a laparoscopic proximal mesorectal excision.

Operation: Identification and Treatment of Complication

During this operation—while dissecting from medial to lateral—the surgeon made a perforation of the left ureter resulting in some leakage of urine. Urologist was called for a cystoscopy and double J-stent. While waiting for the urologist, the intervention was continued by dividing the inferior mesenteric vessels and by dividing the rectum at the proper level by means of endostapler. The urologist went on to perform the cystoscopy and introduced a guide wire through the left ureteral orifice. Using the guide wire, a double J-stent was introduced under laparoscopic vision (Illustration 75.1). The stent went proximal without problems. The colorectal

M.A. Cuesta, M.D.
Department of Surgery, VU University Medical Center, Amsterdam, The Netherlands
e-mail: ma.cuesta@vumc.nl

M.A. Cuesta, H.J. Bonjer (eds.), *Case Studies of Postoperative Complications after Digestive Surgery*, DOI 10.1007/978-3-319-01613-9_75,

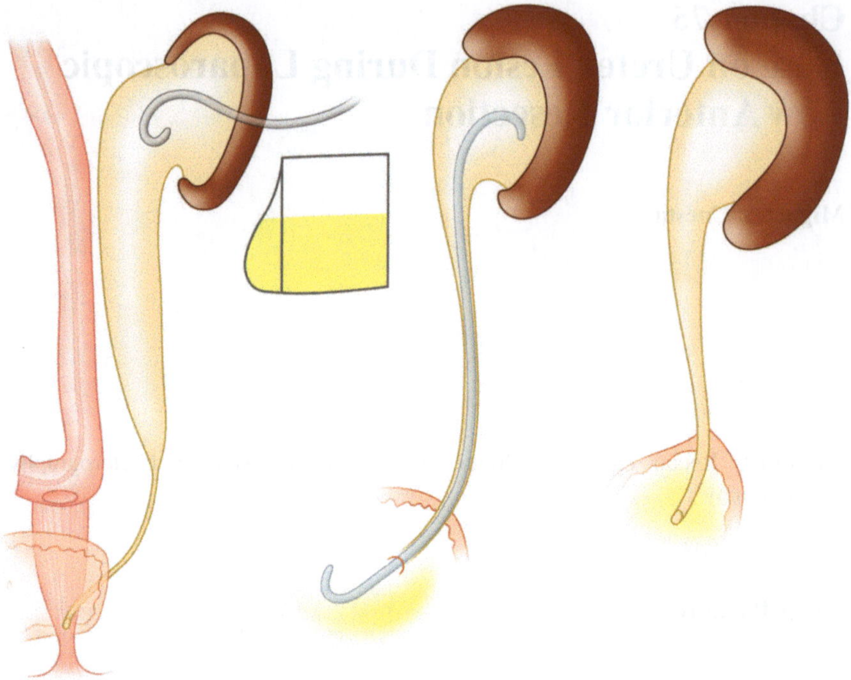

Illustration 75.1 Ureter lesion discovered during the operation should be solved together with the urologist during the operation. Lesions diagnosed in a late period should be treated together with the urologist. Treatment includes from double J-stent and dilatation to percutaneous nephrostomy and eventually nephrectomy

surgeon closed the small ureteral defect by means of two reabsorbable 4.0 stitches. After anastomosis, a drain was left in the pelvis.

Postoperative Course

The postoperative period went without problems, and the patient could be discharged on the 7th postoperative day. At the 4th postoperative week, an ultrasonography of the kidneys showed no dilatation of the left system, and at the 6th week, the J-stent was retired through cystoscopy. After a period of 2 years, neither dilatation of the ureter nor distance metastases have been observed.

Second Patient

Diagnosis and Indication for Surgery

A 59-year-old man experienced rectal blood loss and was diagnosed having a distal rectal cancer staged as T3N1M0.

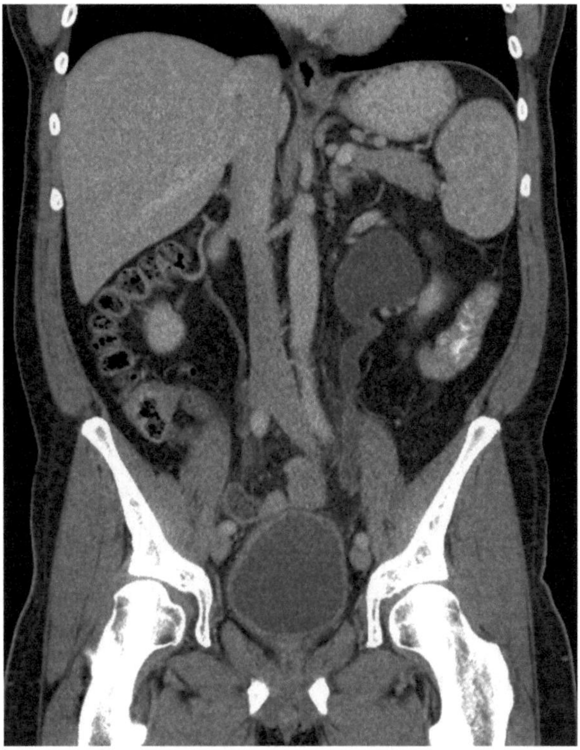

Fig. 75.1 CT scan showing dilatation of the left ureter after a LAR

Operation

After short period radiotherapy (5 × 5 Gy), and after an interval of 6 weeks, a laparoscopic total mesorectal excision (TME) was performed with an end-to-side coloanal anastomosis.

Postoperative Course: Identification and Treatment of Complication

The patient's postoperative period was uneventful, and the postoperative stage was pT2N0. During the first postoperative control at 4 months, no distance metastases were seen, yet there was dilatation of the left ureter (Fig. 75.1). Consultation and retrograde ureterography by the urologist showed a stenosis of the left ureter at the level of the previous dissection. Through a cystoscopy, a guide wire could be passed through stenosis, and a double J-stent was placed (Fig. 75.2a, b). After a period of 2 years during which the patient went through different episodes of ureter dilatation and a recurrence of urinary infections, the urologist decided to perform a left nephrectomy.

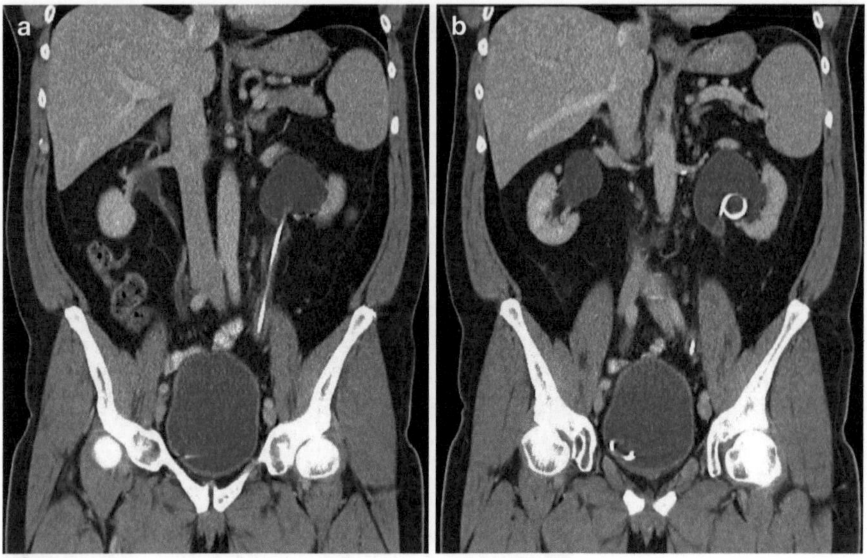

Fig. 75.2 (**a**, **b**) CT scan, dilated system treated by a double J-stent

Discussion

Ureter lesion during surgical interventions is more frequent than reported. It can happen not only on the left side during gynecological or left colon and rectal operations but also at the right ureter during LAR as shown in Fig. 75.3 and managed by a double J-stent or a leak from the left ureter diagnosed during postoperative course because of fever and pain (Fig. 75.4).

It is remarkable that peroperative urological lesions are exclusively reported by gynecologists. Data about urological complications during open and laparoscopic operations, which are performed by colorectal surgeons, are scarcely reported. Ureter lesions and bladder lesions can be recognized during an operation and then repaired, as well as during the postoperative period because of leakage of urine through the drains. Moreover, during follow-up, dilatations of the ureter and of the renal pelvis may be seen caused by late ureter stenosis. This late complication forms a difficult differential diagnosis between recurrent cancer and old ureter lesion by means a clip, hyperthermia, or radiotherapy effect.

World literature published between 1966 and 2003 on ureteral injury during laparoscopic surgery was reviewed [1–4]. A total of 70 reported instances of ureteral injury during laparoscopic surgery were identified. In 18 of the 70 (25.7 %) cases, the initial laparoscopic procedures during which ureteral injury occurred were not described or specified. In cases in which the type of laparoscopic surgery was specified, 14 of the 70 (20.0 %) total cases of ureteral injury occurred during laparoscopically assisted vaginal hysterectomy (LAVH). Ureteral injury was identified

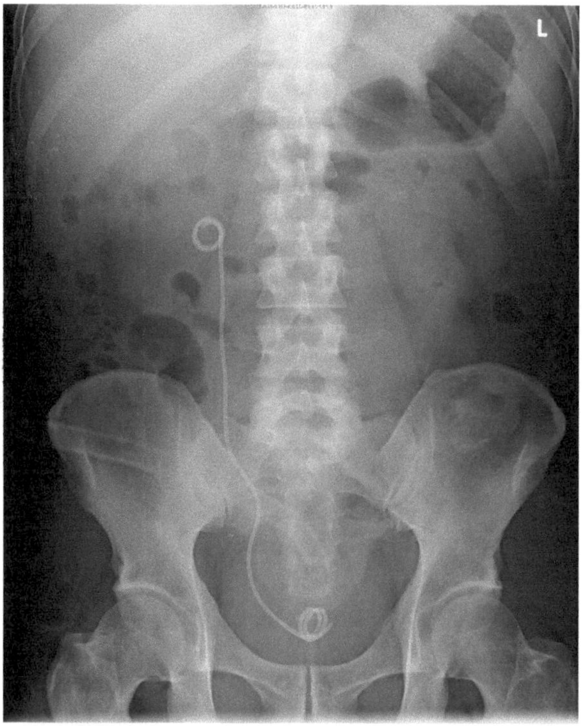

Fig. 75.3 Double J-stent introduced to treat a right ureter lesion during an anterior resection

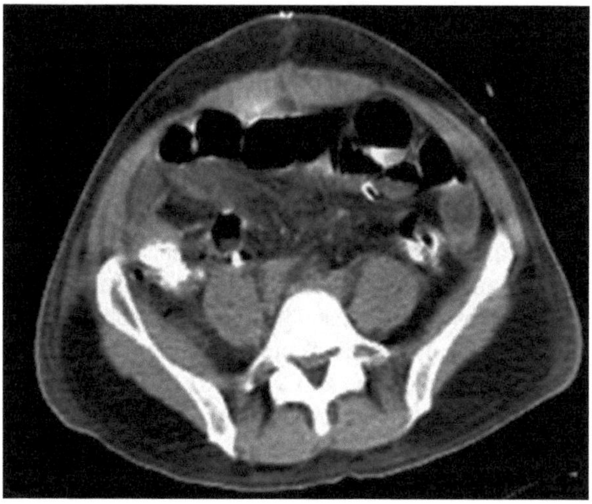

Fig. 75.4 CT scan showing leakage of contrast at the left ureter after an anterior resection

intraoperatively in 6 of 70 (8.6 %) cases; postoperatively in 49 of 70 (70.0 %) cases; and, in 15 of 70 (21.4 %) cases, the time of diagnosis was not specified. In instances in which the types of injury were described, transection occurred most commonly,

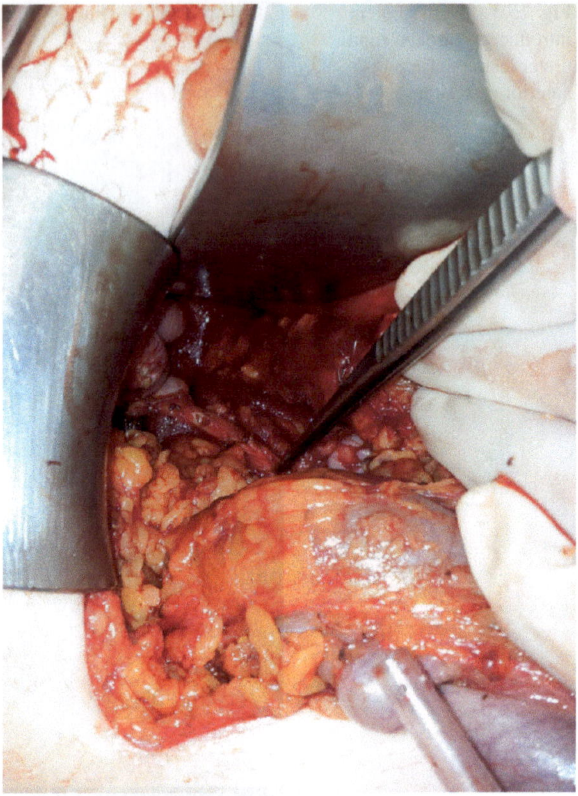

Fig. 75.5 Left ureter lesion, observed after conversion, due to a technical difficult left hemicolectomy for cancer

accounting for 14 of 70 (20.0 %) injuries. The location of ureteral injury was not specified in 46 of the 70 (65.7 %) cases. When location was specified, injuries most often occurred at or above the pelvic brim, accounting for 10 of the total 70 (14.3 %). Electrocautery was involved in 17 of the 70 (24.3 %) cases of ureteral injury, but in 34 of the 70 (48.6 %) cases, the surgical laparoscopic instrument involved was not reported. A laparotomy was used to repair the ureteral injury in 43 of 70 (61.4 %) cases. Laparoscopically assisted vaginal hysterectomy was the leading procedure in which injury occurred, and instruments involved in electrocoagulation were associated with the most injuries incurred during laparoscopic surgery.

Moreover, recently, the COLOR II group published the short-term outcomes of a randomized study comparing the laparoscopic versus the open approached for rectal cancer. Ureter injury has been reported in 1 % of the intervention, equal in both groups [5].

Ureter lesion discovered during the operation should be solved together with the urologist during the operation (Fig. 75.5). Lesions diagnosed in a late period should be also treated together with the urologist. Treatment includes from double J-stent and dilatation to percutaneous nephrostomy and eventually nephrectomy.

References

1. Lent V, Pichlmaier H, Baumbusch F, et al. Urologic errors in surgical procedures. Chirurg. 2008;79:854–8.
2. Soong YK, Yu HT, Wang CJ, et al. Urinary tract injury in laparoscopic-assisted vaginal hysterectomy. J Minim Invasive Gynecol. 2007;14:600–5.
3. Ostrzenski A, Radolinski B, Ostrzenska KM. A review of laparoscopic ureteral injury in pelvic surgery. Obstet Gynecol Surv. 2003;58:794–9.
4. Léonard F, Fotso A, Borghese B, et al. Ureteral complications from laparoscopic hysterectomy indicated for benign uterine pathologies: a 13-year experience in a continuous series of 1300 patients. Hum Reprod. 2007;22:2006–11.
5. Van der Pas MHGM, Haglind E, Cuesta MA, et al. Laparoscopic versus open surgery for rectal cancer (COLOR II): short-term outcomes of a randomised, phase 3 trial. Lancet Oncol. 2013;14(3):210–8.

Chapter 76
Case on Late Ileoanal Pouch Anastomosis Fisteling (Vaginal and Perineal)

Miguel A. Cuesta

Keywords Ileoanal pouch • Fistula • Pouch-vaginal fistula • Perineal fistula • Pouchitis

First Patient

Diagnosis and Indication for Surgery

A 26-year-old man underwent 5 years previously a laparoscopic-assisted panproctocolectomy with an ileoanal pouch anastomosis (IAPA) because of an intractable ulcerative colitis (UC) with a protective loop ileostomy. After 6 weeks, the ileostomy was closed and patient started having frequent stools, was treated by diet and Loperamide until gaining an optimum of 4–6 defecations a day.

Postoperative Course: Identification and Treatment of Complication

Patient was doing well, could work in the construction company of his father, and up until 5 years later, he developed a perineal abscess, which initially drained spontaneously, as well as getting a suprasphincteric fistula (Fig. 76.1a, b). Because of this complication, we considered the presence of an indeterminate kind of colitis or

M.A. Cuesta, M.D.
Department of Surgery, VU University Medical Center, Amsterdam, The Netherlands
e-mail: ma.cuesta@vumc.nl

M.A. Cuesta, H.J. Bonjer (eds.), *Case Studies of Postoperative Complications after Digestive Surgery*, DOI 10.1007/978-3-319-01613-9_76,

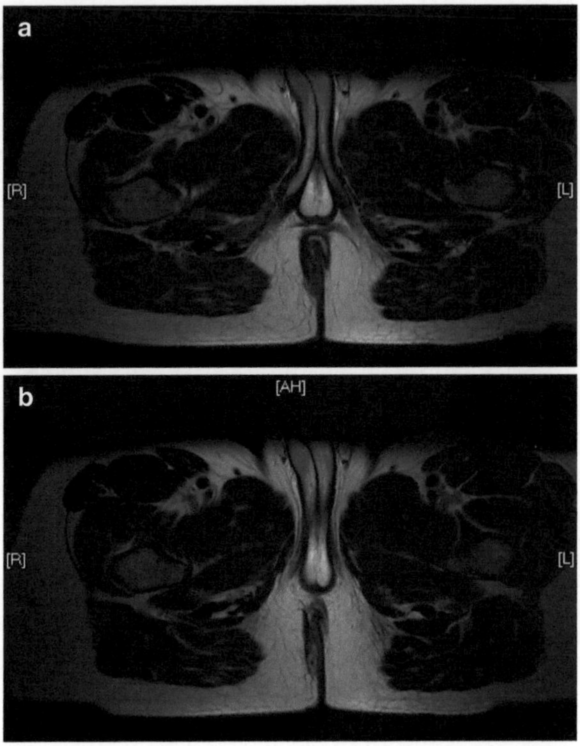

Fig. 76.1 (**a**) MRI showing a suprasphincteric fistula to the pouch. (**b**) MRI, suprasphincteric fistula to the pouch

of a Crohn's disease that had been improperly determined 5 years previously. Review of pathology remained inconclusive. An endoscopy of the pouch showed important pouchitis as treated by antibiotics (Fig. 76.2). The biopsy was negative for granuloma. The fistula was treated conservatively by means of a seton, but leakage from the fistula increased. Thoughts arose about repair, such as closing the fistula by a gracilis muscle plasty or an ileostomy. The patient's desire was very clear "to continue without definitive ileostomy". Two months later, he suddenly became sick with fever and a new perineal abscess. Despite the drainage of the abscess with different tracks, the patient became septic with respiratory insufficiency and he had to be ventilated mechanically for 10 days. A CT scan showed no pelvic abscesses. Because of the extensive perineal infection occurring during this period, we decided to perform a laparotomy with excision of the pouch and creation of an ileostomy (Illustration 76.1). Pathology showed chronic and acute pouchitis without granulomas. They could not typify the findings as Crohn's disease. Steadily but slowly the patient recovered and the perianal fistulas closed. He is currently working again and no signs of Crohn's disease have appeared.

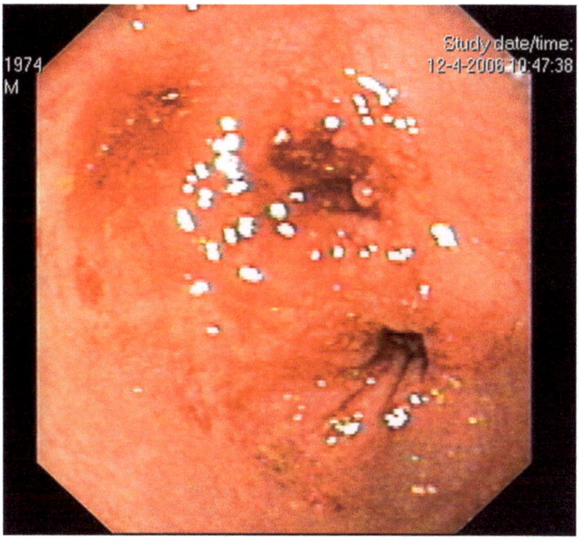

Fig. 76.2 Endoscopy of the pouch showing pouchitis with fistula opening

Second Patient

A 40-year-old lady had previously been treated because of ulcerative colitis by means of panproctocolectomy and IAPA. Seven years later, she experienced small leakages of intestinal contents through her vagina. Patient was referred to discuss with her about the option to close the fistula. After examination, the fistula appeared to be very tiny, localized proximal of the sphincters, leading to small losses through her vagina, and that not on all days. So, we proposed her to close the fistula by means of an interposition of bulbocavernous muscle and Martius plasty protected by a temporarily ileostomy (Illustration 76.1). She refused to undergo the ileostomy because of her limited complaints.

Third Patient

An 18-year-old young man had been referred to us because of intractable ulcerative colitis. He underwent a panproctocolectomy followed by an IAPA and protective ileostomy. After closure of the ileostomy, the patient developed chronic pain at the perianal region and diarrhea. Endoscopy of the pouch showed pouchitis, to be treated conservatively. One year of conservative treatment and analysis followed, in which patient had continuous problems to maintain his weight and do his studies. A second opinion was asked from an experienced surgeon who opened the possibility of chronic infection around the pouch with a 3-cm rectum anastomosed to the pouch. Patient accepted a new operation under this diagnosis.

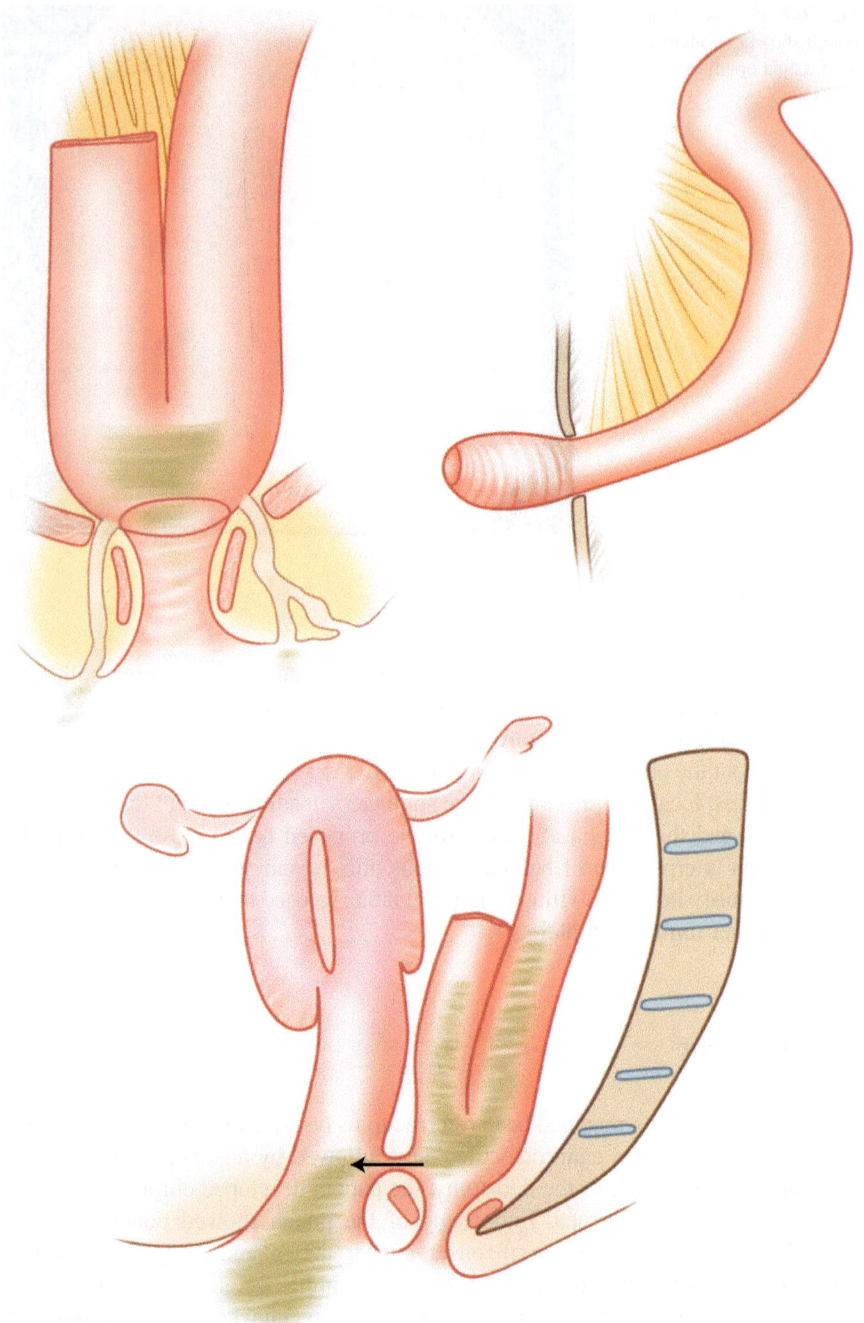

Illustration 76.1 In case of fistulas (*arrow*) forming after IAPA, after an attempt to treat them conservatively, the only real treatment will be to create a definitive ileostomy. Frequently, surgeons will leave the anus of the patient after dismantling the ileoanal anastomosis. This will lead to frequent abscesses at the top of the stump that requires frequent drainage and may lead to chronic sinus and difficult solution

At operation, the pouch was dissected free from the pelvis, the rectal rim shortened, and after regaining enough length the pouch was anastomosed to the anus. No abscesses were found. Cultures were negative. Presacral space was drained. Yet, complaints returned and finally the patient was treated by a definitive ileostomy, successfully commencing with his studies.

Discussion

Indications for panproctocolectomy and IAPA appears to be an intractability of the UC, malignancy, or suspicion for in UC and familial adenomatous polyposis coli (FAP). Some authors will also have performed an IAPA by Crohn's colitis after relapse of the disease for many years. Problems arise when patients start forming fistulas years after an IAPA. Surgeon and gastroenterologist will then immediately think about the possibility of a wrong diagnosis and will ask the pathologist for a review. Intermediate colitis is another possibility here, forming 10 % of all colitis. In case of fistulas forming after IAPA, after an attempt to treat them conservatively, the only real treatment will be to create a definitive ileostomy. Frequently, surgeons will leave the anus of the patient after dismantling the ileoanal anastomosis. This will lead to frequent abscesses at the top of the stump that requires frequent drainage and may lead to chronic sinus and difficult solution.

Lolohea et al have reviewed the incidence and treatment of the ileal pouch anal–vaginal fistula [1]. Fistula between an ileal pouch and the vagina is an uncommon complication and its optimal management has not been determined because of its low incidence. Pouch-vaginal fistula occurs in 6.3 (range, 3.3–15.8) percent of female patients with an ileal pouch-anal anastomosis. Sepsis and technical factors are the most common contributors. Management depends on the level of the fistula, the amount of pelvic scar tissue, and previous treatments. An algorithm for surgical treatment is suggested, including interposition of tissue and ileostomy and definitive ileostomy after excision of the pouch.

Johnson et al. reviewed the outcome and different treatment of these fistula in their institution [2]. They defined treatment success as no recurrence of the fistula anymore with an optimal functioning pouch and no ileostomy. 24 of 619 (3.9 %) women who had primary ileal pouch-anal anastomosis developed a pouch-vaginal fistula. Local and/or combined abdomino-perineal repairs were performed in 22 of 29 patients. Combined abdominoperineal repairs were associated with a higher success rate than that of local perineal repairs, 52.9 vs. 7.9 %, respectively, at 10 years after repair. Overall, 50 % (11/22) of patients who underwent surgical repair of a pouch-vaginal fistula had a successful result with a functioning pouch and no recurrence of the fistula, and 21 % (6/29) of patients required pouch excision. They concluded that the management of pouch-vaginal fistula after ileal pouch-anal anastomosis is associated with a high recurrence rate. Combined abdominoperineal repair appears to offer better results than those of local procedures.

Brown et al. reviewed the outcome of the ileoanal pouch in patients with Crohn's disease and indeterminate colitis [3]. Between 1982 and 2001, 1,270 patients underwent a restorative proctocolectomy: 1,135 had ulcerative colitis, 36 had Crohn's disease, 21 had indeterminate colitis, and 78 had another diagnosis. Pouch complications were significantly more common in patients with Crohn's disease (64 %) and indeterminate colitis (43 %) compared with patients with ulcerative colitis (22 %). Similarly, 56 % of patients with Crohn's disease had their pouch excised or defunctioned, compared with 10 % of patients with indeterminate colitis and 6 % with ulcerative colitis. The functional results in patients with Crohn's disease with a successful pouch were not significantly different from those with indeterminate colitis or ulcerative colitis. Although complication rates may be higher in patients with indeterminate colitis compared with ulcerative colitis, the overall pouch failure rate is similar. On the other hand, more than one-half of patients with Crohn's disease will require pouch excision or diversion. They concluded that it is difficult to identify patients with Crohn's disease who are likely to have a successful outcome after restorative proctocolectomy. Thus, Crohn's disease should remain a relative contraindication to restorative proctocolectomy, whereas ileal pouch-anal anastomosis is an acceptable alternative for patients with indeterminate colitis.

References

1. Lolohea S, Lynch AC, Robertson GB, Frizelle FA. Ileal pouch-anal anastomosis-vaginal fistula: a review. Dis Colon Rectum. 2005;48:1802–10.
2. Johnson PM, O'connor BI, Cohen Z, McLeod RS. Pouch-vaginal fistula after ileal pouch-anal anastomosis: treatment and outcomes. Dis Colon Rectum. 2005;48:1249–53.
3. Brown CJ, Maclean AR, Cohen Z, et al. Crohn's disease and inderterminate colitis and the ileal pouch-anal anastomosis: outcomes and patterns of failures. Dis Colon Rectum. 2005;48:1542–9.

Chapter 77
Case on Anorectal Adenocarcinoma in Colorectal Crohn's Disease

Miguel A. Cuesta and Henri A.H. Winters

Keywords Colorectal Crohn's disease • Adenocarcinoma rectum • TRAM flap

Diagnosis and Indication for Surgery

A 57-year-old man presented, who was known since 15 years to have a colorectal Crohn's disease. Because of complicated perianal fistulas and stenosis in descending colon, a left colonic resection had been performed 10 years previously with creation of a colostomy, leaving 15 cm of rectum as stump. Although fistulas became quite prevalent, yet the patient had minimal complaints for a considerable period of time.

Eighteen months ago he developed pain in the anus and discharge of blood and mucus.

By inspection there was a tumor around the anus with important chronic skin irritation. Study of the rectum was difficult because of supra-anal stenosis and on the CT scan and MRI, imaging suggested the existence of an extensive adenocarcinoma of the distal rectum and anus, without metastases in the lymph nodes of groins (Fig. 77.1a, b). Under anesthesia, biopsies were taken showing adenocarcinoma. A PET CT scan showed a local hotspot but no distance metastases. Decision was taken for doing a long chemo-radiotherapy followed 6 weeks later by a cylindrical abdominoperineal resection with closure of perianal wound by means of a Tranverse Rectus Abdominis Myocutaneous (TRAM) flap. Chemoradiation consisting of daily administration of Capecitabine and 5 days weekly radiation fractions of 2 Gy to a total amount of 50 Gy in 5 weeks.

M.A. Cuesta, M.D. (✉)
Department of Surgery, VU University Medical Center, Amsterdam, The Netherlands
e-mail: ma.cuesta@vumc.nl

H.A.H. Winters
Department Plastic Surgery, VU University Medical Center, Amsterdam, The Netherlands

M.A. Cuesta, H.J. Bonjer (eds.), *Case Studies of Postoperative Complications after Digestive Surgery*, DOI 10.1007/978-3-319-01613-9_77,

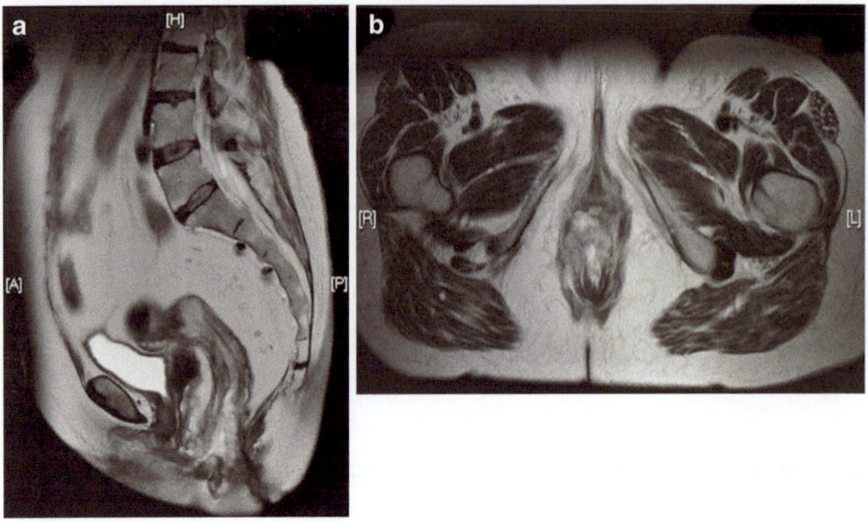

Fig. 77.1 (**a, b**) MRI diagnosis of adenocarcinoma distal rectum and anal area

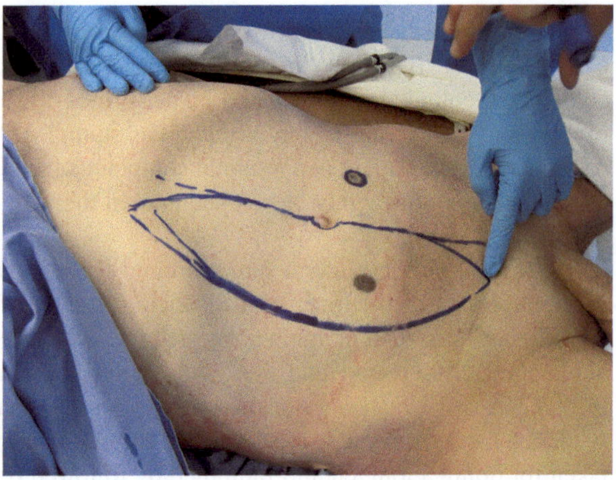

Fig. 77.2 Skin incision for TRAM flap

Operation

Operation was performed together with plastic surgeon. Operation went without complications (Figs. 77.2, 77.3, 77.4, and 77.5b). Pathological examination showed a long adenocarcinoma, radical resected with 10 out of 23 lymph nodes affected by cancer. Resection margins were free.

Six months later, the patient developed an epileptic attack being diagnosed for having two metastases in the left lobe of the brain. Palliation radiotherapy was given, but the patient died 3 months later without signs of local recurrence.

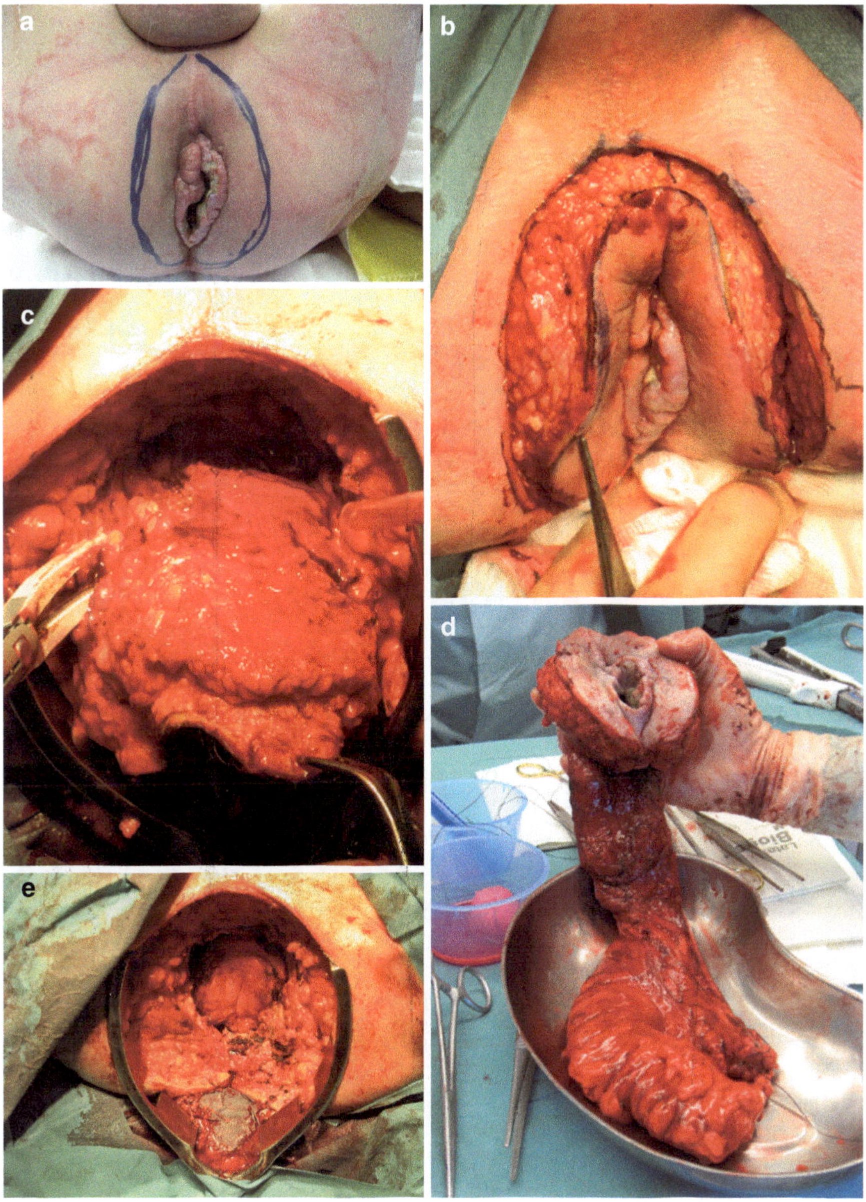

Fig. 77.3 (a,b,c,d,e) External aspect of the tumor and cylindrical APR resection

Discussion

Looking at the history of this patient, it is important to know more data about the risks factors for dysplasia and carcinoma and the incidence for adenocarcinoma of the rectum and anus in Crohn's colitis patients.

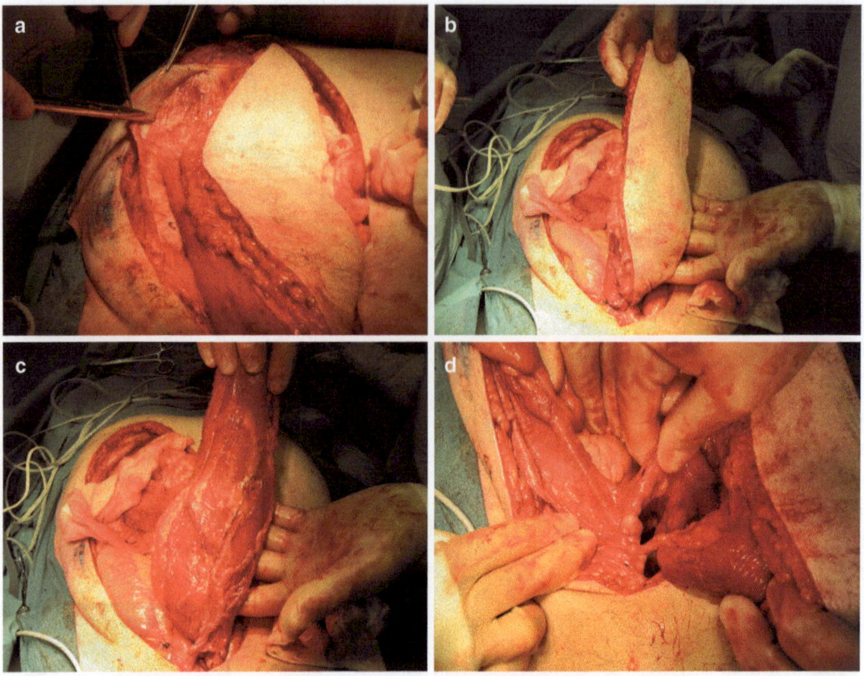

Fig. 77.4 (**a**,**b**,**c**,**d**) TRAM flap creation and vascularization of the flap

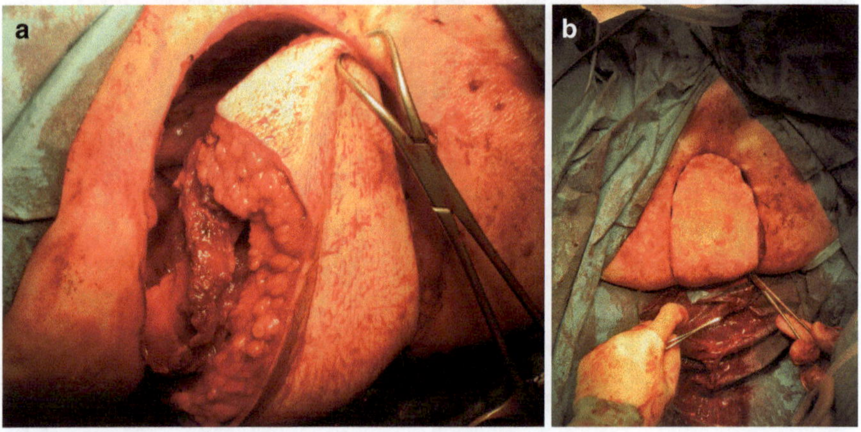

Fig. 77.5 (**a**,**b**) Tram flap closing the perineal wound

Sjodhal et al. studied the incidence of rectal and anal cancer in Crohn's patients in Sweden [1]. During 1987–2000, rectal or anal cancer was diagnosed in 335 Crohn's patients in Sweden (153 males, 182 females). In other words, approximately three Crohn's patients per million inhabitants were diagnosed with rectal or anal cancer each year during that time period, which amounts to 1 % of the total number of cases. Present knowledge from the literature implies that there is an increased risk of rectal and anal cancer only in those Crohn's patients having severe proctitis or severe chronic perianal disease. However, the rectal remnant must also be considered a risk factor. The outcome is the same as in sporadic cancer at a corresponding stage but the prognosis is often poor due to the advanced stage of cancer at diagnosis. They suggest that six high-risk groups should be recommended for annual surveillance after a duration of having Crohn's disease for 15 years including extensive colitis, chronic severe anorectal disease, rectal remnant, strictures, bypassed segments, and sclerosing cholangitis.

Maykel et al. studied the incidence of dysplasia and adenocarcinoma in specimens of patients operated on because of Crohn's colitis, thereby trying to identify risks factors associated with dysplasia and adenocarcinoma [2]. Two hundred twenty-two patients of which 138 females who underwent surgical resection for the treatment of Crohn's colitis were included in the study. There were five cases of dysplasia (2.3 %) and six cases of adenocarcinoma (2.7 %). Three patients with dysplasia and one with adenocarcinoma were diagnosed on preoperative colonoscopy, while the other cases were discovered incidentally on pathologic examination of resected specimens. Factors associated with the presence of dysplasia or adenocarcinoma included older age at diagnosis (38.2 vs. 30.3 years), longer disease duration (16.0 vs. 10.1 years), and the extent of the disease. They concluded that patients having severe Crohn's colitis and requiring surgery are at significant risk for developing dysplasia and adenocarcinoma, particularly when diagnosed at an older age, after a longer disease duration, and with more extensive colon involvement.

References

1. Sjödahl RI, Myrelid P, Söderholm JD. Anal and rectal cancer in Crohn's disease. Colorectal Dis. 2003;5:490–5.
2. Maykel JA, Hagerman G, Mellgren AF, et al. Crohn's colitis: the incidence of dysplasia and adenocarcinoma in surgical patients. Dis Colon Rectum. 2006;49:950–7.

Chapter 78
Case on Recto-Vaginal Fistula After LAR

Cristina Mendez and Miguel A. Cuesta

Keywords Rectal cancer • Low anterior resection • Protective ileostomy • Rectovaginal fistula • Neoadjuvant radiotherapy

Diagnosis and Indication for Surgery Identification of Complication

A 67-year-old female patient with a previous history of hysterectomy because of uterine fibroid was diagnosed having a mid-rectal adenocarcinoma, stage T3N1M0. By CT scan of her thorax and abdomen, no metastases were found, and the patient was proposed for short neoadjuvant radiotherapy, 5 × 5 Gy, followed by low anterior resection after an interval of 6 weeks. Her colon was mechanically prepared. At operation, TME was performed open, without incidences, followed by a mechanical end-to-side anastomosis protected by a temporarily loop ileostomy. On the 5th post-operative day she initially had vaginal loss of blood, and then leakage of fecal material through her vagina developed. By rectal and vaginal examination, the fistula was established at 7 cm from anus, probably at the level of the posterior fornix. A CT scan confirmed the diagnosis (Fig. 78.1a,b,c,d). There were no abscesses. Patient was referred to us for treatment.

C. Mendez, M.D. (✉)
Department of Surgery, Virgen del Rocio, Sevilla, Spain
e-mail: c.mendez10@hotmail.com

M.A. Cuesta, M.D.
Department of Surgery, VU University Medical Center, Amsterdam, The Netherlands
e-mail: ma.cuesta@vumc.nl

M.A. Cuesta, H.J. Bonjer (eds.), *Case Studies of Postoperative Complications after Digestive Surgery*, DOI 10.1007/978-3-319-01613-9_78,

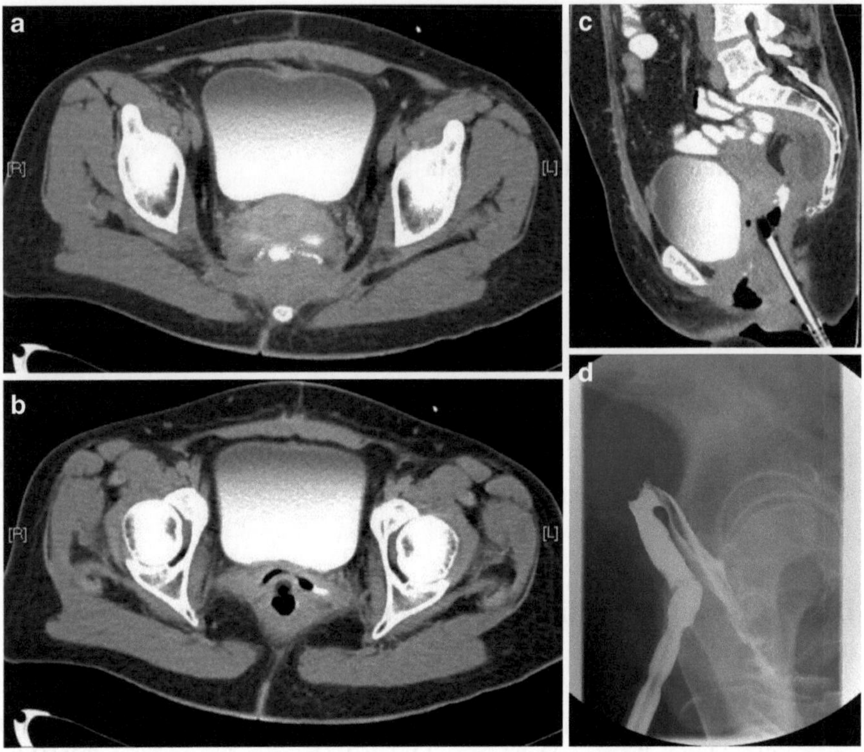

Fig. 78.1 (**a–c**) Imaging by CT scan (and with enema) with rectal contrast the AVF. (**d**) Enema with evidence for recto-vaginal anastomosis

Treatment of Complication: Operation

With assistance of the gynecologist, the patient underwent an exploration under anesthesia. Colposcopy revealed a large fistula of 3 cm between the anterior aspect of the vaginal stump and the anastomosis, located at 7 cm from the anal canal. There was no stenosis of the anastomosis and a proctoscopy showed no recurrence of cancer. Patient had normal sphincters and had no problems with the feces continence. Cancer control by CT scan of thorax and abdomen showed no metastases. A plan was designed to mobilize the splenic flexure through laparotomy, dissecting the descending colon, the fistula, and the rectum distal of anastomosis until the pelvic floor. This was carried out without much fibrosis around the fistula, the fistula was taken down, and the defect in the vagina was closed by the gynecologist. At the level of the pelvic floor the distal rectum was divided, and we decided to perform a pull-through procedure in order to avoid any anastomosis in front of the vaginal suture line. The pull-through procedure was successful and after interposition of omentum between vagina and neorectum, presacral space was drained and the laparotomy was closed. After 1 week, under anesthesia the superfluous loop was shortened and fixed by stitches at the level of the anus (Fig. 78.2). By rectal examination,

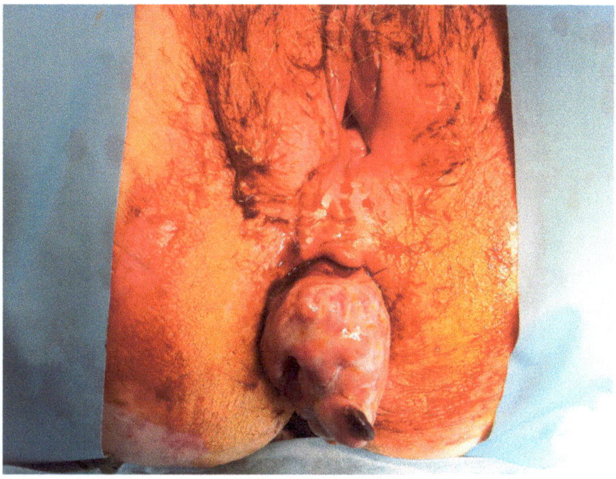

Fig. 78.2 Pull-through before to be shortened

there was no stenosis and the loop was good vital. Patient could go home 2 days later under the proviso that at the outpatient clinic we could by rectal examination treat the tendency towards stenosis. Also, the gynecologist could check the vagina and could observe the healing, thereby administering estrogen crème against atrophy. At last, 3 months after the first operation, the ileostomy could be reversed. Frequent defecation and some grade of soiling took place, treated by active pelvic floor physiotherapy and thereafter remedied by lavage every 2 days. Patient was happy with the solution and is still able to be sexually active.

Discussion

There are three possible causes for the appearance of an anastomosis-vaginal fistula after LAR. First, a lesion on the vagina wall during dissection of the recto-vaginal septum; second, when during the stapled anastomosis a piece of vagina wall is taken with the anastomosis and will develop a fistula; and third—the most dramatic—the introduction of the circular stapler through the vagina and not through the rectum (Illustration 78.1a).

The easiest and most practical solution is to create a definitive colostomy (Illustration 78.1b), but many relatively young women ask for the solution of reconstructing the vagina if so possible, without a definitive stoma. All risks involved have to be shared with patients. Decisions will be taken during the operation. If patient is already incontinent or has soiling, a colostomy is the only solution. In other cases, reconstruction has to be performed, as took place in this patient. A good alternative is to perform a distal stapled anastomosis (Illustration 78.1c). But after this pelvic anastomosis, risks for recurrence of fistula are still present and therefore the coloanal or pull-through is a good alternative with interposition of, e.g., omentum plasty (Illustration 78.1d). Drawback here will be the continence. In the case of frequent defecation or of incontinence, a colon lavage at home may be a good

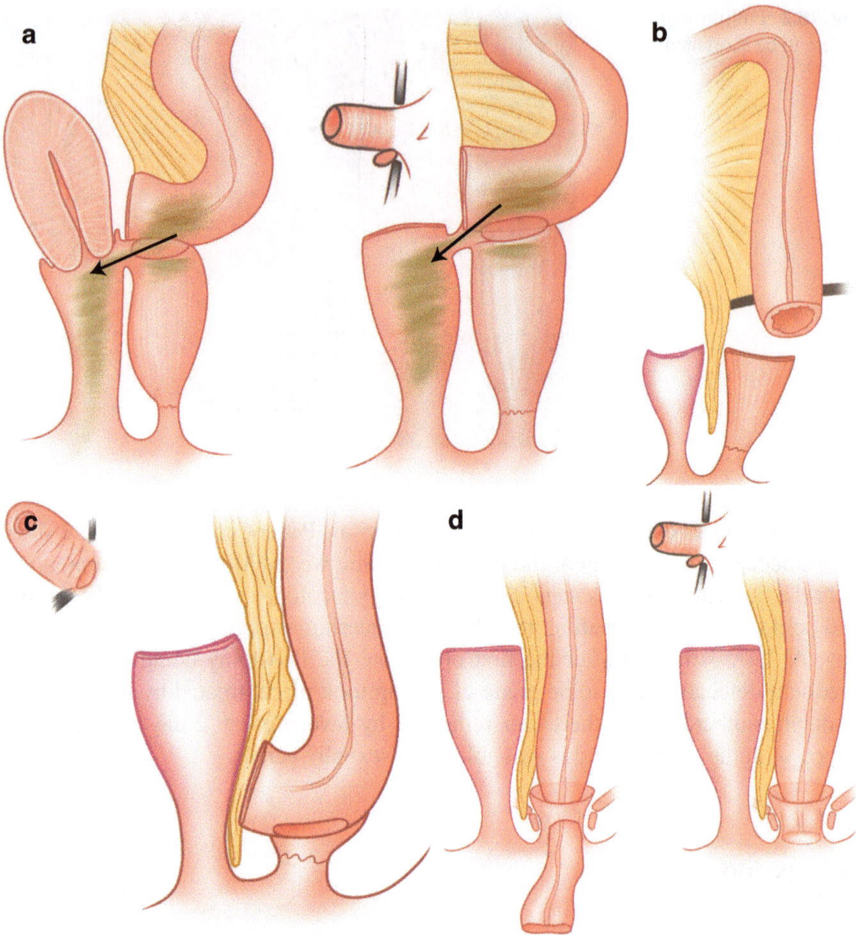

Illustration 78.1 (**a–d**) Different AVF and therapeutic solutions, from definitive colostomy to coloanal anastomosis and pull-through procedure. *Arrow* is the fistula

solution. If patient has the uterus in situ, this should be taken out for the reconstruction.

Matthiessen et al. studied the occurrence and risk factors for this anastomotic-vaginal fistula (AVF) [1]. All female patients, median age 69.5 years, who developed a symptomatic AVF ($n=20$) after anterior resection of the rectum for cancer were identified and compared with those who developed conventional symptomatic leakage ($n=32$) and those who did not leak ($n=338$). Symptomatic anastomotic leakage occurred in 52 (13.3 %) of 390 patients. Twenty (5.1 %) had an anastomotic-vaginal fistula (AVF) and 32 (8.2 %) conventional leakage (CL). Patients with AVF required unscheduled reoperation and defunctioning stoma as often as those with CL. AVF was diagnosed later and more often after discharge from hospital compared with CL. Patients with AVF had lower anastomoses and decreased BMI compared with those with CL. Risk factors for AVF in multivariate analysis were anastomosis <5 cm above the anal verge preoperative radiotherapy and UICC cancer stage IV. Previous hysterectomy was a risk factor neither for AVF nor for CL. They concluded that anastomotic-vaginal fistula forms a significant part of all symptomatic leakages after low anterior resection for cancer in women. Although diagnosed later, the need for abdominal reoperation and defunctioning stoma was not different from patients with CL.

Reference

1. Matthiessen P, Hansson L, Sjödahl R, Rutegård J. Anastomotic-vaginal fistula (AVF) after anterior resection of the rectum for cancer–occurrence and risk factors. Colorectal Dis. 2010;12:351–7.

Chapter 79
Case on Rectovesical Fistula After LAR

Miguel A. Cuesta and R. Jeroen van Moorselaar

Keywords Rectal cancer • Neoadjuvant radiotherapy • Rectovesical fistula • Low anterior resection

Diagnosis and Indication for Surgery Identification of Complication

A 68-year-old man underwent a low anterior resection with a protective ileostomy by open procedure because of mid-rectum adenocarcinoma after a short radiotherapy treatment of 5 Gy 5 days. His postoperative course was complicated first of all by a leakage of the anastomosis (Figs. 79.1 and 79.2) treated by drainage and deviating ileostomy. Secondly he developed fever and urinary tract infection, initially ascribed to usual infection because of the bladder catheter, being treated by antibiotics, as indicated by the culture. Moreover, the aspect of the urine was initially muddy, and the culture included intestinal flora and vegetal fibers (Fig. 79.3). Because of persistent fever, a CT scan with rectal contrast was performed showing a fistula communicating the rectal anastomosis with the bladder (Fig. 79.4). Cystoscopy showed the fistula 2 cm at the level of the left ureter in the trigonum vesicae with staples inside the bladder (Fig. 79.5). Patient was referred for surgical treatment and together with the urologist a laparotomy was planned for taking down the fistula and the stomas.

M.A. Cuesta, M.D. (✉)
Department of Surgery, VU University Medical Center, Amsterdam, The Netherlands
e-mail: ma.cuesta@vumc.nl

R.J. van Moorselaar
Department of Urology, VU University Medical Center, Amsterdam, The Netherlands

M.A. Cuesta, H.J. Bonjer (eds.), *Case Studies of Postoperative Complications after Digestive Surgery*, DOI 10.1007/978-3-319-01613-9_79,

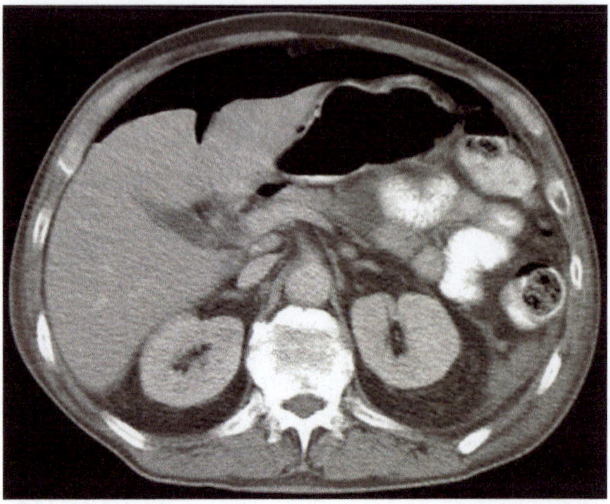

Fig. 79.1 CT scan, leakage of anastomosis with pneumoperitoneum

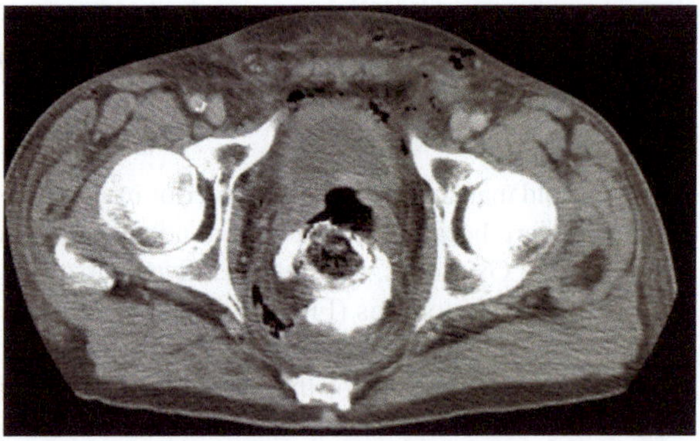

Fig. 79.2 CT scan, leakage of anastomosis LAR

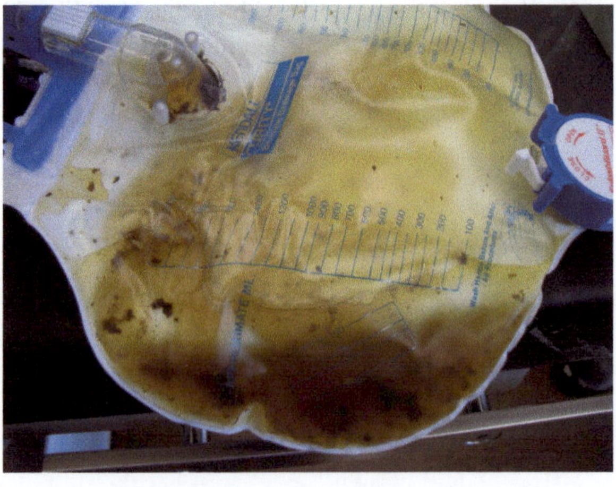

Fig. 79.3 Aspect of the urine

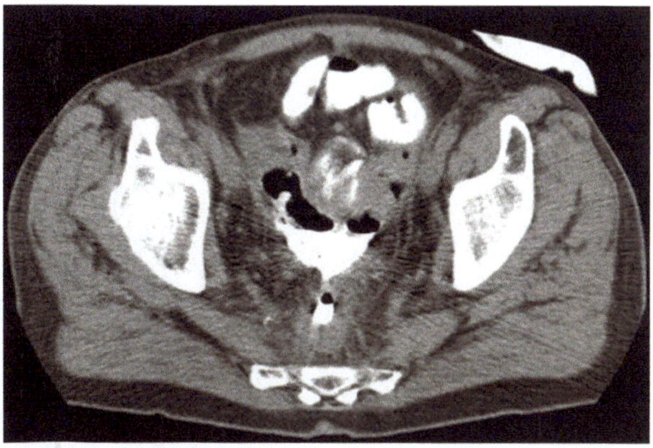

Fig. 79.4 CT scan, rectal contrast showing the fistula into the bladder

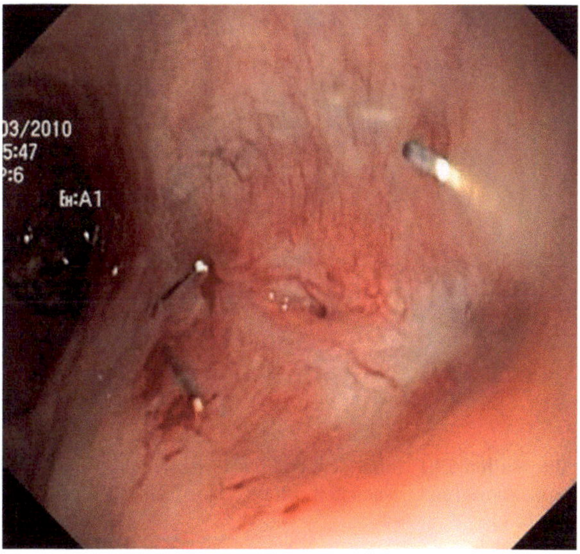

Fig. 79.5 Cystoscopy, showing the fistula, 2 cm from the left ureter with staples

Treatment of Complication: Operation

During the laparotomy, the place of the anastomosis was found because of the stenosis present and the staples. The urologist dissected the bladder from Retzius area and opened the bladder in longitudinal direction. From the inside two ureter catheters could be introduced into the ureters and the fistula localized (Fig. 79.6). The bladder was incised longitudinally up to the fistula and in this way the fistula could be closed in two layers. From there the rest of the rectum was dissected until

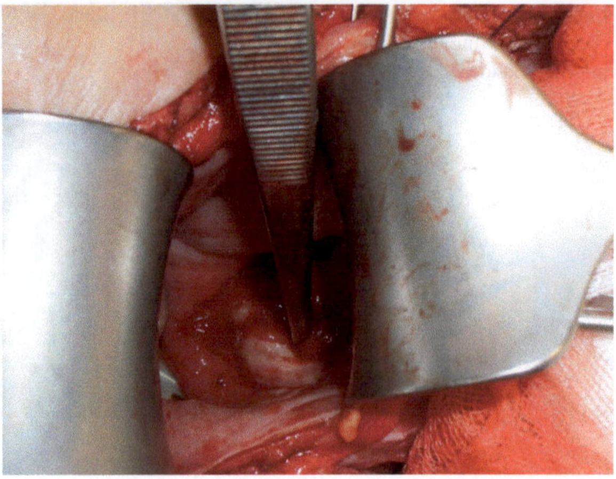

Fig. 79.6 Bladder is open, fistula is visible

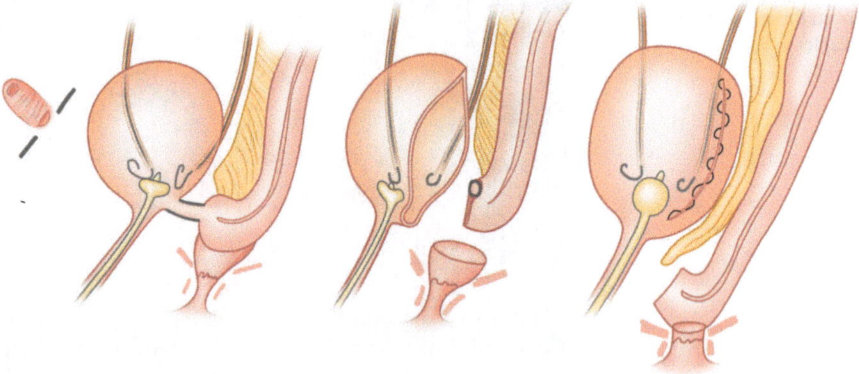

Illustration 79.1 Infrequent complication. Should be solved by means of cystostomy, coloanal anastomosis, and tissue interposition. Once fistula is considered closed, by cystoscopy, ileostomy can be closed

the anal channel and then resected. After mobilization of the splenic flexure, an end-to-side coloanal anastomosis was manually performed transanally and the protective ileostomy was left for deviation of the new anastomosis (Illustration 79.1). The rest of epiplon was interposed between the bladder and the neorectum.

Patient did well and 8 weeks later, after control of the anastomosis, the deviation ileostomy was taken down. Patient is doing very well.

Discussion

This is a very rare complication after TME resection because of rectal cancer. That means that the surgeon has made a lesion of the bladder during anterior dissection at an unusual place [1].

Once diagnosed the complication, it is important to know exactly the location of the fistula. Distance of fistula to the ureter is important for the procedure to follow. If the fistula involves the left ureter, this can be anastomosed in the bladder. For the rectum, a coloanal anastomosis is the only possibility.

Reference

1. Kim CW, Kim JH, Shin VS et al. Complications after sphincter saving resection in rectal cancer patients according to whether chemoradiotherapy is performed before or after surgery. Int J Radiat Oncol Biol Phys. 2010;78:156–63.

Chapter 80
Case on Perineal Problems After APR

Miguel A. Cuesta, Alexander A.F.A. Veenhof, and Juan de Dios Franco

Keywords Abdomino perineal resection • APR • Perineal abscess • Perineal hernia • Rectal cancer

First Patient

Perineal Infection: Diagnosis and Indication for Surgery

A 54-year-old contractor was diagnosed with having a very distal rectal adenocarcinoma, stage T3N1M0. He suffered tenesmus and blood in feces for 4 months before consulting the General Practitioner. The MRI and endosonography showed the external sphincters as not free from the tumor, and we decided to perform a cylindrical laparoscopic APR. Neoadjuvant therapy by 5×5 Gy was given and patient was operated on 6 weeks later. A new MRI before the operation showed an important regression of the tumor.

Operation

The colostomy place was marked and he underwent mechanical colon preparation. The operation occurred without technical problems and perineal defect was closed

M.A. Cuesta, M.D. (✉) • A.A.F.A. Veenhof, M.D.
Department of Surgery, VU University Medical Center, Amsterdam, The Netherlands
e-mail: ma.cuesta@vumc.nl; a.veenhof@vumc.nl

J. de Dios Franco
Department of Surgery, Hospital de Jerez, Cadiz, Spain

M.A. Cuesta, H.J. Bonjer (eds.), *Case Studies of Postoperative Complications after Digestive Surgery*, DOI 10.1007/978-3-319-01613-9_80,

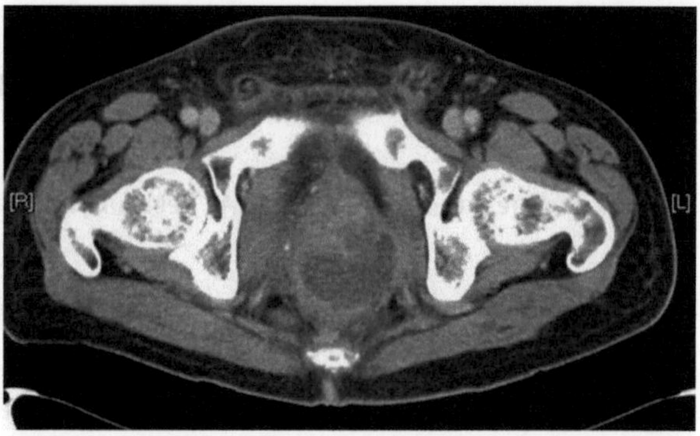

Fig. 80.1 CT scan showing a perineal abscess

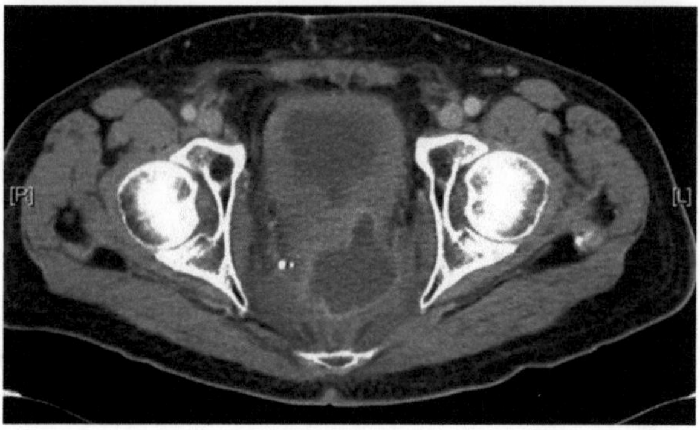

Fig. 80.2 CT scan, recurrent perineal abscess

by using an omental flap, introduced to the pelvis lateral of the colostomy. Pathology of the specimen was pT2N0M0 radical resected with circumferential margins of 1 cm.

Postoperative Course: Identification and Treatment of Complication

Postoperative course was complicated by fever and a perineal wound infection. After drainage of it on the ward, he again developed fever and a CT scan showed abscesses deep in the perineal wound (Fig. 80.1). Under anesthesia, the abscesses were drained and the wound was left open for rinsing. During operation we could see that the omentum left in the pelvis was vital. Two more times during the next 6 months, patient had to be admitted because of recurrent abscesses, these then being drained under anesthesia (Fig. 80.2). At cancer control after 1 year, the CT scan showed two hepatic metastases, being resected. He still feels pain and discomfort at the perineal wound.

Second Patient

Perineal hernia: Diagnosis and Indication for Surgery

A 59-year-old woman with rectal cancer, T3N1M0, underwent in September 2003 a laparoscopic APR with curative intent following neoadjuvant chemoradiotherapy. Preoperative MRI examination already had shown tumor invasion of the surrounding tissue, thus necessitating excision of the posterior vaginal wall along with the tumor. The operation defect was filled with an omentoplasty, and the perineum was closed in layers. No postoperative complications occurred.

Pathology study showed a radically removed pT2N1 adenocarcinoma.

Postoperative Course: Identification and Treatment of Complication

During follow-up, no metastases or local recurrence were found. However, 11 months following surgery the patient complained of a perineal swelling inducing pain and discomfort while sitting. In addition, she developed pollakiuria shortly after. An abdominal CT scan (Fig. 80.3) showed uterus and small intestine protrusion into the small pelvic cavity, thus objectifying a postoperative perineal hernia (Fig. 80.4).

A perineal approach was used to correct the hernia, during which the tissues around the edges and the uterus in retroflexion were approximated and covered by a Vicryl® mesh (Fig. 80.5a). Surgery occurred without complications, as did the patient's recovery. However, the perineal hernia persisted and became progressively symptomatic. A second CT scan showed a recurrent hernia.

Through an abdominal–perineal approach the recurrent perineal hernia was corrected. A Pfannenstiel incision was used to locate the defect in the pelvic floor. It appeared that the small bowel had herniated through a small defect situated behind the uterus and right tuba. After reposition of the small bowel, the defect was closed again by means of a mesh (Fig. 80.5b). No postoperative complications were seen.

Since the last intervention, no recurrent hernia has been observed, and the patient remains recurrence free.

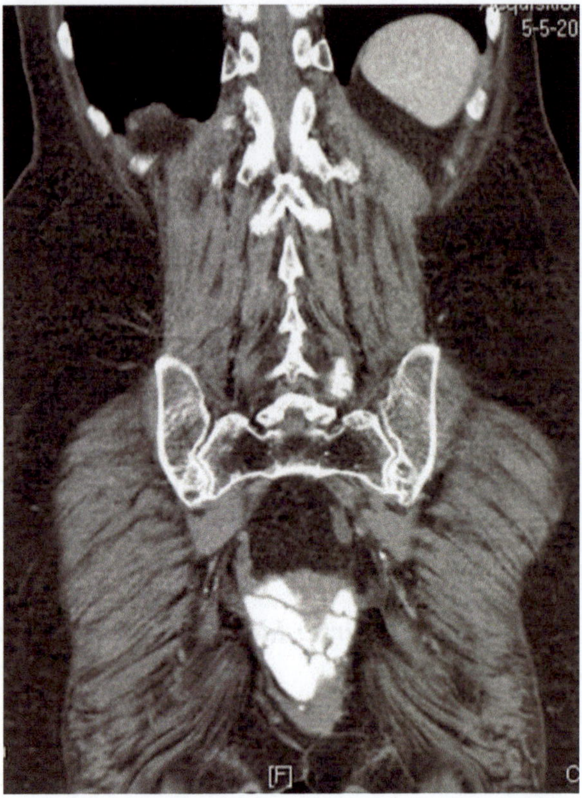

Fig. 80.3 Ct scan, perineal hernia with intestinal contents

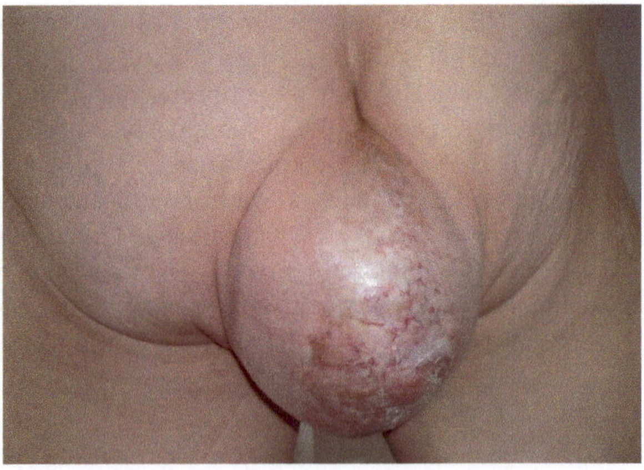

Fig. 80.4 A perineal hernia

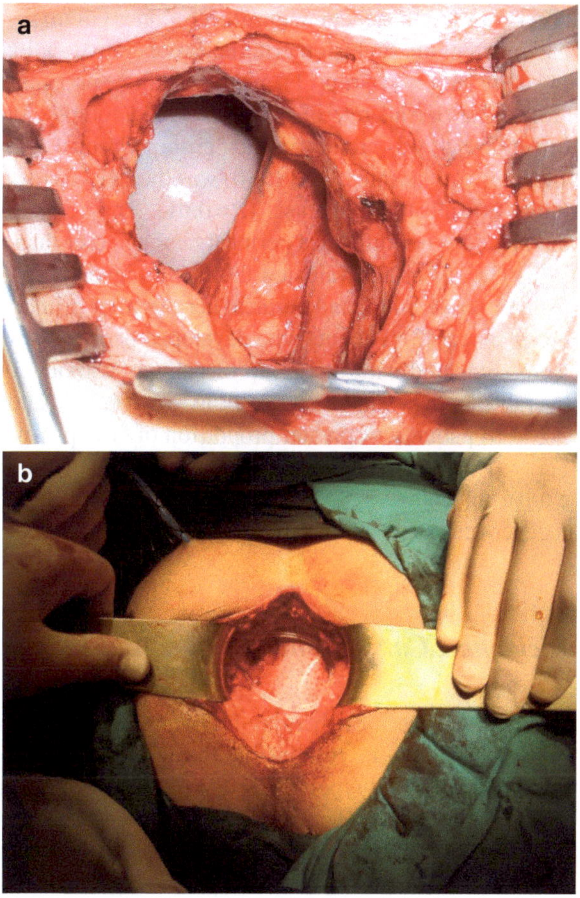

Fig. 80.5 (**a**) first operation, defect in the perineum. (**b**) second operation, defect covered perineal by a mesh

Discussion

The Best Method to Close the Perineal Defect After APR?

After classical APR, the pelvic floor muscles and the skin are approximated and the space drained. But following the more extended cylindrical resection, the question arises how to deal with the defect. Holm et al. advises to close the defect by means of gluteal flap plasty [1]. Another possibility is the use of a mesh to approximate the defect. In our case, the omentum flap as used may be the origin for the problem, due to partial necrosis. We note that contamination of the perineal wound is frequent and in radiated patients may lead to deep wound infections. Zorcolo et al. studied the risk factors for perineal wound complications after abdominoperineal resection (APR), with particular reference to preoperative radiotherapy [2]. Perineal complications were identified in patients who had preoperative long-course radiotherapy

(Group 1) and those who had surgery alone (Group 2). One hundred and fifty-seven patients met the inclusion criteria. Preoperative radiotherapy was performed in 68 (44.7 %) patients (Group 1), and 89 (55.3 %) patients (Group 2) underwent surgery alone. The overall rate of perineal wound complications was 14.8 %. The wound infection rate was similar in each group (Group 1, 10/68, 14.7 %; Group 2, 13/89, 14.9 %;). An elevated BMI (>30) was the only factor correlated with perineal morbidity on univariate analysis ($P=0.01$). They concluded that preoperative radiotherapy does not influence perineal healing other than in patients with obesity [2].

El Gazzaz et al. evaluated the factors involved with perineal wound infection, fistulas, reoperation, and perineal hernias after primary closure after APR for distal rectal cancer [3]. Patients who developed perineal wound complications (Group A) were compared with the group of patients without complications (Group B). The overall rate of wound complications was 16.2 %, and reoperation was required in 5.2 % of patients. A greater proportion of Group A patients had associated comorbidity ($P=0.001$), obesity (0.04), neoadjuvant chemoradiation (0.02), and intraoperative bleeding (0.04). In multivariate analysis, comorbidity was the only independent factor associated with the development of perineal complications [3].

Incidence, Causes, and Treatment of Perineal Hernias

Symptomatic perineal hernias following APR remain rare. Neoadjuvant chemoradiotherapy may be responsible for delayed and difficult healings in the perineal area following this type of surgery. However, no literature is available to support this hypothesis of higher incidences of perineal hernias with the onset of neoadjuvant therapy. Moreover, laparoscopic approach with the creation of less intraabdominal adhesions may play a role in a higher incidence of perineal hernias. The increase use of cylindrical APR operations for distal rectal cancer will need a better closure of the perineal wound by means of muscular plasty or a mesh. Perineal hernias remain a challenging problem, and surgical correction should only be attempted when the hernia becomes symptomatic. So et al. reported no recurrences following the abdominal approach for correction and 5.3 % recurrence following the perineal approach [4]. Although the abdominal approach has a better success rate, better exposure, and conformation on the absence of recurrent disease, this approach is much more invasive. The choice between an abdominal correction or a perineal correction therefore remains a custom-made decision for each individual patient.

Perineal hernias have been described following abdominoperineal resection, sacrectomy, protectomy, and coccygectomy [5]. The latter can be described as some form of intra-abdominal content protruding through the pelvic floor into the perineal area [6]. The true incidence of postoperative perineal hernias is difficult to estimate as the majority remain asymptomatic. However, reported frequencies following APR vary from 0.13 to 0.93 % [4–6]. When perineal hernias become symptomatic, they can cause pain in the perineum due to erosion of skin, bowel obstruction, and urinary problems. Several approaches for symptomatic perineal hernias have been described: abdominal, perineal, or a combination of both.

References

1. Anderin C, Martling A, Lagergren J, et al. Short term outcome after gluteus maximus myocutaneous flap reconstruction of the pelvic floor following extra-levator abdominoperineal excision of the rectum. Colorectal Dis. 2011;13:1463–318.
2. Zorcolo L, Restivo A, Capra F, et al. Does long-course radiotherapy influence postoperative perineal morbidity after abdominoperineal resection of the rectum for cancer? Colorectal Dis. 2011;13:1407–12.
3. El-Gazzaz G, Kiran RP, Lavery I. Wound complications in rectal cancer patients undergoing primary closure of the perineal wound after abdominoperineal resection. Dis Colon Rectum. 2009;52:1962–6.
4. So JB, Palmer MT, Shellito PC. Postoperative perineal hernia. Dis Colon Rectum. 1997;40:954–7.
5. Franklin Jr ME, Abrego D, Parra E. Laparoscopic repair of postoperative perineal hernia. Hernia. 2002;6:42–4.
6. Veenhof AA, vd Peet DL, Cuesta MA. Perineal hernia after laparoscopic abdominoperineal resection for rectal cancer: report of two cases. Dis Colon Rectum. 2007;50:1271–4.

Chapter 81
Case on Tumor Recurrence After TME Because of Rectal Cancer

Suzanne S. Gisbertz and Miguel A. Cuesta

Keywords Rectal cancer • Neoadjuvant therapy • Recurrence rectal cancer

First Patient

Diagnosis and Indication for Surgery

A 26-year-old female student was admitted in the hospital in order to undergo a laparoscopic TME and coloanal procedure after neoadjuvant radiotherapy (5 × 5 Gy) because of a distal rectal well-differentiated adenocarcinoma, 3 cm from the dentate line, staged as T3N0M0 on the MRI, without involvement of the external sphincter or the pelvic floor on the endosonography. For these reasons and considering her age and being childless, it was decided she would undergo a sphincter-saving procedure. Considering her desire to become pregnant in the future, the gynecologist by laparoscopy fixed the right ovary to the abdominal wall outside the radiation field.

Operation

Six weeks after radiotherapy, the patient underwent a laparoscopic TME operation up to the pelvic floor followed by a transanal manual performed coloanal anastomosis side-to-end fashion protected by a loop ileostomy.

S.S. Gisbertz, M.D. (✉)
Department of Surgery, Academic Medical Center, Amsterdam, The Netherlands
e-mail: s.gisbertz@antoniusziekenhuis.nl

M.A. Cuesta, M.D.
Department of Surgery, VU University Medical Center, Amsterdam, The Netherlands
e-mail: ma.cuesta@vumc.nl

M.A. Cuesta, H.J. Bonjer (eds.), *Case Studies of Postoperative Complications after Digestive Surgery*, DOI 10.1007/978-3-319-01613-9_81,

Pathology of tumor was pT2N0M0 with distal resection margin 1.5 cm and a CRM of 5 mm. Postoperative course was uneventful and she went home 7 days later.

Postoperative Course: Identification and Treatment of Complication

At outpatient clinic she relayed her suffering from soiling, thereafter being treated by pelvic floor physiotherapy and neo-rectal lavage yet without complete control of the disturbing soiling. One year later and because of dyspareunia, vaginal examination showed a three ball-like spots located on the left lateral wall of the vagina. Magnetic resonance and PET-CT scan showed the tumors suspected for local recurrence (Figs. 81.1 and 81.2). Exploration under anesthesia, done together

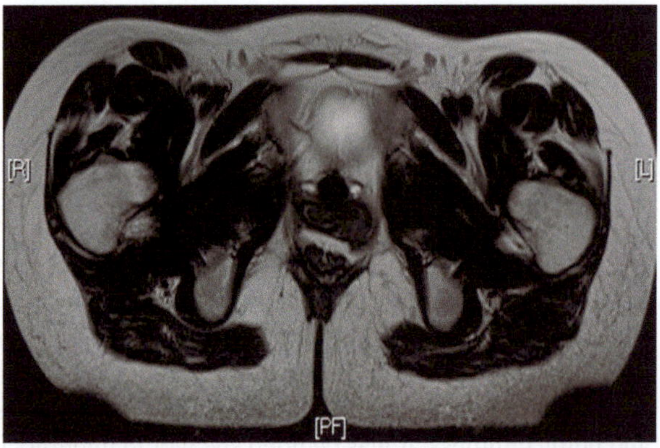

Fig. 81.1 MRI showing local recurrence at the recto-vaginal septum

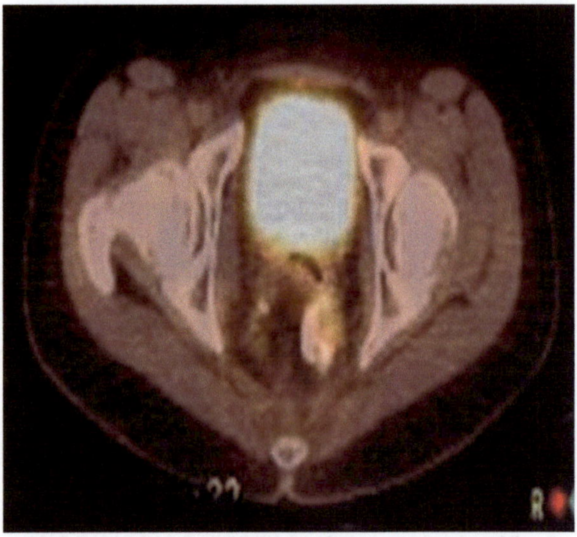

Fig. 81.2 PET positive for recurrent rectal cancer

with the gynecologist, showed the recurrence of growth in the neorectum, being still mobile without ingrowth in lateral pelvic wall. Punction biopsy was taken showing a recurrence of the previously resected tumor. Because no distance metastases were seen on a CT scan, the patient was proposed for surgical intervention to be done together with gynecologist and plastic surgeon. Proposed intervention was to perform a cylindrical APR operation along with 2/3 of posterior vagina and uterus, using the omentum for reconstruction. Postoperatively, pathology showed dubious radicality at one of the margins at the lateral aspect of the specimen, the course being that the patient subsequently was treated by adjuvant chemotherapy. One year after operation, clinical exploration and PET-CT scan showed no recurrence.

Six months later, patient developed pain in the sacral area, and the PET-CT scan showed a local recurrence there. There were no other metastases, and after radiotherapy she was again operated. A sacropelvic resection was performed with intraoperative radiotherapy.

Second Patient

Diagnosis and Indication for Surgery

A 70-year-old female patient was treated by a laparoscopic APR after short radiotherapy (5 × 5 Gy) because of a very distal adenocarcinoma of the rectum and staged as T3N0M0. Pathology staging was pT3N0 with CRM of 3 mm.

Postoperative Course: Identification and Treatment of Complication

After a period of 2 years she developed pain at the os coccygis. On the CT scan and PET scan there was observed a tumor suspect for local recurrence (Figs. 81.3 and 81.4). Exploration under anesthesia confirmed the palpation through the vagina of a hard fixed tumor at the distal part of the sacrum. There were no distance metastases, and the patient was proposed to undergo a re-resection of perineal scar along with posterior vaginal wall and distal sacral part (two or three bodies) by a combined approach through laparotomy and perineum. Through laparotomy it was seen that an intestinal loop was fixed to the tumor, being resected en block with the specimen. The sacrum was divided proximal of the tumor. Pathology showed that even if the tumor appeared to be radically resected, it was difficult to ascertain radicality at the left lateral area. The patient recovered very quickly but remained unable to pass urine spontaneously and so had to catheterize regularly. Six months after she developed a liver metastasis, being PET positive (Fig. 81.5). She underwent a local resection of the metastasis localized at segment 6.

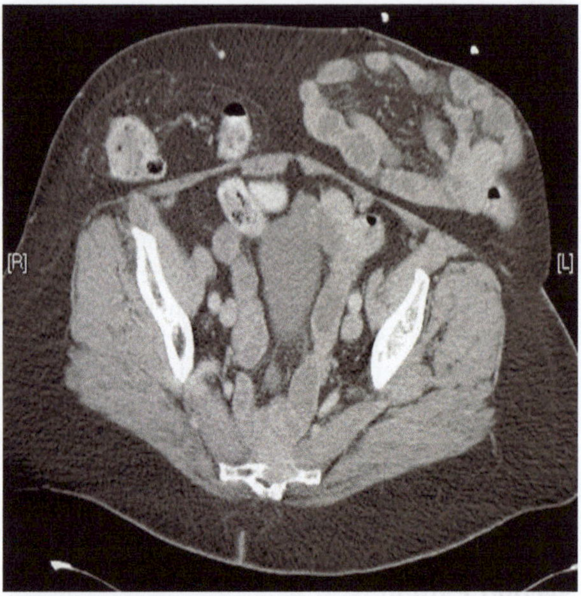

Fig. 81.3 CT scan showing rectal recurrence in presacral area

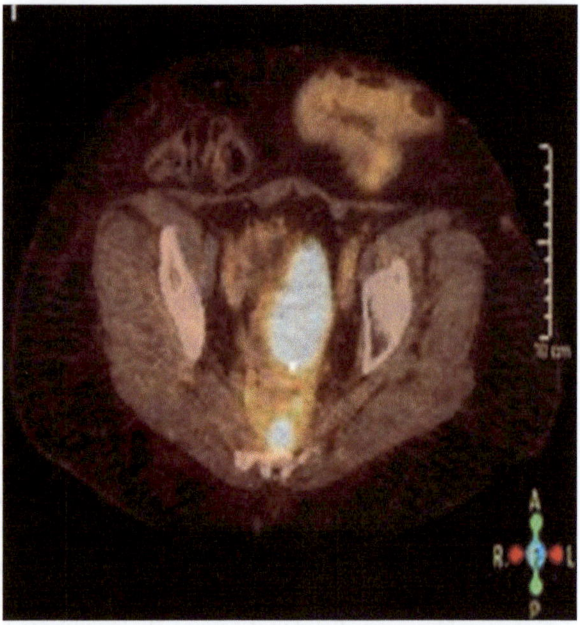

Fig. 81.4 Local recurrence confirmed by PET positive

Discussion

Local recurrence of rectum cancer after surgery has for many years been associated with inadequate operative techniques [1]. The introduction of the TME concept and

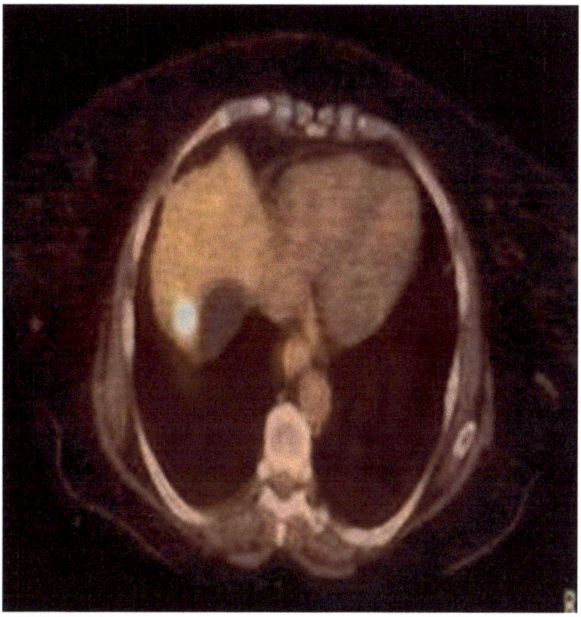

Fig. 81.5 Liver metastasis PET-CT

neoadjuvant chemo-radiotherapy has importantly reduced the local recurrence rate to less than 10 %.

In the Dutch TME trial after a median follow-up of 6 years for surviving patients, the established 5-year local recurrence risk of those patients undergoing a macroscopically complete local resection in case of preoperative radiotherapy was 5.6 %, as compared with 10.9 % in those patients undergoing TME alone. Moreover, overall survival was not different between the two groups (64.2 % and 63.5 %), respectively. Subgroup analysis showed significant effect of radiotherapy in reducing local recurrence risk for patients with nodal involvement, patients with lesions between 5 and 10 cm from anal verge, and for patients with uninvolved CRM margins [2]. Analyzing the patterns of local recurrence in patients included in the Dutch TME trial, Kusters et al. studied 1417 patients of which 713 were randomized into preoperative radiotherapy and total mesorectal excision (RT + TME) and 704 patients into TME alone. Of the 114 patients with local recurrence (LR), the subsites of LR were determined and related to tumor and treatment factors. Presacral local recurrences occurred most in both groups [3]. Radiotherapy reduced anastomotic LR significantly, except when after low anterior resection (LAR) distal margins were less than 5 mm. Abdominoperineal resection (APR) mainly resulted in presacral LR. Thirty percent of the patients had advanced tumors, which resulted in 58 % of all LRs. Lateral LR comprised 20 % of all LRs. Presacral and lateral LR resulted in a poor prognosis, in contrast to anterior or anastomotic LRs with a relatively good prognosis. They concluded that RT reduces LR in all subsites and is especially effective in preventing anastomotic LR after LAR. APR surgery mainly results in presacral LR, which may be prevented by a wider resection (cylindrical type).

Rahbari et al. posed the question, In the era of TME is there still a chance for cure of locally recurrent rectal cancer? [4].

Surgical resection was performed in 92 patients with LR and negative resection margins were achieved in 54 (58.7 %) of these. Recurrent disease was located intraluminal and extraluminal in 35 (38.0 %) patients and 57 (62.0 %) patients, respectively. A total of 19 (20.6 %) patients had extrapelvic metastatic disease at the time of surgery. Perioperative surgical morbidity and in-hospital mortality accounted for 42.4 % and 3.3 %, respectively. On multivariate analysis, partial sacrectomy was associated with surgical morbidity. Three- and five-year disease-specific survival rates were 61 and 47 %. On multivariate analysis, surgical morbidity, presence of extrapelvic disease, and non-curative resection were identified as independent adverse predictors of disease-specific survival. They concluded that surgical resection of local recurrence from rectal cancer in the era TME can be carried out with acceptable morbidity and curative resection rates. Curative resection remains the major prognostic factor.

Dresden et al. studied 147 patients surgically treated because of locally recurrent rectal cancer. Type of surgery was LAR in 54 %, APR in 32 %, abdominotranssacral resection in 26 %, pelvic exanteration in 11 %, and non-anatomic resection in 11 %. Important part of the treatment was the neoadjuvant therapy given in the form of re-irradiation and chemotherapy to the recurrent tumor [5]. Surgery was planned 8–10 weeks after completion of neoadjuvant therapy. Moreover intraoperative radiotherapy (IOERT) was administered in different doses (10–17.5 Gy) according to the outcome of the frozen section during the intervention. They concluded that radical resection is the most significant predictor of improved survival in patients with LR. Neoadjuvant radio-(chemo)therapy is the best option in order to realize a radical resection. Re-irradiation is feasible in patients who already received irradiation as part of the primary rectal cancer treatment.

Concerning the level of sacrectomy and its consequences, distal sacrectomy (S3–S5) has little sequels, whereas the superior S1–S3 has as consequences a neurogenic bladder if the S2 roots are not preserved. Concerning stability of the spine after sacrectomy, this is maintained if the first sacral vertebra is preserved [6].

References

1. Quircke P, Durdey P, Dixon MF, et al. Local recurrence of rectal adenocarcinoma due to inadequate surgical resection. Histopathological study of lateral tumour spread and surgical excision. Lancet. 1986;2:996–9.
2. Peeters KCMJ, Marijnen CAM, Nagtegaal ID, et al. The TME trial after a median follow-up of 6 years. Increased local control but no survival benefit in irradiated patients with resectable rectal carcinoma. Ann Surg. 2007;246:693–701.
3. Kusters M, Marijnen CA, van de Velde CJ, et al. Patterns of local recurrence in rectal cancer; a study of the Dutch TME trial. Eur J Surg Oncol. 2010;36:470–6.
4. Rahbari NN, Ulrich AB, Bruckner T, et al. Surgery for locally recurrent rectal cancer in the era of Total mesorectal excision: is there still a chance for cure ? Ann Surg. 2011;253:522–33.

5. Dresden RC, Gosens MJ, Martijn H, et al. Radical resection after IORT-containing multimodality treatment is the most important determinant for outcome in patients treated for locally recurrent rectal cancer. Ann Surg Oncol. 2008;15:1937–47.
6. Garcia Sabrido JL, Vega D, Calvo F, et al. Tumores sacropelvicos primarios y secundarios. Tratamiento con cirugia radical y radioterapia intraoperatoria. Cir Esp. 2003;73:78–87.

Chapter 82
Case on Complication After Laparoscopic Abdominal Lavage Because of Perforated Diverticulitis

Teresa Sanchez Rodriguez

Keywords Perforated diverticulitis • Peritoneal lavage • Laparoscopy • Hartmann procedure • Peritonitis

Diagnosis and Indication for Surgery

This was a 72-year-old patient who presented with clinical symptoms suggestive of generalized peritonitis. There had been no prior history of abdominal complaints or operations. No changes in the stool pattern. He had a leukocytosis of 23,000 and CRP was 64. Clinical suspicion was of general peritonitis by perforation of a hollow organ. A CT-scan showed features of generalized peritonitis with widespread diverticulitis in the sigmoid and free intra-abdominal fluid and free air (Figs. 82.1 and 82.2). The patient's comorbid conditions were classed as ASA II to III.

Operation

Emergency operation by diagnostic laparoscopy was carried out with intraoperative findings confirming purulent diverticulitis classified according to Hinchey, as stage III disease.

Intravenous fluids and antibiotics were started in the emergency room.

A laparoscopic peritoneal lavage was performed. Pneumoperitoneum was established by open laparoscopy and an umbilical port of 12 mm. Two 5-mm ports were placed in the suprapubic and right-lower quadrants to facilitate manipulation and

T.S. Rodriguez, M.D.
Department of Surgery, Virgen del Rocio, Sevilla, Spain
e-mail: tresasr@hotmail.com

M.A. Cuesta, H.J. Bonjer (eds.), *Case Studies of Postoperative Complications after Digestive Surgery*, DOI 10.1007/978-3-319-01613-9_82,

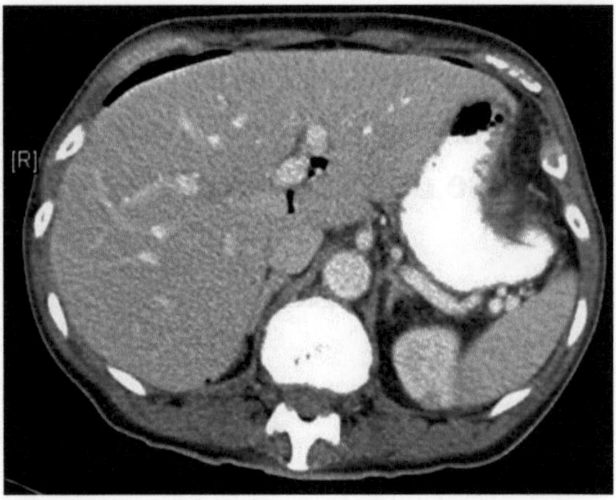

Fig. 82.1 CT scan, diverticulitis

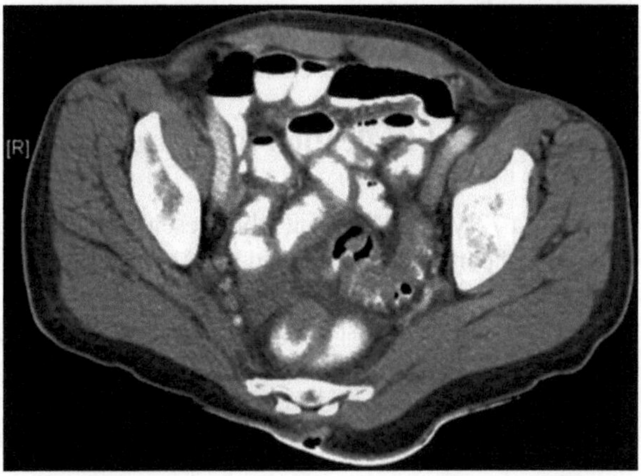

Fig. 82.2 CT scan, pneumoperitoneum

lavage. The peritoneal cavity was examined thoroughly; the inflamed segment of the colon was localized. All purulent fluid was cultivated and aspirated, and the peritoneal lavage was performed in all four quadrants using four liters of warmed saline until the drainage was clear. Two flat drains (Jackson Pratt) were left, in the pelvis through the 5-mm trocars in the lower quadrants.

Postoperative Course: Identification and Treatment of Complication

Patient was admitted to the intensive care ward, being mechanical ventilated. After 24 h, he became hemodynamically unstable with abdominal pain, fever of 38.7 °C, and tachycardia of 126 bpm. Leukocytosis was still present, 23,000 with CRP of 278. As a consequence, we decided to perform an explorative laparotomy. A fecal peritonitis was found, with a diverticulitis perforation in the sigmoid, and a Hartmann's procedure was performed after rinsing the abdomen.

The patient remained in ICU with respiratory support for 3 days. Pneumonia was treated by means of antibiotics and deep wound infection managed with drainage and debridement.

The recovery of the patient was gradual and he could leave the hospital after 4 weeks. Six months later, he recovered definitively after reversal of the Hartmann and a reconstruction of the abdominal wall because of incisional hernia.

Discussion

Diverticular disease of the colon is common in the Western world, with a prevalence of approximately 33 % in patients over 60 years of age. Perforation associated with diverticular disease, as first manifestation of the disease has concurrently increased in prevalence from 2.4 cases per 100,000 in 1986 to 3.8 cases per 100,000 in 2000 [1].

The management of complicated diverticulitis disease in the emergency setting continues to evolve. The great majority of colorectal surgeons have accepted Hartmann's procedure (HP) as the "golden standard." Drawbacks include the need of a colostomy, high morbidity of 30 % with a mortality of 10 %. Additionally significant is that in 20–50 % of those patients undergoing a Hartmann's procedure, the colostomy will never be reversed [2]. Moreover, there are also high complication rates for stoma reversal procedures, with anastomotic leaks ranging from 2 to 30 %. Therefore, other procedures have been studied to approach the perforation, such as primary resection and anastomosis (PRA) with or without protective ileostomy.

Several studies have reported on comparable morbidity and mortality rates after PRA when compared with HP for perforated diverticulitis [3]. Furthermore, wound infection rate has been reported as 9.6 % for PRA versus 24.2 % for HP. Overall anastomotic leakage rate for PRA was 13.9 %, whereas stoma-related complication rate for HP was 10.3 %. Primary anastomosis with a proximal defunctioning stoma (PADS) was shown to result in even better outcomes in terms of anastomotic leakage and wound infection as compared with simple PRA [4]. Yet, due to significant selection bias in their results, only limited conclusions can be drawn from the existing studies.

Until now, truly evidence-based studies have not been performed.

Considering the high morbidity and mortality rates, the role of the laparoscopic lavage introduced by Meyers et al. may be considered as remarkable [5].

Laparoscopic management is a reasonable alternative to the traditionally open resection for Hinchey grade III perforated diverticulitis with generalized peritonitis. Eight patients out of hundred with grade 4 diverticulitis had to be converted to an open Hartmann's procedure. The remaining 92 patients were managed by laparoscopic lavage, with morbidity and mortality rates of 4 and 3 %, respectively. Two patients required postoperative intervention for a pelvic abscess. Only two patients represented with diverticulitis at a median follow-up of 36 months (range 12–84).

This approach has a low mortality rate—despite patient comorbidity and disease severity. Benefits include stoma avoidance and the lower rate of wound complications such as dehiscence and wound infection, with the high risk of incisional hernia. If during laparoscopy a fecal peritonitis is found (Hinchey IV), the patient should undergo a Hartmann procedure.

References

1. Jacobs DO. Clinical practice. Diverticulitis. N Engl J Med. 2007;357:2057–66.
2. Constantinides AV, Heriot A, et al. Operative strategies for diverticular peritonitis. A decision analysis between primary resection and anastomosis versus Hartmann's procedures. Ann Surg. 2007;245:94–103.
3. Outcome Trenti L, Biondo S, et al. Generalized peritonitis due to perforated diverticulitis: Hartmann's procedure or primary anastomosis? Int J Colorectal Dis. 2011;26:377–84.
4. Gooszen AW, Gooszen HG, Veerman W, et al. Operative treatment of acute complications of diverticular disease: primary or secondary anastomosis after sigmoid resection. Eur J Surg. 2001;167:35–9.
5. Myers E, Hurley M, O'Sullivan GC, et al. Laparoscopic peritoneal lavage for generalized peritonitis due to perforated diverticulitis. Br J Surg. 2008;95:97–101.

Chapter 83
Case on Anastomotic Leakage After Taken Down Hartmann Procedure

Niels de Korte

Keywords Diverticulitis • Sigmoid resection • Hartmann procedure • Leakage anastomosis • Peritonitis

Diagnosis and Indication for Surgery

A 70-year-old female patient presented with a 3-month history of abdominal pain, weight loss, and diarrhea. Fifteen years before, a Hartmann procedure had been performed for a perforated diverticulitis. Three months postoperatively the colostomy had been taken down without complications. Her additional history included chronic atrial fibrillation.

A CT angiography was performed on suspicion of abdominal angina, but showed no signs of stenosis in the visceral vessels. There was however evidence of a significant stenotic segment at the level of the anastomosis at the promontory (Fig. 83.1). A contrast enema was performed showing a stenotic segment. A sigmoidoscopy showed no tumor at the level of anastomosis. Because endoscopic dilatations were not effective, patient was scheduled for a resection of the segment.

Operation

A laparotomy was performed through the old scar. On palpation, a stenotic segment of colon was felt at the site of the anastomosis. A resection of the stenotic segment was performed in which the distal part of the resection was about 7 cm proximal of the pelvic floor. The splenic flexure was mobilized to achieve a tension-free anastomosis.

N. de Korte, M.D.
Department of Surgery, Spaarne Hospital, Hoofddorp, The Netherlands
e-mail: ndekorte@yahoo.com

M.A. Cuesta, H.J. Bonjer (eds.), *Case Studies of Postoperative Complications after Digestive Surgery*, DOI 10.1007/978-3-319-01613-9_83,

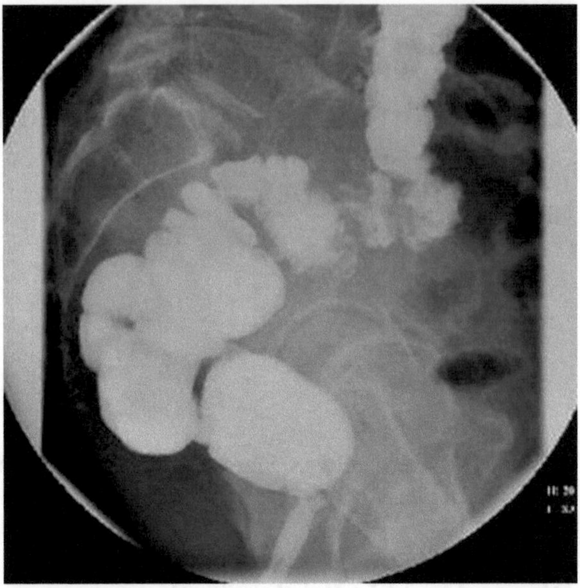

Fig. 83.1 Stenosis at the anastomosis, after take down of a Hartmann procedure

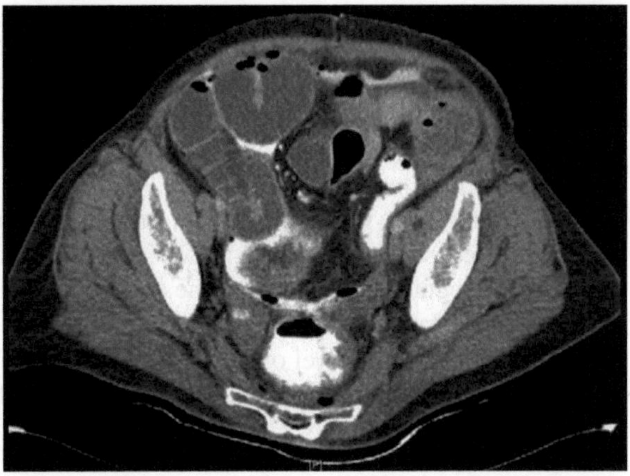

Fig. 83.2 CT scan, leakage of anastomosis with rectal contrast outside the colon

The anastomosis was performed in a side-to-end fashion using the double-stapled technique with a 31 CEEA stapler. A drain was left in the presacral space.

Postoperative Course: Identification and Treatment of Complication

After the 10th postoperative day, the patient developed fever and abdominal pain. A CT scan with rectal and intravenous contrast showed a large amount of air subdiaphragmatic and the evidence of contrast and air leakage at the site of the anastomosis (Fig. 83.2). No abscesses were visible.

Under diagnosis of leakage of the anastomosis, a relaparotomy was performed. During operation, an abscess was found at the site of the anastomosis and an anastomotic leakage of about one-third of the circumference was observed. The anastomosis was taken down and an end-colostomy was created.

The patient developed signs of abdominal sepsis with multiple organ failure. She was admitted to the ICU, mechanical ventilated, and hemodialysis was started because of acute renal insufficiency (ARI). Broad-spectrum antibiotics were iv administered. After 2 days she could we weaned off the mechanical ventilator, and hemodialysis could be stopped after 1 week.

After 14 days, she left the hospital and after 3 months a follow-up at the outpatient department showed she was doing fine. Her colostomy is functioning well. She expressed no desire to attempt restoring bowel continuity.

Discussion

Anastomotic leakage is the most dreaded complication after colorectal surgery. Incidence in the literature varies from 1 to 26 %, with lower anastomosis carrying a higher risk of failure [1]. The literature on the management of anastomotic leakage is scarce and controversial. Historically, the dismantling of the anastomosis and colostomy creation proved to be a safe option, especially in the presence of diffuse peritonitis or ischemia at the level of the anastomosis. The fact that in 70–100 % of these patients the colostomy is never taken down [1, 2] has led to the development of treatment options where the anastomosis is not dismantled. Some series have reported favorable results using the concept of creating a de-functioning stoma above the anastomosis and local drainage [3]. In these series, this is used for patients having small defects in the anastomosis, only local contamination, and no vascular compromise. Closure of the anastomotic defect using Transanal Endoscopic Microsurgery [4] or fibrin glue [5] has been described in small series as having good results.

Summing up, the procedure of choice in treating an anastomotic leakage is influenced by numerous factors including the patient's general condition on reoperation, degree of peritonitis, comorbidity, vascular status of bowel ends, age, and the extent of leakage. In the present case, because of the patient's age, her septic profile at reoperation and the extent of dehiscence, the anastomosis was taken down, creating a definitive colostomy.

References

1. Khan AA, Wheeler JM, Cunningham C, et al. The management and outcome of anastomotic leaks in colorectal surgery. Colorectal Dis. 2008;10:587–92.
2. Maggiori L, Bretagnol F, Lefèvre JH, et al. Conservative management is associated with a decreased risk of definitive stoma after anastomotic leakage complicating sphincter-saving resection for rectal cancer. Colorectal Dis. 2011;13:632–7.

3. Wind J, Koopman AG, van Berge Henegouwen MI, et al. Laparoscopic reintervention for anastomotic leakage after primary laparoscopic colorectal surgery. Br J Surg. 2007;94:1562–6.
4. Beunis A, Pauli S, Van Cleemput M. Anastomotic leakage of a colorectal anastomosis treated by transanal endoscopic microsurgery. Acta Chir Belg. 2008;108:474–6.
5. Testi W, Vernillo R, Spagnulo M, et al. Endoscopic treatment of intestinal anastomotic leakage in low anterior resection of the rectum by using fibrin adhesive. Our experience. Minerva Chir. 2002;57:683–8.

Chapter 84
Case on Complication After Sacrocolpopexy

Chan Yuan

Keywords Vaginal prolapse • Sacrocolpopexy • Bleeding • Rectal perforation • Ileostomy

Diagnosis and Indication for Surgery

A 65-year-old female was operated on because of prolapse of the vagina, causing defecation problems. Twenty years ago she underwent an appendectomy and a hysterectomy because of uterus fibroid 10 years previously.

Operation

A laparoscopic sacrocolpopexy was intended, yet because of multiple adhesions intra-abdominally, a conversion to laparotomy became required. After dissection of the rectum and apex of vagina, a polypropylene mesh was sutured to the vaginal apex and that at the level of the sacrum promontory.

Postoperative Course: Identification and Treatment of Complication

Patient had a difficult postoperative course. Postoperative thrombosis of the left iliac vein occurred and the use of coumarin was started (Fig. 84.1). Because of a bowel obstruction and rectal blood loss, a MRI was performed. A large hematoma

C. Yuan, M.D.
Department of Surgery, VU University Medical Center, Amsterdam, The Netherlands

M.A. Cuesta, H.J. Bonjer (eds.), *Case Studies of Postoperative Complications after Digestive Surgery*, DOI 10.1007/978-3-319-01613-9_84,

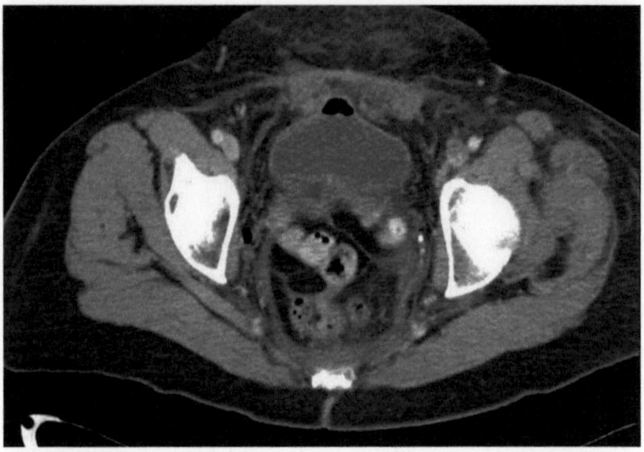

Fig. 84.1 CT scan showing the thrombosis left iliac vein

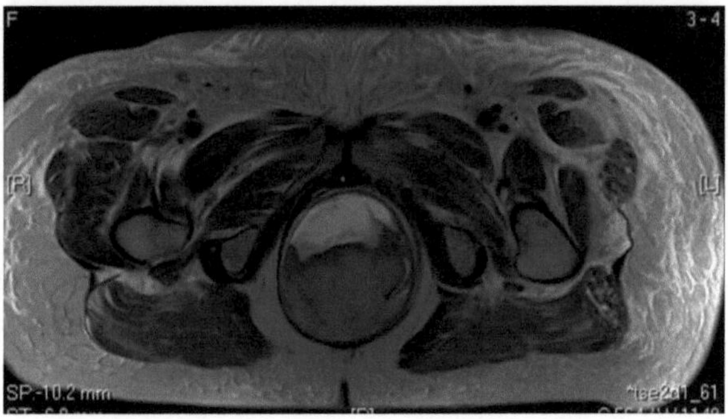

Fig. 84.2 MRI, bleeding in the rectal wall after sacrocolpopexy

was found in the rectal wall, ulcerating through the wall (Fig. 84.2). After 3 days of conservative treatment, a new CT scan showed suspect for rectal perforation (Fig. 84.3); hence, the surgeon decided to perform a relaparotomy. As consequence of the previous operations, extensive adhesions were found in the lower abdomen. Pelvic hematoma was drained and an ileostomy performed to deviate the feces. By palpation it seemed that the perforation caused an important circumferential defect of the rectum. The initial plan was to leave the ileostomy for at least a period of 6 months, so the hematoma and inflammation of the pelvis could subside. Yet, after 3 months the ileostomy was causing important care problems with continuous leakage and high production including dehydration. A proctoscopy showed that at least the last 8 cm of the rectum were normal. Through a laparotomy a rectosigmoid resection of a stenosed and fibrotic traject was performed with a distal colorectal anastomosis, result being the ileostomy closed. To deviate the feces, a colostomy proximal to the anastomosis was created. After 6 months, the control of the anastomosis by enema (Fig. 84.4) showed a good patent anastomosis without leakage, and the colostomy could be closed. After 2 months a stenosis of the anastomosis was found—being digitally dilated under anesthesia. The patient is currently continent for feces and has no recurrence of the vaginal prolapse.

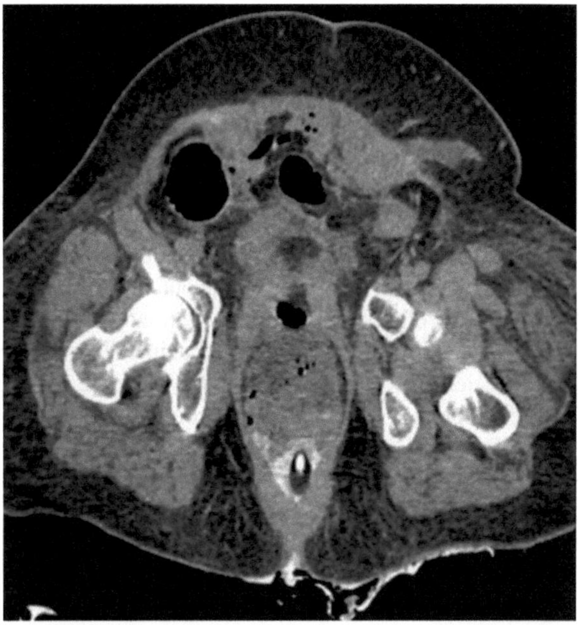

Fig. 84.3 CT scan, rectal wall perforation after bleeding (contrast outside rectum)

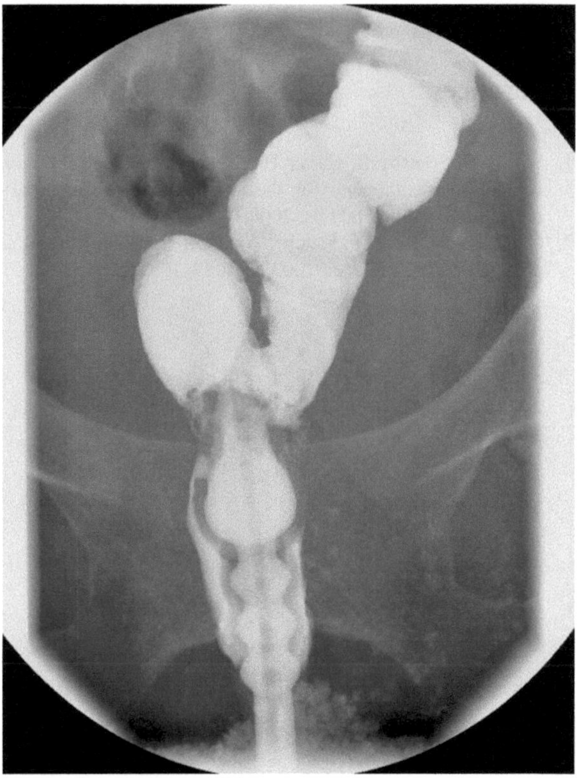

Fig. 84.4 Enema, control of the anastomosis, no leakage

Discussion

An explanation for this complication could probably be that during conversion to laparotomy, a lesion was made at the rectal wall. Treatment with coumarin because of the iliac vein thrombosis could have induced bleeding of a rectal wall leading to rectal perforation. The deviating ileostomy worked properly by diverting the feces, but it was too short and continually caused problems and leaks. After low anterior resection, the anastomosis healed without problems and finally the colostomy could be reversed. Slawik et al. studied the outcome of laparoscopic ventral rectopexy and vaginal sacrocolpopexy [1] for the treatment of recto-genital prolapse in 80 patients and found complications in 21 %: fecal impaction 4 %, wound infection 2 %, bleeding 2 %, leakage 1 %. Ganatra et al. reviewed the current status of laparoscopic sacrocolpopexy for vaginal vault prolapse (VVP) and multicompartmental Pelvic Organ Prolapse [2]. In comparison with the vaginal sacrocolpopexy—up-to-now the gold standard—abdominal sacrocolpopexy (ASC) seems to be superior to VVP for having fewer incidences of recurrent prolapse and less dyspareunia. They reported outcomes from 11 series with more than 1,000 patients. Mean operative time was 158 min with a 2.7 % conversion rate and a 1.6 % early reoperation rate. With a mean follow-up of 24.6 months there was, on average, a 94.4 % satisfaction rate, a 6.2 % prolapse reoperation rate, and a 2.7 % mesh erosion rate.

References

1. Slawik S, Soulsby R, Carter H. Laparoscopic ventral rectopexy, posterior colporrhaphy and vaginal sacrocolpopexy for the treatment of recto-genital prolapse and mechanical outlet obstruction. Colorectal Dis. 2008;10:138–43.
2. Ganatra AM, Rozet F, Sanchez Salas R, et al. The current status of laparoscopic sacrocolpopexy: a review. Eur Urol. 2009;55:1089–103.

Chapter 85
Case on Ischemia–Necrosis of the Sigmoid After Repair of a Ruptured Juxtarenal Aneurysm

Jorg de Bruin

Keyword Aorta aneurysm • Juxtarenal aneurysm • Aortic prosthesis • Renal cooling • Acute renal insufficiency • Sigmoid ischemia

Diagnosis and Indication for Surgery

A 62-year-old patient was presented to our emergency department with nausea, lower back, and abdominal pain. He had a history of hypertension, dyslipidemia, and repair of a traumatic rupture of an Achilles tendon. The pain had started 18 h before presentation and was progressive over time. On physical examination, he was in shock, had tachycardia, and a large pulsatile mass in the abdomen. Ultrasound revealed an aneurysm of 7.2 cm in diameter. Computerized tomography scanning showed a ruptured juxtarenal abdominal aortic aneurysm with a retroperitoneal haematoma (Fig. 85.1).

Operation

The patient was transferred to the operating room and underwent open repair of the juxtarenal aneurysm. The clamp had to be placed suprarenal with renal cooling of both kidneys during the clamping time; however, the anastomosis could be made infrarenal. The anastomosis distally was adjacent to the bifurcation. An aorta-femoral bypass was made on the left side due to stenosis of the iliac segment. Blood

J. de Bruin, M.D.
Department of Surgery, VU Medical Center, Amsterdam, The Netherlands
e-mail: jl.debruin@vumc.nl

M.A. Cuesta, H.J. Bonjer (eds.), *Case Studies of Postoperative Complications after Digestive Surgery*, DOI 10.1007/978-3-319-01613-9_85,

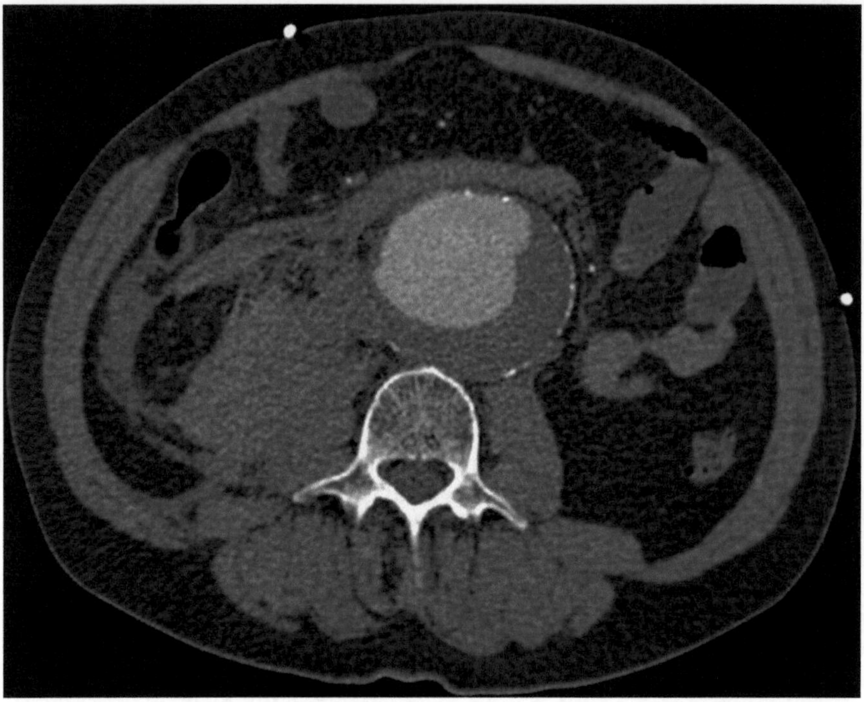

Fig. 85.1 CT scan, juxtarenal abdominal aorta aneurysm

loss was 800 cc. Postoperatively, the patient was transferred to the intensive care unit.

Postoperative Course: Identification and Treatment of Complication

During the first 24 h, the patient developed acute renal insufficiency and remained dependent on noradrenalin. After 48 h, the patient's condition worsened and he developed lactic acidosis with bowel distension. A colonoscopy was performed, under suspicion of sigmoid ischemia, showing ulcerative colitis with ischemia in the sigmoid (Fig. 85.2). Patient was transferred to the operating room and a laparotomy was performed; during the operation, ischemic changes of the sigmoid and left descending colon were seen. A left-sided colectomy was performed, rectal stump closed, and a colostomy was made (Illustration 85.1). The abdomen could not be closed without tension; therefore, a double Vicryl mesh® was used. After the second operation, the patient received two additional interventions to remove contaminated fluids in the pelvic space. Moreover, he had myocardial infarction due to a coronary stenosis; therefore, an angioplasty with coronary stenting was done. Three months after initial surgery, a split skin graft was performed to cover the large abdominal wound.

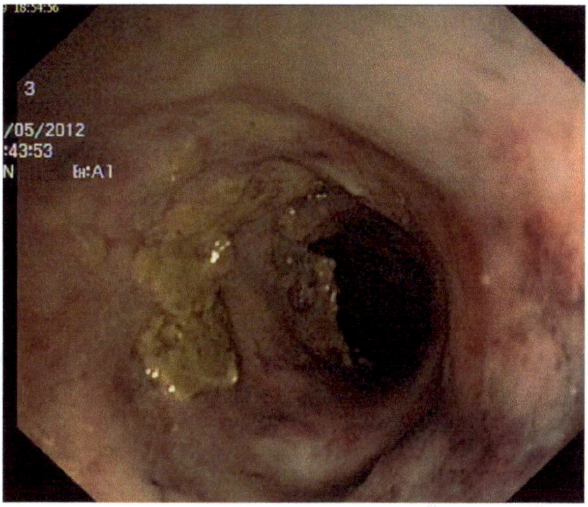

Fig. 85.2 Colonoscopy: ischemia of the sigmoid

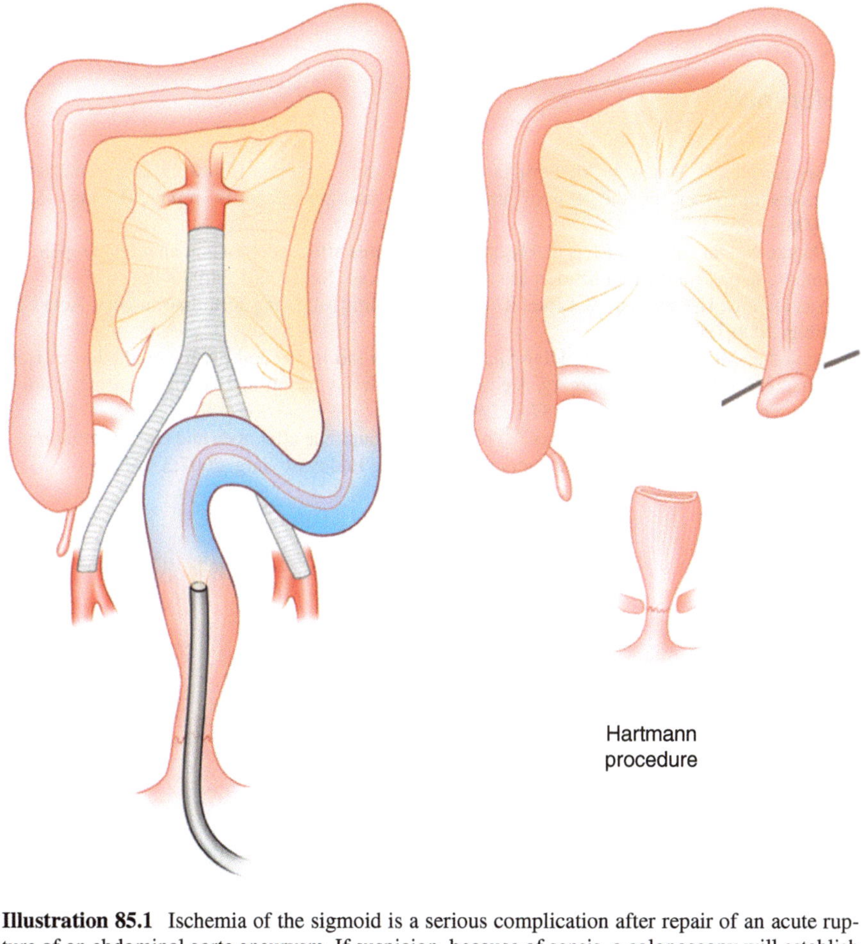

Illustration 85.1 Ischemia of the sigmoid is a serious complication after repair of an acute rupture of an abdominal aorta aneurysm. If suspicion, because of sepsis, a colonoscopy will establish the diagnosis. A sigmoid resection and Hartmann procedure should be done

Discussion

Several risk factors leading to colonic ischemia (CI) after abdominal aortic aneurysm repair have been identified: aneurysm rupture, long duration of operation, and prior renal disease [1]. The incidence of CI has not changed with the introduction of endovascular aortic aneurysm repair [1, 2]. After elective open abdominal aortic aneurysm repair, the rate of incidences vary between 1 and 3 % [2, 3]. However, after ruptured aneurysm, the incidence of clinically significant CI reaches 10 %. Routine postoperative colonoscopy shows higher incidences of ischemic colitis after both elective and ruptured aneurysm repair [4]. A definitive diagnosis is best made by colonoscopy. Diagnosis of CI is strongly associated with poor survival—especially after ruptured abdominal aortic aneurysm repair [5]. In the case of ischemia by colonoscopy and a hemodynamic unstable patient or having high lactate, ischemia should be considered transmural and a laparotomy should be performed. During laparotomy the ischemic part of the left colon or sigmoid has to be resected followed by creation of a left abdomen colostomy (Hartmann procedure).

References

1. Becquemin JP, Majewski M, Fermani N, et al. Colon ischemia following abdominal aortic aneurysm repair in the era of endovascular abdominal aortic repair. J Vasc Surg. 2008;47:258–63.
2. Dadian N, Ohki T, Veith FJ, et al. Overt colon ischemia after endovascular aneurysm repair: the importance of microembolization as an etiology. J Vasc Surg. 2001;34:986–96.
3. Van Damme H, Creemers E, Limet R. Ischaemic colitis following aortoiliac surgery. Acta Chir Belg. 2000;100:21–7.
4. Schiedler MG, Cutler BS, Fiddian-Green RG. Sigmoid intramural pH for prediction of ischemic colitis during aortic surgery. A comparison with risk factors and inferior mesenteric artery stump pressures. Arch Surg. 1987;122:881–6.
5. Acosta S, Lindblad B, Zdanowski Z. Predictors for outcome after open and endovascular repair of ruptured abdominal aortic aneurysms. Eur J Vasc Endovasc Surg. 2007;33:277–84.

Chapter 86
Case on Complications and Approach in Post-radiation Enteritis

Suzanne S. Gisbertz

Keywords Cervix cancer • Radiotherapy • Radiation enteritis • Parenteral nutrition • Laparotomy

First Patient

Diagnosis and Indication for Chemoradiotherapy

A 36-year-old supermarket employee was diagnosed of having a cervix carcinoma stage IIB (Fig. 86.1). The patient was proposed to treat the tumor by chemoradiotherapy, in this case, the external radiotherapy of 23 × 2 Grays in combination with weekly iv. Cisplatin® was given, and between the fourth and sixth week, HDR brachytherapy (2 × 8.5 Grays) at the place of point A of cervix was administered through the Fletcher applications system (Fig. 86.2 and Illustration 86.1a).

Postoperative Course: Identification and Treatment of Complication

The tumor responded optimally to the treatment, but the patient started experiencing abdominal cramps, diarrhea, and weight loss. Suspicion arose of radiation enteritis and this was confirmed by the CT scan. After a period of 3 months, the patient's appetite was decreasing and she had started vomiting. Her abdomen was found distended and in spite of extra nutrition advice, she ended up with a weight of 40 kg. So, she was admitted to the department of gynecology for treatment. Total

S.S. Gisbertz, M.D.
Department of Surgery, Academic Medical Center, Amsterdam, The Netherlands
e-mail: s.gisbertz@antoniusziekenhuis.nl

M.A. Cuesta, H.J. Bonjer (eds.), *Case Studies of Postoperative Complications after Digestive Surgery*, DOI 10.1007/978-3-319-01613-9_86,

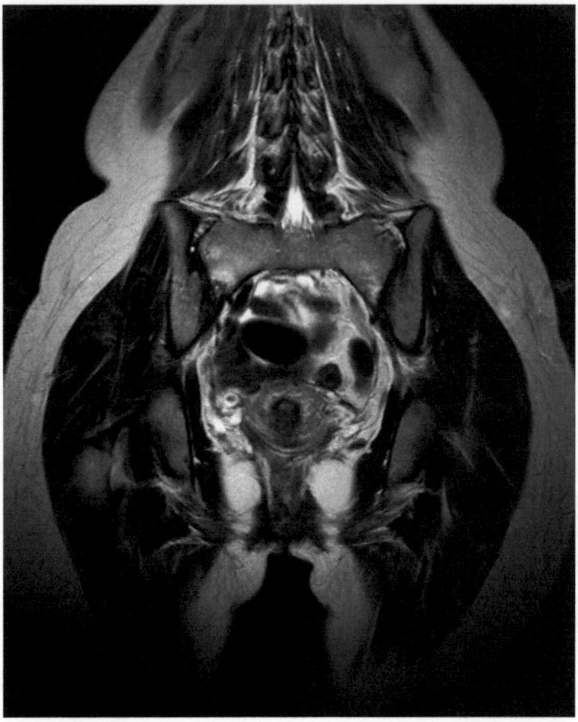

Fig. 86.1 MRI, cervix carcinoma stage 2B

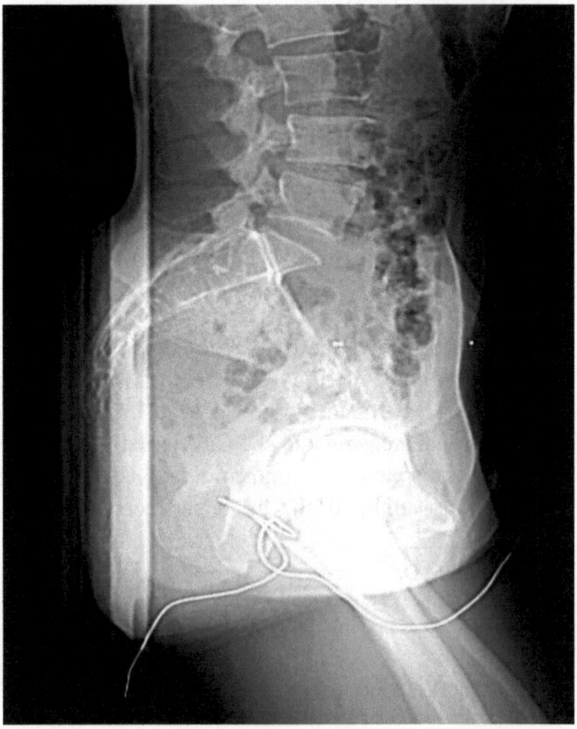

Fig. 86.2 Brachytherapy treatment

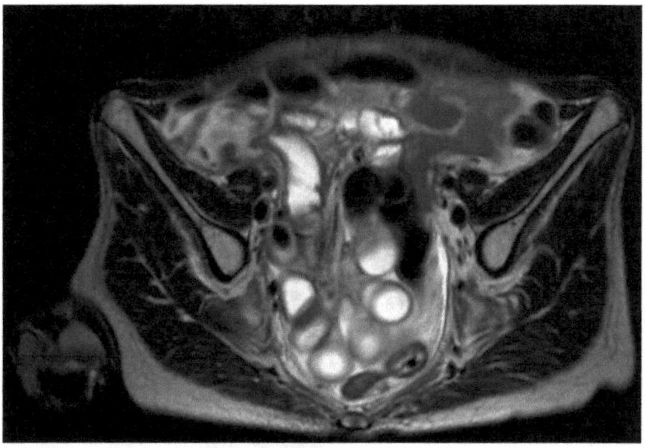

Fig. 86.3 MRI, 9 months later radiation enteritis

parenteral nutrition was started and surgeons were consulted. Exploring the patient and seeing the CT scan, we observed a malnourished young patient having a strong abdominal distension as caused by small bowel and having colonic ileus as caused by stenosis of the sigmoid. Moreover, radiation enteritis of the distal loops of small bowel was observed (Figs. 86.3 and 86.4a, b). The stomach was also dilated. Treatment was started with the TPN, nasogastric tube, and metabolic correction of electrolytes. This situation was considered chronic and in talks with patient and family we advised her to take at least 6–8 weeks of time for improving her general condition and weight before a laparotomy could be planned. Despite her acute disappointment, she accepted this proposal. After the period of 6 weeks her weight now was 47 kg with still abdominal distention and intestinal obstruction. A laparotomy was performed; loops of ileum were covering a proximal rectal perforation of 10 cm at the anterior side. Small bowel was thick but patent. Rectum was dissected distal of perforation and at normal aspect (7 cm from anal verge) was divided by means of stapler device. We decided do not perform a primary anastomosis and an end-colostomy was created outside of the radiation field at the left upper abdomen (Illustration 86.1b). Her postoperative period was uncomplicated, and the patient could be discharged after 10 days without TPN. At gynecological examination, a complete regression of the tumor in the cervix was observed. After a period of 6 months, she suggested taking down the colostomy. Rectal enema was considered normal and the intervention was performed after mobilizing the splenic flexure and transverse colon conveniently (Illustration 86.1b). Small bowel loops were still thick but patent. She recovered very quickly and could be discharged after a week. She is under control of gynecology and surgery. On MRI scan, no rest of the tumor is seen.

Second Patient

Diagnosis and Indication for Surgery

A 44-year-old female patient was diagnosed with rectal cancer. She had been referred by her general practitioner to a local hospital with rectal blood loss. Physical

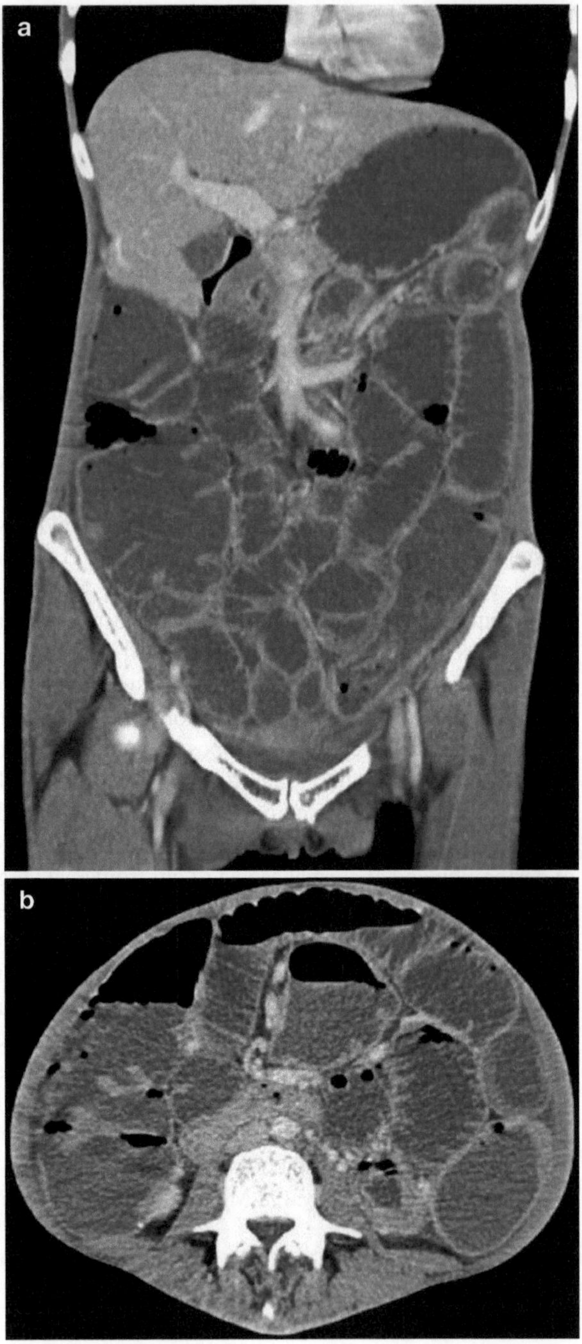

Fig. 86.4 (**a**) CT scan, obstruction at the level of the sigmoid and small bowel ileus. (**b**) CT scan showing intestinal obstruction

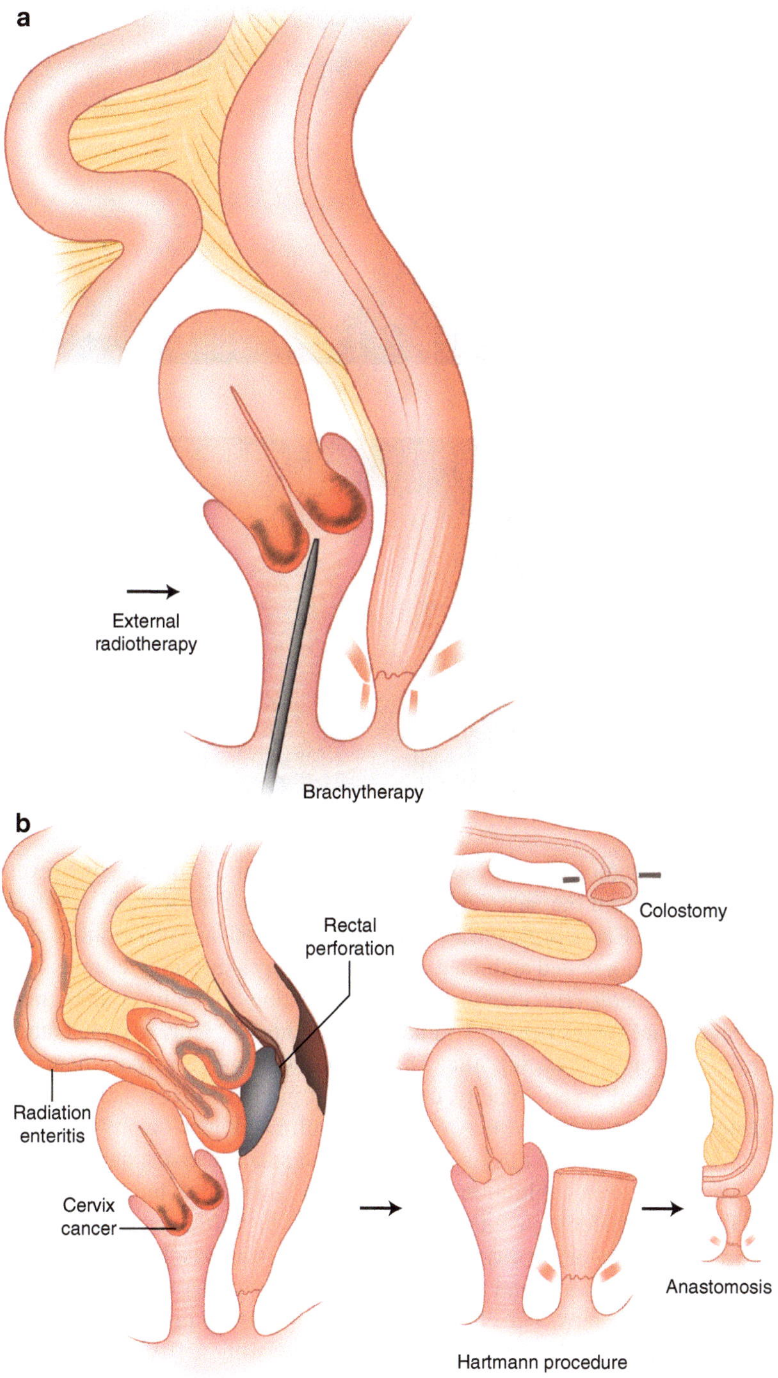

Illustration 86.1 (**a**, **b**) A minority of cases with radiation enterocolitis is managed by a surgical intervention. Most patients can be treated with supportive care such as fluid replenishment and nutritional support. Indications for surgery usually comprise of gastrointestinal obstruction, perforation, or severe proctitis

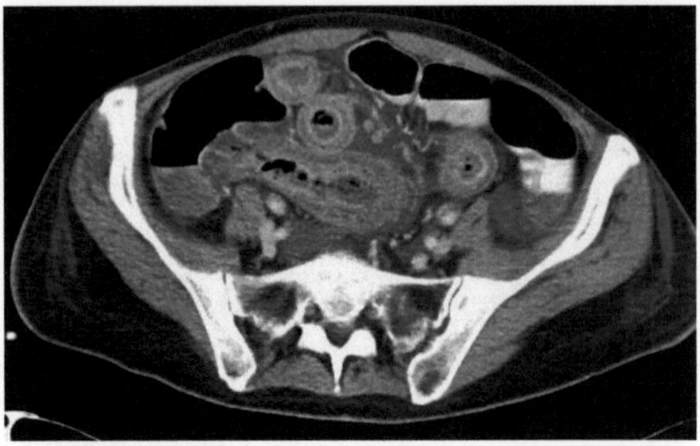

Fig. 86.5 CT scan showing thickened walls of the small intestine, distended colon, infiltration of the mesentery, and free fluid

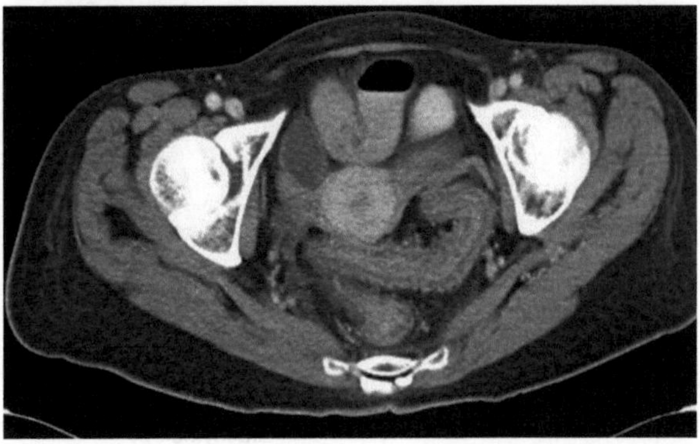

Fig. 86.6 CT scan showing a thickened rectosigmoid loop

examination, including rectal examination, was normal. A colonoscopy revealed a tumor at 10 cm from the anal verge. Biopsies showed a moderately differentiated adenocarcinoma. Endoscopic ultrasound and pelvic MRI staged the tumor as T2N2. CT scanning of thorax and abdomen did not show any signs of metastases. She was treated with neoadjuvant chemoradiation consisting of daily administration of Capecitabine and 5 days per week radiation fractions of 2 Gray to a total amount of 50 Gray in 5 weeks. However, after 18 fractions and in a little more than 3 weeks later she developed severe toxicity, consisting of grade III diarrhea, nausea, vomiting, neutropenic fever, and with a distended, painful abdomen on physical examination. CT scanning showed thickened walls of the small intestine and rectosigmoid loop, distended colon, infiltration of the mesentery, and free fluid (Figs. 86.5 and 86.6). She was transferred to an academic hospital for further treatment. There she was treated with supportive therapy consisting of intravenous fluids, total parenteral nutrition, pain medication, and antibiotics. Seven weeks after the discontinuation of the neoadjuvant therapy, her clinical condition improved in such extent that she could be operated on. She, however, retained low weight (weight 48 kg, length 1.73 m, BMI 16).

Operation Description

A laparoscopic low anterior resection was performed. The rectosigmoidal junction had an inflamed aspect with a thick wall and vascular injection. We therefore chose not to perform an anastomosis; instead a colostomy in the descending colon was created.

Oncologic Stage

The pathological–anatomical investigation revealed a radically removed tumor without lymph node involvement, therefore classified as T1N0M0. Additionally, extensive chemoradiation therapy effects were shown.

Postoperative Course: Identification and Treatment of Complication

The postoperative course of this patient was uneventful; no complications occurred.

One year postoperatively, a colonoscopy of the distal rectum and of the colon via the colostomy was performed, as well as a MRI enteroclysis for visualization of the small intestine, without any signs of radiation enteritis. Mild diversion colitis was seen in the distal rectum. Dissemination investigations did not show signs of metastasis or recurrent disease. Additionally, she gained weight, and her performance status improved to normal levels. On basis of these findings, the continuity was restored with a laparoscopic procedure. This operation was uncomplicated as well.

Discussion

Symptoms of radiation enteritis include nausea, vomiting, colic pain, diarrhea, fever, and additional weight loss; all observed in these two cases [1]. A minority of cases is managed by a surgical intervention. Most patients can be treated with supportive care such as fluid replenishment and nutritional support. Indications for surgery usually comprise gastrointestinal obstruction, perforation, or severe proctitis [4]. It is noteworthy that radiation enteritis and the need for salvage surgery can still be observed until some years after radiation therapy (early versus later radiation enteritis) [1, 2]. Considering the first case with obstruction at the level of the rectosigmoid junction, after getting the patient in a better general and nutritional condition, a resection was made of the proximal rectum with creation of a colostomy. Almost a year later, the colostomy was reversed with success.

Concerning the second patient, no evidence exists for determining the optimal time for surgery after such a severe period of toxic enteral symptoms—especially when considering a colorectal anastomosis. Much depends on the nutritional status of the patient and the extent of the disease. One has to continuously deliberate regarding the need to remove the malignant disease, the risk of morbidity, and even mortality due to the contemplated surgical procedure. Consideration must be taken that most symptoms may have subsided after 2–6 weeks. Furthermore, we take into account that the optimal time for surgery is approximately 6 weeks after chemoradiation therapy [1, 3]. Finally, we note that safely performing an anastomosis in selected cases has been confirmed [1, 4].

References

1. Rodríguez ML, Martín MM, Padellano LC, et al. Gastrointestinal toxicity associated to radiation therapy. Clin Transl Oncol. 2010;12:554–61.
2. Onodera H, Nagayama S, Mori A, et al. Reappraisal of surgical treatment for radiation enteritis. World J Surg. 2005;29:459–63.
3. Lim SB, Choi HS, Jeong SY, et al. Optimal surgery time after preoperative chemoradiotherapy for locally advanced rectal cancers. Ann Surg. 2008;248:243–51.
4. Goligher J. Irradiation proctitis and enteritis. In: Goligher J, editor. Surgery of the anus, rectum and colon. 5th ed. London: Bailliere Tindall; 1984. p. 1047–57.

Chapter 87
Case on Complications Following Cytoreductive Surgery and Heated Intraperitoneal Chemotherapy

Elisabeth A. te Velde and Victor J. Verwaal

Keywords HIPEC • Cytoreductuive surgery and heated intraperitoneal chemotherapy • Complications • Anastomosis leakage • Colon cancer • Peritoneal carcinomatosis

Diagnosis and Indication for Surgery

A 54-year-old male with colorectal cancer was treated with cytoreductive surgery (CRS) in combination with hyperthermic intraperitoneal chemotherapy (HIPEC) because of peritoneal carcinomatosis (Fig. 87.1). A left hemicolectomy was performed with creation of a colostomy and closure of rectal stump and two more small bowel resections.

Identification and Treatment of Complication

After the initial surgery, the postoperative course was complicated by anastomotic leakage and followed by two relaparotomies within a week (Fig. 87.2). Thereafter, a high-output enterocutaneous fistula developed (Fig. 87.3). After 4 months of conservative treatment, take-down of the fistula, abscess drainage, and abdominal wound by means of component separation technique (Ramirez abdominoplasty)

E.A. te Velde (✉)
Department of Surgery, VU University Medical Center, Amsterdam, The Netherlands
e-mail: e.tevelde@vumc.nl

V.J. Verwaal
Department of Surgery, Antoni v Leeuwenhoek Hospital, Amsterdam, The Netherlands

M.A. Cuesta, H.J. Bonjer (eds.), *Case Studies of Postoperative Complications after Digestive Surgery*, DOI 10.1007/978-3-319-01613-9_87,

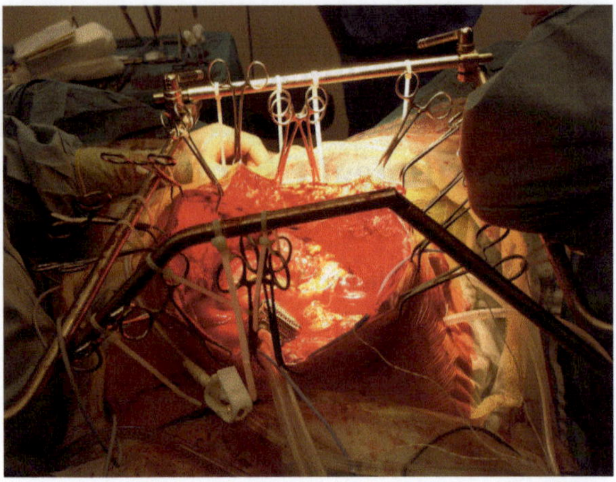

Fig. 87.1 HIPEC procedure

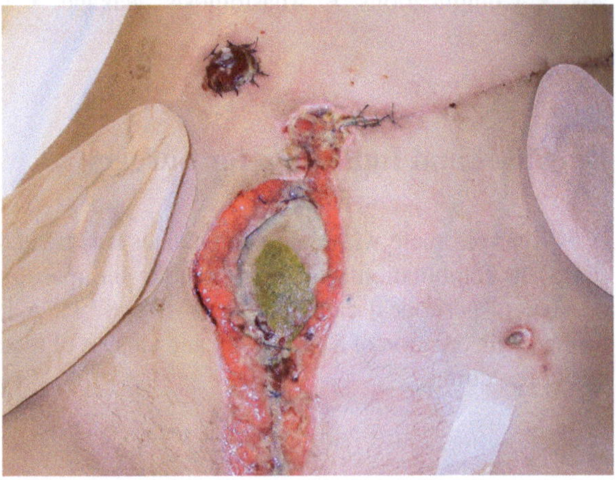

Fig. 87.2 By inspection, necrosis small bowel loop

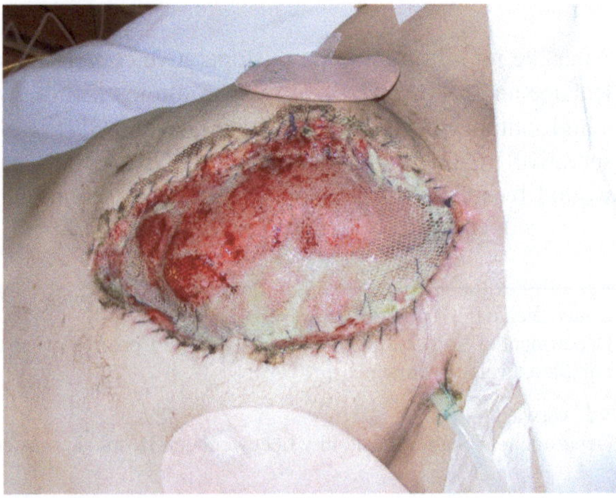

Fig. 87.3 Temporarily closure abdominal wall after multiple laparotomies by means of a mesh

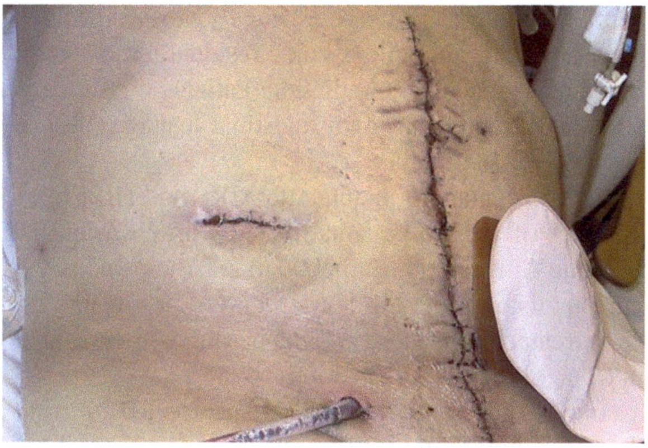

Fig. 87.4 Final aspect after the component separation technique (Ramirez plasty)

were performed (Fig. 87.4). Patient recovered. Two years after this complication, the patient is doing well and without signs of recurrence.

Discussion

Peritoneal metastasis has traditionally been thought of as last stop in metastasis cascade and associated with a poor survival. Commonly, these patients would be treated by systemic chemotherapy, which did not improve their survival significantly—leading to a median survival quotient of approximately 7–12 months. Already, chemotherapy has been studied in the setting of peritoneal metastasis, but only in those patients with measurable lesions; therefore, the effect of chemotherapy on peritoneal metastases is mostly unknown. Patients having metastases that are confined to the peritoneum can be treated with CRS and HIPEC. A prospectively randomized trial has shown that the 5-year survival rate following CRS and HIPEC in a heterogeneous group of patients with peritoneal metastases is equal to that of following surgery for colorectal liver metastases [1]. After a median follow-up of 8 years and provided that a macroscopic radical resection was achieved, a 5-year survival rate of 45 % was reached [2]. Other centers have confirmed this survival rate [3, 4].

Surgical resection of all macroscopic tumor tissue, i.e., resection of all affected peritoneum—including exenteration, adnex extirpation, omentectomy, and peritoneal stripping on indication—is followed by a rinsing with heated (41 °C) chemotherapy (Mitomycin C® or Oxaliplatin®) in order to eradicate all residual microscopic tumor tissue. CRS and HIPEC are associated with high morbidity and mortality rates (15–18 % and 5 %, respectively).

Serious complications following HIPEC are intestinal leakage and fistula. During the resection of all affected peritoneum, the serosa of the intestines is often damaged. These serosa defects should be meticulously repaired and sutured after the rinsing with heated chemotherapy. Patients treated by cytoreductive surgery combined with HIPEC are especially at risk for developing postoperative fistulas, because of possible microscopic residual tumors and due to extensive effect of former surgery and chemoradiation. Patients missing an intact peritoneal surface after CRS and HIPEC and with intestinal leakage often will not have specific clinical signs of peritonitis.

The percentage of fistula after CRS and HIPEC varies between 0 and 26 % [5]. A series of all 306 patients treated with CRS and HIPEC at the National Cancer Institute Amsterdam from 2000 to 2007, revealed 59 patients (19 %) with enterocutaneous fistula. The 30-day mortality rate for this group was 0 %. These patients were treated for pseudomyxoma peritonei in 39 % and for peritoneal carcinomatosis in 61 % of the cases [6].

Importantly, fistulas can lead to postponed adjuvant chemotherapy treatment and therefore might influence prognosis.

References

1. Verwaal VJ, Van Ruth S, De Bree E, et al. Randomized trial of cytoreduction and hyperthermic intraperitoneal chemotherapy versus systemic chemotherapy and palliative surgery in patients with peritoneal carcinomatosis of colorectal cancer. J Clin Oncol. 2003;21:3737–43.
2. Verwaal VJ, Bruin S, Boot H, et al. 8-year follow-up of randomized trial: cytoreduction and hyperthermic intraperitoneal chemotherapy versus systemic chemotherapy in patients with peritoneal carcinomatosis of colorectal cancer. Ann Surg Oncol. 2008;15:2426–32.
3. Hagendoorn J, Van Lammeren G, Boerma D, Van der Beek E, Wiezer MJ, Van Ramshorst B. Cytoreductive surgery and hyperthermic intraperitoneal chemotherapy for peritoneal carcinomatosis from colorectal and gastrointestinal origin shows acceptable morbidity and high survival. Eur J Surg Oncol. 2009;35:833–7.
4. Yan TD, Morris DL. Cytoreductive surgery and perioperative intraperitoneal chemotherapy for isolated colorectal peritoneal carcinomatosis: experimental therapy or standard of care? Ann Surg. 2008;248:829–35.
5. Elias D, Goere D, Blot F, Billard V, Pocard M, Kohneh-Shahri N, et al. Optimization of hyperthermic intraperitoneal chemotherapy with oxaliplatin plus irinotecan at 43 degrees C after compete cytoreductive surgery: mortality and morbidity in 106 consecutive patients. Ann Surg Oncol. 2007;14:1818–24.
6. Burgers PTPW, van der Hoeven JAB, te Velde EA, et al. Kliniek en behandeling van postoperatieve enterocutane fistels na cytoreductieve chirurgie gecombineerd met HIPEC. Ned Tijdschrift v Oncologie. 2009;4:173–81.

Chapter 88
Case on Postoperative Bleeding of a Colorectal Anastomosis

Miguel A. Cuesta

Keywords Colon cancer • Diverticulitis • Laparoscopic resection • Sigmoid • Rectal cancer • Bleeding anastomosis

First Patient

Diagnosis and Indication for Surgery

A 70-year-old man was diagnosed having a proximal rectal cancer staged as T3N0M0 at 13 cm of the anal verge. At that time, he was a healthy person, not taking any particular medicine. It was proposed to perform a laparoscopic low anterior resection.

Operation

The operation went without technical problems and after mobilization of the splenic flexure, a circular stapled side-to-end anastomosis was performed on him. Donuts were held to be intact, and the methylene-blue test showed no leakage taking place.

M.A. Cuesta, M.D.
Department of Surgery, VU University Medical Center, Amsterdam, The Netherlands
e-mail: ma.cuesta@vumc.nl

M.A. Cuesta, H.J. Bonjer (eds.), *Case Studies of Postoperative Complications after Digestive Surgery*, DOI 10.1007/978-3-319-01613-9_88,

Postoperative Course: Identification and Treatment of Complication

At the 1st postoperative day, the patient started passing stools with some clots and at the 2nd postoperative day it became clear that he was passing clots as well as fresh blood. His hemoglobin count decreased 2 points and the surgeon decided to perform a proctoscopy for inspecting the anastomosis. A bleeding was located at the anastomosis, 7-cm of the anal verge, which became treated by adrenalin injection and a clip. The bleeding then stopped.

Second Patient

Diagnosis and Indication for Surgery

A 56-year-old lady was diagnosed having a sigmoid stenosis as caused by recurrent sigmoid diverticulitis. She had been treated conservatively for the past 3 years, but the coming on of colics and constipation induced us to take a decision to operate her. She was at that time still a healthy patient and only took oral medication for her Diabetes Mellitus type 2.

Operation

A laparoscopic sigmoid resection was performed after mobilization of the splenic flexure, with a side-to-end anastomosis. The rectal superior artery was preserved for a better vascularization of the rectum.

Postoperative Course: Identification and Treatment of Complication

Postoperatively, the 1st day she passed stools and clots without a decrease of her hemoglobin rate. The 2nd postoperative day she developed tachycardia and her hemoglobin had decreased three points. We decided to perform an angiography CT-scan, but no blush became visible. A sigmoidoscopy did show a multitude of clots and gastroenterologist could not visualize a bleeding point. Because she was considered hemodynamically unstable, we decided to reoperate. Through an enlarged Pfannenstiel incision, anastomosis was observed and a clot in the anastomosis was found to be present. Furthermore, the anastomosis was resected and a new anastomosis was created in the same fashion. The ensuing postoperative period was uneventful.

Discussion

The point of discussion is what to do about postoperative bleeding?

Customary advice at the moment of anastomosis is to go about inspecting the anastomosis for bleeding and leakage. The problem arising during laparoscopic colorectal surgery is the impossibility of inspecting the anastomosis if the surgeon has not examined a low anastomosis by using a flexible sigmoidoscope.

Shamiyeh et al. have described the use of the intra-operative endoscopy for the assessment of circular stapled anastomosis in laparoscopic colon surgery [1]. The aim of their study was to evaluate the impact of routine intra-operative endoscopy on postoperative complications. They considered two groups of patients, the first group without use of endoscopy and the second group having undergone routine endoscopy. They assessed each circular-stapled anastomosis with a flexible endoscope for evidence of bleeding, integrity of mucosa, and leakage. In the group without endoscopy (253 patients), postoperative anastomotic bleeding was detected in 11 patients (4.3 %) and 7 (2.8 %) of these patients required endoscopic assessment and clipping. In the group involving endoscopy (85 patients), at the time of surgery the endoscopy showed anastomotic bleeding in five patients (5.9 %), which required clipping. Moreover, anastomotic leak was observed in two patients (2.4 %); in one patient the circular staple line was oversewn and in the other patient the anastomosis was redone. Two (2.4 %) patients in the endoscopic group had postoperative anastomotic bleeding requiring re-endoscopy and clipping.

The consideration at hand is that anastomotic bleeding and leakage can be detected at an early stage by intraoperative endoscopic assessment of circular-stapled anastomosis.

Martinez Serrano et al. analyzed the data of 1,389 colorectal procedures [2]. Their findings were that severe postoperative hemorrhage took place in 7 (0.5 %) of all patients. In all the seven patients the anastomosis had been stapled. In six of the seven patients, bleeding resolved with conservative treatment including endoscopy. Only one patient required surgical treatment. No mortality and no anastomotic leaks befell these seven patients.

Linn et al. collected prospectively the data of 143 patients undergoing laparoscopic colorectal surgery with a left-sided stapled anastomosis [3]. Of these, 72 were operated on for benign disease and 71 for a malignant condition. Postoperative anastomotic bleeding occurred in six patients (4 %). All were in the benign pathology group, and all had preservation of the inferior mesenteric artery during surgery. None of the patients required operative intervention for staple line hemorrhage.

Another consideration is that anastomotic bleeding from a stapled anastomosis in laparoscopic left-sided colorectal surgery appears to be an infrequent complication and it may be more common with preservation of the inferior mesenteric artery.

In the series of Malik et al. including 777 patients with severe postoperative bleeding [4], repeated operations were necessary for six patients (0.8 %). In the first three cases involved, conventional reoperation was performed. In the latter three cases, endoscopic therapy (adrenaline injection, diathermy, or endoscopic clipping) was used to control the bleeding. No complications that were either patient or anastomosis related occurred as a result of endoscopic therapy.

References

1. Shamiyeh A, Szabo K, Ulf Wayand W, Zehetner J. Intraoperative endoscopy for the assessment of circular-stapled anastomosis in laparoscopic colon surgery. Surg Laparosc Endosc Percutan Tech. 2012;22:65–7.
2. Martinez Serrano MA, Pares D, Pera M, et al. Management of lower gastrointestinal bleeding after colorectal resection and stapled anastomosis. Tech Coloproctol. 2009;13:49–53.
3. Linn TY, Moran BJ, Cecil TD. Staple line haemorrhage following laparoscopic left-sided colorectal resections may be more common when the inferior mesenteric artery is preserved. Tech Coloproctol. 2008;12:289–93.
4. Malik AH, East JE, Buchanan GN, Kennedy RH. Endoscopic haemostasis of staple-line haemorrhage following colorectal resection. Colorectal Dis. 2008;10:616–8.

Chapter 89
Case on Laparoscopic Approach of Anastomotic Leakage After Laparoscopic Resection

Willem A. Bemelman

Keywords Crohn's disease • Laparoscopic colon resection • Leakage anastomosis • CT scan

Diagnosis and Indication for Surgery

A 32-year-old women with longstanding Crohn's disease of the left colon required surgery because of stenosis in the rectosigmoid of the colon causing obstructive symptoms. Endoscopic investigation had showed a narrowed lumen at 20 cm from the anal verge. Passage of the endoscope was only possible using a pediatric endoscope indicating that the large bowel was segmentally affected from 15 to 35 cm from the anal verge.

Operation

Using a five trocars approach, the affected bowel segment was dissected from medial to lateral creating a wide submesenteric tunnel to mobilize the left colon adequately. At that time, routinely the inferior mesenteric artery was ligated. Nowadays, this is not considered appropriate in benign disease risking compromised vascularization and leaving a large submesenteric window at risk of internal herniation. A close bowel dissection of the mesentery is preferred in benign disease.

At the level of the upper third of the rectum, the rectum was transected using a linear endostapler. The stapled bowel was exteriorized via a small Pfannenstiel incision. The bowel was transected at the upper part of the sigmoid, and the anvil of the

W.A. Bemelman, M.D., Ph.D.
Department of Surgery, Academic Medical Center, Amsterdam, The Netherlands
e-mail: w.a.bemelman@amc.uva.nl

M.A. Cuesta, H.J. Bonjer (eds.), *Case Studies of Postoperative Complications after Digestive Surgery*, DOI 10.1007/978-3-319-01613-9_89,

stapler was inserted in the afferent loop. Using a double stapling technique the anastomosis was completed laparoscopically.

Postoperative Course: Identification and Treatment of Complication

Postoperatively, a full diet was permitted at the first day after surgery. At the 5th postoperative day, she started to vomit, and physical examination showed a distended, but soft abdomen. Initially, she was treated with iv fluids and nasogastric drainage. Because of elevated temperature and C-reactive protein, a CT scan with rectal and intravenous contrast was done the day thereafter. The CT scan revealed limited contrast leakage at the right side of the colorectal anastomosis and signs of small bowel obstruction.

A relaparoscopy was performed using the prior trocar sites. Blunt trocars were inserted. A diffuse purulent peritonitis was found. Extensive laparoscopic rinsing with warm saline was done and gradually the laparoscopic exposure improved. A partially sealed of anastomotic gap of 0.5 cm was found and an internal herniation of the small bowel via the mesenteric gap underneath the afferent colonic loop.

The small bowel was repositioned. A loop ileostomy was fashioned laparoscopically. The loop was opened externally and the efferent bowel loop was cannulated with a Foley catheter. An anesthesia ventilation tube was inserted in the anus. Next the large bowel was lavaged with saline until the lavage fluid coming out of the anus was clear. The fluid leaking through the anastomotic gap was removed by laparoscopic suction. A surgical drain was positioned next to the anastomosis using one of the trocar sites.

Seven days later she could be discharged without any further complication. Four months later the ileostomy could be closed.

Discussion

Anastomotic leakage must be suspected if a patient cannot tolerate a normal diet within a couple of days and has signs of infection. For this reason, earlier diagnosis and reintervention might be expected after a laparoscopic operation. This earlier reintervention might prevent severe generalized peritonitis and systemic sepsis.

Confirmation of a anastomotic leak is best done by CT scan with intravenous and enteral contrast.

During laparoscopic reintervention, the previous trocar wounds are used for insertion of a blunt trocar, e.g., TrocDoc trocar® (Storz; Tubingen, Germany), establishing the pneumoperitoneum [1]. The whole reintervention is performed laparoscopically, and the minilaparotomy used for specimen retrieval at the first operation can be opened only when necessary.

Illustration 89.1 Afferent loop exteriorized as an end stoma

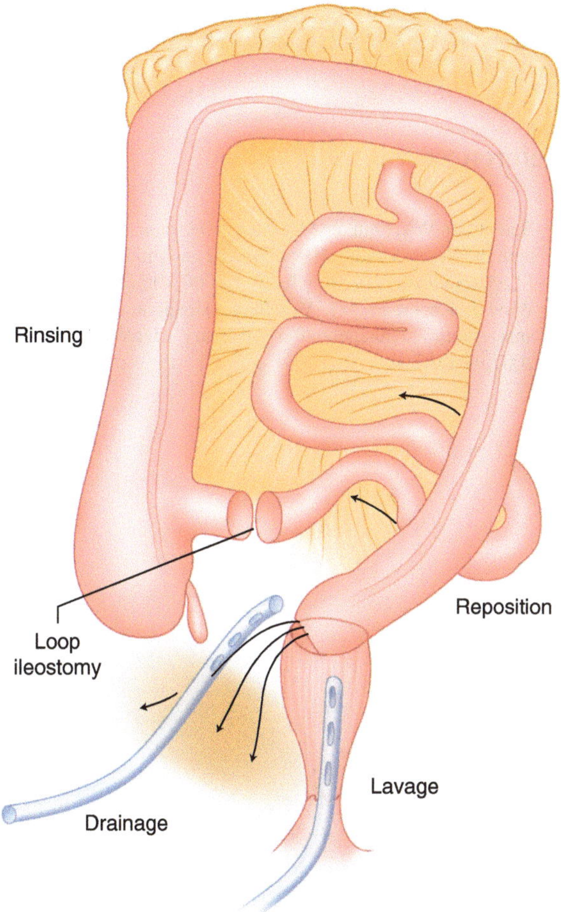

The operative procedure consists of inspection and exploration, then culturing and rinsing the abdominal cavity. Ileoanal, coloanal, and low colorectal anastomoses are diverted by creating a loop ileostomy and irrigation of the rest of the colon. In patients with intra-abdominal located anastomoses with major breakdown, the afferent loop needs to be exteriorized as an end stoma (Illustration 89.1). An end colostomy is created in those with anastomotic leakage after left-sided resections and an end ileostomy is created after right-sided resections.

If longstanding peritonitis with pus pockets and inflammatory adhesions precludes adequate irrigation, an option is to insert a hand port via the (earlier used) Pfannenstiel incision to facilitate irrigation and blunt separation of the bowel loops.

Wind et al. [2] showed that laparoscopic reintervention for anastomotic leakage after primarily laparoscopic surgery is feasible and safe, with no conversions or intraoperative complications observed. They demonstrated that a laparoscopic reintervention tends to be associated with less postoperative morbidity, a faster recovery and fewer abdominal wall complications.

References

1. Bemelman WA, Dunker MS, Busch OR, et al. Efficacy of establishment of pneumoperitoneum with the Veress needle, Hasson trocar and modified blunt trocar (TroDoc): a randomized study. J Laparoendosc Adv Surg Tech A. 2000;10:325–30.
2. Wind J, Koopman AG, Van Berge Henegouwen MI, et al. Laparoscopic reintervention for anastomotic leakage after primary laparoscopic colorectal surgery. Br J Surg 2007;94:1562–6.

Chapter 90
Case on Leakage Distal Anastomosis After Low Anterior Resection with Protective Ileostomy

Marta Gutierrez Moreno, Jurriaan B. Tuynman, and Miguel A. Cuesta

Keywords Rectal cancer • Radiotherapy • Low anterior resection • Laparoscopy • Protective ileostomy • Leakage anastomosis

Diagnosis and Indication for Surgery

A 67-year-old woman was diagnosed of having a mid-rectal carcinoma at 9 cm of the anal verge. By colonoscopy the tumor was biopsied, and two other polyps found and resected at 35 and 55 cm. The two polyps were benign, middle grade of dysplasia, and the rectal tumor adenocarcinoma. On CT scan and MRI, the tumor was staged as T3N1M0 (Fig. 90.1) and proposed to be treated by short scheme radiotherapy of 5×5 Gy to be followed 6 weeks later by LAR. Patient was continent before operation. Complying with recent national studies, no mechanical preparation was administered with exception of two enemas the previous night and another the early morning of operation.

M.G. Moreno, M.D. (✉)
Department of Surgery, Virgen del Rocio, Sevilla, Spain
e-mail: dra_gutierrez_moreno@hotmail.com

J.B. Tuynman • M.A. Cuesta
Department of Surgery, VU University Medical Center, Amsterdam, The Netherlands
e-mail: ma.cuesta@vumc.nl

M.A. Cuesta, H.J. Bonjer (eds.), *Case Studies of Postoperative Complications after Digestive Surgery*, DOI 10.1007/978-3-319-01613-9_90,

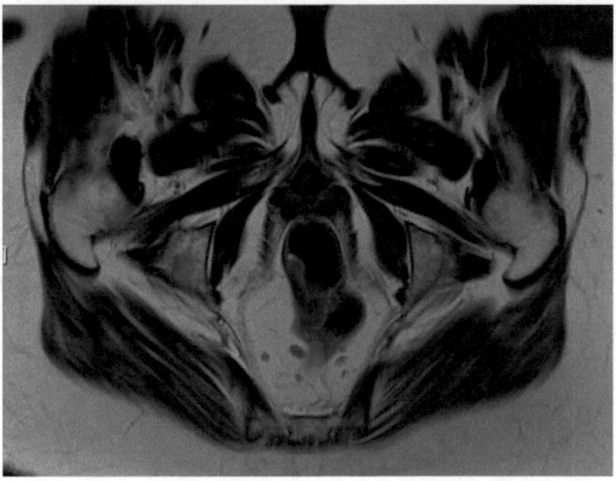

Fig. 90.1 MRI rectum carcinoma

Operation

She underwent a laparoscopic low anterior resection with a side-to-end anastomosis. A protective loop ileostomy was created. No intraoperative complications were noticed. Pathology showed a good response, being pT2N0.

Postoperative Course: Identification and Treatment of Complication

Treated by fast track, the second postoperative day, the patient had flatus and already passed stools. Discharge was planned for the 5th postoperative day, but the patient referred abdominal pain. The next day her condition became worse with fever, tachycardia, and increased CRP values up to 300. A CT scan showed leakage of the anastomosis with fluid collection around the anastomosis and pneumoperitoneum (Fig. 90.2 and Fig. 90.3). Reoperation followed, showing a fecal peritonitis caused by anastomosis leakage, half of circumference on posterior side. Patient was hemodynamically unstable during operation and surgeon decided to dismantle the anastomosis and create a colostomy in the left lower abdomen. Patient was postoperatively septic, she was mechanically ventilated for 4 days, and finally she could step by step be admitted to the normal ward. A long recovery period of 3 months followed. The dehiscent laparotomy wound became a huge incisional hernia. Nine months after the operation, a colorectal anastomosis was performed leaving the ileostomy as protection. Three months later, after control of the anastomosis (Fig. 90.4), ileostomy was closed and the abdominal wall repaired by means of abdominal wall plasty, the so-called component separation technique.

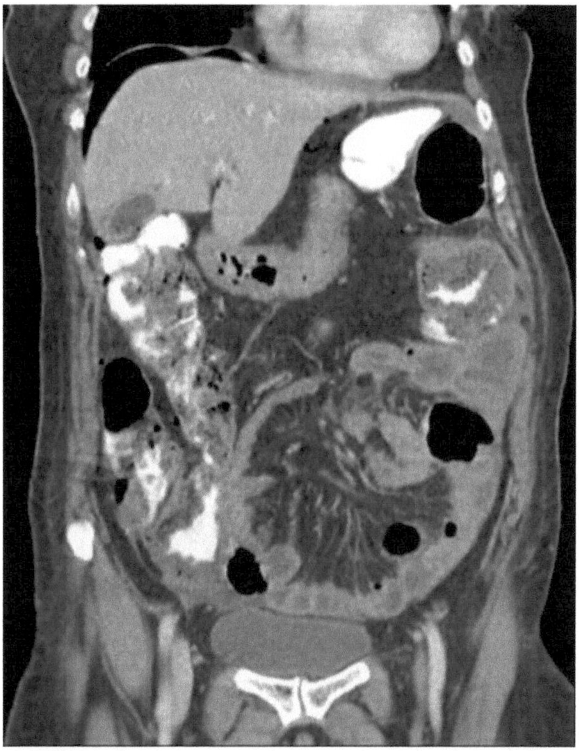

Fig. 90.2 CT scan pneumoperitoneum

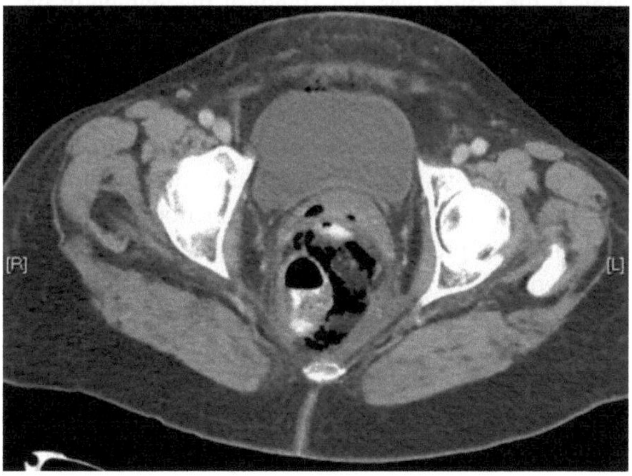

Fig. 90.3 CT scan leakage of the anastomosis

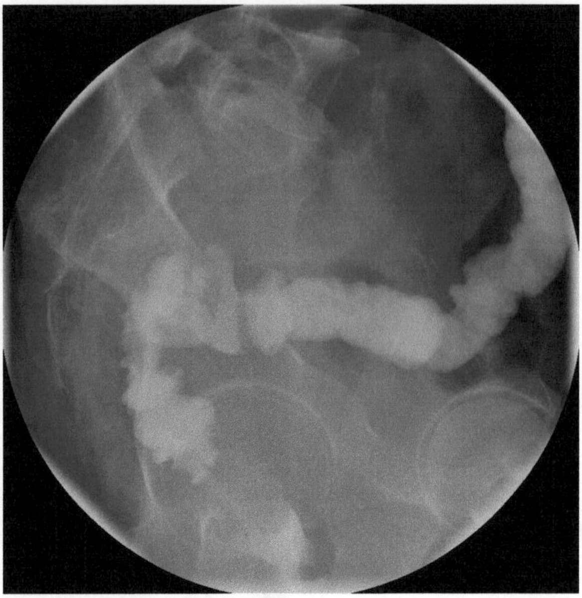

Fig. 90.4 Control enema, anastomosis is patent and there is no leakage

Discussion

Question is what to do with a patient having a leakage after LAR in whom anastomosis was already protected by means of a loop ileostomy? In the patient here presented, the colon was not standard mechanically prepared before operation. It is clear that in this way the colon had remained full of stools. Theoretically, the ileostomy will not protect the low anastomosis from stools once leakage happens.

Three interesting studies shed light on this subject. First, Matthiessen et al. described in a randomized study the value of defunctioning stoma to protect the LAR anastomosis [1]. The study included a total of 234 patients undergoing LAR in two groups with or without defunctioning stoma. In all patients, the colon was mechanically prepared (MBP). A total of 19.2 % of symptomatic leakages were recorded, whereby 10.3 % in the stoma group and 28 % with no-stoma group. Moreover 8.6 % patients needed a reoperation in the stoma group versus 25.4 % in the no-stoma group. Their conclusion was that a defunctioning loop stoma decreased the rate of symptomatic anastomotic leakage and is therefore recommended in low anterior resection for rectal cancer.

Second, the national Dutch study included a total of 1,431 patients to be randomized with and without mechanical preparation for colon and rectum surgery. Primary point of the study was anastomotic leakage, and at the 24th day postoperatively, the rate of leakage was found not to differ between the two groups, of which 4.8 % of those who had mechanical preparation and 5.4 % in those who did not. Patients with mechanical preparation and leakage had fewer abscesses than those not prepared. Moreover, other septic complications and mortality did not differ between the two groups [2]. The conclusion of this study was that classical mechanical preparation can be abandoned.

As a part of this trial, a sub-study was done with 449 patients who underwent a LAR with and without mechanical preparation, whereby 7.6 % leakages were found with MBP and 6.6 % without. There were no differences in protective ileostomies given during initial operation and the only factors related to leakage were the ASA classification and male gender. Conclusion was that MBP has no influence on incidence of anastomotic leakage in low colorectal surgery. Furthermore, omitting MBP in combination with diverting ileostomy was found to have no influence on the incidence of anastomotic leakage, septic complications, and mortality rate [3].

The third study, the French multi-institutional randomized study (GRECCAR study) [4], contrarily dealt with the effect of MBP or of no MBP on the morbidity and mortality of patients undergoing a sphincter-saving rectal resection because of distal rectal cancer. A total of 178 patients, including 89 in both groups, were included in the study. The overall and infectious morbidity rates were significantly higher in no-MBP versus MBP group, whereby 44 % versus 27 % and 34 % versus 16 %, respectively. Regarding both anastomotic leakage and major morbidity rates, there was no significant difference between no-MBP and MBP group: 19 % versus 10 % and 18 % versus 11 %, respectively. Mortality rate (1.1 % versus 3.4 %) and mean hospital stay (16 versus 14 days) did not differ significantly between both groups. This study demonstrated that rectal cancer surgery without MBP was associated with higher risk of overall and infectious morbidity rates without any significant increase of anastomotic leakage rate. Thus, it suggests continuation of MBP before elective rectal resection for cancer.

Another reason for administering MBP in those patients undergoing laparoscopic approach will be the manageability to handle move the colon free of feces during laparoscopic surgery. In spite of contradictory aspects of these trials, it seems logical to give MBP to patients undergoing LAR for rectal cancer with protective ileostomy.

References

1. Matthiessen P, Hallbook O, Rutegard J, et al. Defunctioning stoma reduces symptomatic anastomotic leakage after low anterior resection of the rectum for cancer: a randomized multicenter trial. Ann Surg. 2007;246:207–14.
2. Contant CM, Hop WC, van t' Sant HP, et al. Mechanical bowel preparation for elective colorectal surgery: a multicentre randomized trial. Lancet. 2007;370:2112–7.
3. Van t' Sant HP, Weidema WF, Hop WC, et al. The influence of mechanical bowel preparation in elective lower colorectal surgery. Ann Surg. 2010;251:59–63.
4. Bretagnol F, Panis Y, Rullier E, et al. Rectal cancer surgery with or without bowel preparation: The French GRECCAR III multicenter single-blinded randomized trial. Ann Surg. 2010;252:863–8.

Chapter 91
Case on Leakage Distal Anastomosis After Low Anterior Resection (LAR) Without Protective Ileostomy

Marta Gutierrez Moreno, Jurriaan B. Tuynman, and Miguel A. Cuesta

Keywords Rectal cancer • Radiotherapy • Laparoscopic Low anterior resection • Leakage anastomosis • CT scan • Ileostomy

Diagnosis and Indication for Surgery

A 70-year-old male patient—representative of an Asian enterprise—was diagnosed of having a mid-rectal adenocarcinoma, staged as T3N0M0, hence being treated by neoadjuvant radiotherapy, 5×5 Gy, and proposed to be operated 6 weeks later. On proctoscopy and MRI, the tumor was located at 8 cm from anal verge. He was in very good physical shape and had no known diseases nor any use of medication.

Operation

Operation was performed after a mechanical preparation by using two enemas. A laparoscopic TME was performed after mobilization of splenic flexure and anastomosed end-to-side fashion. Technically, anastomosis was performed without tension and donuts were intact. No protective loop ileostomy was created.

M.G. Moreno, M.D. (✉)
Department of Surgery, Virgen del Rocio, Sevilla, Spain
e-mail: dra_gutierrez_moreno@hotmail.com

J.B. Tuynman • M.A. Cuesta
Department of Surgery, VU University Medical Center, Amsterdam, The Netherlands
e-mail: ma.cuesta@vumc.nl

M.A. Cuesta, H.J. Bonjer (eds.), *Case Studies of Postoperative Complications after Digestive Surgery*, DOI 10.1007/978-3-319-01613-9_91,

Postoperative Course: Identification and Treatment of Complication

The 3rd day after operation, he developed fever, and under diagnosis of pneumonia, a thorax X-ray was performed showing an important pneumoperitoneum (Fig. 91.1a). On the CT scan with rectal contrast a leakage of anastomosis was seen with perianastomotic abscess (Fig. 91.1b). The same day, the surgeon decided to approach him by relaparoscopy. During laparoscopy, a posterior leakage was seen on the lateral aspect of the anastomosis with vital edges, the defect being approximated by stitches. Also, a defunctioning loop ileostomy was created. Postoperative course was complicated again by high fever, worsening of clinical condition, and sepsis. Two days later, a new CT scan showed again the leakage of anastomosis and abscesses in the pelvis with fluid collections in the right abdomen (Fig. 91.1c). After discussion in the multidisciplinary meeting, the surgeon decided to dismantle the anastomosis and create a definitive colostomy on the lower left abdomen.

Subsequently, the patient had two stomas. During the new postoperative period, a new CT scan was performed because of a new period of fever. A large right paracolic abscess was diagnosed and subsequently percutaneously drained (Fig. 91.2). Patient did recover. After a period of 6 months, a new operation was performed to close the ileostomy and repair the incisional hernia. After these operations he went into retirement.

Discussion

Discussion pertains the protective effect of ileostomy (or transverse colostomy) on the LAR anastomosis. The protection effect of stoma is an item already treated in the case 90. Matthiessen et al. reported in their randomized study that patients undergoing LAR with a protective stoma or without a protective stoma experience a significant lower leakage rate (10.3 % versus 28 %) and less necessity for reoperation (8.6 % versus 25.4 %) [1]. Moreover, there is much discussion about the morbidity (and mortality) caused by these protective stomas, and the type of stoma, ileostomy or transverse colostomy [1–3]. It is the general belief that after LAR, especially pertaining to those patients of male gender, smokers, and having undergone neoadjuvant chemoradiotherapy, it is advisable to protect the LAR anastomosis by a loop ileostomy. Probably the best will be to initiate a well-designed randomized trial studying patients randomized for having an ileostomy or not and with MBP or not.

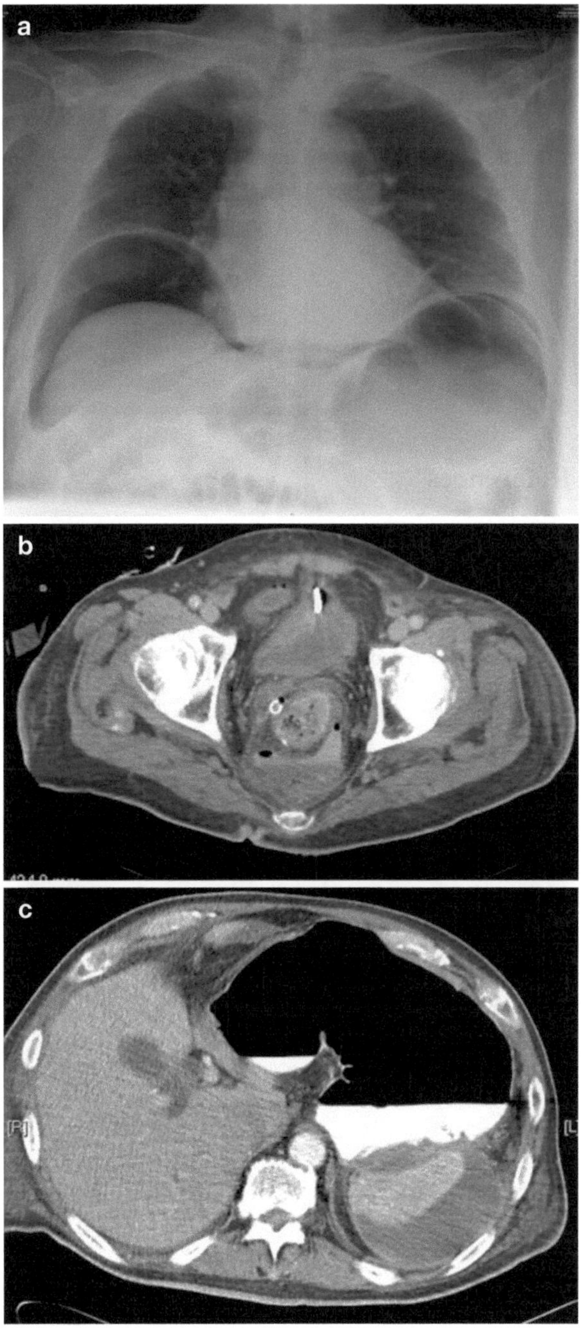

Fig. 91.1 (**a**) Pneumoperitoneum on the abdominal X-ray. (**b**) CT scan, leakage of the colorectal anastomosis. (**c**) CT scan fluid collection in the upper abdomen. Gastric dilatation

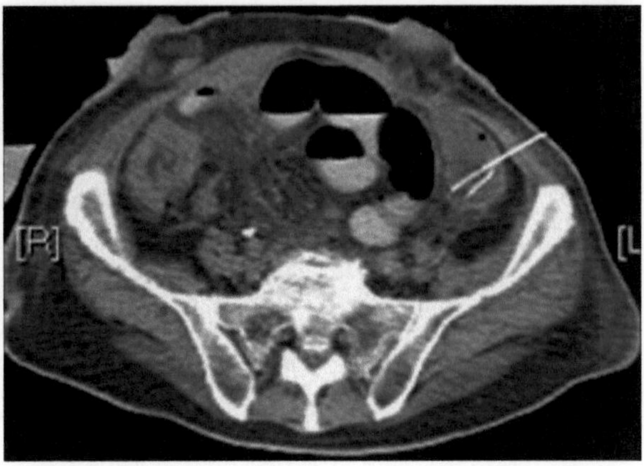

Fig. 91.2 CT scan-guided percutaneous drainage paracolic abscess *left*. Two stomas, ileostomy and colostomy

References

1. Matthiessen P, Hallbook O, Rutegard J, et al. Defunctioning stoma reduces symptomatic anastomotic leakage after low anterior resection of the rectum for cancer: a randomized multicenter trial. Ann Surg. 2007;246:207–14.
2. Giannakopoulos GF, Veenhof AAFA, van der Peet DL, et al. Morbidity and complications of a protective loop ileostomy. Colorectal Dis. 2009;11:609–12.
3. Gooszen AW, Geelkerken RH, Hermans J, et al. Quality of life with a temporary stoma: ileostomy vs colostomy. Dis Colon Rectum. 2000;43:650–5.

Chapter 92
Case on Complications of Ileostomy

Miguel A. Cuesta

Keywords Ileostomy • Stenosis • Prolapse • Torsion • High production

Stenosis

Diagnosis and Indication for Surgery

A 50-year-old technician suffered from having disturbing perineal fistulas and corresponding recurrences for the last 10 years. After the tenth operation, he still experienced soiling by pus as well as anal pain, and so he was referred to our Colorectal Unit. After local exploration at an outpatient clinic, we noticed that the patient had two large external perianal openings with pus pouring spontaneously out of these along the posterior aspect of thigh. We decided before redoing a fistula operation to create a period of rest by constructing a loop ileostomy.

Operation

Loop ileostomy was then created laparoscopically, and during the same operation, two setons were put in the two located fistula tracks.

M.A. Cuesta, M.D.
Department of Surgery, VU University Medical Center, Amsterdam, The Netherlands
e-mail: ma.cuesta@vumc.nl

M.A. Cuesta, H.J. Bonjer (eds.), *Case Studies of Postoperative Complications after Digestive Surgery*, DOI 10.1007/978-3-319-01613-9_92,

Postoperative Course: Identification and Treatment the Complication

The patient developed postoperatively a small bowel ileus with no ileostomy production. The ileostomy was vital and edematous, but difficultly assessed by digital examination. A CT scan showed that a stenosis at the level of fascia caused the intestinal obstruction (Fig. 92.1a, b); its being subsequently locally repaired under anesthesia by enlarging the fascia (Illustration 92.1). After a period of 6 weeks, the

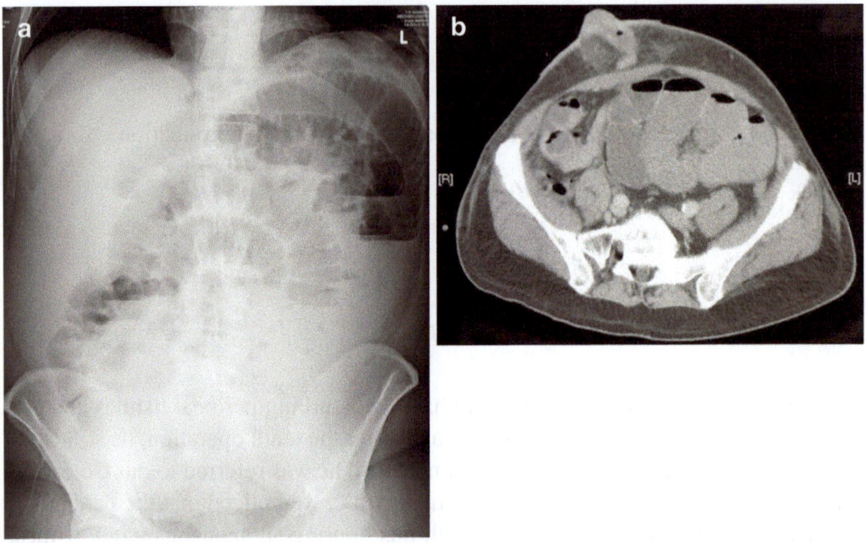

Fig. 92.1 (**a**) Intestinal obstruction. (**b**) CT scan, intestinal obstruction by a stenosis of the ileostomy

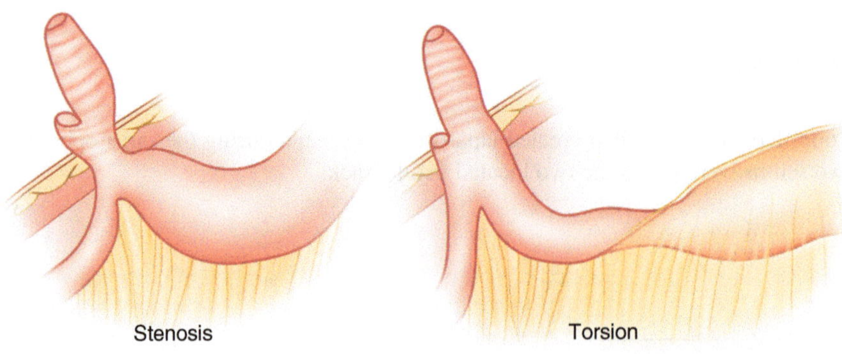

Illustration 92.1 Loop ileostomy was found to be associated with relatively high morbidity, e.g., stenosis and torsions

fistula was treated by mucosa advancement plasty, which healed. After a period of three months, the ileostomy became closed with subsequently still some soiling happening. After 6 years, we again saw the patient with a late recurrence of the fistula, yet without much complaint. Currently, his fistula is being conservatively treated.

Prolapse

Diagnosis and Indication for Surgery

A 58-year-old female high school teacher was seen at the outpatient clinic because of constipation complaints. For the last 10 years she had no spontaneous defecation and so had become completely dependent on taking enemas. She considered herself totally incapacitated, and after a marker study showing location of markers along the whole colon, it was decided to start with a loop ileostomy to treat the constipation and investigate the small bowel function. Proposal was to undertake other treatments in the future, e.g., total colectomy and ileorectal anastomosis.

Patient became so pleased with the optimally functioning ileostomy that she then refused more studies and surgical interventions.

Postoperative Course: Identification and Treatment of Complication

After 10 years, she was seen again at the outpatient clinic and readmitted because of an important prolapsed ileostomy and abdominal distension (Fig. 92.2). The prolapse could be manually reduced and followed by optimal ileostomy production. Shortening repair of the ileostomy was done 3 weeks later. Patient continues to refuse a definitive operation.

Ileostomy Torsion

Diagnosis and Indication for Surgery

A 39-year-old female secretary following a difficult vaginal delivery developed a total perineal rupture, summarily being sutured. Consequentially, she developed a productive low recto-vaginal fistula. Incapacitating as it was, she was proposed to undergo a loop ileostomy to bypass the difficult period leading up to reconstruction of the fistula by means of Martius plasty. Laparoscopically a loop ileostomy was created and the fistula assessed.

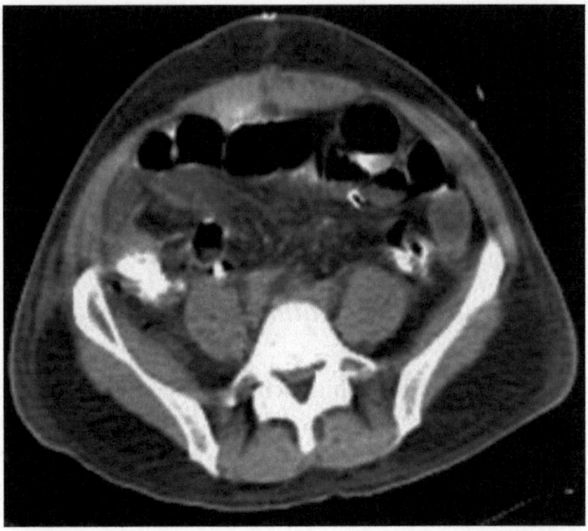

Fig. 92.2 Prolapse of the loop-ileostomy

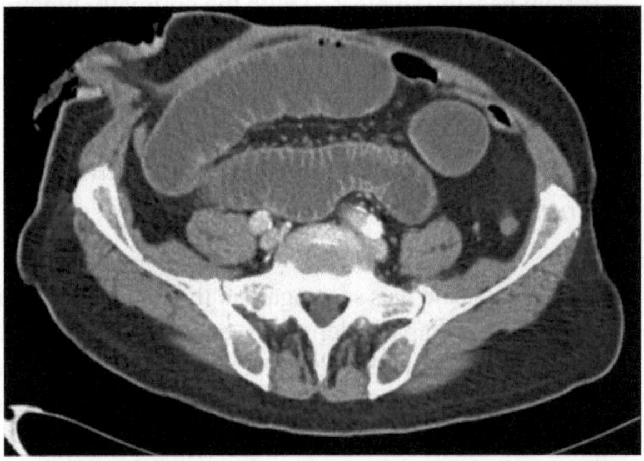

Fig. 92.3 CT scan showing a suspicion for torsion of the ileostomy with intestinal obstruction

Postoperative Course: Identification and Treatment of Complication

Postoperatively for a period of 7 days she passed no stools through a corrected, vital, and patent loop ileostomy. A CT scan showed an intestinal obstruction and the possibility of stenosis or torsion by the abdominal wall (Fig. 92.3), this being corrected by local exploration and laparoscopic control. Ileostomy was found twisted 180 degrees and this torsion was corrected (Illustration 92.1). Ileostomy functioned correctly, the fistula being corrected three months later by means of a Martius plasty with bulbocavernous muscle interposition. After vaginal inspection to control that the fistula was closed could the ileostomy be closed. Patient continued doing well, so that 2 years later a second child was delivered by cesarean section.

High-Output Ileostomy

Diagnosis and Identification of the Complication

A 40-year-old male patient was operated on because of intractable ulcerative colitis by means of total laparoscopic panproctocoletomy, ileoanal pouch anastomosis (IAPA), and protective loop ileostomy. First he developed a paralytic ileus over a period of 10 days, necessitating nasogastric tube drainage and total parenteral nutrition (TPN). Ileostomy was patent by digital examination. On the CT-scan, intestinal loop dilatation was seen and other diagnoses such as torsions or presence of abscesses excluded. After this period, ileostomy production started with a high output between 4 and 6 L per day (Fig. 92.4). This situation continued for a period of 3 weeks in spite of nasogastric tube and somatostatin. An important challenge was the treatment and correction of this metabolic dysfunction by means of oral feeding and TPN, extra liquids supply, and electrolyte correction. The role of Loperamide® was important in order to reduce the ileostomy production. Finally, ileostomy production became normal and he could be discharged. After control of the anastomosis and pouch, the ileostomy was closed 3 months later.

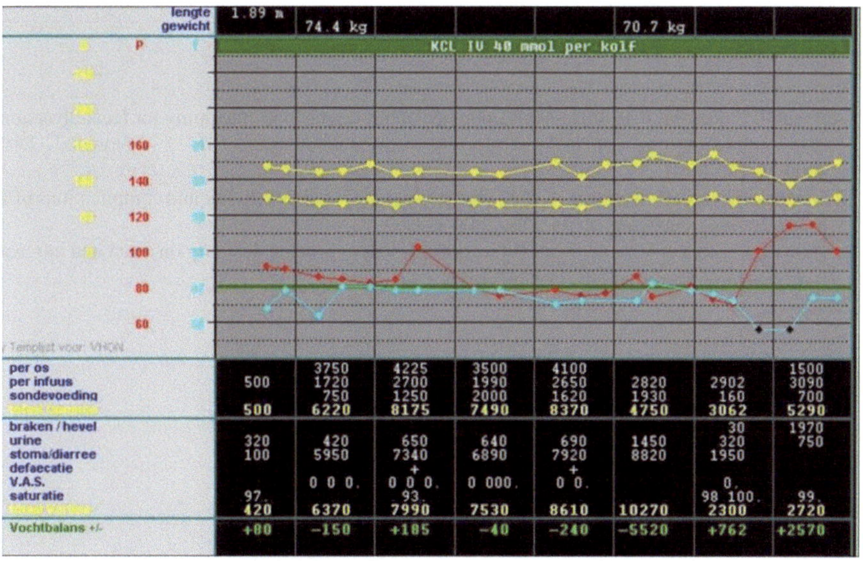

Fig. 92.4 Daily patient's graphic showing high-output production of the ileostomy (under stoma in cc/per day) Rest graphic in Dutch

Discussion

The first point concerns which kind of derivative stoma is better, the loop ileostomy or the loop colostomy. Rondelli et al., did a meta-analysis comparing the loop ileostomy (LI) with loop colostomy as derivative stoma [1]. Twelve comparative studies were included in this analysis, five randomized controlled trials and seven observational studies. They reported on 1,529 patients, 894 (58.5 %) undergoing defunctioning LI. LI reduced the risk of construction of the stoma. Specifically, patients undergoing LI had a lower risk of prolapse and sepsis. Moreover, LI was associated with an excess risk of occlusion after stoma closure and dehydratation. They concluded that this meta-analysis shows that LI is associated with a lower risk of construction of the stoma outcome measures.

The second point concerns the high % of complications observed as consequence of its construction, during the period with the stoma and as consequence of the closure. In our department Giannakopoulos et al. analyzed 119 retrospectively patients with a temporary loop ileostomy [2]. Fifty-nine stoma-related complications were seen in 44 patients (37 %) during the period in which the ileostomy was present. Moreover we found that 34 % of the patients had developed complications after ileostomy closure and only 40 % of patients suffered neither stoma-related complications nor peri-operative complications following ileostomy closure! Furthermore, temporary ileostomy were closed after a median period of 106 days.

High stoma output production with dehydration and impaired electrolytes and renal function was seen in three patients in this series, according with literature [3].

References

1. Rondelli F, Reboldi P, Rulli A, et al. Loop ileostomy versus loop colostomy for fecal diversion after colorectal or coloanal anastomosis: a meta-analysis. Int J Colorectal Dis. 2009;24:479–88.
2. Giannakopoulos GF, Veenhof AAFA, van der Peet DL, et al. Morbidity and complications of a protective loop ileostomy. Color Dis. 2009;11:609–12.
3. Huber FX, Stern J, Hinz U, et al. Effects of restorative proctocolectomy on renal and adrenal function. Dis Colon Rectum. 1999;42:1318–24.

Chapter 93
Case on Necrosis of Colostomy. Retraction and Stenosis

Ramon Gorter

Keywords Colostomy • Ileostomy • Ischemia • Necrosis • Retraction

First Patient

Diagnosis and Indication for Surgery

A 57-year-old healthy man was admitted to our hospital after ingesting 43 cocaine packages. At the time of presentation, 23 packages had already passed with stools. The patient experienced pain in the left lower quadrant of the abdomen, without nausea or vomiting. On physical examination, his blood pressure was 141/66 mm Hg and pulse 80 beats/min. There was local tenderness in the left lower quadrant without rigidity. CT scan was performed, revealing one package in the stomach, the rest in the colon, and also signs of diverticulitis Hinchey 1. The patient was admitted and oral mechanical bowel preparation was started. A gastroscopy was carried out to remove the package from the stomach, yet uneventful. On the third day, patient's condition worsened. His temperature was 38 °C, pulse 120 beats/min, and blood pressure 104/62 mm Hg. His abdomen was distended and painful. A new CT scan revealed intra-abdominal free air and fluids, showing no clear localization of perforation. A laparotomy showed a perforation of the sigmoid probably caused by diverticulitis with a fecal peritonitis. A left hemicolectomy was performed; all cocaine packages were removed from the colon and a colostomy was fashioned on the transverse colon. Pathology report confirmed the diagnosis of perforated diverticulitis.

R. Gorter, M.D.
Pediatric Surgery, VU University Medical Center, Amsterdam, The Netherlands
e-mail: rr.gorter@vumc.nl

M.A. Cuesta, H.J. Bonjer (eds.), *Case Studies of Postoperative Complications after Digestive Surgery*, DOI 10.1007/978-3-319-01613-9_93,

Postoperative Course: Identification and Treatment of Complication

Postoperatively, the patient was admitted to the Intensive Care Unit because of a septic shock for which resuscitation was carried out and broad spectrum antibiotics were started. After surgery, it was noted that the colostomy was ischemic/necrotic. Endoscopy through the stoma revealed necrosis for a length of 4 cm (Fig. 93.1a). It was decided to treat conservatively concerning the ischemic colostomy because the passage of stools was normal and there were no signs of peritonitis. In the following days, retraction of the stoma and stenosis occurred. Patient recovered with extra local care for the retracted colostomy. During outpatient follow-up, the colostomy became stenotic, although it stayed productive with

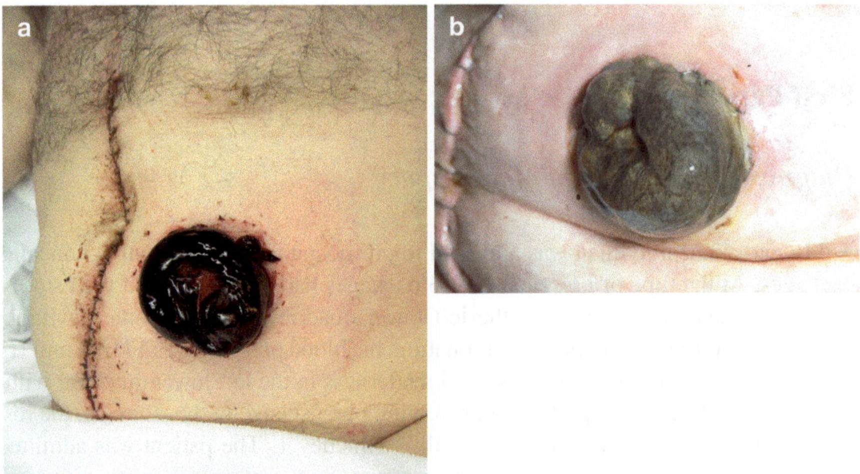

Fig. 93.1 (**a**) Necrosis of a colostomy, 4 cm. (**b**) Necrosis of colostomy, 5 cm

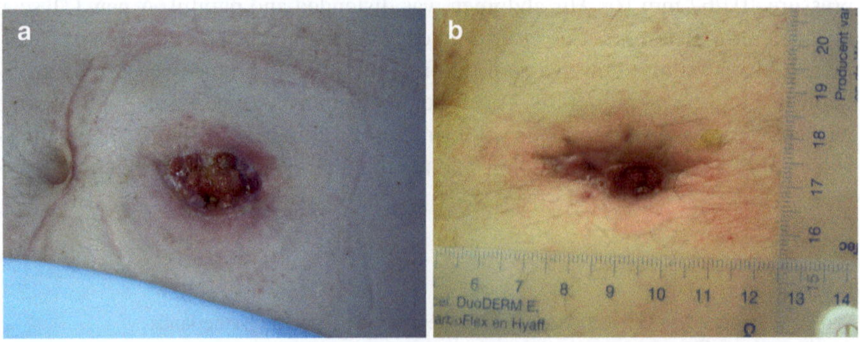

Fig. 93.2 (**a**) Stenosis of colostomy with hyperkeratosis. (**b**) Stenosis of colostomy

oral laxatives. After 6 months, patient had a stenosed colostomy with hyperkeratosis and an incisional hernia (Fig. 93.2a). Operation was planned to reverse the colostomy and repair the hernia. The stenotic track of the colostomy was importantly fixed to abdominal wall. An end-to-side anastomosis was performed after mobilization of splenic flexure and proximal rectum. Abdominal wall was reconstructed by means of a component separation technique (Ramirez plasty). Patient recovered.

Second Patient

Diagnosis and Indication for Surgery

A 74-year-old man was treated in our hospital for a T3N1M0 adenocarcinoma of distal rectum (3 cm of the dentate line).

Operation

After neoadjuvant radiotherapy, 5×5 Gy, a laparoscopic abdominal-perineal resection was performed. Colostomy of the sigmoid was created without any tension, being considered vital after operation. Pathological examination revealed a T3N0Mx adenocarcinoma, radically removed.

Postoperative Course: Identification and Treatment of Complication

Postoperatively the patient developed a deep perineal wound infection, being adequately drained. At day 3, it was noted that colostomy was progressive ischemic, and by endoscopy the ischemia reached 5 cm deep (Fig. 93.1b). Conservatively treated, 1 month later patient developed a colon obstruction based on retraction and stenosis of the stoma. It was decided to place a decompression tube through the stoma for decompression of the colon. In this way, stoma was productive again and patient's condition improved. He was discharged and scheduled for operation, but during the waiting period the stoma had to be regularly dilated by the nurse practitioner (Figs. 93.2b and 93.3). Four months after the initial surgery, colostomy was revised. Laparoscopically approached, the sigmoid was mobilized from adhesions, and after enough length was created by mobilization of splenic flexure, a new colostomy was fashioned. Postoperatively, the new stoma was good, being vital and productive.

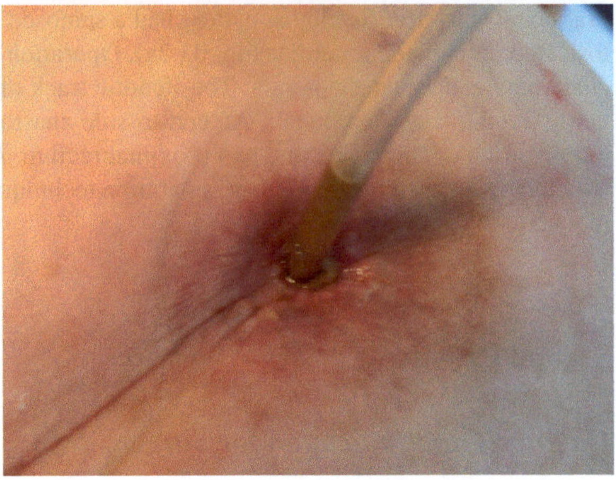

Fig. 93.3 Dilatation and lavage of stenosed colostomy

Third Patient

Diagnosis and Indication for Surgery

A 67-year-old female patient had progressive complaints of fecal incontinence. She had undergone two difficult vaginal deliveries at ages 32 and 39, the last with perineal rupture grade 2. In early years she had been incontinent for gas, but since she had become 52 years of age also for feces. Analyzed for the fecal incontinence, she underwent 5 years before an anterior sphincter repair that was complicated with a wound infection. After recovery, she did pelvic floor biofeedback physiotherapy with some improvement of the incontinence. Nonetheless, in the last 2 years her incontinence had worsened and hence we decided to create a colostomy. A laparoscopic sigmoid colostomy was created with a short rectal stump at the level of promontory.

Postoperative Course: Identification and Treatment of Complication

One day later, the colostomy was ischemic, and because of fever and abdominal pain, she underwent an endoscopy in which 7 cm were found to be ischemic. A new laparoscopy was performed at day 3, and after mobilization of the sigmoid loop, a new colostomy was created after resection of the necrotic/ischemic segment. Colostomy looked vital and productive. Short-term postoperative course went okay, but 6 months later she developed rectal anal complaints of tenesmus and pain. Rectal examination and proctoscopy showed diversion colitis and mucus bezoars, being treated with enemas without success. Complaints were so significant that 1 year later her rectal stump was shortened up to the pelvic floor. Her complaints disappeared, and currently, 1 year later, she is doing well.

Discussion

Colostomy creation is a frequent surgical procedure. It can be temporary or definitive. Different indications exist for colostomy creation, such as distal rectal cancer, complicated diverticulitis, and colon ischemia. However, complications after creation are not uncommon. Most frequent are ischemia/necrosis, stenosis with retraction, prolapse, and parastomal herniation. To prevent these complications, a proper operative technique has to be used. A colostomy should be vital, patent, and small inverted (1 cm) in relation to the skin surface. And, more importantly it is to be created in the proper place, marked beforehand by the surgeon and the stoma nurse at least the day before operation. Complications are more likely to occur in elderly, ASA grade 3 type of patients [1].

Review of the three above presented cases points out that necrosis of the stoma can have significant morbidity and frequently requiring reoperation. Ischemia will develop due to technical problems during inadequate dissection of the mesentery after division of the sigmoid. Surgeons prefer to get a sigmoid loop with less mesentery easy to be fixed to the skin, but in this way a devascularized loop is formed with ischemia as consequence. Another possibility for later ischemia is torsion of the loop or a too small opening through the abdominal wall [2]. Moreover, at the end of the procedure a rectal examination is required in order to be sure that the stoma is not kinked in the abdominal wall. Why ischemia developed in the three cases is not clear. But because no tension is mentioned, probably one of the other above-mentioned factors was not correctly identified. Cottam et al. have published a nationwide audit about stomas in the UK [3]. Of the 256 hospital-based stoma care services within the UK, 93 (36 %) participated. A total of 3,970 stomas were recorded, of which 1,329 (34 %) were identified as problematic. Sixty-two centers reported 45–50 stomas with a range of complications 6–96 %. The loop ileostomy was found to be the stoma that causes most problems. Hence we may regard a stoma of <10 mm to be a predisposing factor for complications and problems are more likely to occur following an emergency procedure.

Pertaining question is: What to do the first postoperative day in the event the colostomy does not look optimal? Examination by means of a glass tube with a lamp can be done to know how deep the vital colon starts. If ischemia is short, 1–2 cm, it can be approached conservatively. In the rest of cases, endoscopy should be done. If there is any suspicion of deep ischemia more than 3 cm or up to the abdominal cavity, reoperation should be done from the beginning in order to have a vital and good productive stoma. Otherwise, a lot of problems and suffering will be the fate of patients and their colostomy. Examples of such suffering affected the first two patients.

References

1. Harris DA, Eqbeare D, Jones S, et al. Complications and mortality following stoma formation. Ann R Coll Surg Engl. 2005;87:427–31.
2. Arumugam PJ, Bevan L, Macdonald L, et al. A prospective audit of stomas–analysis of risk factors and complications and their management. Colorectal Dis. 2003;5:49–52.
3. Cottam J, Richards K, Hasted A, Blackman A. Results of a nationwide prospective audit of stoma complications within 3 weeks of surgery. Colorectal Dis. 2007;9:834–8.

Chapter 94
Case on Parastomal Hernia Complications

Birgitta M.E. Hansson

Keywords Parastomal hernia • Diverticulitis • Leakage • Laparoscopic correction • Open correction • Mesh

Diagnosis and Indication for Surgery

A 66-year-old woman was referred because of a symptomatic parastomal hernia. Five years previously, a Hartmann's procedure had been performed due to acute diverticulitis with perforation and peritonitis. She complained of pain, brought about by stretching of the abdominal wall, a poor fitting of the appliance resulting in leakage, and having peristomal skin irritation. Furthermore, she reported having cosmetic problems. Her quality of life had severely decreased since the hernia had become symptomatic.

Clinical examination showed a huge parastomal hernia in the left lower abdomen. The hernia could not be reduced.

A CT scan was performed to measure the hernia defect and to rule out concomitant incisional hernias since these could not be palpated at clinical examination.

The CT scan showed a hernia defect of more than 5 cm with herniation of small bowel and an incisional hernia in the lower abdomen (Fig. 94.1).

Operation

Due to her growing complaints, a decision was taken to perform a laparoscopic approach and so both hernias were repaired with two separate Gore-Tex dual meshes. The parastomal hernia was repaired according to the technique by

B.M.E. Hansson, M.D.
Department of Surgery, Canisius Hospital, Nijmegen, The Netherlands
e-mail: birgittahanson@hotmail.com

M.A. Cuesta, H.J. Bonjer (eds.), *Case Studies of Postoperative Complications after Digestive Surgery*, DOI 10.1007/978-3-319-01613-9_94,

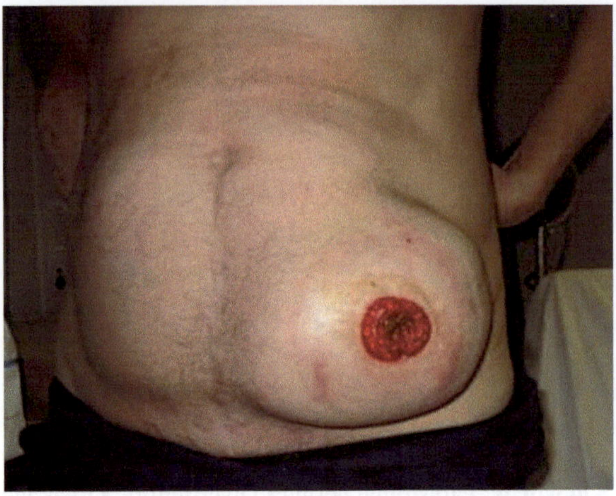

Fig. 94.1 Parastomal hernia

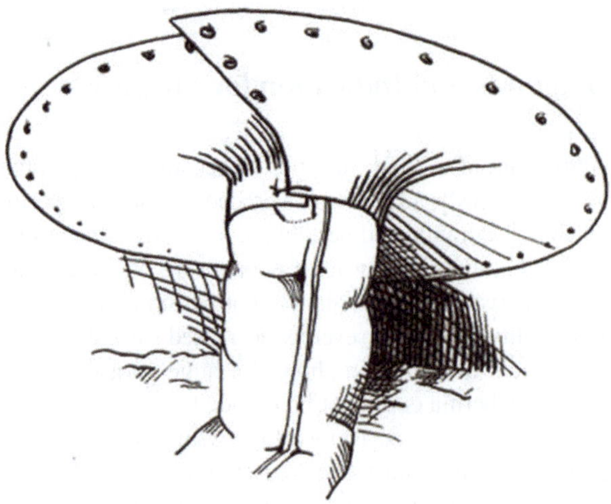

Fig. 94.2 Keyhole method for repair of parastomal hernia

Sugerbaker (Fig. 94.2). For the incisional hernia, the double-crown technique was used. The postoperative course was uneventful. Figure 94.3 shows the postoperative result after application of the Sugerbaker technique.

Discussion

A parastomal hernia is a common complication after stoma formation (Illustration 94.1a). The incidence varies and can be as high as 39 % for colostomies. Risk factors are obesity, chronic cough, medication, the size of the stoma opening being too wide, or the stoma being too lateral (lateral to rectus sheath). A symptomatic parastomal

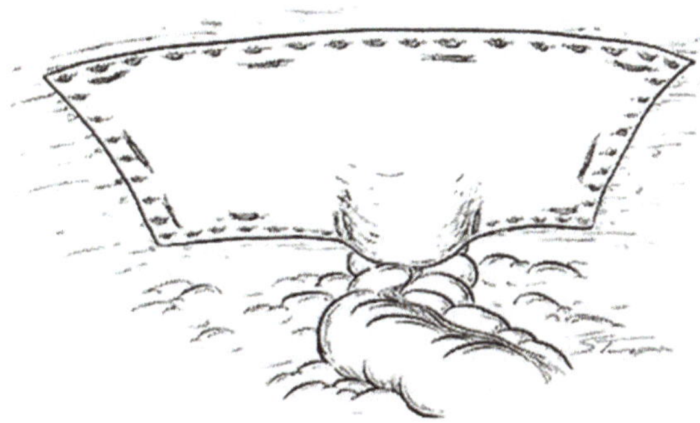

Fig. 94.3 Sugarbaker's non-slit technique of repair of parastomal hernia

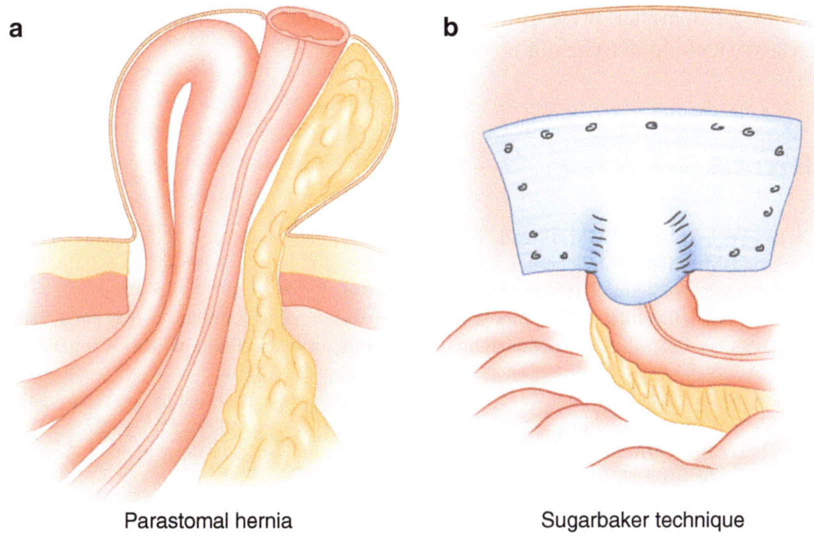

Illustration 94.1 (**a**) A parastomal hernia is a common complication after stoma formation. The incidence varies and can be as high as 39 % for colostomies. Risk factors are obesity, chronic cough, medication, the size of the stoma opening being too wide, or the stoma being too lateral (lateral to rectus sheath). (**b**) Sugarbaker technique

hernia can be treated by relocation of the stoma to a preselected location or by local reinforcement of the abdominal wall with a prosthetic mesh. Stoma relocation involves relaparotomy and replacement of the stoma to the contralateral side. Besides the problem of developing an incisional hernia at the midline or at the old stoma site in 20–30 % of all cases, this technique carries a recurrence rate of up to 36 % [1].

Mesh repair has a lower recurrence rate. Depending on technique and placement, recurrence rates vary between 6.9 and 17.8 %. The overall mesh infection rate is 2.4 % [2]. The mesh can be placed onlay, retromuscular, or intraperitoneal, either by laparoscopy or by open approach.

Review of the literature finds no significant advantage of one approach over the other. Evidence by randomized studies, RCT, is lacking [2].

We personally favor the laparoscopic approach for it has proved to be safe and feasible and it serves minimal damage to the insufficient abdominal wall [3]. A Gore-Tex dual mesh is used to reinforce the abdominal wall. A mesh with or without a slit can be used. The former technique is also called the "keyhole technique."

Unfortunately, this technique has a high recurrence rate due to progressive widening of the central keyhole. Recurrence rates of more than 20 % are reported [2, 4].

The non-slit technique was described by Sugerbaker [5]. Hereby, a mesh is used to cover the hernia opening with an overlap of 4 cm at each side, after the stoma loop is lateralized (Fig. 94.2, Illustration 94.1b). A considerably lower recurrence rate of 11.6 % is reported for this technique [2].

Recently, the use of biological grafts in parastomal hernia repair has been published. However, review of the literature shows no better outcomes as well as the drawback of a higher price [6]. Hence, at this time of writing, we regard the Sugerbaker technique to be our advisable technique.

References

1. Carne PWG, Robertson GM, Frizelle FA. Parastomal hernia. Br J Surg. 2003;90:784–93.
2. Hansson BME, Slater NJ, Schouten van der Velde AP, et al. Surgical techniques for parastomal hernia repair: a systematic review of the literature. Ann Surg. 2012;255:685–95.
3. Hansson BME, de Hingh IHJT, Bleichrodt RP. Laparoscopic hernia repair is safe and feasible: early results of a prospective clinical study including 55 consecutive patients. Surg Endosc. 2007;21:989–93.
4. Hansson BME, Bleichrodt RP, de Hingh IHJT. Laparoscopic parastomal hernia repair using a keyhole technique results in a high recurrence rate. Surg Endosc. 2009;23:1456–59.
5. Sugerbaker PH. Peritoneal approach to prosthetic mesh repair of parastomy hernias. Ann Surg. 1985;201:344–46.
6. Slater NJ, Hansson BME, Buyne OR, et al. Repair of parastomal hernias with biological grafts. A systematic review. J Gastrointest Surg. 2011;15:1252–8.

Chapter 95
Case on Severe Complication After PPH Procedure for Hemorrhoids

Michael F. Gerhards and Jan Peringa

Keywords PPH • Hemorrhopidal prolapse • Hemorrhoids • Procedure for hemorrhoids and prolapse • Rubber band ligation • Rectal perforation • Ileostomy

Diagnosis and Indication for Surgery

A 55-year-old female patient was referred to our hospital because of third-degree hemorrhoidal prolapse. Because former treatment by rubber band ligation (RBL) was not successful, a procedure for prolapse and hemorrhoids (PPH) was proposed. Besides the RBL, no former abdominal nor anorectal procedures were performed.

Operation

After admission in day care, patient was operated under general anesthesia in lithotomy position. All patients are standard given bowel preparation by means of Sodium solution (Fleet™). According to the surgeon, a circular purse string suture was made at 7–8 cm above the dentate line. In accordance with the standard protocol, the PPH01 Ethicon circular stapling machine was introduced, the suture was closed, and a pull through followed. With control of the vaginal wall, and traction on the suture, the stapling machine was closed and resection of the mucosa was performed.

M.F. Gerhards, M.D. (✉)
Department of Surgery, OLVG Hospital, Amsterdam, The Netherlands
e-mail: m.f.gerhards@olvg.nl

J. Peringa, M.D.
Radiology, OLVG Hospital, Amsterdam, The Netherlands

M.A. Cuesta, H.J. Bonjer (eds.), *Case Studies of Postoperative Complications after Digestive Surgery*, DOI 10.1007/978-3-319-01613-9_95,

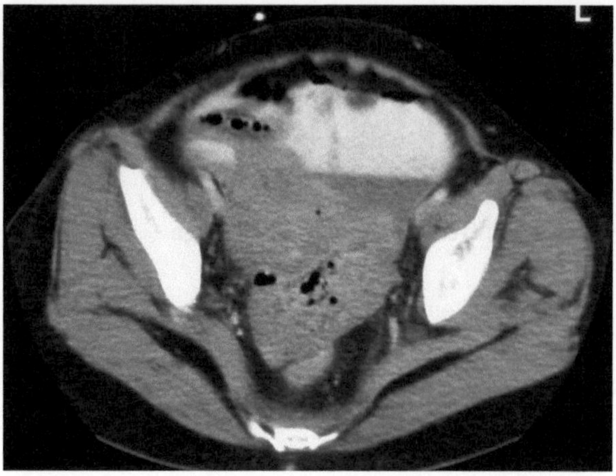

Fig. 95.1 CT scan presented leakage of contrast in the pelvis

Hemostasis was looked after and the procedure was ended uneventful. Patient was sent home in good condition 2 h after the operation.

Postoperative Course: Identification and Treatment of Complication

The same evening patient complained about abdominal pain, nausea, vomiting, and even fever. Patient was referred to the first aid department and physical examination showed high fever, normal tension with high pulse rate, and signs of an "acute" abdomen. Blood test revealed low white blood cells and high CRP. An abdominal X-ray showed a short bowel ileus and eventually a CT scan presented leakage of contrast in the narrow pelvis (Fig. 95.1). Digital rectal examination afterwards showed a defect in the ventral rectal wall. An emergency laparotomy was done and during this procedure the defect was found and closed by primary sutures. De bowel was deviated with a double loop ileostomy, and after extensively rinsing the abdomen, a drain was left in the pelvis and the abdomen was closed again.

The recovery period, with short time admission to the intensive care unit, was prolonged due to persistent fever and signs of sepsis without development of an abscess, ruled out by repeated CT scans. After intravenous treatment with antibiotics, patient was dismissed after 3 weeks. Two weeks later patient is admitted again for 3 days because of abdominal pain, which disappeared spontaneously. Six months later the ileostomy was closed and further recovery was uneventful, and during the last recorded visit to the outpatient clinic, no complaints were persistent. The prolapse has disappeared, no blood loss remained, and spontaneous defecation was possible.

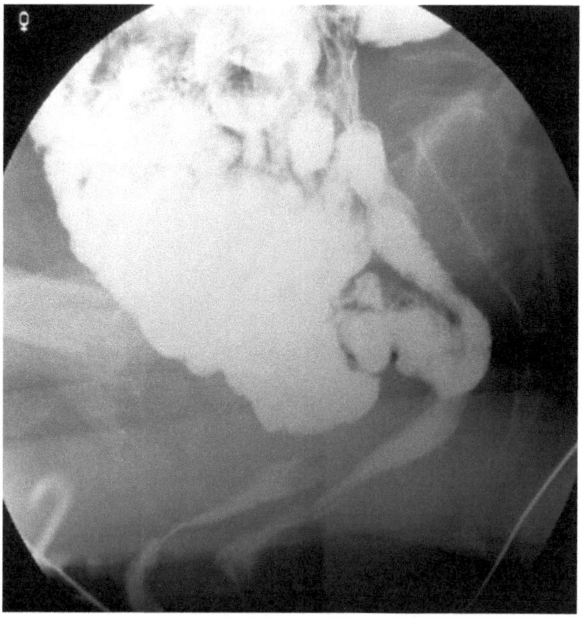

Fig. 95.2 Low recto-uterine pouch on the defecography

Discussion

Procedure for prolapsing hemorrhoids (PPH) carries low postoperative complications; however, it may be followed by unusual and severe problems [1]. Despite bleeding, hematoma, and pain, on the short- and middle long-term follow-up also urgency and fecal incontinence are repeatedly mentioned in the literature. However, in a minority of all cases, more severe complications such as strictures, rectovaginal fistula, total rectal obliteration, and perforation with pelvic sepsis are documented. During analysis of this case, the question remains if we could have prevented the complication, as was quoted by Tjandra et al. In the systematic review on the Procedure for Prolapse and Hemorrhoids (Stapled Hemorrhoidopexy) this group has presented, they reviewed 1,918 procedures and came to the conclusion that these major complications were probably related to technical errors, such as inappropriate placement of a purse string that was too deep or too proximal in the rectum, and as a result, a full thickness rectal anastomosis was performed [2].

In this case, the procedure was performed by a relative inexperienced surgeon (less than 25 PPH's) and by means of a PPH01 stapler. The purse string was probably placed far too high (normal within 2–4 cm above the apex of the hemorrhoids). Furthermore in retrospection, this patient had a relative low recto-uterine pouch (cul-de-sac of Douglas), which was shown during a former defecography, made for outlet symptoms and found during final analysis of this case (Fig. 95.2). The combination of these facts probably resulted in the perforation, which was found on CT scan and during reoperation.

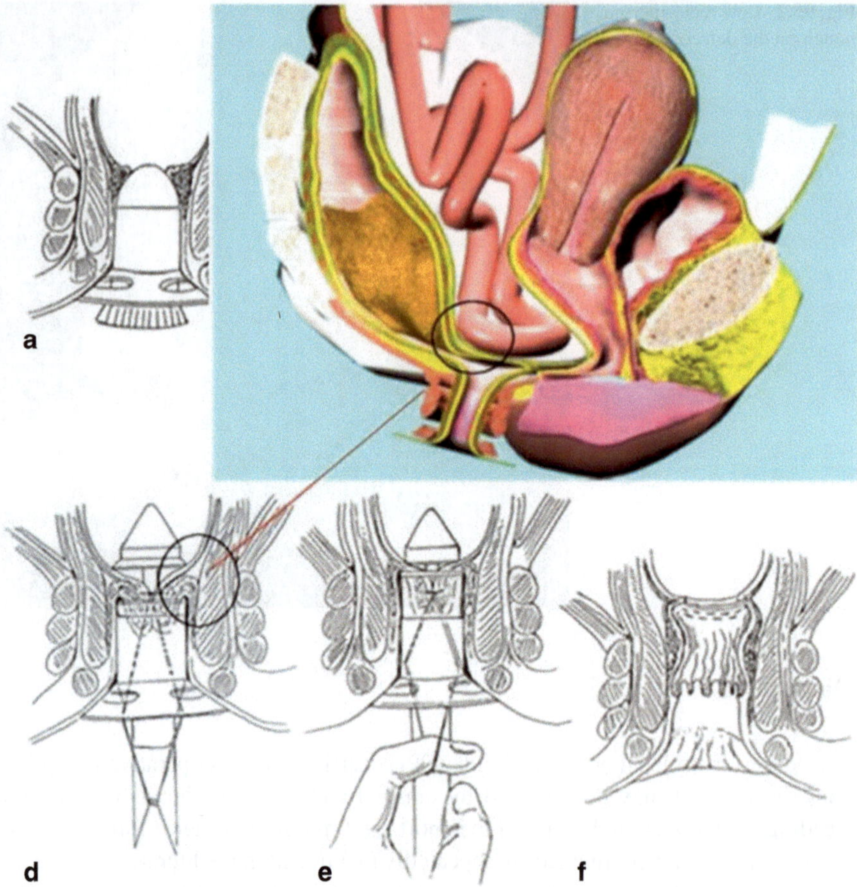

Fig. 95.3 PPH procedure. Purse string was placed too high in this patient

It is difficult to propose the amount of "simple" PPH procedures under supervision, before a surgeon is experienced enough to perform this procedure safely and to recognize technical problems during operation [3]. However, we think that there is an advance in having already experience in stapling machines and also anorectal surgery, as we have encountered by giving site-by-site lessons. In addition, the older PPH01 machine in comparison with the newer PPH03 has a bigger staple closure which can have resulted in an incomplete closure [4]. This problem is repeatedly mentioned after the STARR procedure, during which a complete resection of the rectal wall is exactly aimed [4, 5]. When the defect had been low and pure ventral, it should have resulted in a rectovaginal fistula. When it was more lateral or dorsal, probably the perirectal fat would have covered the problem, as we know from other transanal rectal surgery such as the TEM procedure, and probably without a prolonged postoperative course. In this case, the patient had a low Douglas pouch and the purse string was placed too high (Fig. 95.3), and incomplete closure resulted in a perforation to the free abdominal space, which resulted in sepsis and due to relative late recognition of its possibility, severe consequences for the patient. Surprisingly pathological examination showed no muscle fibers in the specimen, possibly ruling out a full thickness bowel wall resection. In the end, a laparotomy was inevitable, and a diverting ileostomy resulted. In other cases a Hartmann procedure or diverting colostomy was the procedure of choice. It is difficult to conclude which of these procedures is preferable in the acute setting, when stabilizing the patient is the first goal and patients. However, the diverting ileostomy is eventually the easiest procedure to resolve, as is also showed in this case.

In conclusion, we have presented a rare but not uncommon serious complication after an expected regular PPH procedure. This case shows again that in inexperienced hands, stapling machines remain hazardous tools and that a good anamnesis can select difficult patients who are not fit for standard procedures.

References

1. Festen S, van Hoogstraten MJ, van Geloven AA, Gerhards MF. Treatment of grade III and IV haemorrhoidal disease with PPH or THD. A randomized trial on postoperative complications and short-term results. Int J Colorectal Dis. 2009;24:1401–5.
2. Tjandra JJ, Chan MK. Systematic review on the procedure for prolapse and hemorrhoids (stapled hemorrhoidopexy). Dis Colon Rectum. 2007;50:878–92.
3. Jongen J, Bock JU, Peleikis HG, et al. Complications and reoperations in stapled anopexy: learning by doing. Int J Colorectal Dis. 2006;21:166–71.
4. Pescatori M, Gagliardi G. Postoperative complications after procedure for prolapsed hemorrhoids (PPH) and stapled transanal rectal resection (STARR) procedures. Tech Coloproctol. 2008;12:7–19.
5. Sileri P, Stolfi VM, Franceschilli L, et al. Reinterventions for specific technique-related complications of stapled hemorrhoidopexy (SH): a critical appraisal. J Gastrointest Surg. 2008;12:1866–72.

Chapter 96
Case on Complex Recurrent Fistula-in-Ano

Sonsoles Martinez Lopez and Miguel A. Cuesta

Keywords Perianal abscess • Perianal fistula • Recurrence • Fistulotomy • Mucosa advancement plasty • Seton

First Patient

Diagnosis and Indication for Surgery

A female, 45 years of age, was referred to our hospital with previous diagnosis of recurrent perianal abscesses. The patient had reported recurrent symptoms since a year, initially with perianal pain followed by subsequent drainage of purulent contents. On a first physical examination, a left anterolateral perianal fistula was diagnosed. An anal ultrasound was performed confirming a transsphincteric anterior fistula and surgery was proposed.

Operation

During surgery, the fistula was found to be highly transsphincteric, and treatment was initiated after curettage and cleaning with injection of fibrin glue.

S.M. Lopez, M.D. (✉)
Department of Surgery, Gregorio Marañon Hospital, Madrid, Spain
e-mail: sonsolesmartinezlopez@hotmail.com

M.A. Cuesta, M.D.
Department of Surgery, VU University Medical Center, Amsterdam, The Netherlands
e-mail: ma.cuesta@vumc.nl

M.A. Cuesta, H.J. Bonjer (eds.), *Case Studies of Postoperative Complications after Digestive Surgery*, DOI 10.1007/978-3-319-01613-9_96,

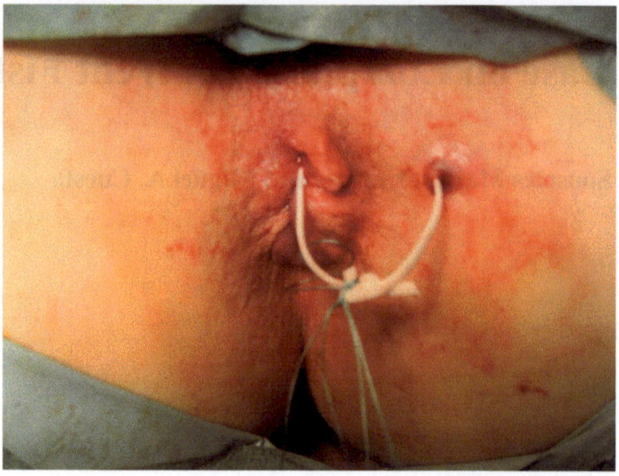

Fig. 96.1 Perianal fistula-in-ano with seton

After 6 weeks, the fistula persisted and a new surgical intervention was planned. During operation, a mucosal advancement flap (MAP) was performed.

Three months after operation, patient continued having discomfort and purulent discharge through the opening in perianal region. Physical examination of perinanal area confirmed the recurrence of the fistula. Complementary tests were performed. An anal endosonography was performed after injection of hydrogen peroxide through the external opening of the fistula. A high transsphincteric fistula was again diagnosed. No secondary tracts or local abscesses were seen. Moreover, using the daily defecation questionnaire, the Wexner Continence Grading Scale, she reported having already a mild grade of incontinence.

With a diagnosis of recurrent anterior perianal fistula, it was proposed to place a loose seton stitch through the track to allow a temporary good drainage of the fistula (Fig. 96.1).

Six weeks later, a fistulotomy was performed, followed by primary sphincter reconstruction and partial closure of mucosa. She was treated postoperatively with high fiber diet. After 8 weeks, at physical examination the wound was found closed. Patient complaints remained about some incontinence for gas. Pelvic floor physiotherapy has been given with acceptable results.

Second Patient

Diagnosis and Indication for Surgery

An obese male patient of 38 years was referred to us because of his fifth recurrent perianal fistula. This patient had a BMI of 38 and had been operated six times, first because of horseshoe perianal abscess 6 years before (Fig. 96.2) and thereafter again five times because of perianal fistula and recurrences. Crohn's disease had

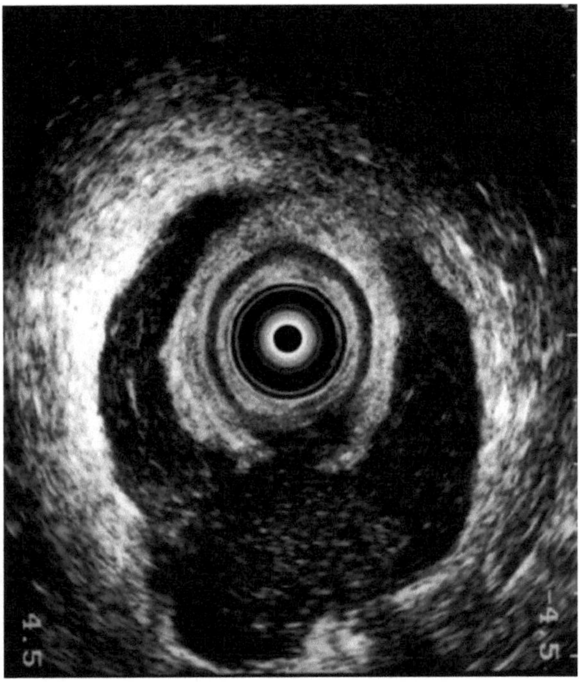

Fig. 96.2 Anal endosonography showing a horseshoe perianal abscess

been excluded 2 years before by means of colonoscopy and MRI enteroclysis. Operations included fistulectomy, mucosa advancement plasty (twice), and seton placement followed by fistulotomy. At the time of referral, he had two posterior fistulas, one at 6 h and the other 9 h, with two different internal openings at the dentate line. Endosonography with H_2O_2 showed two fistula tracks: the one trans-sphincteric and the other suprasphincteric above the level of the puborectalis muscle (Fig. 96.3). Moreover, a defect in both sphincters, internal and external, was visible at the posterior aspect of the anus. Patient told about some incontinence for gas, but not soiling.

Operation

We proposed him an exploration under anesthesia, in which the fistula at 6 h was directly treated by fistulotomy and the suprasphincteric was treated by means of a seton. Six weeks later, a new exploration showed that the amount of tissue in the seton was becoming smaller, but still we decided to wait with the seton and decided not to perform the fistulotomy. This was done 3 months later in which the fistula became more superficial and a fistulotomy was performed. Wound closed by secondary intention in 6 weeks. Patient has soiling and is doing pelvic floor physiotherapy. Patient has been proposed for bariatric surgery.

Fig. 96.3 Anal endosonography showing a posterior extrasphincteric fistula-in-ano

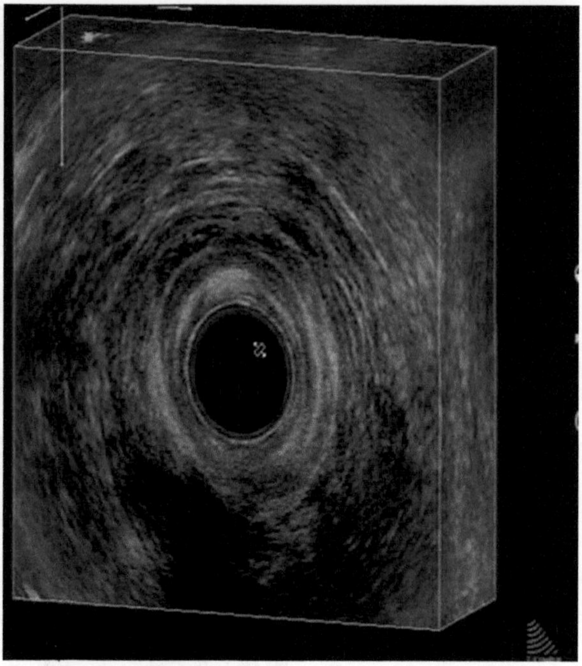

Discussion

Complex perianal fistula is associated with a high morbidity due to its high rate of recurrence and with incontinence, as depending on the surgical technique employed [1–3].

New approaches, such as fibrin glue and anal fistula plug, can involve lower risks of incontinence as compared to classical ones, but may have low and variable healing rates [4, 5].

Classical approaches such as mucosal advancement flap plasty (MAP) are technically difficult in the case of high complex fistula. In addition, fibrotic scar tissue from previous surgery increases the risk of intraoperative problems and postoperative complications occurring. In these complex fistulas, the advanced mucosal flap requires an extensive intra-rectal mobilization to obtain a tension-free closure, with an increased risk of incontinence.

In complex and recurrent perianal fistulas, the fistulotomy with primary sphincteric repair serves as a good technical option having a low recurrence risk (9–14 %) and a low risk of incontinence [1, 4].

New procedures like the anal fistula plug have been recently introduced in order to reduce the soiling and incontinence and the recurrent rates. Van Koperen et al. did a randomized trial comparing the anal plug and the MAP [5]. The results of the anal fistula plug and advancement flap procedures were disappointing in the multicenter setting. There were no significant differences in recurrence (71 % for the plug and 52 % for the MAP), functional outcome, and quality of life between the plug and the advancement flap. They suggested that because the plug is simple to apply and minimally invasive, it can be considered as an initial treatment option for high trans-sphincteric fistulas.

References

1. Holzheimer RG, Siebeck M. Perianal fistulas: developments in the classification and diagnostic techniques, and a new treatment strategy. Eur J Med Res. 2006;11:501–15.
2. Poen AC, Felt-Bersma RJ, Eijsbouts QA, et al. Hydrogen peroxide enhanced transanal ultra-sound in the assessment of fistula-in-ano. Dis Colon Rectum. 1998;41:1147–52.
3. Sloots CE, Felt-Bersma RJ, Poen AC, Cuesta MA. Assessment and classification of never operated and recurrent cryptoglandulair fistulas-in-ano using hydrogen peroxide enhanced trans-anal ultrasound. Colorectal Dis. 2001;3:422–6.
4. van Koperen PJ, Horsthuis K, Bemelman WA. Long-term functional outcome and risk factors for recurrence after surgical treatment for low and high perianal fistulas of cryptoglandular origin. Dis Colon Rectum. 2008;51:1475–81.
5. van Koperen PJ, Bemelman WA, Gerhards MF. The anal fistula plug treatment compared with the mucosal advancement flap for cryptoglandular high transsphincteric perianal fistula: a double-blinded multicenter randomized trial. Dis Colon Rectum. 2011;54:387–93.

Chapter 97
Case on Fecal Incontinence After Delivery

Miguel A. Cuesta

Keywords Childbirth • Fecal incontinence • Episiotomy • Sphincteroplasty • Sacral nerve stimulation • Ultrasonography • Manometry

Diagnosis and Indication for Surgery

A 30-year-old patient delivered her first child, a girl of 3.5 kg, vaginally by lateral episiotomy at the hospital. The next day, mother and baby girl went home without problems. Wound and postpartum evolved normally, but the patient felt that she could not hold her feces properly. After telling this to her GP and gynecologist, some tests were performed. An anorectal function test was carried out. Anal ultrasound showed an anterior defect of the external sphincter (Fig. 97.1), and on the anal manometry, rest pressure was low, 20 mm Hg, and squeeze pressure was normal, 60 mm Hg. Patient was treated initially by means of pelvic floor physiotherapy for 3 months with only slight improvement. After this treatment, the patient remained incontinent for feces and the surgeon was asked to perform a sphincteroplasty, which occurred by overlapping technique. The operation was followed by pelvic floor physiotherapy for a period of 3 months and regulation of the quality of feces by fibers. Despite some improvement, the patient remained incontinent, even though somewhat less so. Finally patient is referred to a specialized center for sacral nerve stimulation treatment.

M.A. Cuesta, M.D.
Department of Surgery, VU University Medical Center, Amsterdam, The Netherlands
e-mail: ma.cuesta@vumc.nl

M.A. Cuesta, H.J. Bonjer (eds.), *Case Studies of Postoperative Complications after Digestive Surgery*, DOI 10.1007/978-3-319-01613-9_97,

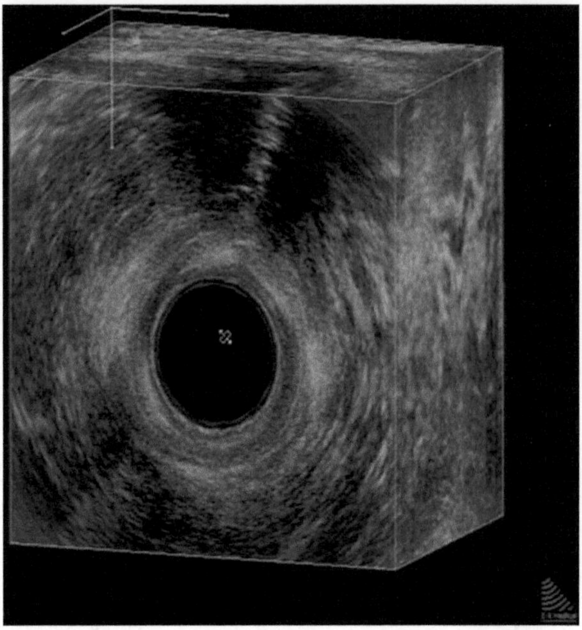

Fig. 97.1 Anal endosonography showing defect in the anterior part of the external sphincter

Discussion

Fecal incontinence can be caused by sphincter lesion, as in this case, or due to neurological damage with intact sphincters. The most frequent cause of fecal incontinence in female patients is related to different grades of sphincter damage caused during pregnancy and delivery. After assessment of the cause, usually conservative treatment follows by pelvic floor physiotherapy (plus biofeedback) and regulation of feces by anti-diarrhea and use of fibers in the diet. If it is an anterior sphincter defect the surgeon is asked to perform a sphincteroplasty by an overlapping technique. In a study performed in our institution 40 % of the women experienced continence after 5 years of the primary repair [1]. But, what to do with the rest of patients without improvement? The possibility to reoperate again, doing a gracilis plasty, or an artificial sphincter is not the solution for this problem; outcomes with these techniques are not good. There is an increasing use of the sacral nerve stimulation, including its use as alternative for the sphincter's repair operations. In the web site of the Harvard Pilgrim Health Care about the sacral nerve stimulation [2], they described the indications and the technology used. "Sacral nerve stimulation is used to treat the symptoms of an overactive bladder, including urinary incontinence. It has also has been approved by the FDA for treatment of fecal incontinence. It involves applying an electric current to one of the sacral nerves via an electrode through the corresponding sacral foramen. The electrode leads are attached to an implantable pulse generator".

Wexner et al. published in 2010 the outcome of a multicenter study about 120 patients with fecal incontinence treated by sacral stimulation [3]. The purpose of this study was to determine the safety and efficacy of sacral nerve stimulation in a large population under the rigors of Food and Drug Administration-approved investigational protocol.

A total of 133 patients underwent test stimulation with a 90 % success rate, and 120 (110 females) of a mean age of 60.5 years and a mean duration of FI of 6.8 years received chronic implantation. At 12 months, 83 % of subjects achieved therapeutic success and 41 % achieved 100 % continence. Therapeutic success was 85 % at 24 months. Incontinent episodes decreased from a mean of 9.4 per week at baseline to 1.9 at 12 months and 2.9 at 2 years. There were no reported unanticipated adverse device effects associated with InterStim Therapy®.

They concluded that Sacral nerve stimulation using InterStim Therapy® is a safe and effective treatment for patients with FI.

References

1. Poen AC, Felt-Bersma RJ, Strijers RL, et al. Third-degree obstetric perineal tear: long-term clinical and functional results after primary repair. Br J Surg. 1998;85:1433–8.
2. Website Harvard Pilgrim Health Care about Sacral nerve Stimulation for fecal incontinence
3. Wexner SD, Coller JA, Devroede G, et al. Sacral nerve stimulation for fecal incontinence: results of a 120-patient prospective multicenter study. Ann Surg. 2010;251:441–9.

Chapter 98
Case on Rectovaginal Fistula Following Delivery

Suzanne S. Gisbertz

Keywords Childbirth • Perineal rupture • Rectovaginal fistula • Ileostomy • Martius plasty

Diagnosis and Indication for Surgery

A 25-year-old female patient was admitted to the gynecology department of a tertiary referral center with a large rectovaginal fistula following delivery. She gave birth to a healthy child in a local hospital 5 days before admittance. Her medical history revealed no previous diseases or operations, except obesity. She was mentally disabled however, and the child was put under her mother's custody. During delivery there was no progress and subsequently an episiotomy and vacuum extraction were performed. During closure of the wound, the gynecologist described a possible "septum" in the vagina, but found no other abnormalities. The young mother was discharged the next day, but after arrival at home discovered that both flatulence and feces escaped through the vagina, leading to fecal incontinence and discomfort. During physical examination a large defect of approximately 4 cm was palpated between the vagina and rectum just above the level of the anal sphincters. A part of the sphincters was not damaged. The perineal area was swollen and painful. She was therewith diagnosed with an obstetric rectovaginal fistula and the indication for surgery was postulated.

S.S. Gisbertz, M.D.
Department of Surgery, Academic Medical Centre, Amsterdam, The Netherlands
e-mail: s.gisbertz@antoniusziekenhuis.nl

M.A. Cuesta, H.J. Bonjer (eds.), *Case Studies of Postoperative Complications after Digestive Surgery*, DOI 10.1007/978-3-319-01613-9_98,

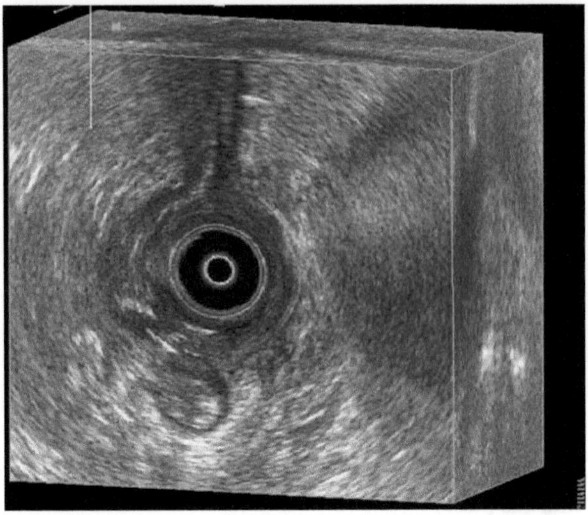

Fig. 98.1 Vaginal endosonography showing a defect between vagina and distal rectum

Operation

It was decided to perform a laparoscopic loop ileostomy as a first-stage operation to deviate the feces and to give the area time to heal. At evaluation under anesthesia, by means of a vaginal endosonography, a rectovaginal fistula was observed with anterior sphincter defect (Fig. 98.1). Local examination confirmed the fistula (Fig. 98.2). A laparoscopic loop ileostomy was created (Fig. 98.3). After 3 months, a Martius flap reconstruction was performed using the left bulbocavernosus flap as interposition and overlapping sphincteroplasty (Fig. 98.4 and Illustration 98.1). Two months after operation, the gynecologist assured us that the fistula had healed and we proceed to close the ileostomy. She is receiving active pelvic floor physiotherapy because of partial incontinence.

Operative Technique of Martius Flap Plasty

The fistula is closed with the interposition of a bulbocavernosus flap according to Martius [1]. For this procedure the flap is obtained from the labia majora and interposed between the rectum and vagina through a vaginal-labial incision (Illustration 98.1). The flap is a muscular graft harvested from either labia majora based on the perineal branch of the pudendal vessels.

The patient is placed in lithotomy position. The posterior vaginal wall is freed from the rectum through a transverse vaginal incision including the opening of the fistula. The fistula defect at the side of the rectum is closed with 3–0 absorbable sutures. An incision between the labium majus and minus is made. The bulbocavernosus muscle is freed and the anterior end of the muscle is transected, preserving the

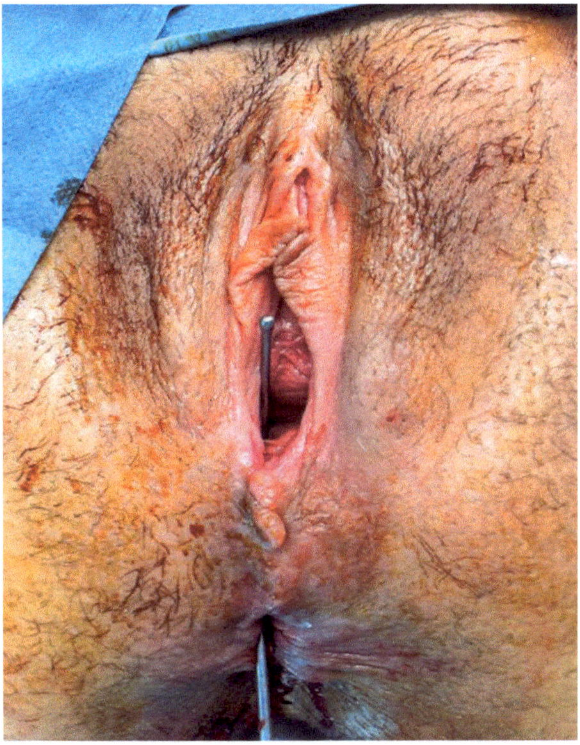

Fig. 98.2 Examination under anesthesia. Rectovaginal fistula

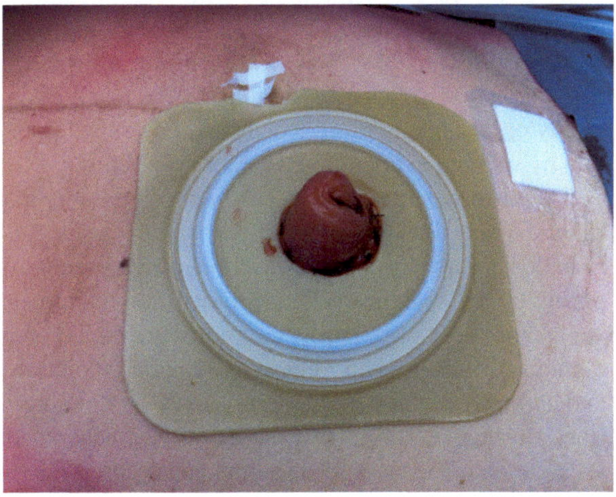

Fig. 98.3 Initial treatment by laparoscopic loop ileostomy

posterolateral vascular pedicle. The flap is transposed to the vaginal through a subcutaneous tunnel. The flap is loosely sutured in place between the vagina and rectum with absorbable sutures over the rectal closure. All wounds are closed in layers after drainage.

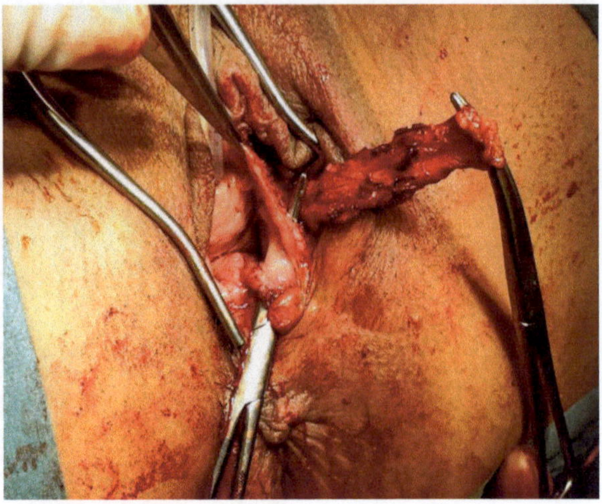

Fig. 98.4 Aspect of operation according to Martius with the bulbocavernosus flap

Discussion

It is noteworthy that the fistula was not discovered during wound closure. Either it was not identified or the ischemia caused by possible prolonged pressure on the rectovaginal septum did not induce necrosis yet. Early discovery, however, would probably not have changed functional outcome. The first step in treatment, especially in the case of large fistula with fecal incontinence or uncontrolled perineal sepsis, is probably always deviation of feces, drainage of abscesses, and local care. Direct reconstructions show disappointing results, with high residual fistula rates [2]. The fistula in this case is probably the result of an inadequately repaired episiotomy or an unrecognized laceration. Prolonged pressure on the rectovaginal septum by vacuum extraction is another possibility.

The most common etiology for rectovaginal fistula is obstetric injury (perineal ruptures, see Illustration 98.1). Other etiologies for rectovaginal fistula include radiation injury, Crohn's disease, operative trauma, infectious diseases, and neoplasm. In the Western world, obstetric injury is rare, occurring in less than 0.1 % of vaginal deliveries [3]. Perineal ruptures are more common in primigravidas, in precipitous births, or when forceps or vacuum extraction is used. Failure to recognize and correctly repair perineal lacerations, or secondary infection of perineal lacerations, further increases the chance of rectovaginal fistula. Prolonged labor with pressure on the rectovaginal septum can produce necrosis and result in rectovaginal fistula.

Treatment is executed in a multidisciplinary setting. Acute primary obstetric fistulas with perineal wound problems should be treated by a feces deviation in order to get an optimal moment for fistula operation. Fistula operation includes layered closure or mucosal advancement flaps. Success rates of 71–100 % have

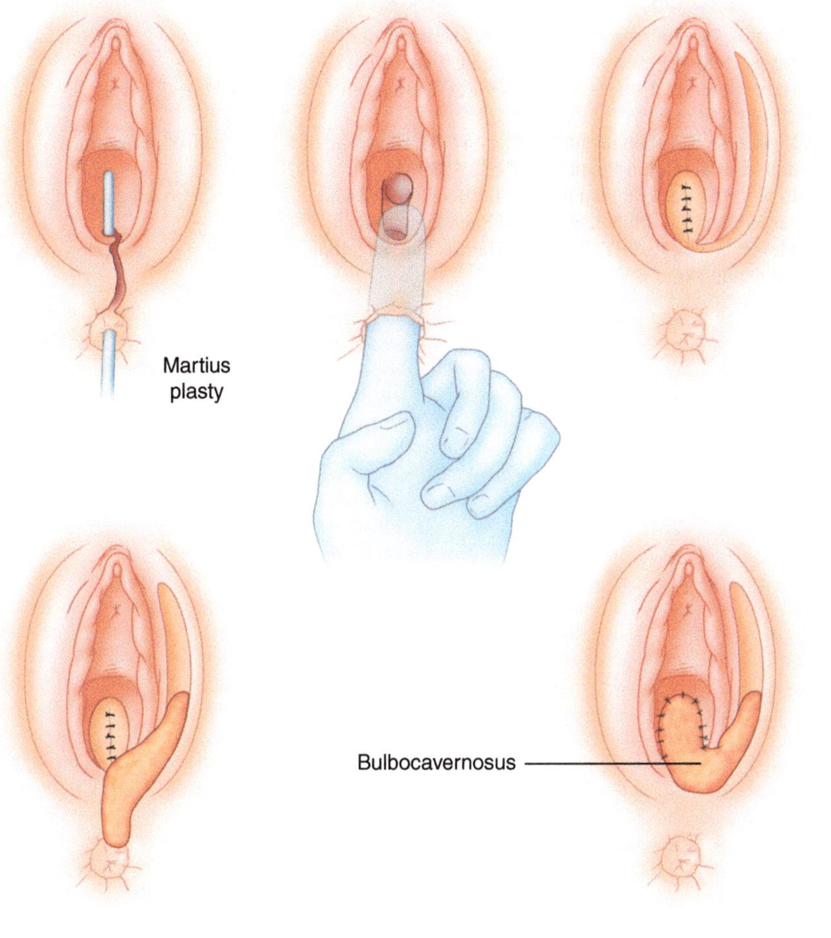

Illustration 98.1 Different steps for the Martius plasty

been described [4]. If there is no inflammation or sepsis, definitive operation can be performed without deviating stoma. Complex rectovaginal fistulas (high fistula, large, recurrent, underlying disease) are more difficult to treat. Tissue interposition with gracilis, sartorius, gluteus maximus, rectus or bulbocavernosus muscle, or omentum have all been described. The Martius flap is the most frequently applied and best documented [5]. This repair protected by a fecal diversion may be the optimal operation. If there is recurrence, permanent or temporary stoma will be maintained for a period of time. In the case of high rectovaginal fistulas a low anterior resection may be needed. Sphincter repair is recommended in all cases of sphincter defects.

References

1. Martius H. Die operative Wiederher-stellung der Volkmmen fehlenden Harnrohre und des Schliessmuskels derselben. Zentralbl Gynakol. 1928;8:480–2.
2. Halverson AL, Hull TL, Fazio VW, et al. Repair of recurrent rectovaginal fistulas. Surgery. 2001;130:753–7.
3. Venkatesh KS, Ramanyam PS, Larson DM, Haywood MA. Anorectal complications of vaginal delivery. Dis Colon Rectum. 1989;32:1039–41.
4. Lowry AC. Rectovaginal fistulas. In: Beck DE, Wexner SD, editors. Fundamentals of anorectal surgery. 2nd ed. Philadelphia, PA: Saunders; 2001. p. 174–86.
5. McNevin MS, Lee PY, Bax TW. Martius flap: an adjunct for repair of complex, low rectovaginal fistula. Am J Surg. 2007;193:597–9.

Chapter 99
Case on Dehiscence/Evisceration of the Abdominal Wall After Laparotomy

Maria Dolores Casado, Gianluca Sciannamea, María Socas, and Salvador Morales-Conde

Keywords Evisceration • Hernia • Mesh

Introduction

Evisceration is a rare (incidence vary from 0.3 to 3.5 %) but very severe complication of abdominal surgery, with a high rate of morbidity and mortality. Risk factors of abdominal wound dehiscence are elderly, immunosuppression, cancer, obesity, hemodynamic instability, diseases increasing abdominal pressure, emergency surgery, bowel surgery, hypoproteinemia, anemia, abdominal trauma, wound infection, vertical incisions, and improper closure techniques. The mortality and the possibility of dehiscence seem to correlate directly with the number of risk factors, so we could minimize the risk of its occurrence. We report two different cases: the first with an evisceration of a median incision and the second with a subcostal one.

First Patient

A 67-year-old man, with obesity, chronic bronchitis, and hypertension arterial, underwent low anterior resection of the rectum with terminal colostomy and resection of two hepatic nodules placed at the segments 2 and 4 due to a metastatic rectal cancer, located at 10 cm from the anal margin.

M.D. Casado, M.D. • G. Sciannamea, M.D. • M. Socas, M.D. • S. Morales-Conde, M.D. (✉)
Department of Surgery, Virgen del Rocio Hospital, Sevilla, Spain
e-mail: smoralesc@gmail.com

M.A. Cuesta, H.J. Bonjer (eds.), *Case Studies of Postoperative Complications after Digestive Surgery*, DOI 10.1007/978-3-319-01613-9_99,

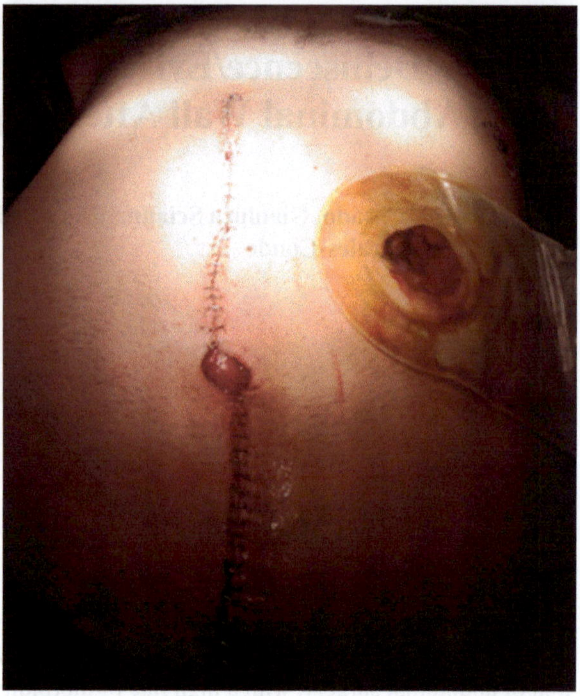

Fig. 99.1 Diagnosis of evisceration by wound inspection

The first postoperative day the patient presented fever, abdominal pain, nausea, and abdominal distension. A CT scan, performed in the same day, did not reveal any complications.

At the third postoperative day the patient presented an important bout of coughing with consequent evisceration and drain of serohematic fluid through the incision; the surgical incision presented wound dehiscence of the middle part of the skin incision, with small bowel exposed through the skin; there was no subcutaneous tissue over the greater part of the fascial defect (Figs. 99.1 and 99.2).

The patient was scheduled for surgery via a laparotomy. Primary closure of the defect was possible, but a polypropylene mesh of 30×30 cm was placed as a suprafascial reinforcement and was fixed with staples (Fig. 99.3). The mesh covered at least 5 cm of normal fascia in all directions around the defect of the fascia. Two suction drains were left in the subcutaneous tissue. Skin was closed with staples. No intraoperative complications occurred, the postoperative course was uneventful, and drains were removed on postoperative day 6, when they drained less than 100 cc of serohematic fluid.

The patient was discharged in the 10th postoperative day; after 3 months, he is asymptomatic, presenting no incisional hernia.

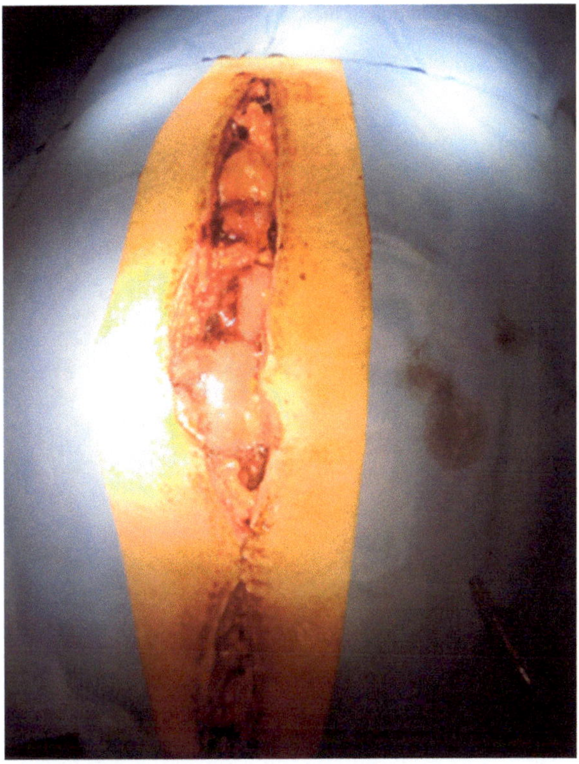

Fig. 99.2 Diagnosis of evisceration after opening the skin

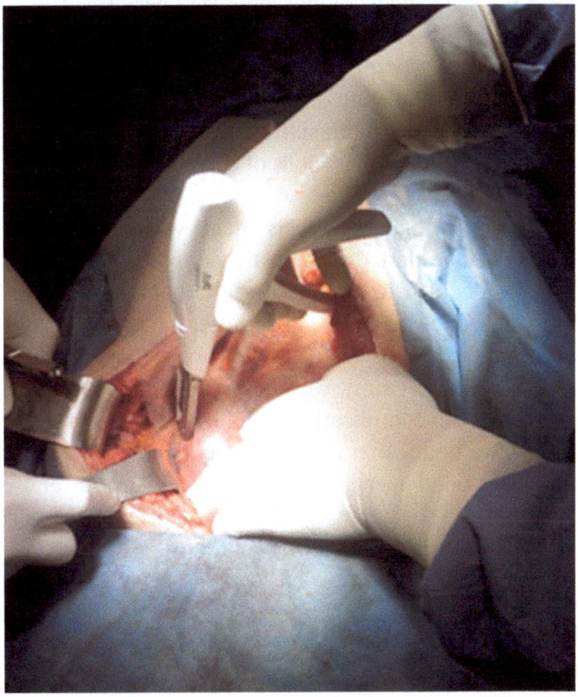

Fig. 99.3 Treatment of evisceration by means of polypropylene mesh stapled to the fascia

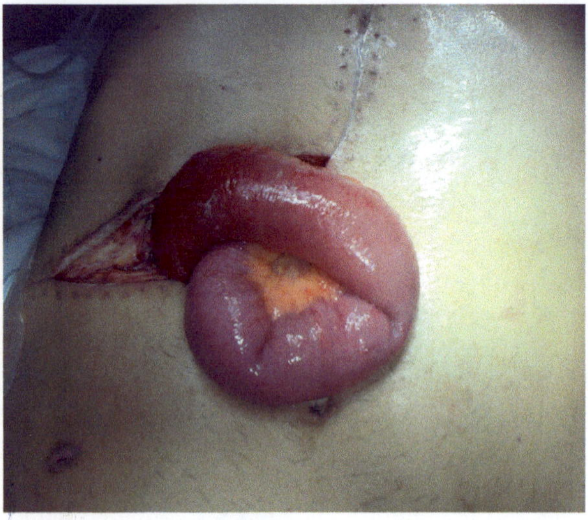

Fig. 99.4 Evisceration of the second patient

Second Patient

An 82-year-old man, heavy smoker (40 cigarettes a day), with a high drinking habit and type II diabetes, was operated in 1981 of a multifocal epidermoid oral carcinoma (T2N1) and he received adjuvant radiochemotherapy. The current history started in April 2010. He suffered an intestinal obstruction characterized by constipation, abdominal distension, and pain.

A CT scan and a colonoscopy were performed.

(a) Colonoscopy showed multiple polypoid lesions all over the colon, with pathology of hyperplasic polyps and a hepatic flexure tumor causing stenosis with pathology of moderate differentiated and ulcerated colon adenocarcinoma. (b) CT scan: great metastatic lesion that occupies nearly all the right liver lobe which is very close to the upper pole of the right kidney. It seems to infiltrate the adrenal gland.

An intracolonic prosthesis (stent) was placed and when the colonic obstruction was solved he started with the neoadjuvant therapy. After a multidisciplinary meeting, we decided to operate first the hepatic metastasis and in a second time the colonic lesion. In January 2011, after finishing neoadjuvant therapy and once being sure that the lesions had a good response to chemotherapy, a right hepatectomy and a right adrenalectomy were performed. The postoperative period was favorable, there were no complications, and he was discharged 8 days after surgery.

Twelve hours after the discharge, the patient came back to the hospital with the surgical wound opened ("J" incision) and the bowel was evident through the wound (Fig. 99.4). The patient said that he had been coughing since he was discharged and suddenly he realized that the wound was wet.

The patient was operated 3 h after his admission. A double running nonabsorbable suture was used to close the abdominal wall. There were no pathological findings in abdominal cavity. We decided not to put a mesh because he was going to be operated in a few weeks of his colon carcinoma.

The postoperative period was favorable and he was discharged 5 days after. We insisted to the patient to leave smoking habit and to wear permanently a strip.

In February 2011 the patient was operated again and a subtotal colectomy and a terminal ileostomy were performed. There were no incidences. During the second postoperative day the ileostomy started working and the oral intake started too.

Discussion

Abdominal wound dehiscence is a rare complication of abdominal surgery. It is most often related to bowel and emergency surgery. Reports usually refer this complication in cirrhotic patients with ascites and elevated intraabdominal pressure, or secondary to severe abdominal trauma.

It is very rare that a subcostal incision become eviscerated. In our case, the fact that the patient was a heavy smoker and the use of neoadjuvant therapy have had a main role in his situation.

The majority of patients who present an evisceration require a relaparotomy, but in case of elderly patients with clinical contraindications a conservative management can be performed of the threatening evisceration with intact skin closure. If the bowels or omentum are eviscerated, surgery is indicated [1].

Repair of the fascial defect, either with mesh or without depending on the case, is imperative to prevent subsequent herniation and recurrent evisceration. Satisfactory results have been reported with the use of this technique to repair eviscerations, but good knowledge of risk factors is mandatory for prophylaxis.

Reference

1. Burger JW, van 't Riet M, Jeekel J. Abdominal incisions: techniques and postoperative complications. Scand J Surg. 2001;91:315–21.

Chapter 100
Case on Recurrence of Incisional Hernia After Large Hernia Repair Using (Low-Weight) Polypropylene Mesh

María Socas, Salvador Morales-Conde, María Sánchez Ramírez, and Antonio Barranco

Keywords Mesh • Hernia • Strength • Trocar • Scan

Lightweight large-porous mesh philosophy takes into consideration all of the recent data regarding physiology and mechanics of the abdominal wall. The new mesh concept reveals an optimized foreign body reaction based on reduction of the amounts of mesh material needed and, in particular, a significantly small area of the large-porous model coming into contact with the recipient hosts tissues Moreover, recent data demonstrate that alterations in the extracellular matrix of hernia patients play a crucial role in the development of hernia recurrence. In particular, long-term recurrences—often occurring months or even years after surgery and implantation of mesh—can be explained by the extracellular matrix hypothesis. However, if the altered extracellular matrix proves to be the weak area, the decisive question becomes whether the amount of material as well as mechanical and tensile strength of the surgical mesh significantly impact the development of recurrent hernia. All experimental evidence and first clinical data indicate the superiority of the lightweight large-porous mesh concept with regard to a reduced number of long-term complications and particularly, an increased comfort, and quality of life after hernia repair.

M. Socas, M.D. • S. Morales-Conde, M.D. (✉) • M. Sánchez Ramírez • A. Barranco
Department of Surgery, Virgen del Rocio Hospital, Sevilla, Spain
e-mail: smoralesc@gmail.com

M.A. Cuesta, H.J. Bonjer (eds.), *Case Studies of Postoperative Complications after Digestive Surgery*, DOI 10.1007/978-3-319-01613-9_100,

Patient

Diagnosis and Indication for Surgery

Female patient aged 49, having BMI 47.7, a history of penicillin allergy, and hypertension, was operated in 2008 for a giant ovarian cyst and subsequently in the same year for a large ventral hernia.

Description of Operation

In this case, at first we repaired a ventral hernia by supra- and infra-umbilical incision by open approach using a polypropylene mesh "UltraPro"—30 by 30 cm, being placed retrofascial and premuscular.

Postoperative Course: Identification and Treatment of Complication

Postoperatively, the patient presented a good evolution and was discharged on the tenth day without incident. During outpatient follow-up, she presented a surgical wound seroma that required weekly cures during 1 month, to which she responded positively and with negative wound cultures.

Eleven months after surgery, the patient had recurrence of the ventral hernia (Illustration 100.1a). The examination revealed a localized defect, an infra-umbilical hernia defect in the midline of 20 by 15 cm. The abdominal CT scan confirmed the presence of a hernia in midline (Fig. 100.1), which led to our decision to reoperate it.

On this occasion, we chose a laparoscopic approach for repair of recurrent ventral hernia. We performed a bilateral laparoscopic approach using a 12-mm trocar and two 5-mm trocars on the left flank and one 10-mm trocar and a 5-mm trocar on the right flank. We found an external defect of 15 by 15 cm and an internal defect of 22 by 12 cm. Important conglomerate adhesions between colon, omentum, and small bowel and multiple defects in the middle of the previous mesh were identified (Fig. 100.2). An e-PTFE mesh of 36 by 24 cm was placed, being fixed with a double crown of tackers and Fibrin Glue (Tissucol spray®), in order to avoid adhesions in the future (Illustration 100.1b).

A year after repair of recurrent of the open incisional hernia, an abdominal CT scan was performed to evaluate the position of the mesh and established there had been no new recurrence (Fig. 100.3).

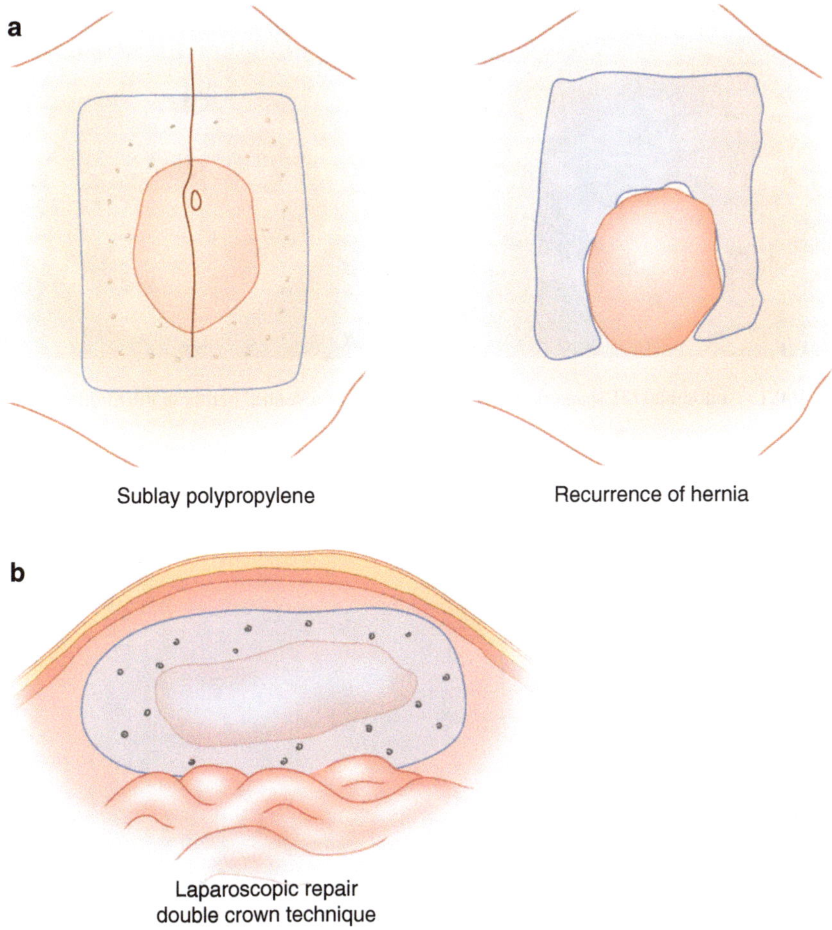

Illustration 100.1 (**a, b**) Low-weight meshes in very large hernias for morbidly obese patients could become a contraindication for open ventral hernia repair. Low-weight mesh may break in the middle and so developing a recurrence. These recurrences require proper repair by laparoscopic approach

Discussion

Laparoscopic repair of ventral hernia is widely accepted for certain indications. One of the advantages of laparoscopic repair is the possibility of detecting those defects unidentifiable by clinical examination, especially in morbidly obese patients. Moreover, the intra-abdominal view also allows detecting meshes previously placed by open approach. For some surgeons, a difficult laparoscopic ventral hernia repair includes also those previously repaired by open approach using a polypropylene mesh. There are indications of an increase of intra-abdominal adhesions to previous

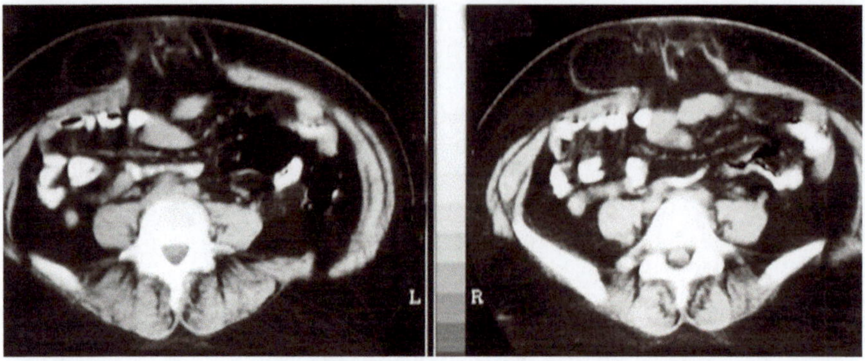

Fig. 100.1 Abdominal CT scan confirmed the existence of a ventral hernia in the midline

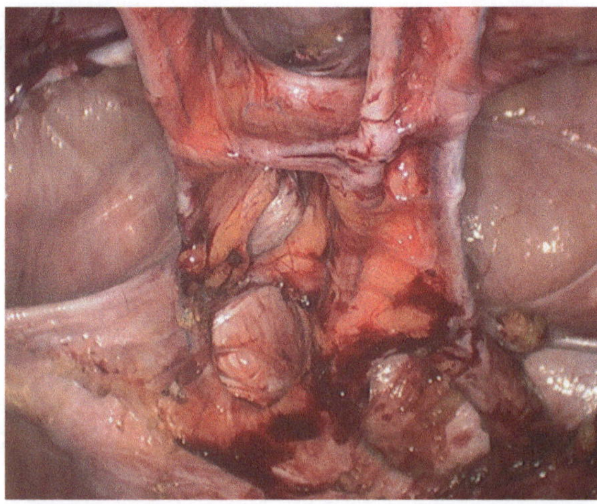

Fig. 100.2 Important conglomerate adhesions between colon, omentum, and small bowel and multiple defects in the middle of the previous mesh

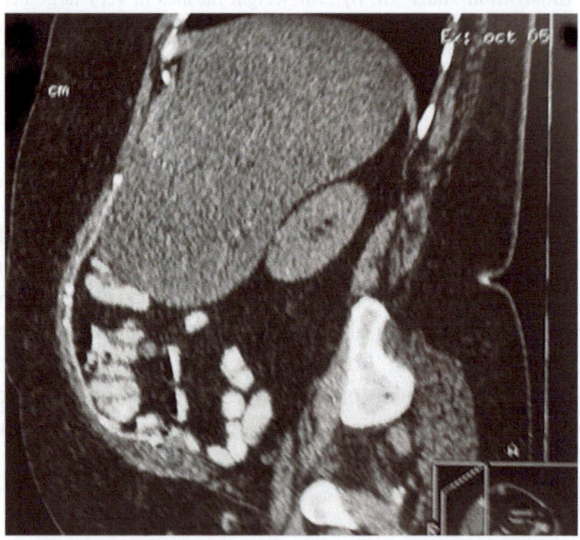

Fig. 100.3 Abdominal CT scan after laparoscopic repair: mesh is in place and no recurrence is observed

placed mesh, even if during previous open surgery the mesh had not been placed in contact with the bowel. Accordingly, the body generates an intense inflammatory response to the prosthetic that results in scar plate formation, increased stiffness of the abdominal wall, and shrinkage of the biomaterial. Reducing the density of polypropylene and creating a "lightweight" mesh theoretically induces the lessening of a foreign-body response, thereby resulting in an improved compliance of the abdominal wall, which causes less contraction or shrinkage of the mesh and hence allows for better tissue incorporation.

Large-pore meshes can be used safely for open primary incisional hernia repair, generating an equal outcome as compared with small-pore meshes in nonobese patients with defects smaller than 10 cm in width, in regard to both recurrence rates and chronic discomfort. In this way, we can conclude that the indications of low-weight meshes in selected cases could be the following: BMI <40 kg/m^2, hernia defects <10 cm, and primary ventral hernia (no recurrence).

This case shows how a previous "lightweight" polypropylene meshes placed preperitoneally could produce dense adhesions. It also demonstrated how the use of lightweight meshes in large hernias for obese patients could lead to breaks in the middle, thereby bringing about a recurrence. This recurrence could be properly repaired with laparoscopy by placing a mesh in contact with the bowel following the double-crown technique.

In conclusion, using low-weight meshes in very large hernias for morbidly obese patients could become a contraindication for open ventral hernia repair. We base this on experiences like ours, given also we already had encountered three similar cases, in which the low-weight mesh had broken in the middle and so developing a recurrence. These recurrences require proper repair by laparoscopic approach [1, 2].

References

1. Morales Conde S. Laparoscopic ventral hernia repair: advances and limitations. Semin Laparosc Surg. 2004;11:191–200.
2. Sharma A, Mehrotra M, Khullar R, et al. Laparoscopic ventral/incisional hernia repair: a single centre experience of 1242 patients over a period of 13 years. Hernia 2011;15:131–9.

Chapter 101
Case on Abdominal Compartment Syndrome

Antonio Barranco, Carlos Bernardos, María Socas, and Salvador Morales-Conde

Keywords Abdominal compartment • Pressure • Support therapy • Fascia • Mesh

The compartment syndrome (CS) is defined as an increase in the pressure inside the abdominal cavity over 12 mmHg. Already known in the nineteenth century, its treatment remains controversial. Recent increasing interest is due to the improvement in surgical techniques over abdominal closure, the availability of damage control surgery, and support measures, leading to a decrease in the associated mortality of CS—even though it still is high in critically ill patients.

Patient

We present a 12-month-old male baby with medical reports as follows: liver transplant, 5 days before complication, due to acute liver failure because of a paracetamol overdose. This young baby had undergone an administration of rectal paracetamol because of high fever and then was reported to the emergency department having general discomfort, high fever up to 40 °C, and progressively low reactivity. The only information available was the administration of an unknown dosage of paracetamol by his parents in a high fever context.

At the time of the admission, the patient looked ill, having an encephalopathic appearance. The test showed signs of liver failure, high levels of transaminases, and an INR up to 9 after receiving vitamin K. The patient was admitted to the Intensive Unit Care (IUC) in order to have support therapy applied while awaiting a liver

A. Barranco • C. Bernardos • M. Socas, M.D. • S. Morales-Conde, M.D. (✉)
Department of Surgery, Virgen del Rocio Hospital, Sevilla, Spain
e-mail: smoralesc@gmail.com

M.A. Cuesta, H.J. Bonjer (eds.), *Case Studies of Postoperative Complications after Digestive Surgery*, DOI 10.1007/978-3-319-01613-9_101,

transplant. After a 36-h stay, a compatible adult donor appeared and then a split-liver transplant was carried out using the left lateral segments (II–III).

Surgery

The problem after the transplant was performed became the impossibility of closing the abdominal wall due to the edema, the bowel dilatation, and a slightly larger liver than appropriate (Fig. 101.1). Obviously, the intra-abdominal pressure (IAP) had not been measured because it was not considered necessary to know that it could become very high. Then a Bogota technique (Fig. 101.2) was performed, attaching the bag to the fascia with a running PDS 2/0 suture. This technique was performed temporally in order to avoid a compartment abdominal syndrome, to recover the

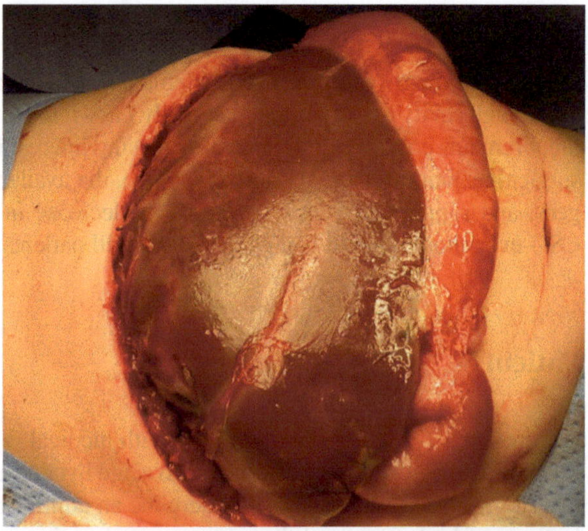

Fig. 101.1 Large size of the liver and bowel dilatation

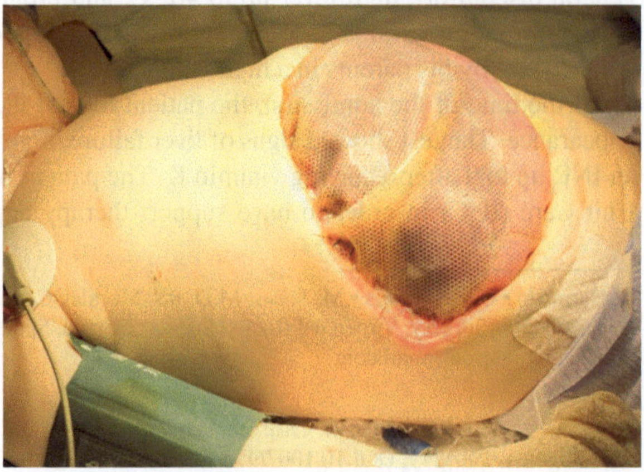

Fig. 101.2 Bogota bag attached to the fascia

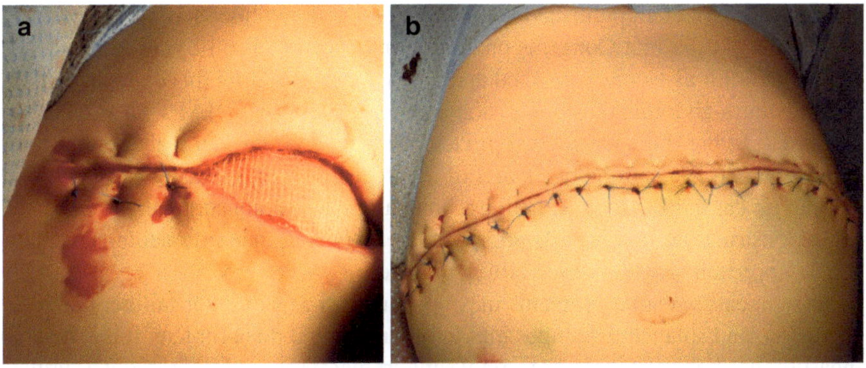

Fig. 101.3 (**a**) Skin closure with interrupted suture. (**b**) Final appearance

patient as fast as possible, and then after few days, to remove the bag and to possibly close the abdominal wall.

Postoperative Course

After 5 days, the patient looked well and a second operation was performed; the film was removed, the fascia was cleaned, and an attempt at closure was done, but unfortunately that failed. The primary closure of the fascia was impossible and only interrupted PDS 2/0 skin stitches were done (Fig. 101.3a). From then on, the postoperative evolution of the patient at the hospital became satisfactory, with a good function of the liver and without complications in the abdominal closure. The patient having a good appearance, an appropriate growth, and not having signs of wound healing complications could after a stay of 24 days be discharged from the IUC. The first postoperative days went satisfactory, the IAP (daily measures) progressively decreased, and there were no problems during his stay. Hence, the patient was discharged from the hospital doing well. After a period of 3 months, the patient underwent a new surgical procedure and the fascia of the muscle was closed tension free by means of interrupted 2/0 Vicryl® stitches and ensuring that there was no intra-abdominal hypertension (IAH) (Fig. 101.3b).

Discussion

The compartment syndrome (CS) is a situation in which the intra-abdominal pressure (IAP) arises to high levels as measured by a urinary catheter inside the bladder and is associated with organ dysfunction and mortality in critically ill patients.

In 1984, Krol et al. published the first series of measurements of the IAP and its definitions. At the first Congress on Abdominal Compartment Syndrome in 2004, several definitions were established and a new age for treating this disease opened.

Now intra-abdominal hypertension (IAH) is defined as IAP>12 mmHg (or 16 cm H_2O), but there are several grades of IAH attending to the abdominal pressure (grades I–IV) and the quickness of its process (acute, subacute, chronic). The CS can be caused by many situations, both surgical and nonsurgical, for example, bowel obstruction, gastric dilatation, pancreatitis, pneumoperitoneum in laparoscopic approach, ascites, hemoperitoneum, etc.

In such cases several problems may appear, such as ventilator failure, low renal perfusion, and splanchnic congestion. In order to avoid this problem, it is crucial to measure the abdominal pressure, apply support measures, and to carry out a surgical procedure to decrease the high pressure inside the abdominal cavity. In summary, an IAP higher than 20 mmHg and a failure of the life support treatment will form an indication for engaging surgical decompression [1].

Reference

1. Schein M, Wittmann DH, Aprahamian C, Condon RE. The abdominal compartment syndrome. The physiological and clinical consequences of elevated intra-abdominal pressure. J Am Coll Surg. 1995;180:745–53.

Chapter 102
Case on Enterocutaneous Fistula Through Previous Laparotomy

María Socas, Salvador Morales-Conde, and Isaias Alarcón

Keywords Laparotomy • Enterocutaneous fistula • Support • Mesh • Wound protection • Nutrition

Enterocutaneous fistula is a dreaded complication following surgery, constituting an abnormal communication between an intestinal segment and the skin. It usually is brought about by drainage wounds but sometimes is brought through the laparotomy wound. The challenge becomes solving the fistula as well as closing the abdominal wall during the same surgical procedure.

Patient

A 54-year-old woman with a previous history of emergency laparotomy presented 2 years previously due to an attempt to suicide, and now was admitted to our emergency unit with complaints of vomiting and a distended abdomen. Abdominal X-ray showed several small bowel fluid levels. After failure of conservative treatment, an exploratory laparotomy was performed. Dense intestinal adhesions were observed as the cause of the occlusion. During adhesiolysis, an accidental intestinal perforation occurred 20 cm from ligament of Treizt. Resection of a 10-cm jejunal segment and mechanic side-to-side anastomosis was performed.

Three days after surgery, the patient presented a leakage in the anastomosis, and a relaparotomy was performed. A direct closure of the leakage was reinforced with

M. Socas, M.D. • S. Morales-Conde, M.D. (✉) • I. Alarcón
Department of Surgery, Virgen del Rocio Hospital, Sevilla, Spain
e-mail: smoralesc@hotmail.com

M.A. Cuesta, H.J. Bonjer (eds.), *Case Studies of Postoperative Complications after Digestive Surgery*, DOI 10.1007/978-3-319-01613-9_102,

Tachosil®. Subsequently, the patient required two more laparotomies due to a recurrence of the leakage and the presence of secondary intra-abdominal abscesses.

In the postoperative period, the patient developed two enterocutaneous fistulae through midline laparotomy with partial skin dehiscence and a high fistula output (more than 1 l/day) (Fig. 102.1).

After 6 months, despite conservative management with total parenteral and also enteral nutrition through a Foley catheter connected to distal fistula, the daily output remained the same. According to the patient's wishes, a new intervention was proposed.

Surgery

A new laparotomy was performed. After dissection of enterocutaneous fistulae, we performed the resection of an 80-cm-sized segment of small bowel (which included both fistulae) and a side-to-side mechanic anastomosis. It became impossible to perform a primary abdominal wall closure due to previous interventions, so a macroporous c-PTFE mesh was placed to cover the fascial defect (Fig. 102.2). The skin was closed where it was possible, and the skin defect over the mesh was covered by vacuum assisted closure (VAC) system using a black sponge (Fig. 102.3).

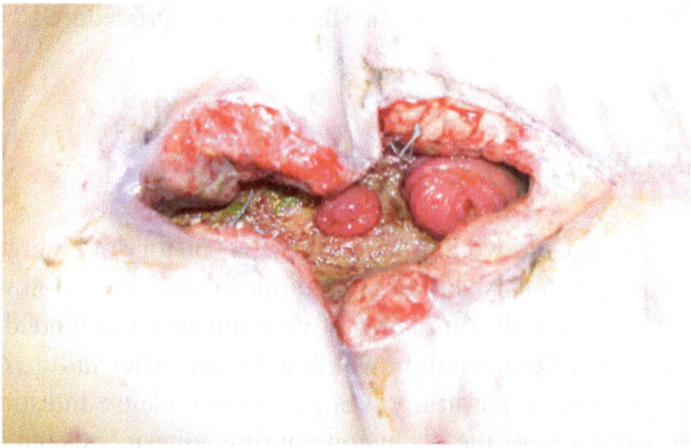

Fig. 102.1 Partial skin dehiscence and a high fistula output

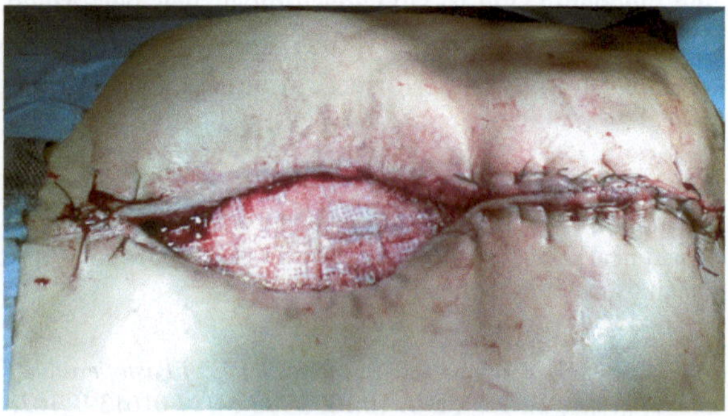

Fig. 102.2 PTFE mesh was placed to cover the fascial defect

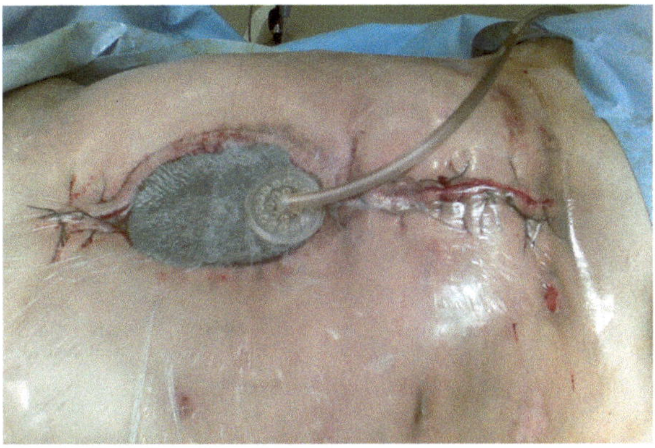

Fig. 102.3 Over the mesh was covered by vacuum assisted closure (VAC)

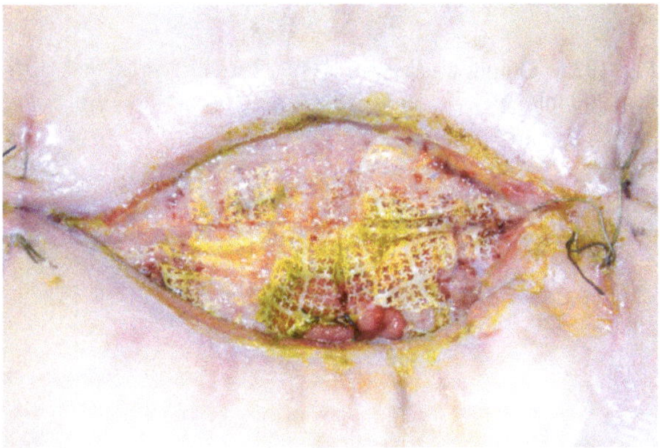

Fig. 102.4 Intestinal content being drained through a tear in the mesh

Outcome

Two days after that last intervention, the VAC output turned intestinal with a daily output of 400 ml. A new intervention was carried out. After removing the VAC system, a partial dehiscence in two different points of previous anastomosis was observed, the intestinal content being drained through a tear in the mesh (Fig. 102.4). A new conservative management was started, now placing a VAC system with a white sponge over the anastomosis exposed through the mesh, and two Kehr tubes were introduced in both dehiscence points to control intestinal leakage (Fig. 102.5). After 8 weeks, the skin condition improved, the mesh was completely integrated, and Kehr tubes output were less than 200 ml/day (Fig. 102.6). Finally, the patient underwent a further laparotomy with intestinal reanastomosis, abdominal closure with Proceed Mesh, and primary closure of skin.

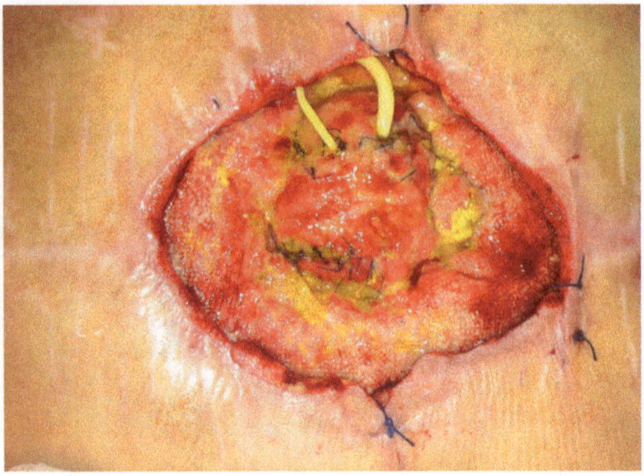

Fig. 102.5 Two Kehr tubes were introduced in both dehiscence points to control intestinal leakage

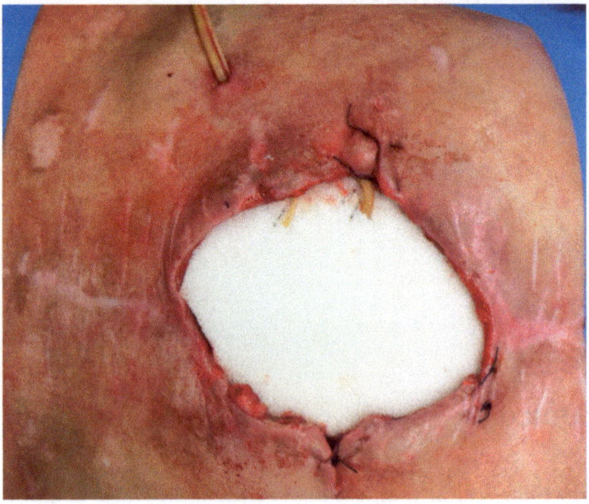

Fig. 102.6 Output was less than 200 ml/day

Conclusion

Closure of enterocutaneous fistulas after multiple laparotomies remains a challenge for patient and surgeons. Aggressive versus initial support measures is still the dilemma [1].

Reference

1. Bjorck M, D'Amours SK, Hamilton AE. Closure of the open abdomen. Am Surg. 2011;77(Suppl 1):S58–61.

Chapter 103
Case on Care and Closure of Open Abdomen Approach

Miguel A. Cuesta and Jurriaan B. Tuynman

Keywords Acute pancreatitis • Organ failure • Open abdomen • VAC therapy • Mesh • Nutrition • Wound manager

First Patient

Diagnosis and Indication for Surgery

A 29-year-old obese female patient known with immunosuppressive disease underwent elsewhere an ERCP because of a suspicion for having CBD stones with colics and alteration of liver enzymes. As a consequence of ERCP without papillotomy, she developed in the course of 2 days a necrotizing acute pancreatitis with multiple organ failure MOF. Patient was intubated and ventilated with a high PEEP of 14 and acute dialysis became necessary because of the acute renal insufficiency. Due to her obesity, with a BMI of 47, ventilation was considered difficult or impossible and an abdominal compartment syndrome was diagnosed. Consequently, surgeon performed a long transversal upper abdomen laparotomy and there a huge fluid collection was drained. Abdomen was left open and temporarily closed by means of a double Vicryl® mesh. The next day feces appeared under the mesh, coming out of the wound. Inspection revealed that the leakage came from the colon, and a reoperation was planned. At relaparotomy, an opening was found in the transverse colon near the splenic flexure. Her upper abdomen was changed as a plastron and surgeon closed the colon distal of perforation by staples. After dissection of the transverse mesentery, the surgeon could create a colostomy at the middle right abdomen. Two

M.A. Cuesta, M.D. (✉) • J.B. Tuynman
Department of Surgery, VU University Medical Center, Amsterdam, The Netherlands
e-mail: ma.cuesta@vumc.nl

M.A. Cuesta, H.J. Bonjer (eds.), *Case Studies of Postoperative Complications after Digestive Surgery*, DOI 10.1007/978-3-319-01613-9_103,

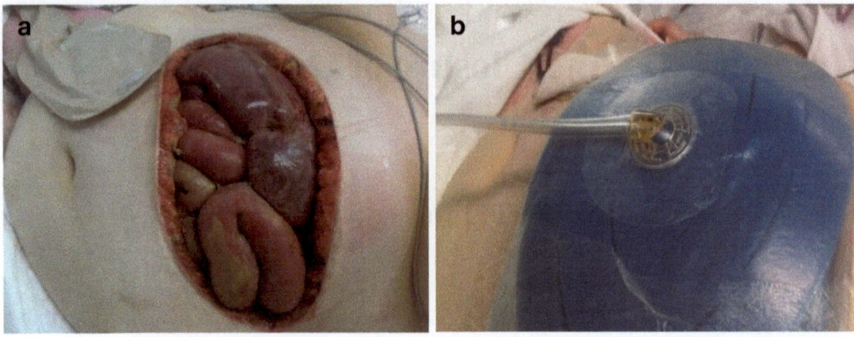

Fig. 103.1 (**a**) Open abdomen procedure with colostomy on the *right side*. (**b**) VAC system applied on the wound

drains were left, one along the colon and the other in the pancreatic area. Abdomen was rinsed and closed temporarily by means of a VAC system (Fig. 103.1a, b). Colostomy remained vital and productive and the wound started to granulate. Ventilation was difficult and a tracheotomy was given. At the same time, clinical condition improved, renal function recovered, and she could be extubated. Eight weeks after admission, in the IC department, patient could go to a revalidation center. She did not wish the VAC system for this period, which was feasible because the wound was smaller with healthy granulating bottom. Polimem® was applied to the surface of the wound.

After a period of revalidation and having gained a BMI of 35 a year later, she underwent a new operation to close the wound and the colostomy.

Second Patient

Diagnosis and Indication for Surgery

A 71-year-old female patient was admitted for an elective treatment of an incisional hernia. In the past she had undergone different surgical interventions, the most important 15 years before, involving the resection of uterus and ovaries because of a low-grade malignant granulosa cell tumor of the right ovary. Due to recurrences of this tumor in the last 15 years she had undergone ten surgical interventions to resect the recurrences. During the last operation, recurrence on the sigmoid was treated by sigmoid resection and definitive colostomy. The incisional hernia developed in the upper part of a middle lower abdomen. Because of the recurrence, the laparotomy scar had already 3 years previously been treated by mesh, yet without success. Patient had multiple complaints of the hernia, experiencing periods of incarceration. At a multidisciplinary session, the surgeon and the gynecologist decided to repair the hernia by a mesh. Important is to say that on the CT scan, it appeared to be a possible recurrence of the known tumor on the left obturator area, yet without pain. Operation was performed and surgeon decided to put a mesh on lay, polypropylene®. On the fourth postoperative day, the patient developed fever and a wound abscess that was drained by retiring some stitches. Next day, at day five, it was clear that intestinal contents were coming out the wound, possibly due to transverse colon or distal ileum. The CT scan revealed no intra-abdominal abscesses.

Patient was treated conservatively, with adequate wound covering and draining system, enteral feeding, Somastotatin, and also psychological support.

The plan was to operate this patient after 6 weeks, but a couple of days before that the patient developed an increasing loss of intestinal contents through the vagina. A new CT scan showed leakage of a small bowel loop to the stump of vagina.

Operation was performed 3 days later (Fig. 103.2a–d); scar with fistulas was excised to enter the abdomen. All loops of the small bowel were dissected free from abdominal wall and pelvis, with care not to damage the colon. Three fistulas were visualized, two of these with trajectories to the abdominal wall and the third to the stump of vagina. A short ileal resection was performed to treat the fistula to vagina; the other two were closed by a horizontal running suture. After inspection and over-inspection to foreclose serosa defects, the tumor was palpated at the obturator region, 5 by 2 cm flat. Abdominal wall was temporarily closed by means of a double Vicryl® mesh sutured to the edges of the fascia. Skin was closed leaving drains behind. Patient recovered slowly, and after 3 weeks she could be transferred to a revalidation center.

Discussion

The pertaining question is: How to treat an open abdomen approach?

Once a preliminary decision has been taken for an open abdomen approach, three different approaches can be followed, depending on whether intestinal leakage is present or not. These are (a) if no intestinal leakage, closing the abdomen temporarily by a reabsorbable mesh and drains; (b) if there is intestinal leakage through the wound, treatment by an adequate receptaculum system like the wound manager with drains may be the ideal solution. It can be opened and closed for inspection, and eventual treatment (Fig. 103.3); and (c) applying a VAC system. It is clear that the VAC system is the best option for an open abdomen without fistulas. This system permits an adequate drainage of the wound and makes the patient manageable. A wound manager with drains may then in the first period be effective. Once this is carried out, the VAC system may then be used to control the open abdomen and thereafter waiting at least for 6 weeks or more for the definitive treatment by laparotomy.

During the definitive treatment by laparotomy, the fistulas and abdominal wall should be closed. A double Vicryl mesh® should be used to temporarily to close the abdominal wall. Later on a definitive closure of the incisional hernia can be accomplished [1, 2].

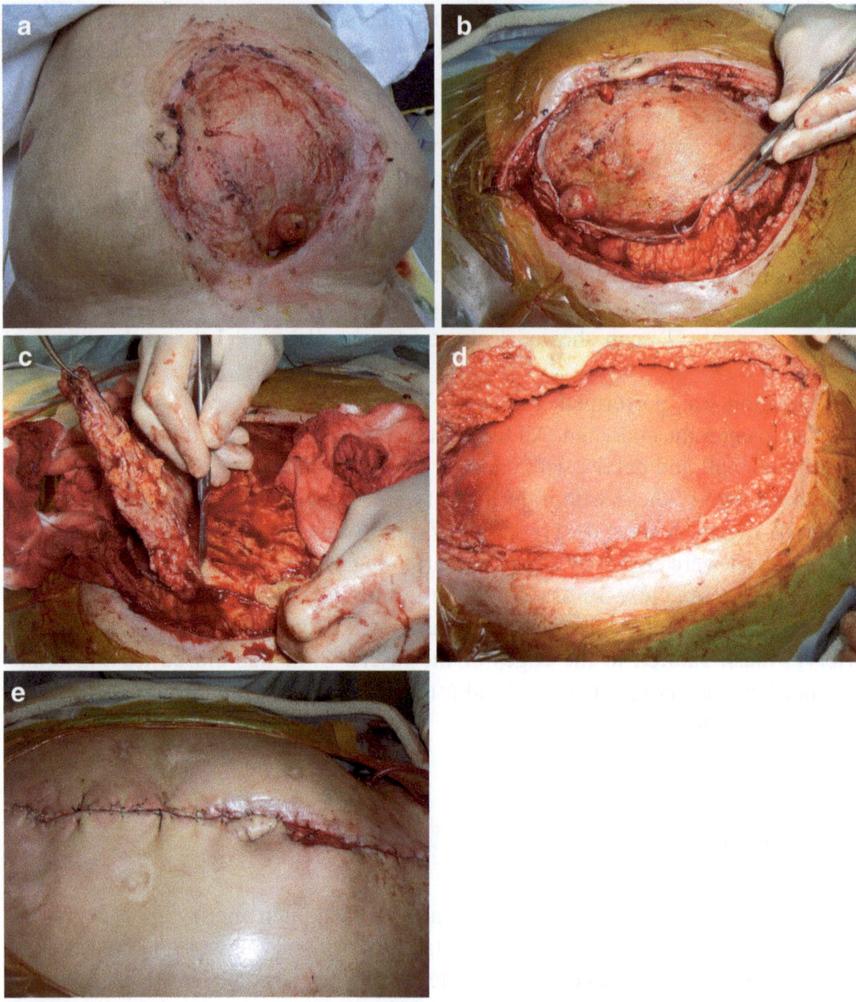

Fig. 103.2 (**a**) Aspect of the scar/wound after abdomen approach treatment with intestinal fistulas. (**b**) Excision of the scar. (**c**) Entry in the abdominal cavity. (**d**) Closure of the scar and fistulas. (**e**) Closure of abdominal wall by means of double Vicryl mesh®

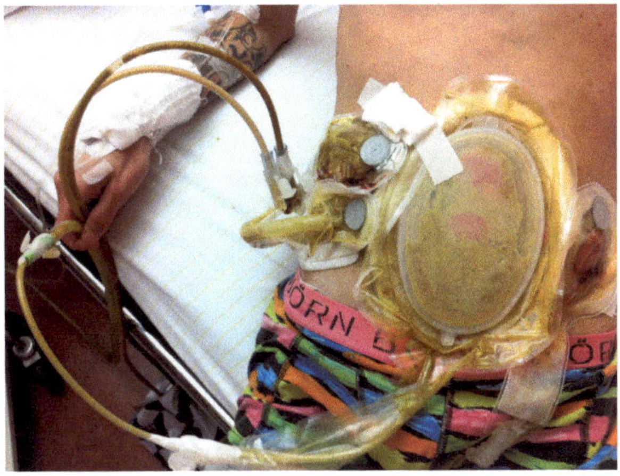

Fig. 103.3 Wound manager for care of an open abdomen approach

References

1. De Waele JJ, Leppaniemi AK. Temporary abdominal closure techniques. Am Surg. 2011; 77 (Suppl 1):S46–50.
2. D'Hondt M, Devriend D, van Rooy F et al. Treatment of small bowel fistulae in the open abdomen with topical negative-pressure therapy. Am J Surg. 2011;202:20–4.

Index

M.A. Cuesta, H.J. Bonjer (eds.), *Case Studies of Postoperative Complications after Digestive Surgery*, DOI 10.1007/978-3-319-01613-9,

D

E

T

MIX
Papier aus verantwortungsvollen Quellen
Paper from responsible sources
FSC® C105338

If you have any concerns about our products,
you can contact us on
ProductSafety@springernature.com

In case Publisher is established outside the EU,
the EU authorized representative is:
Springer Nature Customer Service Center GmbH
Europaplatz 3, 69115 Heidelberg, Germany

Printed by Libri Plureos GmbH
in Hamburg, Germany